Healing, Intention and Energy Medicine

To Laurance S. Rockefeller, whose vision and leadership has left us the legacy of a more holistic life.

For Churchill Livingstone:

Publishing Manager, Health Professions: Inta Ozols
Project Development Manager: Katrina Mather
Design: Jayne Jones

Healing, Intention and Energy Medicine

Science, Research Methods and Clinical Implications

Edited by

Wayne B Jonas MD
Director, Samueli Institute for Information Biology, Corona del Mar, California, and Alexendria, Virginia, USA,
and
Associate Professor,
Department of Family Medicine,
Uniformed Services University of the Health Sciences,
Bethesda, Maryland, USA

Cindy C Crawford BA
Research Assistant, Samueli Institute for Information Biology, Alexandria, Virginia, USA,
and
Department of Family Medicine,
Uniformed Services University of the Health Sciences,
Bethesda, Maryland, USA

Foreword by
Jay Moskowitz PhD
Associate Vice President, Health Sciences Research and Vice Dean for Research and Graduate Education, College of Medicine, Pennsylvania State University, Hershey, PA, USA

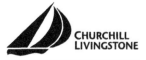
CHURCHILL
LIVINGSTONE

EDINBURGH LONDON NEW YORK OXFORD PHILADELPHIA ST LOUIS SYDNEY TORONTO 2003

CHURCHILL LIVINGSTONE
An imprint of Elsevier Science Limited

First published 2003

ISBN 0443 07237 X

British Library Cataloguing in Publication Data
A catalogue record for this book is available from the British Library

Library of Congress Cataloging in Publication Data
A catalog record for this book is available from the Library of Congress

Note
Medical knowledge is constantly changing. Standard safety precautions must be followed, but as new research and clinical experience broaden our knowledge, changes in treatment and drug therapy may become necessary or appropriate. Readers are advised to check the most current product information provided by the manufacturer of each drug to be administered to verify the recommended dose, the method and duration of administration, and contraindications. It is the responsibility of the practitioner, relying on experience and knowledge of the patient, to determine dosages and the best treatment for each individual patient. Neither the Publisher nor the editor assumes any liability for any injury and/or damage to persons or property arising from this publication.

The Publisher

Transferred to digital print 2007
Printed and bound by CPI Antony Rowe, Eastbourne

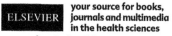

your source for books, journals and multimedia in the health sciences
www.elsevierhealth.com

The Publisher's policy is to use paper manufactured from sustainable forests

Contents

Contributors

David Aldridge Chair of Qualitative Research in Medicine, Universität Willten/Herdecke, Witten, Germany

John A Astin Complementary Medicine Research Institute, California Pacific Medical Center, San Francisco, California, USA

M Allan Cooperstein Independent Clinical/Forensic Psychologist, Willow Grove, PA, USA

Cindy C Crawford Samueli Institute for Information Biology, Department of Family Medicine, Uniformed Services University of the Health Sciences, Bethesda, MD, USA

Jeffery A Dusek Associate Director for Clinical Reseach, Mind Body Medical Institute, Beth-Israel Deaconess Medical Center, Boston, MA, USA

Linda K George Duke University, Durham, USA

Brenda W Gillespie Center for Statistical Consultation and Research, University of Michigan, Michigan, USA

Tim Harlow College Surgery, Collumpton, Devon, UK

David Hufford Professor, Department of Humanities, Pennsylvania State College of Medicine, Hershey, PA, USA

Wayne B Jonas Director, Samueli Institute for Information Biology, Associate Professor, Department of Family Medicine, Uniformed Services University of the Health Sciences, Bethesda, MD, USA

Juliann G Kiang Professor, Departments of Medicine and Pharmacology, Uniformed Services University of the Health Sciences, Bethesda, Maryland; Deputy Chief, Department of Cellular Injury, Walter Reed Army Institute of Research, Silver Spring, Maryland, USA

Gaia LM Kile Complementary and Alternative Medicine Research Center, University of Michigan, Michigan, USA

Ping Y Lu CEO, Burller Information Architects Inc., PO Box 2482, Kensington, Maryland, USA

Edwin May Cognitive Sciences Laboratory, Palo Alto, CA, USA

Michael Mayer The Psychotherapy and Healing Center, Berkeley, CA, USA

Roger Nelson Princeton Engineering Anomalies Research, Princeton, New Jersey, USA

Seán ÓLaoire Menlo Park, CA, USA

Yifang Qian Community Health Network of San Francisco, San Francisco, CA, USA

Dean Radin Institute of Noetic Sciences, Petaluma, CA, USA

Marilyn Schlitz Institute of Noetic Sciences, Petaluma; Institute for Health and Healing, California Pacific Medical Center, CA, USA

Stefan Schmidt Universitätsklinikum Freiburg, Institut für Umweltmedizin und Krankenhaushygiene, Freiburg, Germany

Jane Sherwood Research Nurse Coordinator, Massachusetts General Hospital, Center for the Integration of Medicine and Innovative Technology, Boston, MA, USA

Jerry Solfvin California Pacific Medical Center Research Institute, San Francisco, CA, USA

Andrew G Sparber Nursing and Patient Care Services, Clinical Center, National Institute of Health, USA

Jessica Utts Professor, Department of Statistics, University of California, Davis, CA, USA

Harald Walach Klinikum der Universität, Institut für Umweltmedizin and Krankenhaushygiene, Freiburg, Germany

Sara L Warber Complementary and Alternative Medicine Research Center, University of Michigan, Ann Arbor MI, USA

Xin Yan Chongqing Institute of Traditional Chinese Medicine, Chongqing, Sichuan Province, Peoples Republic of China

Garret Yount California Pacific Medical Center Research Institute, San Francisco CA, USA

Foreword

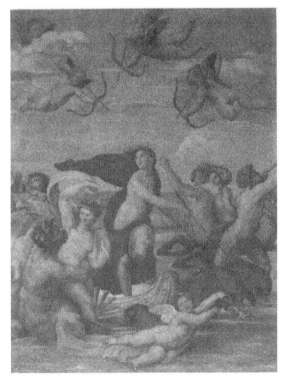

©Massimo Listri/CORBIS

HEALTHCARE IN RENAISSANCE: A CHARIOT DRAWN BY TWO DOLPHINS

When the editors of this wonderful book asked me to write the foreword they indicated that they were seeking someone who was not an expert in the field of spirituality and healing, for that I am not, but they were looking to select, what individuals who perform my duties are called; 'a health scientist administrator.' More specifically, they were seeking a health scientist administrator with interest, not a mere curiosity, in the fields of complementary medicine, spirituality, and healing. The editors were pursuing someone who would or could be willing, most positively, to read the various chapters then help make decisions on a national basis to incorporate or reject the messages being transferred in the dialogues into an academic research and clinical strategy. My goal was to explicitly become an advocate and to assist in developing a national strategy for incorporating spirituality and medicine into future sponsored research initiatives, educational projects, and ultimately, clinical services. In fact, to participate in 'drawing' the blueprint for spirituality and healing in academic medicine! This was a serious and important task placed before me. So, with the knowledge that I would, try, try my best, to fulfill this honor, I proceeded to accept the invitation.

As the Vice Dean for Research of the Penn State College of Medicine, a healthy and growing academic health center, and an Associate Vice President for Health Sciences Research for Penn State University, a research-intense land grant university, one of my responsibilities is to envisage the future of the health research enterprise and to help plan a scientific path for the university in order that the faculty be active participants in the sciences and technologies of the decades to come. This is not simply an exercise of 'crystal ball gazing,' but a program of comprehensive and intense study not unlike the activity of business prognosticators or even hurricane forecasters.

There is ample history of planning for the basis of scientific change. Change in science is illustrated through a plethora of outdated textbooks, many of these only three or four years old, and library stacks full of publications reporting on the acquisition and transfer of new basic and clinical knowledge. In this new technology era, the pace of change is so rapid that as short as a one-year lapse of laboratory work or reading may cause a loss of one's currency in any scientific discipline. There is a constant and increasing flow of new innovations and technologies being conceived, analyzed, and validated, often in human subject studies via clinical trials and demonstration projects. This is an era, however, where there is the ever important environmental factor never seen, to this degree, in centuries of scientific progress – that is an enormous public interest and public advocacy. The public's quest for new cures, treatments, and ways to prevent disease and maintain health is insatiable – it is a quest that drives change through buying and prescribing practices and, many times through federal scientific budget allocations. The National Institutes of Health budget is on course to double its appropriations in five years. This doubling is the result of public engagement. The very positive cases of research funding for AIDS and breast cancer are very well publicized examples of public interest, advocacy, and action.

Without lightening the importance of my mission of producing a foreword for an important document, I decided to provide my impressions, of my recently acquired views, of the future of spirituality and healing in academic medicine, through a visual treat.

Raffaello Sanzio, more popularly known as Raphael, one of the artistic giants of the Renaissance Era, never could have imagined that his fresco entitled, *The Triumph of Galatea*, painted in an Italian palazzo would be discussed in a preface of a Spirituality and Healing compendium almost 500 years after his death.

Why pick a painting by Raphael? Because Raphael was dedicated, to what art critics exclaim, and, I quote 'reconstructing the lost architecture of the eternal city.'[1] In Raphael's case Rome, in ours, the eternal city of Medicine.

Raphael had and, I quote again, 'the love and objectivity to penetrate deeply enough into the art of a past age to give it new life.'[1] I felt, when reviewing the chapters, that the authors addressed both the art and science of spirituality with such a passion that, like Raphael, they are proceeding to 'give it new life.'[1]

I will make analogies of this 'Triumph' with the emergence of this science, and I use this term deliberately, the science of spirituality, the impact of spirituality on both human health and healing, and on the potential for philosophical and empirical changes on the engines of healthcare research can take place in the nation's academic health centers.

A depiction of the Triumph of Galatea illustrates Galatea, the sea-nymph, traveling rapidly across the ocean waves in a chariot drawn by two dolphins. You can almost envisage the rush of her movement and a 'swirling' around her of the fair maidens, sea gods, and cherubs.[2] She alone is free and independent of the swirling human and part human companions.[2] Art critics have described this magnificent piece as one which 'achieves constant movement . . . without letting it become restless and unbalanced.'[2] A message that on our quest for acceptance of spirituality's influence on healing we should be, and I believe, are mindful of. This fresco will help us focus on our thoughts as we transition from fantasy to spirituality.

The journey of spirituality into the practice of medicine and into academic institutions has not, as of today, had the acceleration and movement visualized in this fresco. In fact, if not for books like this one and some dynamic and intellectual leadership of Duke University, The National Institute for Healthcare Research, and the institutions that house the authors, I believe there would not be enough 'momentum' – especially in the university medical centers, to allow the science of spirituality to remain afloat.

This book is a celebration, and I believe an impetus for change.

Why am I optimistic about spirituality's future acceptance in healthcare? Why do I believe conventional medicine has in the last decade embarked on its own renaissance, which will encourage the pursuit of the science of spirituality?

I will answer these questions by examining first the universities and then as a group, individual physicians, scientists, and the public.

First the universities – the time is upon us for the halls of academia, I'll call them, 'coalitions of intellect,' to open their doors to the science of spirituality and its role in healing.

Donald Kennedy, former President of Stanford University, writing a few years ago in an essay entitled *Making Choices in the Research University*[3] indicates that 'directional shifts' will be required if American research universities, and I include academic health centers, are going to meet society's expectations for the new millennium. One reason Kennedy, as do I, believes that the shift will be implemented is because, as Kennedy states so eloquently, and I quote:

Never have our universities lived in a more abruptly changing society. To speak of 'academic rigor' by way of appealing to the disciplinary status quo is self-evidently anachronistic now. We need to open up the rigid cages of institutional thought and custom to new cultures, new alignments, and new problems.[3]

Kennedy does not address the issues spirituality and healing. I, however, believe that spirituality and its effect on healing does apply and the new 'openness' of universities to innovative and non-traditional approaches can help break the academic's *cultural 'rigor mortis'*[3] to new concepts that have not been part of the higher education enterprises' own business plans.

Nannerl O. Keohane, President of Duke University also a proponent of change, writes in an article on *Mission of the Research University*[4] that:

The modern research university occupies a distinctive niche in both space and time, compounded of equal parts of intense nostalgic localism and a generous sense that members of a university are citizens of the world. Yet, universities are also forward-looking, restless, pioneering, attempting to discern and even to control the future.[4]

Richard H. Dean, M.D., the Senior Vice President for Health Affairs at Wake Forest University recently completed an in depth 'Strategy' for distilling the issues and oppor-tunities facing a growing medical center in its effort to achieve and sustain its goal of excellence. In that approach he and the faculty identified key values which included, 'Excellence, Compassion, Innovation and Integrity.' The vision of Wake Forest with relation to the clinical enterprise is to evolve in such a manner that 'we maintain and enhance our position in the market place of healthcare delivery both in reality and in the public's perception.' The public's perception is a concept that we would not have addressed so intensely just one decade ago. Collectively, as change agents, we are opening our institutions to new concepts and ideas. The compassion value is one that relates closely to the contents of this book. The value is articulated in the Wake Forest 'Strategy' as: 'Being aware of, and responsive to, the physical, emotional, *spiritual*, and intellectual needs of others.'

The just cited authors have been the pioneers of this area of change in science and it's time for this pioneering spirit to become contagious. Thus, the writings of these three academic leaders help comfort me, in the reality that the universities are, in fact, open or 'opening' to the concepts that we are studying this day. Thus, the movement will occur – and even if some universities must be pulled, they will attain momentum.

Thus, to the dolphins. Let's call one 'conventional' and the other 'spiritual.' Healing, of the universal patient, in my opinion, must utilize both. The philosophies must move together in parallel. In the past, in fact very recent past, they were going at different speeds and in diverse directions. Would the chariot remain afloat? Certainly not! If we consider the beautiful Galatea as the 'universal, healthy patient' exhibiting a high quality of life looking up to the heavens. That image would certainly change with her conventional and spiritual caregivers moving in different directions at different rates! Just remember the simple formula we learned in physics. Parallelism in this case is important – we need both dolphins – not a merger, but a complementary team approach.

I find many physicians and scientists who are trying to inhibit the pace of our spirituality dolphin, using both doubt and recalcitrance.

I do believe we can overcome this with careful and comprehensive study, validation, and most of all perseverance.

Dr Wayne Jonas, my colleague and friend, like myself, is optimistic and predicts that as current complementary and alternative medicine groups become more 'professional' the therapies and preventive modalities they promote will be adopted into the mainstream.

Now to the doctors, patients, and public.

Dr Edmund Pellgrino, noted ethicist, presents in his writings an earlier image of the physician as a 'benevolent, benign, and authoritarian figure who decided what is best for his/her patients.'[5] That image served society well in a time that was simpler, and when decisions on healthcare did not involve, as they do today, to quote Dr. Pellgrino, a 'host of new value and moral questions'.[6] It more easily fulfilled expectations in a society in which there were fewer educated people who would say, to quote Dr. Pellegrino again, 'Just a moment – I would like to understand what is happening! I want to have a say in what you are going to do'[5] Dr. Pellegrino and I agree to quote him once more: 'A healing decision is one that will make the patient whole again, restore bodily harmony if that is possible, and perhaps even make it better than before the illness occurred.'[5]

A review article published a half decade ago instructs us on the recalcitrance of physicians to move in the directions of society. Consider the dolphin analogy and what this means. Dr Jeffrey S. Levin of the International Center for Integration of Heath and Spirituality writes that surveys show that 80% of Americans believe 'in the power of God or prayer to improve the course of illness'[6] and almost 70% of physicians report patients asking for religious counseling when in the course of terminal illness. 'Yet,' he states, that 'only ten percent of physicians even inquire about the patients beliefs or practices.'[6] A more recent poll of 1,000 American adults, concluded that '79% of the respondents believed that spiritual faith can help people recover from disease' and of these respondents, 63% suggested that physicians should engage in discussions about spiritual faith.[7]

I'll even add another, 'yet,' to Dr. Levin's. Physicians upon graduation from medical school take an oath ultimately derived from the Hippocratic oath and hopefully, in sincere earnestness, not only in a 'ceremonial context' of graduation from four years of rigorous study. The first lines of the oath are:

I swear by all the gods and goddesses, making them my witness, that I will fulfill according to my ability and judgment this oath and this covenant:[8] . . .

An oath to Gods! A rich history of centuries of medicine and by medicine practitioners of covenants with deities. Is this not at least a partial underpinning that should have been sufficient to 'connect' the profession with the issue of religious or spiritual involvement in their patients?

As has been debated over the past few years, I must admit that the issue of spirituality and religion was at times confused and intermingled. Spirituality has been defined as, and I quote: 'the spirit or the soul, as distinguished from the body, what is often thought of as the better or higher part of the mind.'[9] It is a search for the sense of meaning and purpose of life.[9] On the other hand, religion is a 'system of belief, worship, conduct, often involving a code of ethics and philosophy.'[9] I believe that the message today is that organized religion is but one methodology of expressing our spirituality. *Either* is important in the healing process and in the holistic approach to an individual or patient's well-being.

When one is severely ill or near end of life, there is almost always a trilogy of spiritual inputs. In my experience on the hospital ethics committee I have found input from 1) a representative from the patient's family, 2) a religious representative or counselor, and 3) the physician, or other medical care giver.

Since biblical times, frequent prayer has been central to most religions. I am familiar with Jewish religiosity. The Amidah, a prayer recited three times a day, includes a plea 'Heal us O Eternal One and we shall be healed.' Every denomination and religion has a similar prayer. With the patient as one half of a covenant, with the physicians and the patient having interest in the holistic approach to healing, what should the physician's role be?

The American Psychiatric Association has adopted guidelines which suggest that physicians 'should maintain respect for their patient's beliefs' and 'should not impose their own religious, anti-religious, or ideologic systems of beliefs on their patients.' Care should not be a competition of remedies but a congruence. The physician's armamentarium should include every adoring arrow the giver has to offer. Spirituality should, in my opinion, be considered strongly by the physician and other caregivers in the patient's holistic healing process.

But, we know that not all support this view. Sloan, et al, state that 'even in the best studies, the evidence of an association between religion, spirituality, and health is weak and "inconsistent."'[7] The authors conclude that it is premature to promote faith and religion as adjunctive medical treatments. Some may agree. The goal for the advocate for incorporating spirituality into mainstream medicine is to pursue and validate the hypothesis of its value through comprehensive research initiatives.

I conclude with the suggestion that this book should be considered part of the infrastructure in establishing a plan for building acceptance and developing a course for further maturation of the science of spirituality in medicine. I believe that we must establish a national approach for both the academic medicine and the public, based on a series of four basic, and current, premises. Let's review the public interest analogy.

1. Our scientific knowledge base is extraordinary. The opportunity for exciting advances in medicine and healing have never, in our history, been greater than today. The acquisition of new knowledge using molecular biology, functional genetics, non-invasive imaging, and pharmacology and physiology have profound implications for health and healing. I'll insert an editor's note here! It is almost too profound. Will this book's message be heard amidst all of this technological advancement?

2. The pace of application of new science and technology to products is more rapid and more public than ever; gene therapy, telemedicine, and home pregnancy tests. Science and medical advances are now described at the newsstand in *The Wall Street Journal*, *New York Times*, and *Newsweek* sometimes prior to the physician or scientist receiving, by mail, the original scientific report in a Scientific Journal.

3. The country is spiritual. Religious participation is the most common form of voluntary group social activity in the United States.[10] If one combines all other kinds of voluntary group activities they do not exceed involvement in church. We have more houses of worship than ever before.[10] There are organized school prayers at football games in defiance of legislation.

4. American Society is engaged as never before in both body and spiritual health! For the body we have treadmills, fitness clubs, 'thigh busters,' and juice bars. For spirituality we have religious channels on 24 hours a day. Then there's Sunday morning evangelist television. Most importantly, there are conferences in spiritualism and health presented at Harvard, Johns Hopkins, George Washington, and Wake Forest Universities which have begun to inform professionals and the public about how spirituality can be integrated into healthcare.

Why should we be optimistic that our plan will work? It's because these premises are concentric, merging, 'swirling,' science, health, religion, spirituality, and public interest.

The swirl is not random, it is controlled and balanced.

The public is critical to our success.

We need to engage the public with more information from our studies, our conferences, and our opportunities to learn.

Indeed we need to form another era of socio-medical reform. Social reform has a history in this country of transforming medicine and our country. Nineteenth Century reformers advocated sanitation, public hygiene and prevention from infectious diseases. Twentieth century reformers examined social interventions in the health consequences of smoking, violence against women, and more recently school lunches and nutrition.

The twenty-first century public driven reform can be the benefits of social, medical, and spiritual integration of the practice of medicine – a renewed covenant with practitioners and patients that condones treatment that includes both body and soul. Academic medical centers and private medical practitioners should be open to providing the evidence that there is validity to the postulates that are discussed in this book – spirituality does support the healing process.

You, the readers, are also the pioneers, let's explore and discover together – In fact, let's triumph as Galatea does. Allow me to end with a portion of a physician's prayer by Maimodes. Its language is ecumenical.

Illuminate my mind that it recognize what presents itself and that it may comprehend what is absent or hidden . . . for delicate and indefinite are the abounds of the great art of caring for the lives and health of thy creatures.[11]

REFERENCES

1 Oberhuber K 1999. *Raphael, The Paintings*, p. 169
2 Gombrich EH 1957. *The Story of Art*, pp. 234–235
3 Kennedy, Donald, *The Research University in a Time of Discontent*, Making choices in the Research University, The American Academy of Arts & Sciences, 1993, 1994
4 Keohane Nannerl O, *The Research University in a Time of Discontent*, The Mission of the Research University, The American Academy of Arts & Sciences, 1993, 1994
5 Pellegrino Edmund D, MD, 1987. *The Journal of Medical Humanities and Bioethics*, Toward A Reconstruction of Medical Morality, 8: 1, Spring/Summer
6 Levin Jeffrey, Larson David, Puchalski Christina 1997. *JAMA*, 'Religion and Spirituality in Medicine: Research and Education,' 278: 9, September 3
7 Sloan RP, Bagiella E, Powell T 1999. *The Lancet*, Religion, Spirituality, and Medicine, 353, February 20
8 Hippocratic Oath, Translated by Ludwig Edelstein. Reprinted with Permission in: Veatch, RM: Case Studies in Medical Ethics, Cambridge, MA, Harvard University Press, 1977, p 351–352.
9 McKee, Chappel 1992. *Journal of Family Practice*, 35: 2
10 Koenig Harold G 1997. 'Is Religion Good for Your Health?,' *The Haworth Pastoral Press*, New York, NY
11 Freecnar David L, Abrams Judith 1999. Illness and Health in the Jewish Tradition, The Jewish Publication Society Phil., p 160

Jay Moskowitz, PhD
July 2002

Preface

Healing practices that use direct mental or spiritual techniques, such as prayer, ritual, dreamwork, imagery, direct mental intentions, and laying-on of hands, have been part of all known cultures. Despite their universality, little scientific attention has been directed toward investigating these practices or their claims. Here we present a critical summary of spiritual healing, 'energy' medicine and intentionality (intentional mental effort) as an approach to illness, and make recommendations for future research in what we will call simply 'healing.' We address three questions:

1. Are the effects of healing 'real' as examined by high-quality, independently reproduced experiments?
2. How big are the effects of healing interventions?
3. What clinical impact does healing have in real-life clinical situations?

Finally, we address possible next steps for improvement in healing research.

The book consists of critical summaries of current research on healing and healing-related areas by experts, research recommendations for advancement of healing research, and a comprehensive bibliography of current publications on healing. To produce the bibliography we used expert summaries and their citations and additional searches of other sources including a comprehensive literature search. Critical reviews were carried out in six areas:

1. Health correlates of spiritual and religious practices
2. Intercessory or healing prayer
3. 'Energy' healing approaches
4. Therapeutic qigong (Chinese energy healing)
5. Direct mental interaction with living systems
6. Mind–matter interaction studies.

Studies were evaluated with established quality criteria in scientific research. Each area was given an 'evidence level' class A to F (A being the highest with at least three independent, high-quality studies and F being the lowest with expert opinion without high quality research).

SUMMARY OF FINDINGS

We found over 2200 published reports, including books, articles, dissertations, abstracts and other writings on spiritual healing, energy medicine, and mental intention effects. This included 122 laboratory studies, 80 randomized controlled trials, 128 summaries or reviews, 95 reports of observational studies and non-randomized trials, 271 descriptive studies, case reports, and surveys, 1268 other writings including opinions, claims, anecdotes, letters to editors, commentaries, critiques and meeting reports, and 259 selected books. Our findings in each of the six areas are as follows:

Religious practices

Over 75% of 130 studies on the relationship between religious and spiritual practices and health outcomes reported positive associations. However, almost all of this research is observational, with no high-quality randomized controlled trials. There is a positive relationship between religious practices and reduced mortality, better physical health, improved quality of life, and less mental illness and drug abuse. Evidence level was D.

Prayer

Six (46%) of 13 randomized controlled trials on prayer involving 2328 patients reported significant effects on at least one health outcome. The quality of the research was judged as 'fair.' There were three medical conditions in which at least one high-quality randomized clinical trial was done but there were no replications of these trials. Positive effects were reported for patients with acute heart disease, and for patients with HIV/AIDS complications. Negative results were reported for prayer healing of warts and alcoholism. Evidence level was B.

'Energy' healing

Eleven (58%) of 19 randomized controlled trials on 'energy' healing (usually therapeutic touch) involving 1122 patients reported positive effects. The quality of the research was judged as 'fair.' Positive effects have been reported on pain and anxiety in burn patients and institutionalized elderly, respectively, but no high-quality independent replications of these studies were found. Evidence level was B.

Qigong (laboratory research)

Fifty-eight studies (out of 130 reports) examining the biological effects of qigong in the laboratory (on cells and animals) were reviewed. Almost all reported positive effects. The quality of this research was judged as 'poor' and there were no independent high-quality replications on any single model. A summary of the best laboratory study to date on qigong is presented in a section of this book. Evidence level was C.

Qigong (clinical research)

Thirty-three studies (out of 72 reports examining the effects of qigong on high blood pressure) were reviewed. Almost all reported positive

effects. Only five were randomized, however, and the quality of the research was judged as 'poor' with no high-quality replications. One study reported adverse effects. Evidence level was F.

Laboratory research on bioenergy

One hundred and eleven studies were found that were done in the West on laboratory models such as plants, cells, and animals testing the effect of energy and mental healing. Forty-five of these were reviewed as they were randomized with parallel control groups. Average quality of these studies was fair to good. Most were statistically positive. Of the top 10 quality studies evaluated, all but two reported positive effects in favor of the real *vs.* sham bioenergy treatment. Only one independent replication of a high quality study was attempted. Evidence level was B.

Direct mental interaction with living systems (DMILS): electrodermal activity (EDA)

Twenty-four studies involving 636 sessions examined whether individuals could alter electrical conductivity of the skin of another individual at a distance. Nine (37.5%) studies done in four different laboratories were statistically positive. Most studies received 'good' quality ratings but there is no high quality meta-analysis of independent replications. Evidence level was B.

Direct mental interaction with living systems (DMILS): remote staring (RS)

Seven publications describing 13 experiments with 300 sessions examined whether EDA (skin conductance) changed when one individual was staring at another, through a closed-circuit TV. Seven out of 13 experiments were significant ($P < 0.05$). Most studies received 'good' quality ratings but there is no high-quality meta-analysis of independent replications. One attempt at exact replication by two experimenters with different beliefs yielded different results. Evidence level was B.

Research on mind–matter interactions (MMI): individuals

A total of 516 experiments published in 216 articles by 91 different first authors examining attempts by individuals to influence random systems (electronic random event generators; the total of publications cited here is specific to RNG studies) were meta-analyzed. Although the magnitude of the overall effect is small (on average less than 1%) the results are highly statistically significant ($P < 10^{-16}$), have been replicated by multiple independent investigators, and are consistently positive over four decades of research. These studies indicate that there are ways in which mind and matter interact that are consistent with the assumptions of distant and spiritual healing. Evidence level was A.

Research on mind–matter interactions (MMI): groups

About 80 independent tests explored whether random event generator output is altered when associated with group activities that are deeply 'engaging' compared to data taken during 'mundane' group activities in less interesting situations. Overall, these observations report a significant tendency to depart from chance ($P = 2 \times 10^{-16}$). However, no case-controlled or randomized studies have been completed. Evidence level was E.

The impact of healing in a clinical setting

The final summary paper in Section I describes the impact of having spiritual healers become part of a conventional physician group practice. Healing was offered to chronically ill patients who were followed for 6 months after 8–12 healing sessions. The healing treatments resulted in improved symptoms and well-being in about 60% of 87 patients involved in these studies. The practice also had a significant impact on the attitudes of the doctors and healers. In a similar study in which chronically ill patients were offered 'distant healing' by a variety of healers, quality of life improved by over 10 points in those treated compared to those not treated. This

was highly significant both statistically and clinically. Belief in healing and expectation of benefit explained about 25% of the effect.

A graphical summary of the current level of evidence in these areas is presented in Figure 1.

CONCLUSIONS TO HEALING ENERGY RESEARCH PROJECT

Are the effects of mental and spiritual healing 'real?'

There is evidence to suggest that mind and matter interact in a way that is consistent with the assumptions of distant healing. Mental intention has effects on non-living random systems (such as random number generators) and may have effects on living systems. While conclusive evidence that these mental interactions result in healing of specific illnesses is lacking, further quality research should be pursued.

How large are the effects of mental and spiritual healing?

The effect of intention on non-living random systems is small – less than 1%. The effect on some living systems such as the autonomic nervous system and on skin conductance may be larger. The reported effects on illness such as pain and anxiety are still larger; however, better studies show smaller effects. Thus, the true magnitude of these effects is unknown but it is likely smaller than currently reported and probably varies by condition treated.

What impact does spiritual healing have in 'real-life' clinical situations?

Only a few quality studies have examined the impact of spiritual healing in real-life clinical situations. These preliminary studies suggest that chronically ill patients may benefit from spiritual healing. Belief in spiritual healing and expectation of benefit by patients and practitioners contribute significantly to this effect. Some patients and conditions respond better than others.

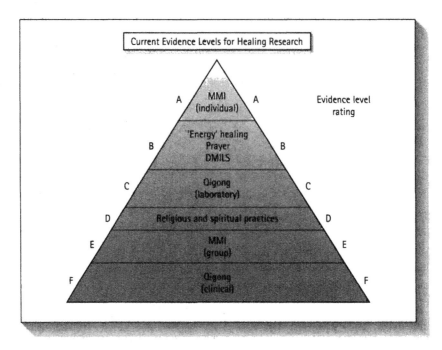

Figure 1 Current evidence levels for healing research. MMI, mind–matter interactions; DMILS, direct mental interaction with living systems. Evidence levels are defined in Table 1.

Table 1 Quality categories and evidence levels

Quality categories

Poor: 0–30% of studies meeting over 60% of maximum quality criteria
Fair: 30–50% of studies meeting over 60% of maximum quality criteria
Good: 50–70% if studies meeting over 60% of maximum quality criteria
Excellent: over 70% of studies meeting over 60% of maximum quality criteria

Evidence levels

A: at least one systematic review or meta-analysis where three high-quality clinical trials or experiments or randomized controlled experiments were found done by independent investigators.
B: at least one properly randomized controlled experiment that rates high quality (>80% of CONSORT criteria).
C: high quality, well-designed controlled experiment without a randomized control comparison group
D: a high-quality, well-designed cohort or case-control analytic study, preferably from more than one center or research group.
E: multiple time series (observational data) with or without intervention
F: opinions of respected authorities, based on clinical experience: descriptive studies and case reports; or reports of expert committees.

RECOMMENDATIONS FOR FUTURE RESEARCH

There are several steps that can improve our knowledge and understanding of healing practices.

1. *Establish consciousness and healing research laboratories.* There is a need for developing centers of excellence with a critical mass of investigators.

These centers should include multidisciplinary expertise in basic science, clinical research, neuroscience, cell biology, mathematics, psychology, theology, physics, computation, statistics and psychophysiology. A number of potential sites currently exist.

2. *Develop a biological model for exploring healing effects.* Laboratory models allow for rigorous and controlled studies needed to test mechanisms

and theories of healing. A bioREG (biological random event generator) is one focus for development. Other models might include a cell biology model of cancer and a neuroscience model examining the neurological correlates of healing and consciousness with technologies such as functional MRI and PET, MEG or qEEG.

3. *Conduct a multicenter healing impact study.* Follow-up studies to those done on healing with chronically ill patients in 'real-life' clinical situations should be conducted. These studies could be done at several sites in order to examine generalizability and have an arm that is blind to treatment in order to examine the role of expectation and belief in healing.

4. *Partner with organizations interested in healing research.* A number of organizations (both public and private) are interested in supporting research on spiritual healing, 'energy' medicine, and intentionality. Partnerships for developing and executing a rigorous and relevant research agenda in healing should be developed.

Wayne B Jonas
Cindy C Crawford
2002

---

[1]The views, opinions and assertions expressed in this book are those of the authors and do not reflect official policy of the Department of the Army, Department of Defense or the US government.

Acknowledgments

Thanks to my wife Susan, my children, Chris, Maeba and Emily and my parents, Henry and Joan for their love and support. Thanks to Marilyn Schlitz, Mitch Krucoff and the organizers of the North Carolina and Hawaii Healing Conferences. Thanks to Ronald A Chez, friend and colleague at the Samueli Institute. Thanks to Henry and Susan Samueli for their continued commitment and support for the Institute and a better world.

WBJ 2002

Thanks to my husband Michael for his endless patience and love. Thanks to the organizers and contributors of our healing conferences. Thanks to the support staff at USUHS for their continued help with materials and references.

CCC 2002

Critical summaries of current research on healing

The health impact of religious and spiritual practices

Linda K. George

This chapter summarizes current epidemiological research on the association of religious and spiritual practices with health and illness.

Why study mental and spiritual healing? There are several compelling reasons: first, healing practices, such as prayer, laying-on of hands, ritual, and mental and psychic healing have been part of every culture since the dawn of mankind; second, these practices continue to fascinate us today; and finally, there is an increasing body of observational evidence that religious and spiritual practices are related to health. Before venturing into the more esoteric investigation of consciousness, spirituality, energy and health effects, it first is necessary to set a foundation from a mainstream research review.

In this chapter, Linda George provides a succinct overview of current epidemiological data on the relationship between religious and spiritual practices and health outcomes. The data consistently show that religious and spiritual practices are associated with better health outcomes, including lower mortality rates. These data cannot determine that such practices are causal – that is, they do not tell us that these practices will lead to better health outcomes. The evidence does, however, compel us to look for such causes. Dr George's thorough description of current scientific thinking on what may contribute to the salutatory effect of religious and spiritual behavior includes social support, dietary habits, lower intake of drugs, smoking and alcohol, the cognitive and physical effects of relaxation from prayer and mediation, increased hardiness from a coherent world view, and other aspects.

Health care practitioners should not be demanding, nor should they prescribe religious practice to their patients or blame illness on a lack of such behaviors. These data are prognostic and not prescriptive. It is not possible to say to what extent spiritual forces or non-local effects contribute to favorable outcomes. Clearly, they do provide important evidence that we should attend to these behaviors in medicine and health care by providing this information in a responsible way to patients who inquire. In addition, we should engage in a fuller scientific investigation of these practices, their causes and their impact on health and disease. **WBJ**

INTRODUCTION: THE EPIDEMIOLOGIC PERSPECTIVE

Social and epidemiologic perspectives on the relationship between religion and health differ substantially from the clinical and experimental perspectives used in the other chapters of this book. The purpose of this chapter is to provide a summary of what social and epidemiologic research has discovered about the links between religion and health. First, however, a few comments that distinguish between this research tradition and those represented elsewhere in this volume are in order.

There are two types of epidemiological studies: population-based studies and clinical studies. Population-based studies focus on defined populations, and much effort goes into defining and representatively sampling the particular population of interest. Most sociological research also uses population-based data. Clinical epidemiology studies, on the other hand, focus on clinical samples, for which sampling is typically much less sophisticated. The research reviewed in this chapter is largely population-based and thus this type of study is our focus of discussion.

Epidemiologists and social scientists study illnesses and the factors that affect risk of illness using naturalistic methods. (Epidemiologists also often perform clinical trials, but when they do this they are evaluating interventions rather than performing epidemiologic studies.) In epidemiologic inquiry, there is no attempt to intervene or to change study participants' usual behaviors and attitudes. This differs sharply from experimental and most clinical research, with important consequences.

Epidemiologic studies offer several advantages relative to experimental and clinical research. Most importantly, there is a known population that is representatively sampled. As a result, findings from social and epidemiologic studies are generalizable to a much greater degree than those generated by other types of research. Any research that recruits participants in the absence of representative (i.e. probability) sampling – and research based on patients from (a) specific health care setting(s) is an important illustration of such sampling – includes selection bias. Personal, economic, social, and health characteristics are significantly related to both whether individuals seek health care and from whom they seek it, creating bias in sample composition. Such bias is largely precluded in population-based epidemiologic studies. A related advantage of population-based studies is that the distributions and relationships observed are the best possible estimates for the population as a whole. Finally, epidemiologic studies have the advantage of capturing behavior, attitudes, and other outcomes as they occur in the 'real world,' in the absence of the artificial conditions of experimental and clinical research. (It is this often strong difference between naturalistic and experimental research that has led to the distinction between efficacy and effectiveness in clinical trials research.)

The major disadvantage of epidemiologic research is that the criteria for causal inference can only be approximated. Without question, controlled experiments are the best method available for meeting the criteria for causal inference. Epidemiologists attempt causal inference and their inferences are often later substantiated in experimental studies. But the inability to assign study participants to levels of the independent variable and to control all possible extraneous factors inherently compromise causal inference in social and epidemiologic studies.

Another disadvantage of epidemiologic studies is the focus on modal population patterns. As a result, important but less common patterns will not be observed. In this review, the links between religious participation and positive health outcomes will be accurately described as consistently observed in epidemiologic studies. However, this does not mean that there are no conditions under which religious participation harms health. It only means that the dominant pattern is one in which religion exerts a salubrious effect on a variety of health outcomes.

The remainder of this chapter is divided into three sections. The first briefly describes major findings from social and epidemiologic studies of the links between religious participation and health. Space limitations do not permit detailed descriptions of the research base and its many complexities; for a review, however, see George et al (2000). The second section of the chapter describes the major focus of current social and epidemiologic research: identifying the mechanisms by which religion affects health. The last section presents some final thoughts about possible links between the findings from social and epidemiologic research and other types of research used to investigate the relationship between religion and health.

THE SOCIAL EPIDEMIOLOGY OF RELIGION AND HEALTH: STATE OF THE EVIDENCE

One of the complexities of summarizing the state of the evidence with regard to the links between religion and health is that both phenomena are multidimensional. In terms of health, a variety of health outcomes have been examined in relation to religious participation. In this chapter, I will briefly review evidence in the areas of mortality, physical illness, disability, and depression. Multiple dimensions of religious participation have been investigated in relation to health. The major ones studied to date include public religious participation (attending religious services), private devotions (time spent in prayer, reading sacred texts, etc.), religious coping (the extent to which individuals use religious beliefs to cope with illness and other stressors), and religious commitment (the importance or centrality of religion in a person's life). Not all the dimensions of religious experience

have been investigated with regard to every health outcome.

Mortality

Perhaps the strongest, and methodologically most compelling, evidence of a link between religious involvement and health is observed in the area of mortality. Numerous population-based studies have demonstrated that, with other predictors of mortality, including health, statistically controlled, public religious participation is strongly predictive of survival (Hummer et al 1999, Koenig et al 1999, Oman & Reed 1998, Rogers 1996, Strawbridge et al 1997). Indeed, in our study of a representative sample of older adults in central North Carolina, regular attendance at religious services was associated with an 8-year survival advantage, compared to attending services less than once a week (Koenig et al 1999). Bryant & Rakowski (1992) reported similar findings for a sample of older African Americans. We also found significant survival advantages among those who attended religious services regularly in a clinical sample of 1010 older veterans hospitalized for serious physical illness (Koenig et al 1998a). Multiple dimensions of religious experience have been investigated. Without question, public religious participation is the dimension most strongly linked to survival, although a recent study reports that time spent in private devotion also has a strong and significant protective effect (Helm et al 2000). These studies are especially compelling from a methodologic perspective because all of them are longitudinal and the temporal order of the religion–mortality relationship is clear.

Physical Health

A large body of research has examined the links between religious participation and physical health. Conceptually, it is important to distinguish between illness onset and the course and outcome of illness. To the extent that religious involvement reduces the risk of illness onset, it has a *preventative* effect; to the extent that religious involvement is associated with a more favorable illness course and/or outcome (e.g.

recovery), it has a *therapeutic* effect. It is important to know whether religious participation has both these effects or whether the effects are primarily preventative or therapeutic.

Research to date reports a relationship between religious participation and numerous physical illnesses, including coronary disease and heart attacks, emphysema, cirrhosis and other kinds of liver disease (see, for example, Comstock & Partridge 1972, Medalie et al 1973), hypertension (see, for example, Larson et al 1989, Levin & Vanderpool 1989), and disability (Idler & Kasl 1992). In all these studies, the relationship observed was that of less illness among religious participants. Although multiple dimensions of religious experience are associated with lower risk of physical illness and disability, the strongest and most consistent evidence is exhibited by public religious participation. Unfortunately, these are cross-sectional studies, in which religious participation and health status were measured at the same time. Consequently, we cannot know the causal order of the variables of interest – it may be that religious participation protects health or unhealthy people may be less likely to participate in religious behaviors. Thus, overall we know little about the effects of religious involvement on the onset of illness, although associations with the prevalence of illness are plentiful.

Another body of research examines the effects of religious participation on the course and outcome of physical illness. Fortunately, the majority of this research is longitudinal (i.e. religious involvement at a given point in time is used to predict the subsequent illness course). Most research to date suggests that religious involvement is associated with better illness course. This pattern has been observed for better health and longer survival after heart transplant (Harris et al 1995), reduced mortality following other cardiac surgeries (Oxman et al 1995), and reduced risk of both non-fatal and fatal repeat heart attacks (Thoresen 1990). Our studies of recovery from physical illness have focused on clinical populations with a variety of serious physical illnesses for which study participants were hospitalized. We, too, have found that religious involvement is associated with quicker and more complete

recovery (Koenig et al 1998a, 1998b). There also is prospective evidence that religious involvement predicts a better, less severe trajectory of disability (Idler & Kasl 1997, Koenig & George 1998).

Several dimensions of religious experience are significant predictors of illness course. Religious coping exhibits the strongest associations, although religious commitment and public religious participation also predict better illness course and outcome. The dominance of more private forms of religious participation for illness recovery may reflect the fact that those who are seriously ill are unable to attend religious services.

Mental Health

Research indicates that religious involvement is also robustly related to mental illness. Indeed, it appears that the effects of religion on mental health outcomes are stronger than for physical illness outcomes, although the effects of religion on mortality are equally as large. Unfortunately, as is the case for physical illness, there are few studies of the effects of religious participation on the onset of mental illness. Most studies of representative samples of community-dwelling adults are cross-sectional. Thus, the associations are between the religious participation and the prevalence of mental illness and the causal order underlying the relationship is unclear. Specifically, religious involvement is associated with lower prevalence of anxiety disorders (Koenig et al 1993a, 1993b), major depression (Koenig et al 1997, Meador et al 1992), alcohol and drug abuse and dependence (Amodeo et al 1992, Francis 1994, Gorsuch 1993, Koenig 1994), and psychological distress (Braam et al 1998, Brown et al 1992, Ellison 1995). As is true for prevalence studies of other health outcomes, attending religious services is the dimension of religious experience most strongly related to mental health.

Research on the effects of religion on the course and outcome of mental illness has been restricted to depressed patients – specifically, seriously medically ill older adults with co-morbid depression. Although there is only one study to date, religious involvement, especially religious coping, increased the odds of recovery from depression and decreased the amount of time between diagnosis and recovery (Koenig et al 1998c).

RELIGION AND HEALTH: THE SEARCH FOR MECHANISMS

For epidemiologists and social scientists, the driving issue in this field is the search for the mechanisms that explain the typically salubrious effects of religious participation. This issue is of critical importance for two reasons. First, it is axiomatic that the purpose of science is to explain relationships, not merely describe them – and, regardless of any personal beliefs, scientists, as scientists, must reject as untestable the hypothesis that divine intervention accounts for the health benefits of religious involvement. Second, if we can identify the mechanisms by which religious participation benefits health, we may be able to 'package' those mechanisms in other ways. This is important because not all individuals find religious participation palatable.

Thus far, studies designed to identify the mechanisms that underlie the relationships between religion and health have employed the strategy of examining social and behavioral factors that (a) have proven to be significant predictors of health outcomes in other research traditions and (b) might be facilitated or strengthened by religious participation. Three such potential mechanisms have received most attention thus far: health behaviors, social bonds, and psychosocial resources.

Health Behaviors

One mechanism by which religious involvement promotes health and longevity may be health behaviors. That is, religious participation may encourage effective health practices (for example avoidance of tobacco, alcohol in excess, illegal drugs, and promiscuous sexual activity) and those health practices may, in turn, protect and promote health. It should be noted that, in the studies reviewed below, health behaviors were consistently significant predictors of mortality and morbidity. The issue is not whether health behaviors are associated with health outcomes –

they are, and robustly so. The question at hand is whether health habits also explain why religious participation, especially attending religious services, promotes health.

Evidence to date concerning the extent to which health behaviors mediate or explain relationships between religious involvement and health outcomes has been mixed. Five studies examined the extent to which health behaviors explained the effects of attending religious services on mortality. Three of the studies reported that health behaviors explained a small, but statistically significant portion of the relationship between religious service attendance and mortality (Hummer et al 1999, Oman & Reed 1998, Strawbridge et al 1997). In the other two studies, health behaviors failed to significantly reduce the service attendance–mortality relationship (Koenig et al 1999, Koenig et al 1998a). Despite differences in statistical significance across studies, the pattern is more consistent than discrepant. Health behaviors explain, at most, a small part of the relationship between public religious participation and mortality.

Idler and colleagues investigated the extent to which health behaviors explain the relationship between public religious participation and disability. In all three studies, health practices explained a small, but significant proportion of this relationship (Idler 1987; Idler & Kasl 1992, 1997).

Evidence is also inconclusive for the relationship between religious participation and depression. Three studies addressed this issue. Two report that health behaviors explain a small, but significant proportion of the relationship between attending religious services and depression (Idler 1987, Musick et al 2000). The other study failed to find significant mediating effects (Koenig et al 1997).

It appears that a small part of the relationships between public religious participation and health outcomes may be explained by the fact that on average those who attend religious services have better health habits than those who do not. Nonetheless, health behaviors are far from being the only factor that can account for the health benefits of religious participation.

Social Bonds

Another possible explanation for the relationship between religious participation and health is social bonds. That is, social ties, especially the receipt of tangible and intangible forms of social support, are known to promote health and, especially, help mitigate the effects of stress on health. It may be that religious participation benefits health because it plays a role in developing and sustaining high-quality social ties. Again, it should be noted that in all the studies reviewed here, social bonds were significant predictors of mortality and morbidity. The issue at hand is whether social bonds are also a mechanism by which religion affects health.

Evidence so far indicates quite clearly that social bonds are not a mechanism by which religious participation protects and promotes health. Two dimensions of social ties have been investigated in multiple studies: social interaction (i.e. the amount of time spent with members of one's social network) and social support.

Studies of the potential mediating role of social interaction focused on two health outcomes: mortality and disability. Six studies examined the extent to which social interaction explained the relationship between attending religious services and mortality. In all six studies, social interaction had no mediating effects (Bryant & Rakowski 1992, Goldman et al 1995, House et al 1982, Hummer et al 1999, Koenig et al 1999, Oman & Reed 1998). The same pattern applies to studies of public religious participation and disability (Idler 1987, Idler & Kasl 1992).

Results are almost as consistent for studies examining the mediating effects of social support. These studies looked at two health outcomes: mortality and depression. Three studies examined the extent to which social support explained the relationship between attending religious services and mortality (Hummer et al 1999, Koenig et al 1998a, 1999). In all three studies, social support failed to significantly mediate the effects of service attendance on mortality. Seven studies examined the degree to which social support explained the relationship between attending religious services and depression among community-dwelling adults. Only one study reported that social support explained part of this relationship (Sherkat & Reed 1992). The other six studies failed to find that social support significantly mediated the relationship between public religious participation and depression (Braam et al 1998, Commerford & Reznikoff 1996, Ellison 1995, Koenig et al 1997, Musick et al 1998, Musick et al 2000). A further two studies examined the extent to which social support explained the effects of religious participation on recovery from depression in clinical samples. Again, no significant mediating effects were observed (Koenig & George 1998, Koenig et al 1998c).

Psychosocial Resources

Psychosocial resources refer to cognitive and affective states that can variously help or hinder effective behavior and well-being more broadly. The major psychosocial resources examined in research on religion and health include self-esteem, a sense of mastery or self-efficacy, and feelings of optimism and hope. There is substantial evidence that a solid sense of self-worth and competence, as well as a generally positive outlook, are associated with better health, especially mental health (see George 2001 for a recent review). Several investigators have hypothesized that religious participation may enhance these psychosocial states which, in turn, benefit health.

However, very few studies have tested this hypothesis. Three examined the mediating role of psychosocial resources; the health outcome in all three was depression or psychological distress. The results were mixed. Two reported that psychosocial resources explained a small, but statistically significant proportion of the relationship between religious participation and depression/distress (Commerford & Reznikoff 1996, Krause 1992). The third study failed to find significant mediating effects (Braam et al 1998). This issue clearly requires additional research, but evidence to date does not suggest that psychosocial resources are the dominant means by which religious involvement protects and promotes health.

Other Possible Mediators

The primary potential mechanisms hypothesized to explain the relationships between religious participation and health clearly have not met expectations. Although they may explain small proportions of the links between religion and health, other mechanisms remain unestablished. This section briefly describes three other possible explanatory factors, each of which has received some theoretical attention but not been adequately empirically tested.

World views

By 'world views' we mean the organized systems of beliefs that form the taken-for-granted assumptions upon which our understanding of the world rests. As such, they are fundamental cornerstones of our identity. Antonovsky's concept of 'sense of coherence' (1980) is often used as an illustration of a world view. According to Antonovsky, individuals possess a sense of coherence if they see the world as predictable, manageable, and meaningful, with the latter being especially important. Sense of coherence has been demonstrated by Antonovsky and others to predict better health and longer survival. It is possible that one of the ways in which religion promotes health is by providing and sustaining deeply-ingrained belief systems that give meaning to life, especially to aspects of life that may lack meaning in secular society. To date, there have been no tests of the extent to which sense of coherence or other world views mediate the relationship between religious involvement and health. This is a high priority for future research.

Belief/expectancy

Another route by which religious participation may promote health is the power of belief or expectancy. That is, commitment to the belief that one is aligned with a higher power that has the ability to make one 'whole' may benefit health. There is ample research evidence that strong beliefs can generate substantial effects. The best example is probably the placebo effect – the fact that patients who receive an inert substance which they believe to be medication frequently demonstrate improvements in health. It is becoming increasingly clear that the placebo effect is more than a methodological nuisance complicating experimental design. Rather, it is a testimony to the power of belief itself to change things (Benson & Friedman 1996). One pathway by which religion promotes health may be by strengthening a conviction that a higher power is bestowing health and healing. This is an extremely difficult hypothesis to test empirically, but the theoretical case for it is intriguing.

Distal and proximal dimensions of religion

A final possible explanation for the relationship between religious involvement and health may require looking more closely at various dimensions of religion. Pargament (1977) provides a strong argument for this strategy. He posits that some dimensions of religious experience are causally more proximal than other more distal factors. For example, he hypothesizes that religious coping may explain, in whole or in part, the relationship between attending religious services and health outcomes, and his empirical evidence supports this hypothesis (Mahoney et al 1999). According to this hypothesis, attending religious services increases the extent to which members of the congregation use religious coping in the face of stress and challenge; religious coping, in turn, is associated with better health outcomes. This line of reasoning is important because it reminds us that there may be something unique (or relatively unique) about religion that promotes health, rather than religion serving merely as a vehicle by which social and behavioral resources affect health.

FINAL THOUGHTS

The research described in this chapter is in the epidemiologic and social science tradition. From this perspective, a field of research begins by demonstrating that there is a relationship between variables of interest; in this case, one or more dimensions of religious experience and one or more health outcomes. There is now strong evidence that several dimensions of religious involvement are robustly related to multiple health outcomes. These relationships indicate that religious participation is associated with lower risk of physical illness, mental illness, disability, and mortality. In addition, religious experience is associated with faster and more complete recovery from both physical and mental illness.

The next step in this research tradition is to demonstrate that the relationship is not spurious (i.e. is not simply the result of the variables of interest being highly correlated with other variables). The relationships reported above have withstood that test. All of the studies cited that reported significant relationships between dimensions of religious involvement and health outcomes were multivariate studies in which potential confounding factors were statistically controlled. Certainly the specific set of control variables included in the empirical models differed across studies – and one could argue that no single study included the full range of potential confounding factors. Nonetheless, an impressive array of known and suspected predictors of mortality and religious participation have been studied. The multivariate models have been sufficiently appropriate and extensive to convince me that the observed relationships between religious involvement and health are real and meaningful. This does not mean that every study finds relationships between religious involvement and health that withstand the demands of statistical controls, but the vast majority do.

The third step in this research tradition – after robust and non-spurious relationships are established – is to identify the mechanisms that explain the observed relationships. This is where research on the health benefits of religious participation is now largely centered. To date, the search for mechanisms has been unsuccessful. We know that health behaviors, social ties, and psychosocial resources explain little, if any, of the relationship between religious participation and health outcomes. These three hypothesized explanatory factors share a common scientific status: they were extracted from other research

on social and behavioral factors and health. The obvious assumption was that one or more factors that we already know to be broadly related to health is the pathway by which religion affects health. Health behaviors, social ties, and psychosocial resources are robust predictors of physical health, mental health, disability, and mortality; however, they do not explain why religion protects and promotes health.

From the perspective of social epidemiology, the major challenge confronting the field is to identify the mechanisms that account for the salubrious effects of religion on health, given that the obvious candidates have been eliminated. At least two other strategies can be pursued. First, the field can 'break out of the box' of the standard paradigm of social/behavioral factors and health and look for new kinds of possible explanations. Current theorizing about the potential value of examining world views and beliefs/expectancies fall under this strategy, as do efforts to use proximal religious factors to explain more distal religious variables.

Second, selection effects must be considered more thoughtfully and extensively than they have been as yet. 'Selection effects' refers to variables that are causally prior to the independent variable of interest and that may account for observed relationships between independent and dependent variables. In this context, we would look for variables that predict why some individuals are embedded in religious communities and others are not. It may be those variables, rather than religious participation itself, that are causally related to the health outcomes. Taking selection effects seriously is important for other reasons. As shown in other chapters in this volume, a great deal of interest and effort is going into developing and testing various forms of religious or spiritual interventions. If the patterns observed in naturalistic research are a result of selection effects rather than religious participation, the theoretical justification for such interventions would be severely undercut. If, for example, religious participation is strongly predicted by a set of personality traits and it is those traits that account for the health benefits of religion, the appropriate target of intervention would be personality traits rather than religious or spiritual interventions.

It is unclear to me how much social and epidemiologic perspectives offer – at this point, at any rate – to investigators working in other paradigms such as clinical trials. At minimum, social and epidemiologic research must be credited with establishing the existence of a meaningful relationship between religious involvement and health outcomes. Hopefully this research tradition also offers other relevant findings, and unless the results of investigating the links between religion (or spirituality) and health are at least compatible across research paradigms, the chances of developing an integrated science of religion and health are slim.

REFERENCES

Amodeo M, Kurtz N, Cutter H S G 1992 Abstinence, reasons for drinking, and life satisfaction. International Journal of Addictions 27: 707–716

Antonovsky A 1980 Health, stress, and coping. Jossey-Bass, San Francisco

Benson H, Friedman R 1996 Harnessing the power of the placebo effect and renaming it 'remembered wellness.' Annual Review of Medicine 47: 193–199

Braam A W, Beekman A T F, Knipscheer C P M, Deeg D J H, van den Eeden P, van Tilburg W 1998 Religious denomination and depression in older Dutch citizens: patterns and models. Journal of Aging and Health 4: 483–503

Brown D R, Gary L E, Greene A D, Milburn N G 1992 Patterns of social affiliation as predictors of depressive symptoms among urban blacks. Journal of Health and Social Behavior 33: 242–266

Bryant S, Rakowski W 1992 Predictors of mortality among elderly African Americans. Research on Aging 14: 50–67

Commerford M, Reznikoff M 1996 Relationship of religion and perceived social support to self-esteem and depression in nursing home residents. Journal of Psychology 130: 35–50

Comstock G W, Partridge K B 1972 Church attendance and health. Journal of Chronic Diseases 25: 665–672

Ellison C G 1995 Race, religious involvement, and depressive symptomatology in a southeastern U.S. community. Social Science and Medicine 40: 1561–1572

Francis L J 1994 Denominational identity, church attendance, and drinking behavior among adults in England. Journal of Alcohol and Drug Addiction 39: 27–33

George L K 2001 The social psychology of health. In: Binstock R H, George L K (eds) Handbook of aging and the social sciences, 5th edn. Academic, San Diego

George LK Larson DB, McCullough ME, Koenig HG 2000 Spirituality and health: What we know, what we need to know. Journal of Social and Clinical Psychology 19: 102–116

Goldman N, Korenman S, Weinstein R 1995 Marital status and health among the elderly. Social Science and Medicine 40: 1717–1730

Gorsuch R L 1993 Religious aspects of substance abuse and recovery. Journal of Social Issues 25: 65–83

Harris R C, Dew M A, Lee A 1995 The role of religion in heart-transplant recipients' long-term health and well-being. Journal of Religion and Health 34: 17–31

Helm H M, Hays J C, Flint E P, Koenig H G, Blazer D G 2000 Does private religious activity prolong survival? A six-year follow-up study of 3,851 older adults. Journal of Gerontology: Medical Sciences 55A: M400–M405

House J S, Robbins C, Metzner H L 1982 The association of social relationships and activities with mortality: prospective evidence from the Tecumseh community health study. American Journal of Epidemiology 116: 123–140

Hummer R A, Rogers R G, Nam C B, Ellison C G 1999 Religious involvement and U.S. adult mortality. Demography 36: 273–285

Idler E L 1987 Religious involvement and the health of the elderly: some hypotheses and an initial test. Social Forces 66: 226–238

Idler E L, Kasl S V 1992 Religion, disability, depression, and the timing of death. American Journal of Sociology 97: 1052–1079

Idler E L, Kasl S V 1997 Religion among elderly disabled persons II: Attendance at religious services as a predictor of the course of disability. Journal of Gerontology: Social Sciences 52B: S306–S316

Koenig H G, George L K 1998 Depression and disability outcomes in depressed medically ill hospitalized older adults. American Journal of Geriatric Psychiatry 6: 230–247

Koenig H G, Ford S M, George L K, Blazer D G, Meador K G 1993a Religion and anxiety disorder: an examination and comparison of associations in young, middle-aged, and elderly adults. Journal of Anxiety Disorders 7: 321–342

Koenig H G, George L K, Blazer D G, Pritchett J, Meador K G 1993b The relationship between religion and anxiety in a sample of community-dwelling older adults. Journal of Geriatric Psychiatry 28: 65–93

Koenig H G, George L K, Meador K G, Blazer D G, Ford S M 1994 The relationship between religion and alcoholism in a sample of community-dwelling adults. Hospital and Community Psychiatry 45: 225–231

Koenig H G, Hays J C, George L K, Blazer D G 1997 Modeling the cross-sectional relationships between religion, physical health, social support, and depressive symptoms. American Journal of Geriatric Psychiatry 5: 131–145

Koenig H G, Larson D B, Hays J C et al 1998a Religion and survival of 1010 male veterans hospitalized with medical illness. Journal of Religion and Health 37: 15–29

Koenig H G, Pargament K I, Nielsen J 1998b Religious coping and health status in medically ill hospitalized older adults. Journal of Nervous and Mental Disease 186: 513–521

Koenig H G, George L K, Peterson B L 1998c Religiosity and remission from depression in medically ill older patients. American Journal of Psychiatry 155: 536–542

Koenig H G, Hays J C, Larson D B et al 1999 Does religious attendance promote survival? A six-year follow-up study of 3,968 older adults. Journal of Gerontology: Medical Sciences 54A: M370–M376

Krause N 1992 Stress, religiosity, and psychological well-being among older blacks. Journal of Aging and Health 4: 412–439

Larson D B, Koenig H G, Kaplan B H, Levin J S 1989 The impact of religion on men's blood pressure. Journal of Religion and Health 28: 265–278

Levin J S, Vanderpool H Y 1989 Is religion therapeutically significant for hypertension? Social Science and Medicine 29: 69–78

Mahoney A, Pargament K I, Jewell T et al 1999 Marriage and the spiritual realm: the role of proximal and distal religious constructs in marital functioning. Journal of Family Psychology 13: 321–338

Meador K G, Koenig H G, Turnbull J, Blazer D G, George L K, Hughes D C 1992 Religious affiliation and major depression. Hospital and Community Psychiatry 43: 1204–1208

Medalie J H, Kahn H A, Neufeld H N, Riss E, Goldbourt U 1973 Five-year myocardial infarction incidence II: association of single variables to age and birthplace. Journal of Chronic Disease 26: 329–349

Musick M, Koenig H G, Hays J C, Cohen H J 1998 Religious activity and depression among community-dwelling older elderly persons with cancer: the moderating effect of race. Journal of Gerontology: Social Sciences 53B: S218–S227

Musick M, Blazer D G, Hays J C 2000 Religious activity, alcohol use, and depression in a sample of elderly Baptists. Research on Aging 22: 91–116

Oman D, Reed D 1998 Religion and mortality among the community-dwelling elderly. American Journal of Public Health 88: 1469–1475

Oxman T E, Freeman D H, Manheimer E D 1995 Lack of social participation or religious strength and comfort as risk factors for death after cardiac surgery in the elderly. Psychosomatic Medicine 57: 5–15

Pargament K I 1997 The psychology of religion and coping. Guilford Press, New York

Rogers R G 1996 The effects of family composition, health, and social support linkages on mortality. Journal of Health and Social Behavior 37: 326–338

Sherkat D E, Reed M D 1992 The effects of religion and social support on self-esteem and depression among the suddenly bereaved. Social Indicators Research 26: 259–275

Strawbridge W J, Cohen R D, Shema S J, Kaplan G A 1997 Frequent attendance at religious services and mortality over 28 years. American Journal of Public Health 87: 957–961

Thorsen C E 1990 Long-term 8-year follow-up of recurrent coronary prevention. International Society of Behavioral Medicine, Uppsala, Sweden

2

Intercessory prayer and healing prayer

John A Astin

This chapter summarizes the randomized controlled trials on distant intercessory prayer and its effects on clinical outcomes.

Prayer is one of the most widely practiced behaviors by individuals, families, and communities during illness or crisis. Surveys indicate that nearly 90% of patients with serious illness will engage in prayer for the alleviation of their suffering or disease. There are thousands of varieties of prayer, each with its own cultural context and ritual. While the cognitive effects of relaxation and lowered anxiety are obvious benefits to the person praying, most individuals believe there are additional effects on those being prayed for, either through direct mental influence or via divine mediators. Are there also effects from prayer on those not doing the praying? Can distant effects of prayer be examined in controlled research?

In this chapter, John Astin examines these questions using standard systematic review methods for the evaluation of controlled trials on clinical illness. He finds that the quantity and quality of research on prayer is too limited to draw definitive conclusions. Yet, some high quality studies have reported positive effects. A major problem is that there are no accepted standards for how to conduct a quality prayer study or what to measure – two items addressed in later chapters in this book. Higher quality studies and studies examining mechanisms and contributing factors to these effects are two strategies for improving our understanding of prayer in health care.   **WBJ**

INTRODUCTION

Despite positive findings in a number of studies suggesting that intercessory prayer and other forms of distant healing may be potentially effective therapeutic modalities, this area of research remains highly controversial as shown by a recent (and at times heated) exchange of letters and editorials in the *Archives of Internal Medicine* (Dossey 2000, Hamm 2000) and *Annals of Internal Medicine* (Atwood 2001, Courcey 2001, Kaptchuk 2001). The present review was carried out in order to help clarify the nature and extent of the apparently conflicting findings in the literature by extending and elaborating upon the results of a recently published systematic review by Astin et al (2000) examining the efficacy of 'distant healing.' Astin et al reported positive treatment effects (on at least one outcome variable) in 57% of the 23 randomized trials reviewed and concluded that, despite inconsistent results and methodological limitations in a number of the studies, the findings were quite compelling and that at minimum, additional research in the areas of distant healing and intercessory prayer were called for. The objective of the present review and reanalysis of selected data from the Astin et al (2000) study was to further investigate all available randomized clinical trials (RCTs) testing the efficacy of intercessory prayer and healing prayer/distant healing (excluding therapeutic touch) as a treatment for any medical condition.

Method

A comprehensive literature search was conducted to identify studies of intercessory prayer or healing prayer (for example, distant or distance healing); see Astin et al (2000) for a detailed description of the search methods employed. While numerous studies have been carried out in these areas (for example, in his review of spiritual healing, Benor (1990) identified 130 controlled investigations), only studies that met the following criteria were included:

1. Random assignment of study participants
2. Placebo control condition

3. Publication in peer-reviewed journals (excluding published abstracts, theses, unpublished articles, etc.)
4. Clinical (rather than experimental) investigations
5. Use of human subjects suffering from any medical condition.

The methodological quality of the studies was assessed using the criteria outlined by Jadad et al (1996) and the indicators of trial quality detailed in the CONSORT (consorted standards of reporting trials) statement (Begg et al 1996). As noted by Astin et al (2000), a meta-analytic approach was initially considered but subsequently abandoned when the heterogeneity of the trials (both in outcome and in terms of type of intervention) became apparent. Nevertheless, effect sizes were calculated in an effort to provide some quantitative measure of the magnitude of clinical effects. Effect sizes were calculated using Cohen's *d* (Cohen 1988), weighted for sample size. Hedges' correction was applied to all effect sizes (Hedges 1982). In studies where multiple outcomes were reported, a single outcome was chosen for the effect size calculation based upon: first, having shown a significant change following the treatment, and/or, second, being the primary outcome measure in cases where there were either several or no significant treatment effects observed. When it was not clear precisely which of several outcomes was considered primary, the outcome was selected at random.

Results

Fourteen studies met the chosen criteria: they were Abbot et al (2001), Beutler et al (1988), Braud & Schlitz (1983), Byrd (1988), Collipp (1969), Greyson (1996), Harkness et al (2000), Harris et al (1999), Joyce & Welldon (1965), Miller (1982), O'Laoire (1997), Sicher et al (1998), Walker et al (1997), and Wirth et al (1993). The main reasons for exclusion were: lack of randomization, no adequate placebo condition, use of non-human experimental subjects and/or non-clinical populations, and not being published in peer reviewed journals or being abstracts. These 14 trials involved a total of 2448 study participants. Methodological details and results are summarized in Table 2.1.

Six trials (43%) showed a significant treatment effect on at least one outcome in those patients being sent prayers or distant healing (Braud & Schlitz 1983, Byrd 1988, Harris et al 1999, Miller 1982, Sicher et al 1998, Wirth et al 1993).

Effect sizes were calculated for eight studies. Across these trials, there was a pooled or averaged effect size of 0.30 ($P = 0.003$). A chi-square test for homogeneity was significant ($P < 0.01$), suggesting heterogeneity in the observed effect sizes (although it is not clear from this analysis what was the actual source of the observed heterogeneity). A 'fail-safe N' of 36 was calculated which represents the number of studies with zero effect that there would have to be to make the pooled effect size results non-significant. This number suggests that it is less likely the significant findings are due to some 'file-drawer effect' (i.e., the selective reporting and publishing of only positive results), although this remains a possibility. Box 2.1 summarizes the principal outcomes and effect sizes for the eight trials. It also includes information on whether distant healers/intercessors were experienced (for example professionals) or lay persons (see Discussion section).

Methodological issues

Mean scores on the Jadad scale (Jadad et al 1996) for the 14 trials reviewed was 4.1 (out of 5), suggesting moderate to high methodologic quality. (This finding is in part a function of our stringent inclusion criteria since only studies that were both randomized and placebo-controlled were considered, and these are two of the four factors assessed in this quality rating scale.) Trial quality was also assessed using criteria outlined in the CONSORT statement (Begg et al 1996). There was considerable variability in scores on this indicator. Out of a total of 13 possible factors we examined, the mean CONSORT criteria score across trials was 6.3. Not surprisingly there was a tendency for earlier published studies to score considerably lower on the CONSORT criteria (originally published in 1996) as many of these factors are only now being included in the standard conduct and write-up of randomized controlled trials. There was, in fact, a significant correlation between overall quality of the trials (combining CONSORT and Jadad scale criteria) and year of publication at 0.65 ($P = 0.012$). Based on these combined scores, the trials with highest methodological quality (>12/18) were those by Abbott et al (2001), Harkness et al (2000), Sicher et al (1998), Greyson (1996), Walker et al (1997), Harris et al (1999), and Braud & Schlitz (1983). There was a non-significant trend in the direction of higher quality trials showing lower effect sizes ($R = -0.47$; $P = 0.24$) overall.

Looking at individual items from the CONSORT statement, certain factors did quite well while others faired quite poorly. For example, > 71% of the trials we reviewed had clearly stated hypotheses, discussed inclusion/exclusion criteria, stated method and rationale for analyses, and discussed potential sources of bias. However, in only three of the 14 studies was a power analysis performed, and only four trials

Box 2.1 Effect sizes ($N = 8$)

Study	Outcome	Effect size	Experienced healers
Beutler et al (1988)	Blood pressure	0.53	Y
Byrd (1988)	Byrd hospital course	0.26	N
Collip (1969)	Mortality	0.78	N
Greyson (1996)	Depression	0.31	Y
Harkness et al (2000)	Warts	−0.03	Y
Harris et al (1999)	MAHI CCU* score	0.13	N
	Byrd hospital course	0.06	
Miller (1982)	Systolic blood pressure	0.78	Y
Sicher et al (1998)	Illness severity	0.96	Y

*MAHI CCU, Mid-America Heart Institute Coronary Care Unit.

Table 2.1 Randomized, placebo-controlled trials of intercessory prayer and healing prayer

Author(s) (year)	Design	Sample size	Experimental treatment	Control intervention	Results	Comments	Quality score (out of 18)
Abbott et al (2001)	Four-armed randomized double blind controlled trial	105 chronic pain patients	Spiritual healing (both face-to-face and behind one way mirror)	Simulated face-to-face healing and no healing	Comparing distant healing to control, no treatment effects were observed on any outcome measure with the exception of a higher preponderance of 'unusual' subjective experiences during treatment for distant healing group		11
Beutler et al (1988)	Double blind – three parallel groups	120 patients with hypertension	Laying on of hands (12 healers, 20 minutes/week for 15 weeks)	Healing at a distance; usual care	No treatment effects	Unclear what precisely healers did; acute rise in diastolic after laying-on of hands	9
Braud & Schlitz (1983)	Single blind (within and between subject)	32 subjects with high levels of autonomic arousal	Distant mental influence (intention to decrease arousal with ten 30-second sessions)	No-influence control conditions	10% reduction in galvanic skin response between control and influence sessions	No effect in subjects with initially low galvanic skin response levels	12
Byrd (1988)	Double blind – two parallel groups	393 coronary care patients	Prayer in Christian tradition (3–7 intercessors per patient until patient released from hospital)	Usual care (no placebo necessary)	Treatment group required less ventilatory support, antibiotics or diuretics	Outcomes combined into 'severity score' (to handle multiple comparisons) was lower in treatment group	7
Collipp (1969)	Triple blind – two parallel groups	18 leukemia patients (children)	Daily prayer (15 months)	Usual care (no placebo required)	Higher death rate in control (90% level)	Heterogeneity of groups makes findings inconclusive – no inclusion criteria	3
Greyson (1996)	Double blind	40 patients with depression	Distance healing (LeShan technique)	Usual care	No treatment effect	May have been underpowered	12

Study	Design	Sample	Intervention	Control	Results	Comments	Score
Harkness et al (2000)	Double blind	84 patients with warts	6 weeks of distant healing ('channeling of energy') by 10 healers	No treatment (no placebo necessary)	No significant treatment effect on size or number of warts	Appears as if baseline values were not controlled for in analysis	15
Harris et al (1999)	Double blind – two parallel groups	990 coronary care patients	Remote intercessory prayer (Christian tradition) for 28 days	Usual care (placebo not necessary)	Significant treatment effects for summed and weighted coronary care unit score – no differences in length of hospital stay	No differences observed when the summed scoring system developed in Byrd study was used – unclear whether baseline differences were adequately controlled	13
Joyce & Welldon (1965)	Double blind – two parallel groups	48 subjects with psychological or rheumatic disease	Prayer in Christian or Quaker tradition – patients received 15 hours of daily prayer for 6 months	Usual care (no placebo required)*	No significant differences in clinical or attitude state	Inclusion/exclusion criteria not stated; heterogeneous patient groups; results of only 16 pairs available	10
Miller (1982)	Double blind – two parallel groups	96 subjects with hypertension	'Remote mental healing' in Church of Religious Science tradition	No treatment (no placebo necessary)	Decrease in systolic blood pressure in treatment group	Unclear how many subjects lost to follow-up – results only given for 4/8 healers; use of medication not controlled for	3
O'Laoire (1997)	Double blind	406 healthy subjects	Non-directed and directed intercessory prayer	No prayer	No significant treatment effects on any outcome (self-esteem, anxiety, depression)		8

Continued

Table 2.1 *Continued*

Author(s) (year)	Design	Sample size	Experimental treatment	Control intervention	Results	Comments	Quality score (out of 18)
Sicher et al (1998)	Double blind – two parallel groups	40 AIDS patients	Distance healing (40 healers from different spiritual traditions – each patient treated by 10 healers)	Usual care (no placebo necessary)	Healing group had fewer new AIDS defining illnesses, lower illness severity, fewer doctor visits and hospitalizations and improved mood	Mood changes may have been due to baseline differences – no apparent statistical adjustment for multiple comparisons	15
Walker et al (1997)	Double blind – two parallel groups	40 patients in alcohol abuse treatment	Prayer (for 6 months)	Usual care (placebo not necessary)	No treatment effect	Insufficiently powered	12
Wirth et al (1993)	Double blind – crossover study	21 patients with bilateral asymptomatic impacted third molar having surgery	Distance healing (Reiki, LeShan), 15–20 minutes, 3 hours post operation	No treatment (placebo not necessary)	Treated group showed decrease in pain intensity and greater pain relief post operatively		11

*In all of the prayer studies, a placebo was unnecessary as patients were unaware whether they were being prayed for or not.

discussed any efforts to conceal group assignment (allocation concealment), which, research suggests, tends to inflate effect size estimates. While 61% of the trials reported baseline differences between treatment and control groups, only three studies (23%) statistically controlled for these differences (e.g. using ANCOVA (analysis of co-variance)). Thirty-five percent of trials clearly stated what the primary and secondary outcome measures were while in only seven of the 14 studies was sufficient summary data provided (e.g., to calculate effect sizes, reanalyze data, replicate findings, etc.). Finally, while issues of bias affecting internal validity were discussed in a majority (71%) of studies, issues related to generalizability and external validity were only adequately discussed in one study (O'Laoire 1997).

In summary, taking the above methodological limitations and difficulties into consideration, we believe the current level of evidence for intercessory prayer and healing prayer should be regarded as 'moderate' based on the qualitative rating criteria suggested by Slavin (1995) ('moderate' being defined as evidence from one relevant, high-quality RCT and one or more relevant, low-quality RCTs with generally consistent outcomes).

Discussion

In this systematic review of 14 randomized controlled trials examining intercessory prayer and healing prayer, six studies (43%) showed a positive treatment effect on at least one outcome. An overall significant effect size of 0.30 was found for eight of these trials although this result must be interpreted with caution owing to the heterogeneous nature of the outcomes assessed. Quality of the trials was quite variable, with approximately 50% of studies being deemed to have moderate to strong methodological quality while four (28%) could be considered of poor quality (evidencing less than 50% of the methodological criteria we examined). Papers published more recently were significantly more likely to be of higher quality and there was a non-significant trend in the direction of lower quality trials reporting higher effect sizes.

As noted, the scientific investigation of areas such as intercessory prayer and healing prayer is a controversial one. This can be explained in part by two factors. First, such studies suggest the incorporation into medicine of practices (for example, prayer) at least tangentially if not directly related to religion and spirituality. Rightly or wrongly, the integration (as well as study) of prayer in health care has been questioned on ethical, philosophical, and theological grounds (Posner 2000, Sloan et al 1999, Sloan et al 2000, Thomson 1997). Second, the investigation of distant healing techniques may be resisted (in some cases vigorously) by those who find even the suggestion that such practices may be efficacious threatening to long-held personal beliefs (such as world views, paradigms) regarding the nature of human beings, human consciousness, and the universe at large.

DIRECTIONS FOR FUTURE RESEARCH

In their recent systematic review, Astin et al (2000) summarized a number of the methodological challenges inherent in research on healing prayer and distant healing, including: the difficulty of obtaining 'pure' control groups; the need to assess psychosocial factors known to interact with health outcomes; small sample sizes potentially resulting in insufficient statistical power; and the importance of assessing the beliefs and expectations of both patients and investigators and their possible effect upon/interaction with healers' intentions and the degree of effectiveness. Below we elaborate further on some of these points and also discuss a number of additional observations and factors to consider in the studies we reviewed and in terms of future research efforts in these areas:

1. It has been suggested that the degree of healer/intercessor experience may be one crucial factor in determining the magnitude or strength of any observed distant healing effect; for example, the effect sizes in the study by Sicher et al (1998), which used experienced healers, were significantly larger than those found in either the Byrd (1988) or Harris et al (1999) studies. In the present review, we found no clear pattern suggesting that experienced healers produced

more consistently positive or stronger healing outcomes than lay healers, although it remains for future research to examine this interesting question. Related issues include:

    a. to what extent might there be some type of dose–response relationship in distant healing (e.g., is more intensive or frequent prayer better than less prayer? is there any ideal length of time for a distant healing intervention to be initially or maximally effective?)

    b. the specific content of the prayers/distant healing affirmations and the extent to which these do or do not correlate with actual outcomes (e.g., whereas Braud & Schlitz (1983) found that specific mental intentions produced quite specific physiological outcomes, no clear effect was observed for the specific outcomes focused upon by the intercessors in either the Byrd or Harris et al studies (Posner 2000)).

2. It would seem important to assess the beliefs and expectations of patients, as well as their degree of openness or receptivity to healing prayer (and whether such beliefs change at all following such interventions). In addition, as has been done by some investigators, it is important to examine (*post hoc*) whether patients thought they were in the treatment or control group and the extent to which such beliefs may in some way act as important mediating variables, ultimately influencing clinical outcomes (Sicher et al 1998).

3. As noted, only 35% of the studies in our review clearly or adequately stated what the primary and secondary hypotheses and outcomes were. As has been the case in both the Byrd and Harris et al prayer studies, critics (Posner 2000) have argued that reported positive findings are questionable in part because what were reported as statistically significant outcomes did not clearly reflect (i.e., only loosely matched) the authors' originally stated hypotheses. For example, although Harris et al reported that they were attempting to replicate Byrd's findings and stated that their results did in fact lend support to those of Byrd, they failed to find a significant distant healing effect on the hospital course measure used in the original Byrd study. Future

research must therefore state very clear hypotheses and utilize well-validated and reliable outcome measures that directly examine the investigators' stated hypotheses. In addition, it is important that researchers limit the number of outcome measures employed and/or adjust for multiple statistical comparisons as this has been an additional (and often valid) criticism leveled at some of the prayer studies.

4. The issue of informed consent remains a controversial one in this type of research. For example, although Harris et al argued (effectively to their human subjects review board) that informed consent was not necessary in their study since any potential harm from the intervention was unlikely, others have questioned the ethics and validity of this position (Goldstein 2000).

5. Publication bias (the tendency for journals and researchers to only publish positive findings) is certainly an important issue as evidence suggests that such biases are quite common and can significantly alter the results of meta-analyses and systematic reviews (Sutton et al 2000). With this in mind, the interpretation of positive findings such as those reported here and by Astin et al (2000) regarding the potential efficacy of distant healing must be interpreted with some caution. However, it should also be kept in mind that reverse publication bias, particularly in controversial areas such as prayer and distant healing, is also a distinct possibility as suggested by the recent study by Resch et al (2000), showing a bias by journal reviewers against manuscripts dealing with a non-traditional medical approach (homeopathy).

6. An unresolved yet critical issue relevant not only to distant healing but also to all medical research is determining what constitutes 'sufficient' evidence regarding the efficacy of a particular intervention. For example, in terms of the intercessory prayer research (and the field of parapsychology in general), there has been considerable debate regarding what an adequate P value should be that would enable one to safely conclude that any observed distant healing effects cannot be attributed to chance alone (Posner 2000, Sandweiss 2000). In this regard, some have argued that 'extraordinary claims demand extraordinary evidence.' However, this seems tantamount to

creating precisely the kind of research double standard that some in the biomedical community have accused the alternative medicine community of perpetuating (Angell & Kassirer 1998). It is important to bear in mind that the decision that 1/20 or 1/100 or 1/10 000 constitutes 'adequate' assurance that one's findings are not the product of mere chance is an arbitrary one, just as the standard of $P < 0.05$ is a fairly arbitrary – albeit nearly universally agreed upon – statistical probability cut-off point. One of the great difficulties with P values in general is that they are primarily focused on safeguarding researchers against committing type I errors (erroneously concluding there is an effect when there is not). However, although setting more stringent P values decreases the chances that one will commit such false-positive errors, it also increases the likelihood of committing type II errors (falsely concluding that one's intervention has no effect when in fact it does). The challenge in the case of the distant healing research (if one takes the summary findings from

this and the earlier Astin et al systematic review) is to strike an often difficult balance between on the one hand not overstating the potential implications of the positive findings while at the same time not underplaying their potential importance and significance.

CONCLUSIONS

Methodological limitations notwithstanding, using Slavin's 'best-evidence' synthesis (Slavin 1995), we conclude that there is at present moderate scientific evidence supporting the efficacy of various distant healing/intercessory prayer approaches in medicine. Additional well-designed, large-scale randomized trials are now needed, however, to confirm or refute these preliminary findings. Furthermore, given the heterogeneity of outcomes assessed to date, it is not possible at present to determine which specific health-related problems are most likely to respond to such healing interventions.

REFERENCES

Abbot N C, Harkness E F, Stevinson C, Marshall F P, Conn D A, Ernst E 2001 Spiritual healing as a therapy for chronic pain: a randomized clinical trial. Pain 91: 79–89

Angell M, Kassirer J P 1998 Alternative medicine – the risks of untested and unregulated remedies. New England Journal of Medicine 339: 839–841

Astin J A, Harkness E, Ernst E 2000 The efficacy of distant healing: a systematic review of randomized controlled trials. Annals of Internal Medicine 132: 903–910

Atwood K C 2001 The efficacy of spiritual healing. Annals of Internal Medicine 134: 1150

Begg C, Cho M, Eastwood S. et al 1996 Improving the quality of reporting of randomized controlled trials: the CONSORT statement. Journal of the American Medical Association 276: 637–639

Benor D 1990 Survey of spiritual healing research. Complementary Medical Research 4: 9–33

Beutler J J, Attevelt J T, Schouten S A et al 1988 Paranormal healing and hypertension. British Medical Journal 296: 1491–1494

Braud W, Schlitz M 1983 Psychokinetic influence on electrodermal activity. Journal of Parapsychology 47: 95–119

Byrd R C 1988 Positive therapeutic effects of intercessory prayer in a coronary care unit population. Southern Medical Journal 817: 826–829

Cohen J 1988 Statistical power analysis for the behavioral sciences, 2nd edn. Erlbaum Associates, Hillsdale NJ

Collipp P J 1969 The efficacy of prayer: a triple-blind study. Medical Times 97: 201–204

Courcey K 2001 Distant healing. Annals of Internal Medicine 134: 532–533

Dossey L 2000 Prayer and medical science: a commentary on the prayer study by Harris et al and a response to critics. Archives of Internal Medicine 160: 1735–1737

Goldstein J 2000 Waiving informed consent for research on spiritual matters? Archives of Internal Medicine 160: 1870–1871

Greyson B 1996 Distance healing of patients with major depression. Journal of Scientific Exploration 10: 447–465

Hamm R M 2000 No effect of intercessory prayer has been proven [letter; comment]. Archives of Internal Medicine 160: 1872–1873

Harkness E F, Abbot N C, Ernst E 2000 A randomized clinical trial of distant healing for skin warts. American Journal of Medicine 108: 448–452

Harris W S, Gowda M, Kolb J W et al 1999 A randomized controlled trial of the effects of remote intercessory prayer on outcomes in patients admitted to the coronary care unit. Archives of Internal Medicine 159: 2273–2278

Hedges L V 1982 Estimation of effect size from a series of independent experiments. Psychological Bulletin 92: 490–499

Jadad A R, Moore R A, Carroll D et al 1996 Assessing the quality of reports of randomized clinical trials: is blinding necessary? Controlled Clinical Trials 17: 1–12

Joyce C R B, Welldon R M C 1965 The objective efficacy of prayer: a double-blind clinical trial. Journal of Chronic Disease 18: 367–377

Kaptchuk T J 2001 Distant healing. Annals of Internal Medicine 134: 532–533

Miller R N 1982 Study on the effectiveness of remote mental healing. Medical Hypotheses 85: 481–490

ÓLaoire S 1997 An experimental study of the effects of distant intercessory prayer on self-esteem anxiety and depression. Alternative Therapies in Health and Medicine 36: 38–53

Posner G 2000 Another controversial effort to establish the medical efficacy of intercessory prayer. Scientific Review of Alternative Medicine 4: 15–17

Resch K I, Ernst E, Garrow J 2000 A randomized controlled study of reviewer bias against an unconventional therapy. Journal of the Royal Society of Medicine 93: 164–167

Sandweiss D A 2000 P value out of control. Archives of Internal Medicine 160: 1872

Sicher F, Targ E, Moore D 2nd, Smith H S 1998 A randomized double-blind study of the effect of distant healing in a population with advanced AIDS: report of a small scale study. Western Journal of Medicine 169: 356–363

Slavin R E 1995 Best evidence synthesis: an intelligent alternative to meta-analysis. Journal of Clinical Epidemiology 48: 9–18

Sloan R P, Bagiella E, Powell T 1999 Religion spirituality and medicine. Lancet 353: 664–667

Sloan R P, Bagiella E, VandeCreek L et al 2000 Should physicians prescribe religious activities? New England Journal of Medicine 342: 1913–1916

Sutton A J, Duval S J, Tweedie R L, Abrams K R, Jones D R 2000 Empirical assessment of effect of publication bias on meta-analyses. British Medical Journal 320: 1574–1577

Thomson K S 1997 Miracles on demand: prayer and the causation of healing. Alternative Therapies in Health and Medicine 3: 92–96

Walker S R, Tonigan J S, Miller W R, Corner S, Kahlich L 1997 Intercessory prayer in the treatment of alcohol abuse and dependence: a pilot investigation. Alternative Therapies in Health and Medicine 36: 79–86

Wirth D P, Brenlan D R, Levine R J, Rodriguez C M 1993 The effect of complementary healing therapy on postoperative pain after surgical removal of impacted third molar teeth. Complementary Therapies in Medicine 1: 133–138

3

Direct mental interactions with living systems (DMILS)

Stefan Schmidt

This chapter summarizes the current research on the effects of intention and attention on biological systems with a focus on autonomic reactivity in humans.

Consciousness, in the form of attention and intentional activity, accompanies all treatments, whether conventional, complementary or spiritual. Thus, examining the influence of conscious activity on living systems can allow us to better understand a mechanism that may underlie all healing interactions. Because research on clinical conditions can be complex and variable, laboratory experiments provide a means of examining the effects of consciousness under more controlled conditions.

By measuring the electrical activity on the skin, a dynamic measure of a person's autonomic arousal, autonomic nervous function can be objectively assessed. A conscious activity such as prayer and meditation has a calming effect on this electrodermal activity (EDA). Does conscious activity have a similar effect on the autonomic function of another person, even when the other person is separate from and unaware of when this mental activity is occurring? In this chapter, Stefan Schmidt critically summarizes research on this phenomenon. He reviews the studies in which one person tries to intentionally calm or arouse another person who is isolated and unaware of these attempts, and studies in which only paying attention (staring) at another person influences their EDA.

These data indicate that non-local effects may occur from the interaction of a healer's conscious activity influencing the physiology of the patient. This may be one mechanism for healing which occurs during the placebo effect, spiritual and mental healing, and in all medical care. Although statistically significant, the magnitude of these effects are fairly small (Cohen's $d = 0.16$). The data are also not without flaws, and Dr Schmidt makes several recommendations for improvement in this research.   **WBJ**

INTRODUCTION

Direct mental interaction in living systems (DMILS) represents an experimental paradigm in parapsychology that was developed in the mid-1970s. Experiments are designed to investigate whether there is an interaction between two people who are spatially separated. This interaction is operationalized as covariation between the intentions of one person and the physiological reactions of the other person.

This chapter outlines the procedure of a typical DMILS experiment. This experiment is then related to healing energy research (HER), in order to find a set of appropriate questions on DMILS research from a HER perspective. Using these questions as a basis, the chapter then describes a systematic literature review of DMILS which can provide answers. Furthermore, this systematic literature review also describes the most recent knowledge of DMILS research in general.

DMILS: AN EXPERIMENTAL PARADIGM

DMILS is a laboratory experiment. Usually, three people – two participants and an experimenter – are needed to conduct a DMILS session, although the experimenter can also combine the two roles of agent and experimenter. The two participants have different tasks and are often referred to as 'sender' or 'agent' and 'receiver'. This description is helpful to describe the experiment although it is also somewhat misleading as it entails certain implications of information transfer which are not necessary for the experiment to be successful. Therefore I will use the

terms in a preliminary way. (Possible misunderstandings are addressed below.)

The two participants are physically separated from each other to prevent any conventional means of communication. At least one of the participants (i.e. the receiver) has to be housed in an acoustically and, ideally, also electromagnetically shielded chamber. Several physiological measures are recorded from the receiver such as electrodermal activity (EDA), respiration, heart rate, blood pressure, or ECG (electrocardiogram). During the experimental session the receiver's task is simply to maintain a wakeful but relaxed and open state. The agent is placed in front of a monitor which displays an extract of the physiological recording taken from the receiver, to keep the agent informed of the level of arousal or activation of his counterpart (feedback condition). The agent's task is to activate or to calm the receiver from a distance. Therefore the session time is divided into several epochs usually lasting between 30 and 60 seconds. During each of these periods one of two conditions (e.g. 'calm' or 'activate') is displayed as a word on the screen of the monitor to the agent, requesting the agent to perform in any way that might lead to the appropriate reaction in the receiver. The sequence of the epochs is randomized and balanced. Often the epochs are interspersed with rest intervals. The agent is not restricted in the method used to activate or calm the receiver, and various strategies, including imagery or physical methods, are allowed (Figure 3.1).

For evaluation, the physiological data are summed up according to the two different conditions, for example ten 1-minute 'calm' epochs might be compared with ten 1-minute 'activate' epochs. Under the null hypothesis the same amount of activity or arousal is expected in both conditions. If the physiological activity differs significantly in the intended direction (more activation during activate epochs) one can speak of a so-called DMILS effect.

DMILS FROM A HEALING PERSPECTIVE

From a parapsychological perspective, the purported DMILS effect can be interpreted in many

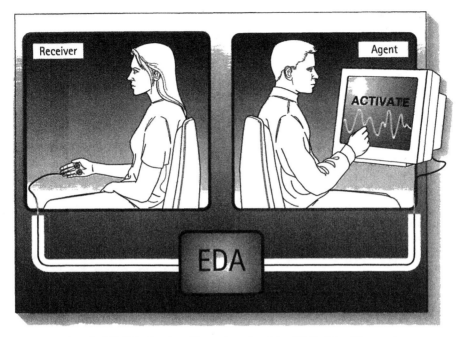

Figure 3.1 A typical DMILS situation. Electrodermal activity (EDA) data of the receiver are fed back to the agent. The agent tries to change the physiological activity of the receiver by means of intention.

ways. This is due to the fact that almost nothing is known about the way in which parapsychological or Psi effects are mediated. There are several competing theories (see, for example, von Lucadou 1995, May et al 1995, Millar 1978, or Stokes 1997, for an overview), but they are all more or less rough models that cannot provide detailed information about the functioning of these effects. There is also no dominant theory or model that is accepted by a majority of the researchers in this field.

The basic mechanism of these effects is as yet unknown; nor do we know which constituents are needed or how this system, consisting of at least two people and certain laboratory equipment, is organized.

As a result, differing interpretations and explanations are possible. The most common interpretation is that the sender, as the 'active' part, is influencing the receiver's physiology. However, this is only the most obvious interpretation, resulting from the way the experiment is described and the fact that the receiver is called a 'receiver' and not, for instance, a 'remote viewer' or an 'observer.' It might also be true that the

receiver acts subconsciously as a remote viewer, who, perceiving the conditions from the sender's monitor, influences his or her own physiology accordingly. With that interpretation the sender is not needed. It might also be that the experimenter foresees the best moment to start the experiment with the natural fluctuation of more and less activation in the receiver just falling in the corresponding epochs. This is why the acronym DMILS stands for distant *interaction* in living systems. In some way there might be an unconventional interaction within the whole experimental system, or between parts of it, that can be seen in the recorded data.

From a healing perspective, DMILS can be seen as a research paradigm of the very mechanism underlying a distant healing process. The DMILS set-up has some parallels to a distant healing situation. There is a sender or a healer who tries to change the physical or physiological state of a healee or receiver from a distance by intentional means. This is why the DMILS paradigm is of major importance for any healing research that takes into account the possibility of distant healing. The DMILS set-up can provide us with an answer to the very basic question as to whether it is in principle possible for an organism to react physiologically in accordance with a remote intention. In other words, is there a mechanism independent from any healing context that is responsible for effects of distant intention and that might also be used in a distant healing situation? If one assumes that DMILS experiments and distant healing rely on the same effect, then the DMILS laboratory is an excellent setting to study this effect under controlled conditions. These investigations can address three areas: proof-, process-, and model-oriented research.

Taking this analogy into account, healing research can pose the following questions to the laboratory:

- Is there empirical evidence for an effect of distant intention that might also apply to distant healing (proof-oriented)?
- Are there conditions that improve or diminish the size of the effect (process-oriented)?
- Are there further empirical results that help us understand distant healing in a theoretical sense or that help us generate an appropriate model of distant healing (model-oriented)?

SYSTEMATIC LITERATURE REVIEW

Methods

The literature review presented here is the first step of a meta-analysis in preparation. The meta-analysis will include all DMILS studies and remote staring studies (a related paradigm, see below) with EDA as dependent variable, since EDA is by far the most included variable in DMILS research. Some studies report several different psychophysiological variables including EDA as dependent variable; I know of only one study on human DMILS that measured blood pressure rather than EDA, but to my knowledge this study was never published.

For this review all studies using a non-human target system, for example gerbils (Braud 1979), fish (Braud et al 1979), blood conserves (Braud 1990), or enzymes (Bunnell 1999), have been

excluded. Also excluded were all studies having behavioral measurements as dependent variables such as a concentration task (Brady & Morris 1997, Braud et al 1995), control of muscle tremor (Braud et al 1989) or ideomotoric reactions (Braud & Jackson 1982). Moreover, the data set does not include studies with prerecorded targets; in these studies the psychophysiological data are already recorded when a participant tries to interact with them (e.g. Radin et al 1998). These studies can be considered as a separate category that has been recently addressed by Braud (2000).

The studies were retrieved as follows: we included all the publications mentioned in a meta-analysis of EDA-DMILS studies published by Schlitz & Braud in 1997. We conducted an additional literature search for EDA-DMILS studies from 1996 up to 2000 in the following journals: *Journal of Parapsychology, Journal of the American Society for Psychical Research, Journal of the Society for Psychical Research, European Journal of Parapsychology, Journal for Scientific Exploration,* and the *Proceedings of the Annual Convention of the Parapsychological Association.* We also searched for so-far unpublished material for the meta-analysis, but the seven studies we found are not included in this literature review. Two EDA-DMILS studies by Braud & Schlitz have never been published but will be included as their overall results are presented in various overviews (e.g. Braud & Schlitz 1989a, Braud & Schlitz 1991, Schlitz & Braud 1997).

Results

Data set

In summary, 22 studies published as single papers or in overviews from 1978 to 1999 were found (Table 3.1). They form a data set of 24 single experiments with an overall number of 636 sessions, conducted in four different laboratories (San Antonio, Edinburgh, Las Vegas, and Freiburg). As the various sessions in different experiments were of different length one might also count the number of epoch pairs (e.g. calm–control, activate–control, or calm–activate) to assess the size of the entire data set. There were 6842 such pairs. The number of sessions within these studies varied

Table 3.1 Overview of all DMILS experiments by author(s), year of publication, numbers of sessions performed, additional hypotheses tested, level and direction of significance testing and according effect size (r).

Experiment	Author(s)	Year	Target system	N[1]	Additional hypotheses	Significance	Effect size (r)
1	Braud	1978	EDA	10		$P = 0.02$ 2t	0.72
2	Braud	1978	EDA	10		$P = 0.01$ 1t	0.70
3	Braud et al	1979	EDA (SRR)	10	Gifted sender	$P = 0.04$ 1t	0.56
4	Braud	1979	EDA (SRR)	10		n.s. 1t	−0.25
5a	Braud & Schlitz	1983	EDA (SRR)	16	Participants with labile EDA	$P = 0.014$ 1t	0.53
5b	Schlitz & Braud	1985	EDA (SRR)	16	Participants with stable EDA	n.s. 1t	−0.02
6	Braud et al	1985	EDA (SRR)	15	Senders were healing practitioners	n.s. 2t	0.16
7	Braud et al	1985	EDA (SRR)	24	Feedback vs. no feedback	$P = 0.04$ 2t	0.35
8	Braud et al	1985	EDA (SRR)	32	Blocking vs. no blocking	n.s.	0.20
9	Braud et al	1985	EDA (SRR), HR, skin temperature, muscle tension, respiration	30	Specificity vs. generality	n.s.	0.08
10	Braud & Schlitz	1989b	EDA (SRR)	40	Model of intuitive data sorting (IDS) pilot study	n.s.	0.03
11a	Braud & Schlitz	1989b	EDA (SRR)	32	IDS disfavoring condition	$P = 0.019$ 1t	0.40
11b	Braud & Schlitz	1989b	EDA (SRR)	32	IDS favoring condition	n.s. 1t	−0.09
12	Braud & Schlitz	n.p.[2]	EDA (SRR)	30	Direction of influence	n.s.	0.08
13	Braud & Schlitz	n.p.	EDA (SRR)	16	Modulation of magnitude	n.s.	0.32
14	Delanoy & Sah	1994	EDA (SRR)	32		$P = 0.043$ 1t	0.31
15	Radin et al	1995	EDA (SRR)	16		n.s. 1t	0.27
16	Wezelman et al	1996	EDA (SCL), HR, BVP	11	Healing rituals	n.s.	0.08[3]
17	Rebman et al	1996	EDA (SCL), HR, BVP	16	Healing rituals	$P = 0.0004$ 1t	0.37[3]
18	Delanoy & Morris	1998	EDA (SCL)	36	Experimenter trainees	n.s. 1t	0.16
19	Schneider et al	2000	EDA (SCL)	40	Personal vs. neutral experimenter interaction	n.s. 2t	0.17
20	Watt et al	1999	EDA (SCL)	32	Blocking vs. cooperating	n.s. 1t	−0.01
21	Watt et al	1999	EDA (SCL)	50	Blocking vs. cooperating	$P = 0.038$	0.25
22	Delanoy et al	1999	EDA (SCL)	80	Biological related pairs vs. close related pairs	n.s. 1t	−0.04

[1] Number of sessions.

[2] Not published

[3] Instead of the number of sessions, the number of epoch pairs was taken as N to calculate r as the original test statistic was based on that number.

EDA, electrodermal activity; SRR, skin resistance response; SCL, skin conductance level; HR, heart rate; BVP, blood volume pulse. n.s., not significant; 1t, one-tailed test; 2t, two-tailed test.

from 10 to 80, the length of an epoch pair from 40 to 120 seconds (without interspersed rest periods), and the number of epoch pairs per session from 5 to 16.

Significance

Nine of the 24 experiments yielded significant results according to their hypotheses. This means that 37.5% of the experiments had significant results compared to the 5% that would have been expected by chance.

Effect sizes for EDA

In a procedure similar to that used by Braud & Schlitz (1991, 1997) we calculated an effect size for the results of the EDA data of each experiment. This effect size is Rosenthal's r (Rosenthal 1991). It is free of any distribution assumptions and can be used with various test statistics, including non-parametric ones. In this case two different test scores were employed, t-scores stemming mostly from single-mean t-tests and z-scores stemming from the non-parametric Wilcoxon test. The formulas were $r = z / \sqrt{N}$ and $r = \sqrt{t^2/(t^2+df)}$. For N we took the number of sessions per experiment. For the studies performed by Wezelman et al (1996) and Rebman et al (1996) we took the number of epoch pairs as N, as this was their unit for statistical evaluation. One problem with calculating Rosenthal's r in that way is that one cannot calculate a confidence interval (CI) for the effect size. Although Rosenthal provided a formula for the calculation of r's variance (Rosenthal 1994), this formula presupposes normal distribution and is only recommended for data stemming from parametric test statistics.

The effect size of the 24 experiments ranged from $r = -0.25$ to $r = 0.72$, with negative results indicating an outcome opposite to the expected direction. The mean was at $r = 0.22$ with a standard deviation (SD) of 0.25. The 95% CI of the mean ranged from 0.11 to 0.32 and was significantly different from zero. Figure 3.2 shows the effect sizes for the single experiments.

As can be seen from the graph, the largest effect sizes were obtained within the first five experiments. They are all relatively small with 10 (1, 2, 3, 4) or 16 (5a, 5b) sessions. Therefore, it might be interesting to calculate an effect size weighted by the number of sessions. As expected, the effect size drops down to $r = 0.16$, and a similar result of $r = 0.17$ is obtained if the studies are weighted by the number of epoch pairs.

The large range of effect sizes might indicate that not all the data are estimates of the same effect. This can be assessed by applying a statistical model to this sample and looking for possible moderators of the effect size. We are planning to do this in the meta-analysis mentioned above, but for a preliminary investigation of the characteristics of that sample we applied a test of homogeneity proposed by Rosenthal (1991, pp. 73–74). It yielded a $\chi^2 = 29.76$ with $d.f. = 23$. The corresponding P value was $P = 0.15$, proving the sample to be homogenous on this test.

Dependent variables other than EDA

Only three studies in this data set record physiological measures other than EDA. These are: heart rate, peripheral skin temperature, frontalis muscle tension, and breathing rate in experiment 9, and heart rate and blood volume pulse in experiments 16 and 17. In experiment 9 the authors found some differential results for the heart rate, but all variables showed no overall effect. In experiment 16 the results for heart rate and blood volume pulse were not significant. The same was true for the blood volume pulse in experiment 17, while the heart rate was significantly lower ($P = 0.01$) in the experimental condition.

In a recent pilot study (Schmidt et al 2001) we explored the relationship between a DMILS effect in EDA and respiration. The data showed that irregularities in respiration (sudden changes in the rhythm) accounted for substantial parts of the EDA-DMILS effect found in the study.

Different laboratories

The DMILS studies were all conducted in four laboratories. The Mind Science Foundation in San Antonio accounted for 50.8% of all sessions,

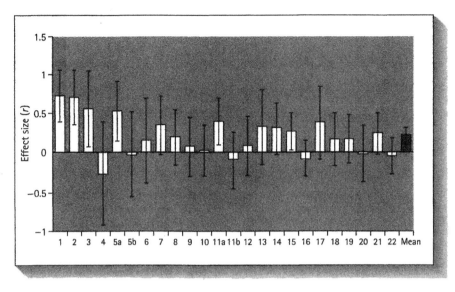

Figure 3.2 Graphical display of effect size (*r*) of all 24 single experiments including overall unweighted mean effect size. Error bars represent the 95% confidence interval.

Edinburgh for 33%, Freiburg for 11.9% and Las Vegas for 4.2%. While research activities have stopped in Texas and Nevada, the European laboratories still conduct DMILS research. Approximately 400 unpublished sessions have recently been conducted in those two laboratories. This unpublished data set has more than 60% of the size of the data set presented in this review.

A comparison of effect sizes by laboratory shows that San Antonio has a mean of *r* = 0.25 while the other three laboratories are within the range *r* = 0.15 to *r* = 0.17.

Methodological Quality of the Studies

EDA

As EDA is the only dependent variable in most of the DMILS experiments, its measurement by state-of-the-art techniques is crucial. To assess whether the published DMILS studies meet the proposed standard procedures published by a committee of the Society of Psychophysiological Research in 1981 (Fowles et al 1981), we evaluated all publications according to these guidelines (Schmidt & Walach 2000). This analysis revealed that none of the DMILS studies met these standards. DMILS researchers have mostly neglected

the knowledge provided in psychophysiological literature. For example, none of the measurements in the experiments reviewed used an appropriate electrode gel, needed for the recording of EDA signals. Most of the studies did not report their methods in detail, which made it more difficult to judge whether inappropriate measurements had invalidated the data. For the discussion of possible artifacts due to these methodological shortcomings the next topic is of special importance.

Intraindividual design

For all discussions of methodological shortcomings the DMILS design holds one big advantage. DMILS always deals with intraindividual differences. Every test statistic calculated on DMILS data compares experimental and control epochs of the *same* participant. As these epochs are presented in a changing sequence, this means that any shortcoming holds for both the experimental epoch and the according control or comparison epoch. By taking the differences between these epochs, all eventual artifacts will be filtered out. This means methodological inappropriateness can always result in not finding an effect that might be there, but it is hard to imagine that a weak methodology will result in finding a DMILS effect that would not have been found with a better one.

This argument of the advantages of the intraindividual comparison relies strongly on one fact, namely the balanced and randomized sequence of the epochs.

Balanced and randomized sequence

The sequence of the (usually 10) epoch pairs have to fulfill three criteria to guarantee an artifact-free comparison of the epochs:

1. There must be the same number of epochs of each kind and, of course, all epochs have to have the same length.
2. The sequence of the experimental and control epochs must be randomized.
3. The sequence of the epochs must be balanced in a way that does not lead to any effects due to the natural variation of the recorded variable.

While point 1 is trivial and point 2 is obvious, point 3 is crucial. Consider the following example of a receiver becoming more and more tired – and therefore less activated – in the course of a 20-minute recording period. If the 10 activation and 10 calm epochs are presented in sequence as, for example, AACAAACAACAC-CACCCACC, one will find a DMILS effect even if nothing extraordinary happened. This is because the sequence is unbalanced and contains more activation periods at the beginning of the session than at the end. The same is true of any repeating pattern within the data that correlates by chance with a rhythmic pattern of the receiver's physiology. A balanced and randomized sequence of the epochs is, therefore, crucial. Wiseman & Smith (1994, p. 475) found that even a sequence that looks pretty much balanced at first glance may lead to spurious findings. Therefore the data of this review were checked to see if the description of the procedures guaranteed a balanced design.

All experiments took care to ensure a basically balanced design with the exception of the first four. We excluded these from the analysis and calculated an unweighted and a weighted (by session) mean effect size on the remaining 20 studies. The unweighted effect size dropped to $r = 0.17$ with a smaller standard deviation of SD = 0.18 and 95% CI ranging from $r = 0.09$ to $r = 0.26$. The weighted effect size is $r = 0.15$, which is more or less the same as before.

Selection of participants

Most study subjects were unselected participants. Due to the intraindividual design there is no need to randomize participants into different groups or to match them. Moreover, as the focus of interest in the DMILS experiment is to explore whether there is *in principle* a hitherto unexplained interaction between two separated people, DMILS experiments do not necessarily rely on a representative sample. It might even be possible that only some gifted people are able to perform above chance in DMILS experiments. Under this premise a representative sample may not find an existing effect.

On the other hand, representative samples are needed for any research asking process-oriented questions on interindividual differences that could be generalized to the population. This might be an important point for future research, but from the perspective of today's situation there is no need for representative samples.

Statistics

In a recent analysis we (Schmidt et al 2000) compared different statistical evaluation strategies in DMILS experiments. Because of the complicated structure of the data this is not a trivial problem. Any strategy must deal with three problems: the first is parameterization and accumulation of the epochs; the second concerns intraindividual comparison of experimental and control epochs; and the third the accumulation of the data from all sessions to a score that allows for statistical testing of the whole experiment.

Our analysis revealed that the predominant statistical method used in DMILS research so far, the so-called percent influence score (PIS; Braud & Schlitz 1991, p. 5), has a severe lack of statistical power for some kinds of data. This presumably means that some DMILS effects in the data have not been found due to inappropriate methods.

Process-oriented Results

A variety of different process-oriented hypotheses were tested in various DMILS experiments. Table 3.1 also presents an overview of all process-oriented hypotheses.

There is no agreed process-oriented knowledge for the DMILS set-up in the sense that any process-oriented hypothesis was replicated at least once successfully. There are several reasons for this. The problem is that for some so-far unknown reason some DMILS experiments yield significant results and others do not. The logical consequence of that fact is the search for unknown moderators which will result in testing different process-oriented hypotheses. Thus, quite a lot of different hypotheses have been tested, but there have been very few replications of positive findings. Furthermore, the absence of a hypothesized DMILS effect in general makes the situation even more difficult, for in this case one cannot draw any conclusion on the process-oriented hypothesis to be tested.

A complete mapping of all process-oriented findings would be rather extensive. A good overview can be found in Schlitz & Braud (1997). This chapter therefore focuses only on the results that are of relevance from a healing perspective.

In experiment 3, a so-called gifted person, Matthew Manning, acted as a sender in 10 sessions. The study yielded a significant result ($p = 0.04$, two-tailed) with a large effect size of $r = 0.56$. The study had more of an exploratory character. There was no comparison between 'gifted' and 'non-gifted' senders; that means the effect does not depend necessarily on the special sender. Furthermore, as stated above in the section on the methodological quality of the studies, the randomization in experiment 3 was not balanced; thus, the effect could also be due to inappropriate randomization.

In experiment 6, Schlitz and Braud employed as senders three healing practitioners with experience in Reiki. Each acted as a sender in five sessions. The study did not reveal any significant result.

Experiments 16 and 17 addressed explicitly the analogy between DMILS and some aspects of traditional healing. The authors stated that 'the DMILS experiment itself is actually a modern version of the same principles that underlie certain traditional magical healing rituals that fall into the general category of magic' (Wezelman et al 1996, p. 2). Accordingly they prepared their set-up similar to a traditional (voodoo) healing situation. The senders were called 'healers', and their chamber was a darkened room illuminated by a golden candle. Ritual objects such as a doll with personal belongings of the receiver were placed on black cloth within the cabin. The results of these experiments are hard to interpret as the authors did not define precisely what should be regarded as a relevant outcome of their studies. They present various P values by different statistical evaluation methods. For this review we chose to take the cumulative difference between the control and the experimental condition at the end of the 60 second epochs. This was not significant for EDA in the 54 pairs of epochs compared in experiment 16. In experiment 17, the same statistic for 78 epoch pairs yielded a highly significant z-score of $z = 3.3$ ($P = 0.0004$, one-tailed). Nevertheless, the data allow only for limited conclusion regarding the healing context as there was no comparison condition.

Results on Model Testing

Another line of DMILS research might be to develop a theoretical model that explains the supposed DMILS effect, so that single hypotheses can be derived from the model and tested empirically. As stated above, one problem in parapsychological research is that there is no predominant or agreed model that could explain findings such as DMILS effects.

There is only one study that tests a theoretical assumption known by the name of intuitive data sorting (IDS). According to this model, a predecessor of the DAT (decision augmentation theory) model (see May et al 1995, May et al 1996), 'the influencer or experimenter psychically, yet unconsciously, scans the future electrodermal activity stream of the subjects and begins an experimental session at a time that maximizes the degree of fit between the ongoing electrodermal activity and the prescribed schedule of influence and control epochs' (Braud & Schlitz 1989b, p. 290). Braud & Schlitz therefore varied the degrees of freedom for the sender to start the epochs in the experiments 11a (low) and 11b (high). They expected a higher DMILS effect in experiment 11b under the assumption of the IDS model. In fact the opposite was true; experiment 11a scored significantly, whereas 11b did not.

REMOTE STARING: A DMILS RELATED PARADIGM

In parapsychological research there is an experimental paradigm that is very similar to the DMILS set-up. It was also promoted by Braud and colleagues (Braud & Schlitz 1991, Braud et al 1993a, Braud et al 1993b) and is normally referred to as 'remote staring'. It was designed to investigate whether one person can detect another person staring at him or her.

In some experiments a person stares at participants through a one way mirror. Participants are then asked whether they perceived a gaze or not (Baker 2000, Colwell et al 2000, Schwartz & Russek 1999). Braud and colleagues used a different method. Instead of assessing the person's conscious knowledge by asking him or her verbally, they assessed the EDA and compared autonomic arousal for staring and non-staring periods.

The procedures in these experiments are more or less the same as those used in the DMILS experiments described above, but the sender is now referred to as the 'starer', while the receiver is called the 'staree'. Instead of seeing the EDA feedback on a monitor the starer can look at the staree by means of a closed-circuit television system. The observation effect is measured by intraindividual comparison of epochs in which the starer is gazing at the monitor (experimental condition) with epochs in which he or she is looking elsewhere.

The similarity to the DMILS set-up is obvious. Instead of having an intention to activate or calm his or her counterpart, the starer is observing the person in the other chamber. The intentional condition is operationalized in a slightly different way, but nevertheless this experiment also investigates the relationship between an intentional state in one person and resulting physiological changes in another person. Therefore, the remote staring data set may provide additional knowledge of the questions of interest from a healing perspective.

Study Retrieval

We included all experiments that studied the detection of a remote observation with physiological measurements as dependent variables. Retrieval strategies were the same as for DMILS studies. We included all remote staring studies from the meta-analysis by Schlitz & Braud (1997) and performed an additional search of the parapsychological literature from 1996 to 2000.

Results

We found seven publications (including conference proceedings) describing 13 experiments with 300 sessions (Table 3.2). Studies were conducted in four different laboratories: San Antonio, Palo Alto, Sausalito, and Hertfordshire.

Of the 13 studies, seven were significant ($P < 0.05$) with an eighth experiment being marginally significant at $P = 0.06$.

The effect sizes ranged from $r = 0.07$ to $r = 0.57$. The mean unweighted effect size was $r = 0.33$ (SD = 0.16), the 95% CI ranged from 0.255 to 0.405 and was significantly different from zero. The weighted (by the number of session) effect size was $r = 0.31$.* Figure 3.3 shows the effect sizes of the experiments.

An interesting question is whether the starees were aroused or calmed by the remote observation. Of the eight experiments with significant results, four show an effect of arousal and four an effect of calming. They are all displayed as

---

*By the time this chapter went into print we descovered that due to the undirected hypotheses in this experimental paradigm sampling errors did not cancel earch other out as expected. The effect sizes reported are therefore confounded with sampling error. A correction procedure would reduce them by approx. 0.15 to approx. $r=0.18$ and $r=0.16$ respectively.

Table 3.2 Overview on all remote starting experiments, by author(s), year of publication, numbers of sessions performed, special hypotheses tested, level and direction of significance testing and according effect size (r).

Experiment	Author(s)	Year	Target system	N	Specialty	Significance	Effect size (r)
1a	Braud et al	1993a	EDA (SRR)	16		$P = 0.018$ 2t	0.57
1b	Braud et al	1993a	EDA (SRR)	16	Connectedness training	$P = 0.048$ 2t	0.49
2	Braud et al	1993b	EDA (SRR)	30		$P = 0.06$ 2t	0.34
3	Braud et al	1993b	EDA (SRR)	16		$P = 0.05$ 2t	0.47
4	Schlitz & LaBerge	1997	EDA (SCR)	24		$P < 0.036$ 1t	0.36
5	Schlitz & LaBerge	1997	EDA (SCR)	24		$P < 0.014$ 1t	0.44
6	Wiseman & Smith	1994	EDA	30	Several observers for each receiver	n.s. 1t	0.26
7	Wiseman et al Wasserman & Hurst	1995	EDA	22	Gender pairing, distance	n.s. 1t	0.14
8	Wiseman et al	1995	EDA	20	Gender pairing	n.s. 1t	0.20
9a	Wiseman & Schlitz	1997	EDA (SRL)	16	Experimenter Schlitz	$P = 0.04$ 2t	0.51
9b		1997	EDA (SRL)	16	Experimenter Wiseman	n.s. 2t	0.11
10a	Wiseman & Schlitz	1999	EDA (SRL)	35	Experimenter Schlitz	$P = 0.05$ 2t	0.33
10b		1999	EDA (SRL)	35	Experimenter Wiseman	n.s. 2t	0.07

EDA, electrodermal activity; SCR, skin conductance response; SRR, skin resistance response; SRL, skin resistance level; SCL, skin conductance level n.s., not significant; 1t, one-tailed test; 2t, two-tailed test

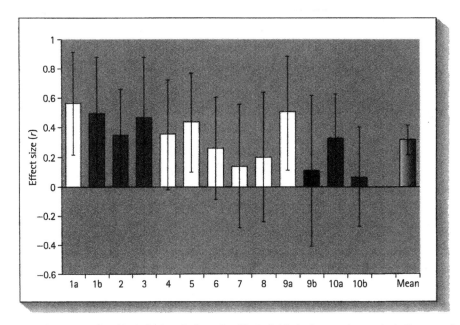

Figure 3.3 Graphical display of effect size (*r*) of all 13 single experiments including overall unweighted mean effect size. Error bars represent the 95% confidence interval. Filled bars represent calming effects, empty bars arousal effects (experiment 9b could not be classified).

positive effect sizes in Figure 3.3, as only effect sizes opposite to the hypothesized direction are displayed as negative. Most of the significant tests applied in remote staring are two-tailed. To map this difference in activation the bars in Figure 3.3 are either filled (calming) or empty (arousal), with experiment 9b being unclear of the direction of the effect. But it is important to mention that this classification is somewhat preliminary as the often incomplete description of the EDA methodology does not allow a clear interpretation in terms of calming or activation.

It might be interesting to note that experiments 1a and 1b are two halves of one study with the same set-up. While in the first experiment participants (starees) were untrained, participants in experiment 1b had taken part in 20 hours of connectedness training, 'engaging in intellectual and experiential exercises involving feelings of interconnectedness with other people and dealing with their own psychological resistance to merging with others' (Braud et al 1990, p. 20). The experiment yielded a significant arousal when the untrained participants were stared at, while the trained participants calmed down when observed.

Experimenter Effects

In contrast to the DMILS data set, the remote staring data set yielded a process-oriented result that was successfully replicated. This is related to often heard rumors within parapsychology that some researchers are highly successful while others never find *Psi*. After Braud and colleagues had presented their first findings on the remote staring effect, several others tried to replicate them. While Schlitz (together with LaBerge) was successful in two replications (4, 5), Wiseman and colleagues found only non-significant results in three experiments (6–8).

To find out whether these results are related to the experimenter or to other differences in the set-up, they decided to conduct an experiment together, both using the same equipment and procedures in the laboratory of the University of Hertfordshire where Wiseman is employed (experiments 9a, 9b). While the 16 participants introduced and observed by Schlitz showed a significant overall result, the 16 participants cared for by Wiseman performed at chance. The same was true for a larger replication (35 sessions each) that was conducted in Schlitz's laboratory in Sausalito, California. In both cases the difference between the experimenters was not large enough to reach a level of significance but both studies stated clearly that with Schlitz as experimenter participants performed better than chance.

DISCUSSION

Let us turn back to the questions posed from a healing perspective to the data of the DMILS data set. The first question was whether there is any empirical evidence for an effect of remote intention measured in terms of physiological changes. The answer is yes. The published DMILS data set containing more than 600 sessions shows a small to medium mean effect size that differs significantly from zero. This situation remains more or less the same when the effect sizes are weighted by the size of the study. A preliminary test proved the data set to be homogenous.

If there is such strong evidence for *Psi* the logical consequence is to investigate whether the effect can be explained in any other way that does not rely on a parapsychological and previous unexplained concept. The assessment for the methodological quality of the studies in this review showed that there are indeed some methodological insufficiencies, especially for the applied EDA methods and statistics. But it is difficult to imagine how these shortcomings might have led to artificial DMILS effects. From my perspective most of the insufficiencies reported would result in not finding effects even if they were present, rather than the other way round. The reason for this is the intraindividual comparison that is calculated in every single DMILS experiment. It was pointed out above that here randomization plays a vital role. By excluding all studies with inadequate randomized sequences it could be demonstrated that the remaining studies still have a significant mean effect size of $r = 0.17$.

There have been various alternative hypotheses to explain the data, such as experimenter fraud, sensory cueing, or cheating participants, discussed in the literature (see, for example, Schlitz & Braud 1997, Wiseman & Schlitz 1997). Although this seems very implausible it could only be checked by a set of independent replications. As the group of parapsychologists doing DMILS research is very small there is a lack of independent publications. There are only four laboratories which have carried out DMILS research, and all their experience, (tacit) knowledge and staff can be traced back to the beginnings in San Antonio where Braud started the DMILS set-up. Braud visited Edinburgh in the early 1990s and taught, among others, Delanoy, Morris and Radin how to perform a DMILS experiment. Delanoy and Morris then started the Freiburg laboratory, Radin the one in Las Vegas. So, although there is a lack of independent replication, the fact that all four laboratories found more or less the same effect sizes is a preliminary argument against alternative explanations such as sensory cueing or cheating participants.

The review of the remote staring studies can be regarded as a kind of validation data set for the DMILS data set. The design is almost the same. However, the way the intention is operationalized is slightly different in a way one could describe as less overt. The mean effect size for remote staring is noticeably higher (see footnote on p. 32) than the one for DMILS but the confidence intervals share an interval from $r = 0.255$ to $r = 0.30$. One cannot judge from these results whether remote staring effects are different from DMILS effects, but the remote staring results clearly confirm the findings reported for DMILS.

Regarding the second question on process-oriented research that might help to understand a healing situation, the situation is disappointing. While the overall DMILS effect is quite stable in various experiments, very little is known about the conditions necessary to increase or decrease the effect.

The only process-oriented result that survived a first replication concerns the experimenter effect and stems from remote staring studies. It looks as though the finding of a remote staring effect is related to a certain person. One problem with this result is that Schlitz and Wiseman had served several functions in their experiments. Both were principal investigators (organizing the whole study), experimenters (interacting with the participants), and starers. Therefore one cannot draw a firm conclusion from this finding, but it is one of the most promising research lines within the actual DMILS and remote staring activities.

Another line of process-oriented research is just about to start. This will ask questions about the relationship between effects in EDA and other psychophysiological systems. So far nobody has addressed the question how EDA is more activated or calmed in a DMILS session. I would call this line of research differential EDA research. Preliminary results such as exploring the variance of the EDA (Watt et al 1999), comparing different EDA parameters, or assessing the relationship between EDA and respiration (Schmidt et al, 2001) indicate that this will help a great deal in our understanding of what happens within the physiology of the receiver. The Freiburg laboratory plans additional EEG mapping during DMILS experiments (Plihal 2000) and interesting results can be expected from that work.

As far as the third question on theoretical understanding and modeling of the DMILS situation is concerned, not much can be said in terms of empirical evidence confirming certain models. The only test applied so far failed. As stated before, there are several good candidates for a theory explaining *Psi* effects, but except for the efforts made by Braud & Schlitz (1989b), so far no one has applied them to the DMILS laboratory in deriving and testing hypotheses.

CONCLUSIONS

DMILS studies provide an interesting data set showing that effects of remote intention can be found within electrodermal activity in laboratory situations. However, the field faces limited resources, and interest from mainstream science is also limited. As a consequence, so far only four different laboratories have investigated DMILS while the number of researchers working with this set-up is no greater than 20. Currently only two laboratories are actively conducting research. Therefore, there is a severe lack of independent replications. The strong proof-oriented findings call for an extension of that research. By extension I mean:

1. to extend from EDA to other physiological and behavioral measures
2. to extend the research into the mainstream psychophysiological research by promoting the DMILS findings to researchers in that field
3. to extend theoretical understanding of the situation by applying and testing different models in experimental situations
4. to extend the process oriented understanding of the supposed effect by testing promising moderator variables and by conducting differential research on EDA.

ACKNOWLEDGMENTS

My work was generously supported by the Institut für Grenzgebiete der Psychologie und Psychohygiene e.V. The DMILS meta-analysis was supported by a grant from the Institute of Noetic Sciences. I am grateful to Harald Walach, Rainer Schneider, and Deborah Lawrie for helpful comments on the paper and for correcting my faulty English. I am also grateful to Ulrike Biedermann for her help with the literature.

REFERENCES

Baker R A 2000 Can we tell when someone is staring at us. Skeptical Inquirer 24: 34–40
Brady C, Morris R L 1997 Attention focusing facilitated through remote mental interaction: a replication and exploration of parameters. Parapsychological Association 40th Annual Convention. Proceedings of presented papers, pp. 73–91. Parapsychological Association, Durham, NC

Braud W G 1979 Conformance behavior involving living systems. In: Roll W G (ed) Research in parapsychology 1978. Abstracts and papers from the 21st annual convention of the parapsychological associaton, 1978, pp. 111–115. Scrarecrow Press, Metuchen, NJ
Braud W G 1990 Distant mental influence of rate of hemolysis of human red blood cells. Journal of the American Society for Psychical Research 84: 1–24

Braud W G 2000 Wellness implications of retroactive intentional influence: exploring an outrageous hypothesis. Alternative Therapies 6: 37–48

Braud W G, Jackson J 1982 The use of ideomotor reactions as Psi indicators. Parapsychology Review 13(2): 10–11

Braud W G, Schlitz M J 1989a A methodology for objective study of transpersonal imagery. Journal of Scientific Exploration 3: 43–63

Braud W G, Schlitz M J 1989b Possible role of intuitive data sorting in electrodermal biological psychokinesis (Bio-PK). Journal of the American Society for Psychical Research 83: 289–302

Braud W G, Schlitz M J 1991 Conscious interactions with remote biological systems: anomalous intentionality effects. Subtle Energies 2: 1–46

Braud W G, Davis G, Wood R 1979 Experiments with Matthew Manning. Journal of the Society for Psychical Research 50: 199–223

Braud W G, Schlitz M J, Schmidt H 1989 Remote mental influence of animate and inanimate target systems. Parapsychological Association 32nd Annual Convention. Proceedings of presented papers, pp. 12–25. Parapsychological Association, Durham, NC

Braud W G, Shafer D, Andrews S 1990 Electrodermal correlates of remote attention: autonomic reaction to an unseen gaze. Parapsychological Association 33rd Annual Convention. Proceedings of presented papers, pp. 14–28. Parapsychological Association, Durham, NC

Braud W G, Shafer D, Andrews S 1993a Further studies of autonomic detection of remote staring, new control procedures, and personality correlates. Journal of Parapsychology 57: 391–409

Braud W G, Shafer D, Andrews S 1993b Reactions to an unseen gaze (remote attention): a review, with new data on autonomic staring detection. Journal of Parapsychology 57: 373–390

Braud W G, Shafer D, McNeill K, Guerra V 1995 Attention focusing facilitated through remote mental interaction. Journal of the American Society for Psychical Research 89: 103–115

Bunnell T 1999 The effect of 'healing with intent' on pepsin enzyme activity. Journal of Scientific Exploration 13: 139–148

Colwell J, Schröder S, Sladen D 2000 The ability to detect unseen staring: a literature review and empirical tests. British Journal of Psychology 91: 71–85

Fowles D C, Christie M J, Edelberg R, Grings W W, Lykken D T, Venables P H 1981 Publication recommendations for electrodermal measurements. Psychophysiology 18: 232–239

May E, Utts J M, Spottiswoode S J P 1995 Decision augmentation theory: toward a model of anomalous mental phenomena. Journal of Parapsychology 59: 195–220

May E, Utts J M, Spottiswoode S J P 1996 Decision augmentation theory: applications to the random number generator. Journal of Scientific Exploration 9: 453–488

Millar B 1978 The observational theories: a primer. European Journal of Parapsychology 2: 304–332

Plihal W 2000 Arbeitsprogramm. Abteilung Experimentelle Studien am Institut für Grenzgebiete der Psychologie und Psychohygiene e.V. (unpublished)

Radin D I, Machado F R, Zangari W 1998 Effects of distant healing intention through time and space: two exploratory studies. Parapsychological Association 41st Annual Convention. Proceedings of presented papers, pp. 143–161. Parapsychological Association, Durham, NC

Rebman J M, Radin D I, Hapke R A, Gaughan K Z 1996 Remote influence of the autonomic nervous system by a ritual healing technique. Parapsychological Association 39th Annual Convention. Proceedings of presented papers, pp. 133–147. Parapsychological Association, Durham, NC

Rosenthal R 1991 Meta-analytic procedures for social research, revised edn. Sage, Newbury Park

Rosenthal R 1994 Parametric measures of effect size. In: Cooper H, Hedges L V (eds) The handbook of research synthesis. Russell Sage Foundation, New York, pp. 231–244

Schlitz M J, Braud W G 1997 Distant intentionality and healing: assesing the evidence. Alternative Therapies in Health and Medicine 3: 62–73

Schmidt S, Walach H 2000 Electrodermal activity (EDA) – state of the art measurement and techniques for parapsychological purposes. Journal of Parapsychology 64: 139–162

Schmidt S, Schneider R, Binder M, Bürkle D, Walach H 2001 Investigating methodological issues in EDA-DMILS: results from a pilot study. Journal of Parapsychology 65: 59–82

Schwartz G E, Russek L G S 1999 Registration of actual and intended eye gaze: correlation with spiritual beliefs and experiences. Journal of Scientific Exploration 13: 213–229

Stokes D M 1997 The nature of mind: parapsychology and the role of consciousness in the physical world. McFarland, Jefferson

Von Lucadou W 1995 The model of pragmatic information (MPI). European Journal of Parapsychology 11: 58–75

Watt C A, Ravenscroft J, McDermott Z 1999 Exploring the limits of direct mental influence: two studies comparing 'blocking' and 'co-operating' strategies. Journal of Scientific Exploration 13: 515–535

Wezelman R, Radin D I, Rebman J M, Stevens P R 1996 An experimental test of magical healing rituals in mental influence of remote human physiology. Parapsychological Association 39th Annual Convention. Proceedings of presented papers, pp. 1–12. Parapsychological Association, Durham, NC

Wiseman R, Schlitz M J 1997 Experimenter effects and the remote detection of staring. Journal of Parapsychology 61: 197–207

Wiseman R, Schlitz M J 1999 Experimenter effects and remote detection of staring: an attempted replication. Parapsychological Association 42nd Annual Convention. Proceedings of presented papers, pp. 471–479. Parapsychological Association, Durham, NC.

Wiseman R, Smith M D 1994 A further look at the detection of unseen gaze. Parapsychological Association 37th Annual Convention. Proceedings of presented papers, pp. 465–478. Parapsychological Association, Durham, NC

DMILS STUDIES

Braud W G 1978 Allofeedback: immediate feedback for a psychokinetic influence upon another person's physiology. In: Roll W G (ed) Research in parapsychology 1977. Abstracts and papers from the 20th Annual Convention of Parapsychological Association, 1977, pp. 123–134. Scarecrow Press, Metuchen, NJ

Braud W G 1979 Conformance behavior involving living systems. In: Roll W G (ed) Research in Parapsychology 1978. Abstracts and papers from the 21st Annual Convention of the Parapsychological Association, 1978, pp. 111–115. Scrarecrow Press, Metuchen, NJ

Braud W G, Schlitz M J 1983 Psychokinetic influence on electrodermal activity. Journal of Parapsychology 47: 95–119

Braud W G, Schlitz M J 1989a A methodology for objective study of transpersonal imagery. Journal of Scientific Exploration 3: 43–63

Braud W G, Schlitz M J 1989b Possible role of intuitive data sorting in electrodermal biological psychokinesis (Bio-PK). Journal of the American Society for Psychical Research 83: 289–302

Braud W G, Schlitz M J 1991 Conscious interactions with remote biological systems: anomalous intentionality effects. Subtle Energies 2: 1–46

Braud W G, Davis G, Wood R 1979 Experiments with Matthew Manning. Journal of the Society for Psychical Research 50: 199–223

Braud W G, Schlitz M J, Collins J, Klitch H 1985 Further studies of the Bio-PK-effekt: feedback, blocking; specificity/generality. In: White R A, Solfvin J (eds) Research in parapsychology 1984. Abstracts and papers from the 27th Annual Convention of the Parapsychological Association, 1984, pp. 45–48. Scarecrow Press, Metuchen, NJ

Delanoy D L, Morris R L 1998 A DMILS training study utilising two shielded environments. European Journal of Parapsychology 14: 52–67

Delanoy D L, Sah S 1994 Cognitive and physiological PSI responses to remote positive and neutral emotional states.
Parapsychological Association 37th Annual Convention. Proceedings of presented papers, pp. 128–138. Parapsychological Association, Durham, NC

Delanoy D L, Morris R L, Brady C, Roe A 1999 An EDA DMILS study exploring agent-receiver pairing. Parapsychological Association 42nd Annual Convention. Proceedings of presented papers, pp. 68–82. Parapsychological Association, Durham, NC

Radin D I, Taylor R K, Braud W G 1995 Remote mental influence of human electrodermal activity: a pilot replication. European Journal of Parapsychology 11: 19–34

Rebman J M, Radin D I, Hapke R A, Gaughan K Z 1996 Remote influence of the autonomic nervous system by a ritual healing technique. Parapsychological Association 39th Annual Convention. Proceedings of presented papers, pp. 133–147. Parapsychological Association, Durham, NC

Schlitz M J, Braud W G 1985 Reiki-plus natural healing: an ethnographic and experimental study. PSI-Research 4: 100–123

Schlitz M J, Braud W G 1997 Distant intentionality and healing: assessing the evidence. Alternative Therapies in Health and Medicine 3: 62–73

Schneider R, Binder M, Walach H (2000) Examining the role of neutral and personal experimenter participant interaction: results from an EDA-DMILS experiment. Journal of Parapsychology 64: 181–194

Watt C A, Ravenscroft J, McDermott Z 1999 Exploring the limits of direct mental influence: two studies comparing 'blocking' and 'co-operating' strategies. Journal of Scientific Exploration 13: 515–535

Wezelman R, Radin D I, Rebman J M, Stevens P R 1996 An experimental test of magical healing rituals in mental influence of remote human physiology. Parapsychological Association 39th Annual Convention. Proceedings of presented papers, pp. 1–12. Parapsychological Association, Durham, NC

REMOTE STARING STUDIES

Braud W G, Shafer D, Andrews S 1993a Further studies of autonomic detection of remote staring, new control procedures, and personality correlates. Journal of Parapsychology 57: 391–409

Braud W G, Shafer D, Andrews S 1993b Reactions to an unseen gaze (remote attention): a review, with new data on autonomic staring detection. Journal of Parapsychology 57: 373–390

Schlitz M J, LaBerge S 1997 Cover observation increases skin conductance in subjects unaware of when they are being observed: a replication. Journal of Parapsychology 61: 185–196
Wiseman R, Schlitz M J 1997 Experimenter effects and the remote detection of staring. Journal of Parapsychology 61: 197–207

Wiseman R, Smith M D 1994 A further look at the detection of unseen gaze. Parapsychological Association 37th Annual Convention. Proceedings of presented papers, pp. 465–478. Parapsychological Association, Durham, NC

Wiseman R, Smith M D, Freedman D, Wasserman T, Hurst C 1995 Examining the remote staring effect: two further experiments. 38th Annual Parapsychological Convention. Proceedings of presented papers, pp. 480–490. Parapsychological Association, Durham, NC

4

Research on mind–matter interactions (MMI): individual intention

Dean Radin
Roger Nelson

This chapter summarizes 40 years of experiments on mind–matter interactions with random number generators by multiple investigators under various conditions.

A fundamental assumption underlying the concept and claims of mental and spiritual healing is that the intention of the healer can directly influence physical events. 'Directly' means without an intervening physical or psychological intervention such as a pill, needle, knife, or word. This claim requires that the mental activity of the healer correlate with physical changes in the environment external to the healer.

While there are claims of miraculous healings throughout history, it is not possible to study these events in a scientific way since they are not consistent or frequent. However, some physical events do occur in regular and predictable ways and if quality scientific evidence indicated that such systems could be influenced, this would be evidence that mind and matter interact in a way that make mental and spiritual healing more plausible. Such a system would need to be simple and easily performed to allow study by independent observers and to create control conditions that investigate alternative explanations other than direct mind–matter interaction. The simplest, most studied and controllable system currently available is the random event generator (REG).

A REG can be any system that behaves in a random way. For example, dice throwing or flipping a coin are random systems. On average, 100 coin flips will generate 50 heads and 50 tails. If you let 100 balls fall down a properly balanced tray with evenly spaced pins, approximately half will fall to the right of center and half to the left. In the 1970s Robert Jahn, then Dean of the School of Engineering at Princeton University, and others began to study REG behavior to determine if mental activity – specifically the intention of an individual – could influence these expected and usual behaviors in such systems. Jahn and his colleagues developed electronic devices that could generate hundreds of random events (similar to coin flips) in a second and record these electronic random events on a computer. This allowed for easily collected and calculated data to be generated for use in mind–machine interaction studies.

The flexibility of electronic REGs has made possible a large number of experiments and numerous individuals and groups have now conducted experiments over more than 40 years. There have been steady improvements in study design, so that standard protocols are now used by more people. This chapter describes this research and quantitatively summarizes its results. Of all the research described in this book, the REG data set is the only one in which there are experiments that meet all of the standard quality criteria and as such are considered fully adequate as evidence. **WBJ**

A META-ANALYSIS OF MIND–MATTER INTERACTION EXPERIMENTS FROM 1959 TO 2000

Introduction

Underlying the concept of 'distant healing' is an assumption that goes beyond the present understanding of mind–body interactions within a given body, as in the discipline of psychoneuroimmunology. Distant healing requires some form of mind–matter interaction (MMI) at a distance. While not widely known to the medical and scientific mainstream, a substantial empirical literature has addressed whether MMI is possible in principle by studying the effects of mental intention on inanimate physical systems. These studies, conducted by researchers around the world for nearly a century, have examined MMI effects on, for example, morphological changes in thin strips of metal (Hasted & Robertson 1980, Randall & Davis 1982, Sasaki & Ochi 1982), the distribution of metallic and plastic balls (Cox 1974, Forwald 1977, Nelson et al 1983), temperature changes in well-shielded environments (Schmeidler 1973, 1984), the statistical behavior of spinning coins (Binski 1958, Thouless 1945), latencies in radioactive decay (Chauvin & Genthon 1965, Ollmar & Tengstrand 1976), and perturbations in sensitive magnetometers (Puthoff & Targ 1976) and interferometers (Jahn 1982).

While many of these studies produced interesting results, by far two classes of MMI experiments have been conducted most often. The first involves tossing dice while intending certain die faces to appear, the second involves mental interaction with random numbers. In dice experiments, individuals typically toss one or more dice while wishing for pre-specified faces to appear. In most of the published studies the dice were held in cups, or were tossed by a machine to avoid the possibility of manual manipulation. The statistical evaluation was based on the number of resulting matches to the target face compared to the number of dice tossed. A meta-analysis found 73 relevant experiments, published between 1935 and 1987, reflecting the efforts of 52 different principal investigators (Radin & Ferrari 1991). Most (74%) of these studies were conducted in the 1940s and 1950s. The publications describe a total of 2.6 million dice-throws in 148 experiments, and just over 150 000 dice-throws in 31 studies where no mental influence was applied to the dice (as a control test).

This set of dice experiments produced a small overall effect (an average of 1.2% over chance expectation), but statistically this was more than 18 standard errors from chance. The control results were well within chance expectation. Examination of 10 factors of methodological quality showed that variations in reported study designs were not correlated with the outcomes, and that experimental quality significantly improved with time. In addition, the 'file-drawer' or selective reporting problem could not plausibly explain the results.

A second class of MMI experiments began in 1959. These involved mental influence of random numbers generated by truly random number generators (RNGs). RNGs are electronic circuits designed to produce a sequence of random bits at the press of a button. After generating a sequence of, say, 100 bits, the number of 1s in the sequence might be provided as feedback. A single 'run' in such an experiment might consist of an observer being asked to mentally intend an RNG to generate, in two successive button presses, a high number (i.e. the number of 1 bits was greater than chance expectation of 50), and then a low number (less than 50). This may be followed by a control condition in which no directional intention is applied. An experiment might consist of a group of individuals, each contributing 100 such runs, or one individual contributing several thousand runs. Outcomes of these experiments are often statistically expressed in terms of z scores, or standard normal deviates from chance. For meta-analytic purposes, outcomes in these studies were evaluated one-tailed (i.e. looking for deviations from chance in the direction of the pre-defined mental intention). Thus reported z scores are recorded for trials defined as high-aim, whereas sign-reversed z scores are recorded for trials defined as low-aim.

A 1989 meta-analysis of RNG experiments located 597 experiments and 235 control studies. These were described in 152 articles, published between 1959 and 1987, by 68 different principal investigators (Radin & Nelson 1989). Of these 597 experiments, 258 were reported in a long-term RNG study from the Princeton Engineering Anomalies Research (PEAR) laboratory, which also reported 127 of the control studies.

The overall statistical outcome was small in magnitude (the equivalent of a 0.9% shift of the 50% chance expected ratio of 1s to 0s in a binary RNG), but this shift of the mean was more than 12 standard errors from chance. As in the dice studies, no significant effects could be attributed to variations in experimental quality, and the file-drawer problem could not plausibly explain

these results. This chapter updates the RNG literature and compares pre- and post-1987 results.

Results

A literature review found 64 new publications describing 176 RNG experiments that were not retrieved in the earlier meta-analysis (for convenience this will be referred to as MA-1989).[1] Of these 176 experiments, 84 were reported up to and including 1987 and 92 after 1987. The new publications included a description of the 20-year PEAR RNG program, thus the 258 PEAR laboratory experiments reported separately in MA-1989 were collapsed into a single datapoint for the purposes of the present (MA-2000) analysis. This resulted in combining 339 non-PEAR experiments from the MA-1989 database along with 176 new studies, for a total of 515 studies reported by 91 different principal investigators in 216 publications. Figure 4.1 shows the number of RNG experiments reported annually from 1959 to 2000.

The RNG experiments in MA-1989 were independently assessed for methodological rigor by the first and second author on a quantitative 16-point scale.[2] For MA-2000 methodological quality was judged based on a subjective five-point scale by the second author. To allow a pooled examination of the effects of experimental quality across all experiments, the MA-1989 16-point quality scores were transformed into equivalent 5-point scores.

Besides the quality score, for each experiment the total number of random samples (referred to as N) and the statistical outcome were recorded (in the form of z scores). Experiments reported only as non-significant, without further details, were assigned z scores of 0. The value of N across all RNG studies ranged from a low of 312 individual random events to a high of 390 million random events. The total N was just over 1.4 billion.

---

[1]See the chapter Appendix for a description of the new analysis.

[2]These included factors such as the presence or absence of control tests, use of failsafe equipment, redundant data recording, data permanently archived, data selection prevented by protocol or equipment, fixed run lengths, and tamper resistant hardware.

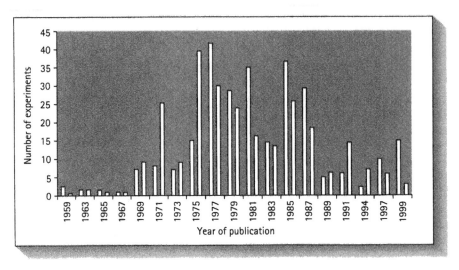

Figure 4.1 Number of RNG experiments published annually.

The average effect size per random event over these 515 studies, expressed in terms of a percentage over chance expectation assuming a binary RNG, was 0.7%. Overall this cumulated to 16.1 standard errors from chance ($P \ll 10^{-50}$). Figure 4.2 shows the chronological history of this cumulative z score.[3]

Figure 4.3 shows the cumulative mean z score for 423 studies reported up to and including 1987 ($\bar{z} = 0.73$, combined $z = 15.1$), and for the 92 post-1987 studies ($\bar{z} = 0.61$, combined $z = 5.86$). A t-test for the difference in the terminal mean z scores is not significant ($P = 0.48$), indicating that experiments published after MA-1989 continue to provide similar evidence for MMI effects.

Approximately 50% of the 515 studies (259) were reported by 10 of the 91 investigators. Their average z score was $\bar{z} = 0.96$ (combined $z = 15.5$). For the remaining 81 investigators, $\bar{z} = 0.46$ (combined $z = 7.3$). Of that group, 23 authors reported a single RNG study, $\bar{z} = 0.65$ (combined $z = 3.1$). This suggests that the overall non-chance result was not attributable to peculiar methods employed by a small group of investigators.

Estimating the file-drawer effect

While a 16 standard error effect is impressively significant, it is likely that some of this effect can be attributed to selective reporting practices. This is because authors tend not to write up – and editors tend not to publish – experiments reporting statistically non-significant results. This publication bias inflates a meta-analytic assessment of a set of studies, as a meta-analysis is based upon published (or otherwise retrievable) reports.

In the worst case, published articles are composed only of significant studies, (i.e. where the outcomes are reported as $P < 0.05$ or $z > 1.645$). In this case, the file-drawer distribution would be composed only of non-significant studies, (i.e. where $P > 0.05$ or $z < 1.645$ (Scargle 2000)). To assess the effects of this worst-case model, a set of 10 000 z scores was generated[4] and the mean of the distribution below $z = 1.645$ was determined. This value was $\bar{z}' = -0.105$. From this we can determine how many studies averaging $\bar{z}'$ would be required to bring the combined statistical outcome down from the observed 16.1

---

[3]z scores were combined by Stouffer's method.

[4]Using the Microsoft Excel 2000 random number generator routine for a normal distribution.

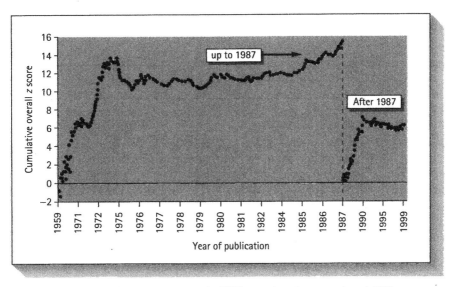

Figure 4.2   Cumulative *z* score for RNG experiments pre- and post-1987.

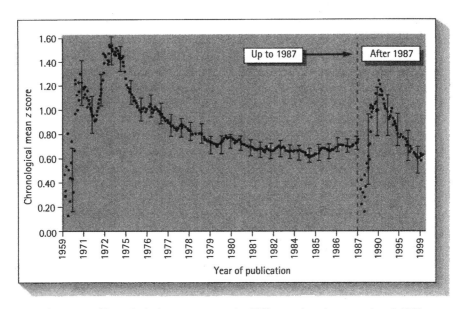

Figure 4.3   Chronological mean *z* scores for RNG experiments pre- and post-1987, with one standard error bars.

standard errors to just above significance (i.e. to $z < 1.645$).

The answer is 2610 studies. This is a ratio of 5.1 unpublished, non-significant, and slightly negative studies to each experiment retrieved in the meta-analysis. Following Rosenthal (1991), we may call the observed meta-analytic result 'robust'

with respect to the selective reporting problem.[5] Note that this worst-case scenario for the file-drawer estimate assumes that each of the 91 authors reporting at least one RNG study had

---

[5]Rosenthal recommended a 5 to 1 ratio for calling a combined effect robust.

also conducted an additional 29 non-significant studies averaging $\bar{z} = -0.105$.

A more realistic model for the file-drawer effect can be formed by examining the actual distribution of 515 z scores (Fig. 4.4). The anomalous spike of observed studies at $z = 0$ is due to the fact that some studies reported only as non-significant were conservatively assigned $z = 0$ in the meta-analysis.

Figure 4.4 also shows a substantial surplus of z scores starting at $z = 1.65$, which is precisely what we would expect from a selective reporting bias. However, we also see a surplus of z scores starting at $z = -2$. This indicates that when experiments proved to be significantly negative, at $P < 0.05$, two-tailed (i.e. at $z < -1.96$), they also tended to be published. This is supported by the fact that at $z \leq -2$ the observed number of studies (39) is far more than the expected number, $P \approx 10^{-10}$. This suggests that a more realistic model for the file-drawer is a z score distribution bounded by the ranges $-1.96 < z < 1.65$.

The average z for a distribution truncated in this fashion, determined by examining a distribution of 10 000 random z scores, is $\bar{z}' = -0.046$. Again we should ask how many studies averaging $\bar{z}'$ would be required to bring the overall statistical outcome down to $z < 1.645$. The answer is 5240, or a ratio of 10.2 unpublished to each published experiment. This would have required each of the 91 authors to have conducted approximately 58 studies,

averaging $\bar{z} = -0.046$, and not to have published any of them. This seems implausible.

Another way to assess the file-drawer effect is to examine the combined statistical result of observed studies falling within the presumed file-drawer range of $-1.96 < z < 1.65$. There were 320 such studies, with a combined statistical effect of 2.59 standard errors from chance ($P < 0.005$). In other words, the cumulative effect of all published non-significant studies is in itself significantly positive. This again indicates that the distribution of observed studies is genuinely shifted beyond chance and that the overall result is not due to a selective reporting problem. The next question is whether design flaws might have been responsible for the observed result.

Quality assessment

If there were a negative correlation between measures of methodological quality and experimental outcomes, it would imply that apparently significant results were actually due to flaws in experimental design. Alternatively, significant studies tend to be reported in more detail than non-significant studies, in which case we might expect to see a positive correlation between study quality and outcomes. If instead no correlation were observed between quality and study outcomes, then it would suggest that methodological quality was not a

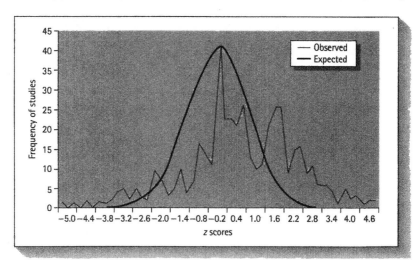

Figure 4.4 Distribution of observed and chance-expected RNG experiments.

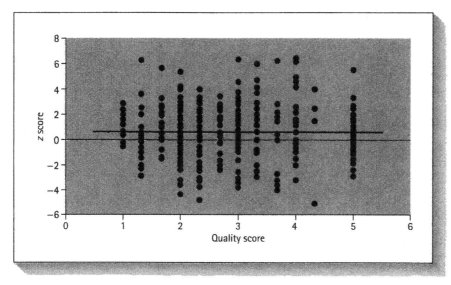

Figure 4.5 Relationship between quality and z score.

significant factor in producing the non-chance results.

Figure 4.5 plots the correlation between experimental quality and reported z scores. Table 4.1 shows that this correlation is non-significant ($P = 0.255$). The same correlation versus effect size (defined as the percentage over chance expectation of 50% for a binary RNG) is also non-significant ($P = 0.109$). Thus, the outcomes of the RNG studies were not due to variations in design quality. Figure 4.6 shows that experimental quality substantially improved with time.

DISCUSSION

The experiments discussed in this chapter were considered in the context of evaluating claims of distant healing effects. The results of this meta-analysis support the existence of genuine mind–matter interaction effects, which in turn supports the plausibility of distant healing.

A common assumption about RNG experiments is that MMI effects 'operate' on individual random events. If this assumption were true, then the statistical results would increase proportionally with $\sqrt{N}$, where N is the number of bits per experiment. That is, the correlation between $\sqrt{N}$ and z should be positive. Indeed, the number of random events used per experiment has significantly increased over the years ($r = 0.35$, $P = 10^{-15}$), reflecting both an increase in the speed with which bits can be generated in modern RNG circuits, and the expectation that more bits per experiment would lead to more significant results.

However, the observed correlation between $\sqrt{N}$ and z is $r = -0.015$, $P = 0.36$. This means the statistical effects observed in these experiments are effectively independent of sample size, and cannot be explained as simple, linear, force-like mechanisms. Thus, if MMI effects in RNG experiments legitimately model similar effects in living systems, then it is likely that distant healing effects also cannot be explained as simple causal process.

Table 4.1 Relationships between study quality and z scores, and quality *vs.* effect size. There are 490 studies listed for the correlation with effect size, as 25 experiments were insufficiently detailed to determine sample size and could not be included in the correlation.

Parameter	Quality *vs z*	Quality vs effect size per bit
r	0.029	−0.056
t	0.659	−1.234
N	515	490
P	0.255	0.109

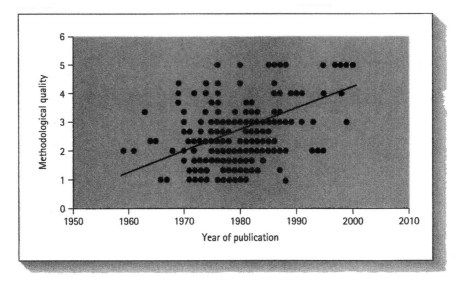

Figure 4.6   Relationship between year of publication and experimental quality, $r = 0.502$, $P = 10^{-34}$.

Further indication that a novel approach will be required to explain these effects are experiments strongly resembling RNG studies, but involving pre-recorded random bits rather than bits generated in real-time. Those studies show significant cumulative results similar to those reported here (Bierman 1998). This implies that some MMI effects, perhaps including those claimed for distant healing, may involve acausal processes.

CONCLUSION

Meta-analysis of 515 RNG experiments conducted by 91 researchers over a span of 41 years indi-cates the presence of a small magnitude, but statistically highly significant and repeatable mind–matter interaction effect. The overall results cannot be attributed to chance, selective reporting problems, or variations in design quality. These studies indicate that there are ways in which mind and matter interact that support the plausibility of distant intentional healing. Because modern RNG experiments can be conducted under tightly controlled laboratory conditions at relatively low cost, they may serve as a convenient model to help us better understand the relevant conditions and mechanisms of distant healing.

REFERENCES

Bierman D J 1998 Do psi phenomena suggest radical dualism? In: Hameroff S, Kaszniak A, and Scott A (eds) Toward a science of consciousness II. MIT Press, Cambridge MA

Binski S 1958 Performance by a single subject in exploratory PK experiments. Zeitschrift fur Parapsychologie und Grenzgebiete der Psychologie 2: 30–40

Chauvin R, Genthon J-P 1965 An investigation of the possibility of PK experiments with uranium and a geiger-counter. Zeitschrift fur Parapsychologie und Grenzgebiete der Psychologie 8: 140–147

Cox W E 1974 PK tests with a thirty-two channel balls machine. Journal of Parapsychology 38: 56–68

Forwald H 1977 A PK experiment with a single ball rolling on a decline. European Journal of Parapsychology 2: 4–14

Hasted J B, Robertson D 1980 Paranormal action on metal and its surroundings. Journal of the Society for Psychical Research 50: 379–398

Jahn R G 1982 The persistent paradox of psychic phenomena: an engineering perspective. Proceedings of the IEEE 70: 136–170

Nelson R D, Dunne B J, Jahn R G A 1983 Psychokinesis experiment with a random mechanical cascade. Technical note PEAR 83002, Princeton Engineering Anomalies Research, Princeton University, School of Engineering/Applied Science

Ollmar S, Tengstrand G 1976 PK on radioactive decay. Research Letter 7: 23–26

Puthoff H E, Targ R 1976 A perceptual channel for information transfer over kilometer distances: historical perspective and recent research. Proceedings of the IEEE 64: 329–354

Radin D I, Ferrari D C 1991 Effects of consciousness on the fall of dice: a meta-analysis. Journal of Scientific Exploration 5: 61–84

Radin D I, Nelson R D 1989 Evidence for consciousness-related anomalies in random physical systems. Foundations of Physics 19: 1499–1514

Randall J L, Davis C P 1982 Paranormal deformation of nitinol wire: a confirmatory experiment. Journal of the Society for Psychical Research 51: 368–373

Rosenthal R 1991 Meta-analytic procedures for social research, rev. edn. Sage, Newbury Park CA

Sasaki K S Ochi Y 1982 Observation of the deformation of pure aluminum plates by psychokinesis. Journal of the Psi Science Institute of Japan 7: 7–13

Scargle J D 2000 Publication bias: the 'File-Drawer Problem' in scientific inference. Journal of Scientific Exploration 14: 91–106

Schmeidler G R 1973 PK effects upon continuously recorded temperature. Journal of the American Society for Psychical Research 67: 325–340

Schmeidler G R 1984 Further analyses of PK with continuous temperature recordings. Journal of the American Society for Psychical Research 78: 355–362

Thouless R H 1945 Some experiments on PK effects in coin spinning. Proceedings of the Society for Psychical Research 47: 277–281

APPENDIX

Roger Nelson

The RNG literature was first examined in 1987 for a meta-analysis ultimately published in 1989 (Radin & Nelson 1989). Though our search at the time was reasonably thorough, we did not locate all the relevant papers, and in the meantime many more RNG studies have been conducted. Dr Fiona Steinkamp, at the Institut für Grenzgebiete der Psychologie und Psychohygiene (IGPP) in Freiburg, Germany, has undertaken a comprehensive update and extension of the original RNG meta-analysis, and she provided us with a complete set of papers which were not included in the 1987 survey, or were published later.

A preliminary meta-analysis of these additional papers was prepared as part of a presentation of the state of the art of mind–matter interaction research at the Science and Spirituality in Healing conference in Winston-Salem, NC, October 26–29, 2000. This update of the RNG meta-analysis is less formal than the 1987 effort and should be regarded as an approximation that can later be compared to the more exacting analysis intended by the IGPP team. In particular, the quality assessment for this effort used a five-point subjective rating scale, rather than the quantitative count of specific methodological features we had originally employed. The ratings were based on the same methodological criteria as in the 1987 analysis although the features were not explicitly counted. Judgements were made independently for each paper without consideration of possible implications for the intended use in various correlational studies. The relationship of study quality to effect size in the new body of experiments will eventually be treated more rigorously by the IGPP group, but we felt it was important to provide a preliminary estimate of quality to address this important meta-analytic question.

The new database includes a total of 65 additional articles describing RNG studies and five papers discussing a new experimental variant called FieldREG. The latter studies examine correlations between RNG outputs and implicit variations in attention within groups of people rather than explicit assignment of intention in individuals.

The new experiments were reported by 36 principal authors and include published articles, technical reports, theses, reports in proceedings, and abstracts in journals or books. The total of 70 papers includes 183 RNG studies and 22 FieldREG studies, for a total of 205 reported outcomes. Some 27 of these papers, comprising 67 studies, were found with publication dates prior to 1987, which had not been discovered in the search at that time. Most of those were from conference proceedings or non-English-language journals.

It is important to note that the great majority of the post-1987 database were process-oriented experiments, in which two or more conditions (identified as separate studies in our meta-analytic database) were compared. This means that some of the conditions were not expected to produce anomalous deviations because the intention of the experiment was to compare differences among conditions rather than the simple effects of intention on RNG behavior. The present meta-analysis was not designed to address questions about underlying processes. Rather, we wished to assess the cumulative evidence for consciousness-related anomalies in the RNG literature. Therefore, a decision was made at the outset to disregard the implicit intentions embedded in complex, process-oriented experimental designs, and to regard each study or data subset in the same way, as if the participants always intended to achieve an anomalous effect in the direction of nominal intention. This is a conservative approach because it ignores predicted differential effects, and it penalizes any successful effort to reduce deviation as may be required in certain experimental conditions.

5

Research on mind–matter interactions (MMI): group attention

Roger Nelson
Dean Radin

This chapter summarizes experiments from an ongoing program examining correlations of collective coherent group attention with random number generators.

After the development of electronic REGs (described in Chapter 4), it was noticed that non-random behavior sometimes occurred during group activities when no intention was being directed at the machine. It seemed that when a group was intensively focused, as during concerts and sports events, REGs deviated from chance patterns more often than during chaotic and unfocused group events, for example, in the middle of a city street or library. REG deviations also seemed to occur during intense group activities such as psychodrama more often than during more mundane activities, for example in a lecture or committee discussion. These observations led the Princeton Engineering Anomalies Laboratory and several other groups to launch a series of systematic investigations into the effect on REG deviations during focused or 'profound' group activities compared to more chaotic or 'mundane' activities. This chapter describes and statistically analyzes the results of those experiences.

Collective healing rituals, often performed in groups, are a common approach to healing in many societies. Healing rituals such as the group Shoshoni healing ceremony described in the chapter have also been among the group activities related to healing in which REG deviations occur more often than chance. If healing is associated with coherent group attention and does not require any intention toward the REG, this implies a model of healing interaction between individuals rather than a sender–receiver model of healing transmission to a patient. It also indicates that the REG is not measuring intention, but rather an effect generated on a more general level of conscious attention. This implies that a collective healing interaction between healer and patient alters the environment, rather than an individual healer altering the machine or the patient directly. This also implies that the REG is not a receiver, but a detector of coherence.

A major deviation in a worldwide network of REGs monitored from Princeton University occurred during the September 11, 2001 terrorist attacks in the United States when world attention was focused on the events in New York, Pennsylvania and Washington. These data are not incorporated into this chapter. Detailed descriptions of the REG behavior during and after this event, with various interpretations of the data, are available at the website: http://noosphere.princeton.edu/terror.html.   **WBJ**

FIELDREG EXPERIMENTS AND GROUP CONSCIOUSNESS: EXTENDING REG/RNG RESEARCH TO REAL-WORLD SITUATIONS

Introduction

In Chapter 4 we describe a meta-analysis of 41 years of individual mind–matter interaction (MMI) experiments in which the output of a random event generator (REG)[1] serves as the target for the participant's intention to affect a sensitive physical system. Here we discuss a variant called FieldREG which uses the same technology for an extension of the laboratory research into field applications. These may be thought of as 'group' MMI experiments. Similar equipment and software serve to record data, but in this case we look for effects of consciousness in the absence of

intention or attention to the device itself. The protocol is equally rigorous as an experimental design, but instead of manipulating conditions, the FieldREG protocol samples pre-existing conditions. This research program helps link the laboratory MMI research to studies of real-world applications of healing intention in clinical practice. The connections to healing are at this point largely by extrapolation, but there have been some relatively direct efforts to see whether the healing situation may generate anomalies in FieldREG data. Here we describe the paradigm and give some examples suggesting that the REG technology may respond to the structuring influence of something we might tentatively call a 'consciousness field' such as is envisioned by many healers.

In the laboratory research, an electronic REG produces streams of random numbers which might be envisioned as a high-speed sequence of coin flips. The REG output is well defined and the distribution of results is calibrated to conform to precise statistical expectations. In an experiment, a participant holds prescribed intentions in mind, and wills or wishes the REG device to produce departures from chance expectation. Somewhat surprisingly, since we do not know how to explain such departures, people often succeed at this task, so that the results show small but statistically significant deviations. Meta-analysis leaves little doubt that this is a repeatable finding, despite the miniscule size of the effect and its high variability.

In 1993, a continuously running version of the REG experiment was set up in the Princeton Engineering Anomalies Research (PEAR) laboratory, with the option to conduct intention-based experiments, but with the primary goal of assessing data collected during other time-periods. Index entries could be made to identify the presence of people in the room, demonstrations, special events or meetings, and independent experiments using other equipment, with the intention of looking for possible correlations. This experiment led naturally to the idea of bringing an REG into the field, to take data in circumstances that have an identifiable impact on the consciousness of the people involved. We wished to determine whether situations that

---

[1]The term random number generator, or RNG, as used in Chapter 4, is equivalent.

deeply engage people might elicit a group consciousness defined by unusual resonance or coherence which, in turn, might have a detectable effect on the REG. Early explorations supported this expectation, and led to a formal, predictive experimental protocol. We were able to establish that most of the events and gatherings chosen for FieldREG applications could be segregated into two categories which successfully discriminate the data. The first, situations which promote deep engagement, interpersonal resonance, or coherent group interaction, tended to yield anomalous data showing relatively consistent departures from chance expectation. In contrast, mundane, day-to-day situations and those which have a chaotic nature or competitive aspects tended to produce only random fluctuations (Nelson et al 1996).

Methodology

To facilitate this line of research, miniaturized REG devices were constructed for use with laptop computers, and later, palmtop computers. Software was designed to allow continuous, time-stamped data recording with indexing to register the timing of particular events. Other researchers, notably Radin and Bierman, developed variants on the theme, with different methodologies but a similar purpose (Radin et al 1996, Bierman 1996). The FieldREG paradigm differs in important ways from the laboratory experiment, most notably, as mentioned earlier, in having no assigned intentions. Participants in a group where FieldREG data are being recorded are not instructed to try to affect the machine, and indeed they typically pay no attention to it or may even not know that such data are being collected. The REG is used as if it were a monitoring instrument that is expected to be sensitive to the degree of interpersonal resonance or coherence that might be present in a group.

Although continuing exploration is needed to broaden our perspective, the early work allowed us to develop true, hypothesis-based experiments using two main categories for predictions. These serve the functions of the standard treatment and control conditions in variable-manipu-

lation experiments. In the FieldREG protocol we do not manipulate conditions, but instead draw fixed samples from two existing, pre-defined categories of conditions. The equivalent of a treatment condition is created by the *a priori* identification of 'resonant' situations that are predicted to produce non-random behavior in REG data taken in that environment. In contrast, 'mundane' situations are predicted to show no deviations from expectation, and they serve a function that is analogous to a control condition (Nelson 1997, Nelson et al 1998). In most applications, the segregation into these two categories is made by identifying separate venues where data will be taken. In some cases, it is possible to acquire data in both conditions by identifying separate periods of time as 'active' *vs.* 'control' data within an application. For example, Radin and colleagues rated parts of a holotropic breathwork workshop for high *vs.* low coherence, and compared the corresponding REG deviations (Radin et al 1996).

A large database of FieldREG applications, categorized predictively as either resonant or mundane, has been collected by the PEAR group, as well as by Radin and his colleagues. The difference in outcomes is stark, with only the former category showing consistent deviations of the means to larger values in the pre-specified data segments. In the PEAR database, the increase in the variance of the means compounds over 28 independent replications to a probability of 2.2×10^{-6}. In 12 mundane situations, by contrast, there is a modest reduction in the variance measure, with a cumulative probability of 0.91. A further set of 40 explorations in venues for which we had not developed an adequate database for predictive categorization showed a significant increase in variance overall ($P = 0.002$), with considerable differences among several subsets grouped by common characteristics. In addition to the 'mundane' control data, the FieldREG protocol is supported by two additional measures of expected behavior for the REG. Large database calibrations are analyzed to determine the quality of the random source, according to specified criteria that ensure behavior indistinguishable from chance expectation under normal, non-experimental conditions. In addition, a resampling procedure is employed in which data segments corresponding to the active, experimental data are extracted from surrounding, inactive data. The resampling typically is repeated 1000 times, to produce an empirical 'chance' distribution against which the active data can be compared.

EXAMPLES RELEVANT TO HEALING

The following examples, with graphic displays of the data, provide a sense of the structuring effect on nominally random sequences seen in situations that promote engaged group consciousness. These are selected for their relevance to the topic of healing, though in most cases the connection is indirect. The examples suggest that FieldREG studies of actual intentional healing would be interesting and instructive, and imply

that our prediction should be for positive anomalous deviations during healing sessions.

Small Group: Direct Mental and Healing Interactions (DMHI)

In a small, intimate working group, members may become so engaged in their common task that they give up some of their individual identification and integrate into the group, creating a 'group consciousness.' In an early application, at a 1993 meeting of a group discussing direct mental and healing interactions (DMHI), the FieldREG data contained several striking segments, as shown in Figure 5.1 (Nelson et al 1996). One of the 12 meeting sessions, marked in the figure by vertical lines, showed a trend that was extremely unlikely to be mere chance fluctuation, with odds of 500 to 1. With the appropriate correction for multiple analysis the deviation

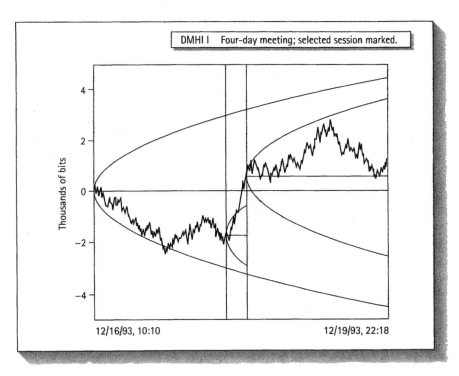

Figure 5.1 FieldREG data taken during a 4-day meeting of a group of researchers working to develop methods for assessing the effects of conscious intent to change physiological measures. The purpose was to create robust experiments that would provide useful perspectives on non-local or intentional healing. The marked segment identifies a selected 2-hour session in which there was an unusually high degree of resonance between the speaker and the rest of the group.

remains unlikely with odds of 40 to 1. It is tempting to speculate that the combination of an interesting topic, which we all felt was profoundly important, with a charismatic presentation produced a real group consciousness. Though they are temporary, such integrated and mutually engaged states of consciousness are noteworthy and readily identifiable in retrospect. The FieldREG data appear to provide an additional, objective confirmation of this perception.

Holotropic Breathwork

In a field experiment with related methodology, Radin and colleagues collected data at a day-long workshop focused on personal growth and healing techniques. It involved active training in holotropic breathwork, a powerful technique which strongly holds the participants' attention (Radin et al 1996). Data were gathered over a total of 7 hours during the workshop, and were segregated into periods of high and low group coherence as rated by the experimenters. The cumulative odds against chance for the high-coherence data grew to about 1000 to 1 over the course of the workshop, while the low-coherence

data, serving as a control condition, indicated there was nothing unusual about the REG device or the analysis methodology. Figure 5.2 shows the progressive divergence of the active data from theoretical expectation and from the well-behaved control data.

Shamanistic Healing at a Sacred Site

While most of the applications in the FieldREG program of research over the past several years have been concerned with group consciousness in a very broad spectrum of situations, several have addressed directly the possibility that healing practices and intentions may affect REG devices. The idea is based on conceptual similarities which are apparent in the descriptions. We find that periods of interpersonal resonance and engagement are correlated with anomalous deviations in FieldREG data, and this is compatible with the suggestions healers often make that their work is enabled by deep interconnections. An opportunity to meet and work with a Shoshone medicine man at Devils Tower in Wyoming resulted in support for the suggestion that a healing intent *per se* might correlate with

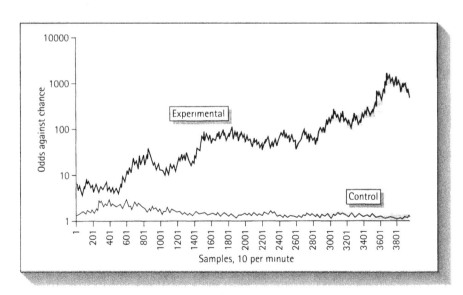

Figure 5.2 Data collected during a holotropic breathwork personal growth workshop. The upper curve, labeled experimental, shows a clear trend which culminates in a significant probability of 0.002. The lower curve shows data taken during a control period of the same length following the workshop.

anomalies in the FieldREG data (Nelson et al 1998). The Shaman in this example has a personal mission to heal the sacred places of the American Indians, and to help protect them against modern developments and destructive forces. He conducted a healing ceremony at a 'power' spot he had located, and cooperated with our scientific methodology by conducting a second, 'sham' ceremony with much the same outward appearance at a control location determined by one of our small group. The first situation yielded a strong and steady cumulative deviation (the odds against chance were about 200 to 1) over the 20 minutes of the healing ceremony, while the arbitrarily located control ceremony produced data indistinguishable from random expectation. Figure 5.3 shows the data from the healing ceremony.

Kom Ombo Temple, Egypt

In another example representing healing practices in the context of a sacred site, data were gathered in the holy of holies of an Ancient Egyptian temple at Kom Ombo (Nelson 1997). This was a place dedicated to the goddess of healing, and the ancient records describe rituals involving passing through a tunnel which still exists in the ruins. Several members of our tour group took advantage of the opportunity and created a semblance of the ritual during our visit. The FieldREG data corresponding to the time we were in the holy of holies and thinking deeply about the implications of a temple like this one showed a strong and persistent deviation (Fig. 5.4) that is statistically significant, with a chance probability of less than 1 in 100.

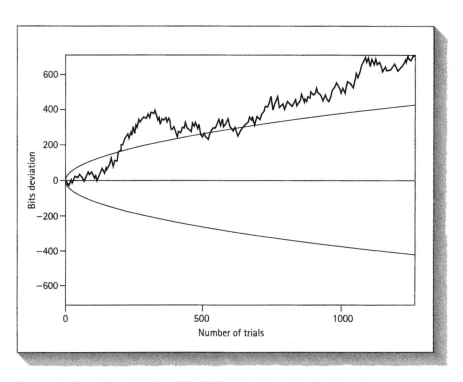

Figure 5.3 Cumulative deviation of FieldREG data during a 20-minute healing ceremony performed by a Shoshone Shaman at Devils Tower, Wyoming. The horizontal line shows the expectation for the random walk described by the accumulating deviations, and the parabolic envelope shows the locus of the 0.05 probability for so large a deviation as the database increases.

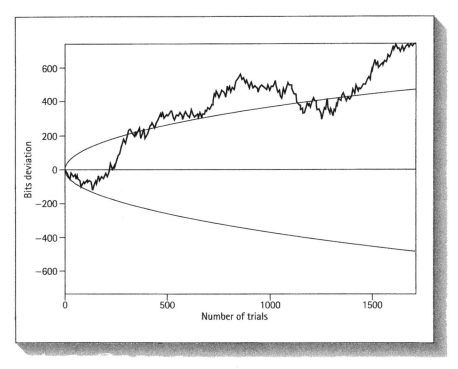

Figure 5.4 FieldREG data taken during a 22-minute ritual performed in the holy of holies of the Temple of Healing in Kom Ombo, Egypt, by a small group interested in the spiritual practices of the Ancient Egyptians. The parabola shows the 5% significance level, and the jagged line shows the data, which culminate in a probability against chance of 0.009.

A Mundane Example

The cases shown in the previous examples are selected for their conceptual relevance to healing. It happens that they all are applications in which a strong deviation occurred, and a comparison context may be of some value. Most academic conferences are characterized by a congenial atmosphere, but not by deep, widely shared engagement. Figure 5.5 shows data collected during a typical academic conference, in this case a meeting of the Society for Scientific Exploration (SSE), which is a gathering of scientists and researchers from a broad range of disciplines, all of whom share a commitment to open-minded examination of issues at the growing frontiers of science. The meeting presentations are on topics which tend to be rejected as unscientific by the wider scientific community, and the SSE provides a forum in which such topics, including non-local healing, for example, will be given a respectful

hearing. Though the meeting has a cooperative and collaborative quality, it is multifaceted and diverse, and does not have the intense, shared focus that characterizes resonant situations. The graph in Figure 5.5 is typical for academic meetings, which we categorize as mundane gatherings, with no strong trends to distinguish the data from the random expectation. This is given as an example of the 'control' condition in the FieldREG protocol.

HEALERS IN PRACTICE

At least two studies are currently under way to collect FieldREG-style data in the presence of healers working with clients in clinical situations. In one case the data are being gathered in a number of different treatment contexts with several healers. In the other, a well-known healer is participating in a long-term experiment, by hosting a FieldREG in his treatment room and

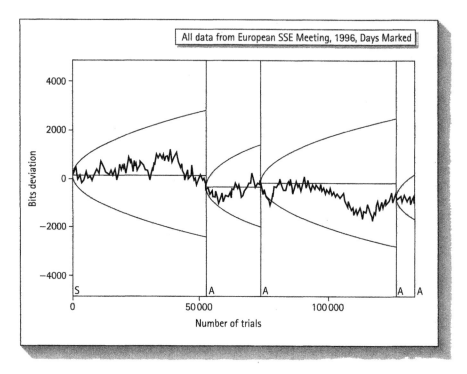

Figure 5.5 Cumulative deviation of FieldREG data during the European meeting of the Society for Scientific Exploration in October, 1996. The vertical lines mark the separate days. The horizontal lines show the expectation for the random walk described by the accumulating deviations, and the parabolic envelopes show the locus of the 0.05 probability for so large a deviation as the database increases.

marking the times of sessions with his clients. Neither of these studies is complete, so we can report only informal results. Preliminary assessments show promise but also considerable complexity, in that our simple in-going expectation of consistent deviations during the healing session is probably not correct. Instead, there appears to be a broader or more general effect on the environment.

DISCUSSION AND CONCLUSION

Tentatively, we propose that emotionally engaging situations are the source of an 'active information field' which may be actualized as reduced entropy in appropriately designed random physical systems. The REG technology allows an assessment of structure in a nominally random data stream during identified periods of time, displaying it as changes in the statistical distribution of the data. In practice, we predict that a profoundly engaging common interest can create a group consciousness that functions as a source of structuring information. The labile REG device acts as a potential sink for such information if it is available.

The FieldREG results are striking, especially in terms of their overall consistency relative to the closely related laboratory REG experiments. Within the category that is predicted to produce deviation, the reliability is sufficient to produce an effect size that is more than twice that found in the meta-analysis of the REG database. With regard to the actual source of the effect, we can exclude artifacts with the same confidence as we have in the laboratory experiments. On the other hand, we cannot assert confidently that the source is a 'consciousness field' generated by the group in question. Although we say that there is no intention directed toward the REG, or toward wishing for high scores, the experimenter almost certainly does have, at least unconsciously, an intention or wish for the experiment to be interesting. Similarly, there may be other contextual aspects to the FieldREG experiment which should be considered as relevant to understanding how this might work. Clearly we have much to learn about this relatively new perspective on the subtle and surprising reach of consciousness.

There is a certain wisdom embodied in long-standing customs and practices. For all of history we have prayed, and we have practiced healing. This is a qualitative background against which we should find results from REG and FieldREG experiments less surprising, and it should help us to develop this prospective source of both theoretical and practical insights for the study of consciousness.

REFERENCES

Bierman D 1996 Exploring correlations between local emotional and global emotional events and the behavior of a random number generator. Journal of Scientific Exploration 10: 363–373

Nelson R D 1997 FieldREG measurements in Egypt: resonant consciousness at sacred sites. Technical note 97002, Princeton Engineering Anomalies Research, School of Engineering/Applied Science, Princeton University, Princeton NJ

Nelson R D, Bradish G J, Dobyns Y H, Dunne B J, Jahn R G 1996 FieldREG anomalies in group situations. Journal of Scientific Exploration 10: 111–141

Nelson R D, Jahn R G, Dunne B J, Dobyns Y H, Bradish G J 1998 FieldREG II: consciousness field effects: replications and explorations. Journal of Scientific Exploration 12: 425–454

Radin D I, Rebman J M, Cross M P 1996 Anomalous organization of random events by group consciousness: two exploratory experiments. Journal of Scientific Exploration 10: 143–168

6

Non-sensory access to information: remote viewing

Jessica Utts
Edwin May

This chapter summarizes the quantity, quality, and results of a systematic, 20-year investigation into human ability to access information via means other than traditional mechanisms.

In health care, assessment is as crucial as treatment. Medicine is replete with descriptions of master diagnosticians who could assess a patient's condition and prognosis with extremely subtle cues, such as a smell, a shade of color or a light touch. Healers in many cultures claim to make assessments by intuition, sometimes even remotely from the patient. Are there data examining the ability of individuals to access information without known means of information access or sensory cues? If so, this might be another avenue of investigation for as yet unexamined methods used by expert diagnosticians and healers.

Studies on intuitive diagnosis are few and of variable quality. There are, however, two extensive data sets which examine whether individuals have the ability to detect information via non-sensory means. The research described in this chapter was sponsored primarily by the US government over the past 30 years. This program examined factors that might contribute to this ability, including selection of skilled individuals, training techniques to enhance non-sensory access to information and systematic scoring methods for determining accuracy of that information access. Jessica Utts, a statistician, and Edwin May, a physicist who conducted much of this research for the US Government, review and analyze these data. Further research with similar methods may help us understand mechanisms whereby clinicians access information that enhances their diagnostic abilities.   **WBJ**

INTRODUCTION

Anecdotes about anomalous distant communication have persisted throughout history. These anecdotes include stories about information transmitted from one person to another (commonly known as telepathy), from a non-living source to a person (commonly known as clairvoyance), and from the future to the present (commonly known as precognition). In the latter part of the 20th century the US government supported the scientific study of these types of phenomena, neutrally called 'anomalous cognition' (AC). In particular, numerous studies focused on 'remote viewing' in which an individual (the receiver) was asked to describe an unspecified remote location, photograph, etc. (the target). The target was sometimes viewed by another person (the sender) but was more often simply specified on paper or in a computer. Sometimes the target was not designated until after the remote viewing description had been recorded. Thus, the assumed mode of transmission encompassed all three of the common types: telepathy, clairvoyance, and precognition.

The results of the remote viewing experiments were overwhelmingly supportive of some kind of anomalous information acquisition (Utts 1996). The mechanism through which the information is acquired is still not understood, but researchers have recently discovered some interesting relationships between successful AC and other factors. Further investigation of these relationships may lead to discoveries about how anomalous cognition works.

The purpose of this chapter is to review what is known about remote viewing and related 'free-response' psi experiments, and to link that information with intuitive medical diagnosis. There are two ways in which the current remote viewing results, and the relationships between remote viewing success and other variables, may impact intuitive medical diagnosis. First, these results

lead to suggestions about how intuitive diagnosis may be enhanced. Second, they invite an exploration of research questions involving intuitive diagnosis that may help to solve the mystery of how anomalous cognition works.

REMOTE VIEWING
Procedure

The scientists who conducted anomalous cognition experiments for the US government coined the term 'remote viewing' to avoid the use of emotionally- and context-laden terms such as 'psychic' and 'telepathy'. Unfortunately, since the declassification of the government studies in 1995, the term 'remote viewing' has itself been widely used by organizations with methods and claims that differ substantially from the scientific study of remote viewing conducted by researchers. Therefore, it is worth reviewing the standard remote viewing protocol used in the experiments discussed in this chapter. A standard remote viewing session in which there is no sender would be done either as follows, or using some slight variation of this outline:

• A receiver (also known as a subject) and a monitor (or experimenter) are isolated in a remote and sensory-shielded room in the laboratory.

• About 5 minutes later, at a pre-arranged time and a location distant from the receiver's room, an assistant randomly selects one of a large, predefined set of possible target photographs. The time is pre-arranged so that the assistant does not have any contact with the receiver after the target has been selected, avoiding possible subtle transmission of information about the target through normal means. Thus both the receiver and the monitor are blind to the target choice.

• Under the guidance of the monitor, the receiver spends the next 15–20 minutes trying to describe the target. The description usually involves sketches and narratives written on several sheets of paper. The monitor's role is to make sure the receiver records all impressions and to help guide the receiver through the process, much like a coach may guide an athlete. Experienced receivers do not require a monitor.

- When the receiver thinks he or she has finished, the session comes to an end. The monitor then makes a copy of the description and locks the original in a safe location.
- The receiver is then shown the target photograph and the copy of his or her description for feedback.
- When a series of sessions is completed an independent member of the laboratory staff, who was not involved in the experimental process to that stage, judges the results. (The judging process is described below.)

There are in addition numerous security measures not included in the brief description given above but they can be found in other sources such as Utts (1996) and May (1996). As protocols have changed to reflect new technology and new research questions, these security measures have been periodically reviewed and approved by an advisory board consisting of a prestigious multidisciplinary team of scientists, including expertise on detecting fraud.

Judging, Effect Size, and Quality Measure

Two common methods are used to judge remote viewing and to assess the quality of the material produced. The standard method of assessment is rank-order judging; this proceeds as follows:

- Before an experiment begins, a large pool of targets is assembled, and grouped into sets of five.[1] The five targets in each set are as dissimilar as possible, for reasons that will become clear. Some experiments used photographs as targets, others used short video segments and others used physical locations.
- For each session, a target set of five is randomly selected, and then one of the five is randomly chosen to be the target for that session. The remaining four targets in the set are used as 'decoys' for the judging process.

---

[1]Five is used here for illustrative purposes, but some experiments use target sets of four.

- A judge who has no prior knowledge of what transpired in a session is given the five targets from the set for that session, as well as the description provided by the receiver.
- The judge's task is to rank the five target possibilities as to how closely they match the description. The target possibility that matches the response best is ranked 1, and so on. All target possibilities must be assigned a rank, with no ties.
- The useable data value from each session consists only of the rank assigned to the correct target. By chance, that rank could be any of the numbers from 1 to 5 with equal likelihood. The term 'direct hit' is used if the correct target receives a rank of one.
- The results of an entire experiment are summarized by either counting the number of direct hits, or by summing the rank assigned to the correct target across all sessions in the experiment. This summary measure is then compared to what would be expected by chance, and an average effect size (described below) for the entire experiment is computed.

To illustrate this procedure, an AC response from a novice receiver is shown in Figure 6.1.

It would be very difficult indeed to identify what the target photograph might be from just looking at the response in Figure 6.1. Fortunately, the analyst need only to decide which of the five target photographs best matches this response, even if the match is not particularly good. Figure 6.2 shows the set of five judging photographs, only one of which is the intended target.

Upon close inspection, it is possible to find elements in the response in Figure 6.1 that match something in each of the five photographs in Figure 6.2. So, particularly with novice receivers, the rank-order is very much a subjective task. In this case the analyst chose the windmills as the best match and the coast, waterfall, desert, and city as the second through fifth best match, respectively. As it turns out, the windmills photograph was the intended target, so this trial would receive a rank number of 1, or in other words, would be a direct hit.

This novice example was chosen from a 24-trial formal series conducted in an industrial setting.

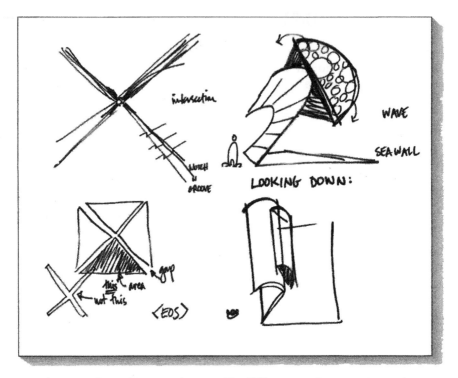

Figure 6.1 A complete anomalous cognition (AC) response from a novice receiver.

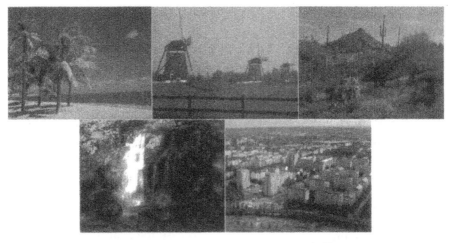

Figure 6.2 Judging pack for the response shown in Figure 6.1.

The effect size for the study was 0.530 ± 0.204, which corresponds to a P value of 0.0046.

In general, the statistical term 'effect size' denotes the amount by which the average results for one unit (person, session, etc.) differ from what would be expected by chance, or the amount by which the average results for two groups differ from each other. The difference is standardized using common statistical procedures so that effect sizes may be compared across experiments that use different types of measurements. If results are at chance, or if two groups are comparable, the average effect size will be 0. By convention, it is generally accepted that an effect size around 0.2 is small, around 0.5 is medium and around 0.8 is large. A medium effect size is said to be visible to the naked eye of an astute observer, while a large effect size should be evident to any observer. As an example, a difference of slightly over 1 inch in the mean heights of two groups of adults reflects a medium effect size, while a difference in mean heights of 2 inches reflects a large effect size.

While the use of rank-order judging is statistically straightforward, it does not provide a discriminating measure of the quality of the remote viewing. A remote viewing description that has just enough information to choose the correct target out of a set of five possibilities receives the same amount of 'credit' as one that is a perfect drawing of the target. Therefore, another measure has been developed to measure the quality of the remote viewing, called the 'figure of merit' (May et al 1990). The figure of merit is based on matching the response to a long list of possible target elements, ranging from shapes and colors to specific features such as buildings and waterfalls. Mathematically, it is a combination of the degree to which target elements were included in the response, and response elements were part of the target. Thus, to receive a high figure of merit a response must be an efficient description of the target. The figure of merit is not as easy to evaluate statistically, because there is no independent information about how large it would be by chance. It can be used as a differential measure, by computing a figure of merit for the response matched to the actual target and matched to all other targets in the large pool. However, the resulting probability measure depends on the size of the target pool. The figure of merit is nonetheless a good measure to use for correlating remote viewing quality with other quantitative variables, as will be seen subsequently.

EVIDENCE FOR ANOMALOUS COGNITION

In science, the strength of evidence for any phenomenon, relationship, and so on rests on independent replications by a variety of scientists.

Situations involving natural or measurement variability rely on statistical evidence, and it is important to compare the results of experiments to what would be expected to happen by chance, after random variation is taken into account. The four criteria generally considered to be important requirements for evidence of something real, rather than just chance variation are:

1. Strong statistical evidence based on P values, confidence intervals, Bayesian methods or other well-accepted statistical models (see Chapter 17 for an explanation of these terms)
2. Replication of the statistical evidence by various researchers
3. Elimination or numerical compensation for possible artifacts and confounding variables
4. Systematic changes in response when external variables are changed.

A number of publications have summarized the strong evidence for anomalous cognition and show that the evidence clearly meets the first three requirements (see, for example, Utts 1996, Radin 1997a, Bem et al 2001), and the evidence continues to accumulate (see for example Alexander & Broughton 2001). In addition to remote viewing studies, the preponderance of evidence for anomalous cognition derives from ganzfeld experiments, discussed elsewhere in this volume (Ch. 7). The ganzfeld experiments are similar to remote viewing experiments except that the receiver is placed in a special sensory-isolated state, and the description is verbal instead of written. In ganzfeld experiments the receiver usually does the judging, and there are four choices (the actual target and three decoys) rather than the five choices commonly used in remote viewing experiments. Therefore, by chance the success rate (the hit rate) should be about 25%. Instead, the hit rate for almost 3000 standard ganzfeld sessions that have been conducted to date is about 32%. If chance alone is responsible, the odds of a hit rate that extreme are less than one in 10^{-15} (see Ch. 7). The effect sizes for remote viewing and ganzfeld experiments are similar. We will refer to the collection of remote viewing and ganzfeld experiments as 'free-response' psi experiments, or as studies of anomalous cognition.

There are also a number of separate publications examining systematic changes in the quality of anomalous cognition as a function of other variables, addressing the fourth criterion for evidence. Of course the strongest evidence is provided by an explanation and understanding of how and why a phenomenon occurs, but once that barrier is overcome there is no longer any need for statistical evidence. The current status of anomalous cognition is that the statistical evidence, including systematic changes with other variables, is overwhelming. Hopefully this evidence can be developed into an enhanced understanding of nature, consciousness, or whatever mechanism is involved through further experimental and theoretical work.

FACTORS CORRELATED WITH ANOMALOUS COGNITION

There have been a number of intriguing findings relating anomalous cognition performance to other factors. In this section, seven of these findings are summarized and discussed.

A Classical Model for Transmission of Information

As these findings are reviewed it is useful to have a framework for discussing and connecting them. For lack of a better model, we will use a classical framework of information transmission, in which it is assumed that there is a source, a method of transmission and a detector.

This framework may not be correct, but it explains most other known situations in which information is transmitted, so it is a good place to start. For example, as you read these words you acquire information. We can assume that the source is the print you are reading, the method of transmission involves light striking the words and being transmitted to your eyes, and the receptor includes your eyes and brain. We can't be completely sure this model is correct; for instance, perhaps the source is that you are reaching into the past and tapping my brain or computer as I write these words. But it is the nature of science to assume the most parsimonious explanation. If eventually the evidence cannot be fit into this classical information transmission framework, that is useful knowledge and the inconsistencies can lead to a new framework.

The correlated factors we examine can provide clues to what might constitute each of the three parts of the classical system. However, as will be increasingly evident, we can already reject the model that assumes anomalous cognition works by transmitting a message through time and space, as we know it.

The seven results are presented first, followed by a discussion of how they fit with the classical model of transmission. As you read each of the seven findings, think about whether they seem to be related to the source, the method of transmission, the receptor, or some combination.

Time and Distance

The most striking aspect of the first two physical correlates is their *lack* of relationship with successful anomalous cognition. Neither time nor distance between the source and the receptor seem to change the quality of the information received. The lack of correlation with time includes results for which the target was generated after the remote viewing session took place.

Numerous studies have been done in which there was a large physical distance between the target and the receiver. Jahn & Dunne (1987) and Dunne et al (1989)[2] reported remote viewing results for which the target and receiver were separated by the Atlantic Ocean, with one in Princeton, New Jersey, and the other in Europe. In much of the remote viewing work done for the US government at SRI International and at Science Applications International Corporation (SAIC), the targets and remote viewers were separated by up to several thousand miles, for

---

[2]Hansen et al (1992) have raised methodological concerns about some of these experiments but the effect sizes are similar to most other anomalous cognition experiments, so it is unlikely that those concerns completely account for the results.

instance, with the target in California and the remote viewers on the East Coast of the United States (e.g. Puthoff & Targ 1976). There is a striking consistency between the results of these experiments and results when the target and receiver are in close proximity. Therefore, whatever the method of transmission, ordinary earthbound distances do not seem to dampen it.

Even more puzzling are results showing that anomalous cognition works well when the receiver produces results *before* the target has been generated. In other words, the transmission of information does not appear to follow the arrow of time as we know it. Dunne et al (1989) reported remote-viewing results for which the target was generated as much as 150 hours after the remote viewing description was provided. There are many other sources of data in parapsychology that seem to support a precognitive model of information transfer (see for example Honorton & Ferrari 1989, May et al 1995, Radin 1997b).

Senders and Sender–Receiver Pairs

Anecdotes from throughout history indicate that people who are biologically close, such as parent and child, are more prone to experience telepathy. However, it is logical to assume that people who know each other well are more likely to know what might be going through each other's minds using normal methods of inference. Therefore, it is interesting to test whether the relationship between the sender and the receiver makes a difference in anomalous cognition experiments.

There is weak evidence from ganzfeld studies supporting the idea that biologically close sender–receiver pairs are likely to be successful, but spouses are not. Alexander & Broughton (2001) summarize two studies they conducted in which they measured the relationship between the sender and receiver, and the corresponding hit rates. The data are summarized in Box 6.1. Notice that friends and spouses as senders did not result in successful sessions in this small set of sessions, with hit rates of 16% and 20%, respectively, while parent/child and sibling pairs were very successful, with hit rates of 44% and 75%. Remember that chance predicts a 25% suc-

Box 6.1 Sender–receiver relationships and hit rates (from Alexander & Broughton 2001)

Relationship	N trials	N hits	% hits
Lab assigned	47	15	31.9
Friend	76	12	15.8
Spouse	25	5	20.0
Parent/child	32	14	43.8
Sibling	8	6	75.0

cess rate. Taken together, the biologically linked pairs had a 50% hit rate (20 hits, 40 trials), for an exact binomial *P* value of 0.001.

However, there is more substantial evidence showing that anomalous cognition works well without any sender at all. In fact in the same study, Alexander & Broughton report that no sender was used in 13 trials, resulting in six hits, or 46%. A ganzfeld experiment at the University of Edinburgh (Morris et al 1995) consisted of 97 sessions in which there were approximately equal numbers of sessions conducted under three conditions. In one condition there was a sender and the receiver knew this was the case. In the other two conditions it was randomly determined at the last minute whether or not there would be a sender, and this was unknown to the receiver. A hit rate of 25% was expected by chance but the hit rate was 34% both when there was a known sender and when there was no sender. The hit rate was 28% when there was a sender but the receiver did not know if there would be one. The overall results were statistically significant with a hit rate of 33%. An experiment carried out at SAIC (Lantz et al 1994) used experienced remote viewers and had each one complete 20 sessions with a sender and 20 without a sender. The remote viewers were blind to the sender condition, in other words they did not know when there was a sender and when there was not. The experiment was successful and there was no statistical difference in results for the two conditions.

How can the results from the biologically close sender–receiver pairs in the ganzfeld be reconciled with the results showing that a sender does not seem to be necessary? Two possibilities warrant mention. First, perhaps the receiver is more comfortable revealing the mental images going through his or her mind when they know the person listening is their parent, child or sibling. (In ganzfeld experiments with a sender, the sender typically hears the audio stream produced by the receiver.) Second, perhaps the population in which both parent and child or two siblings are willing to participate in anomalous cognition experiments is somehow special. If there is a biological basis for anomalous cognition, both ability and interest may run in families. The number of sessions with biological pairs is still relatively small, so another possibility is that the results are simply due to chance, despite the small P value. Further experiments are needed to determine if that is the case.

Characteristics of Good Receivers

Some individuals appear to be better receivers than others in anomalous cognition experiments. In the remote viewing experiments at SRI and SAIC, a select group of individuals were used in many experiments, and their results were consistently better than 'unselected' receivers (May et al 1988, Utts 1996). However, despite attempts to find characteristics that differentiated these individuals from others, nothing emerged that was particularly different about them.

In contrast, in ganzfeld experiments two findings related to the receivers have been replicated. Rather than testing a small set of specific individuals, ganzfeld researchers use volunteer participants, many of whom participate in only one session. Systematic recording and examination of information about these participants has allowed researchers to identify a class of individuals who seem to perform better than others (Honorton & Schechter 1987, Honorton 1997, Alexander & Broughton 2001). In particular, receivers who practice a mental discipline such as meditation or yoga do particularly well. Honorton (1997) reported a 34% hit rate for $N = 220$ trials in which the receivers had ever practiced a mental discipline, exact $P = 0.002$. Alexander & Broughton (2001) found 12 hits in 28 trials (43%, exact $P = 0.029$) for current practitioners, and 16 hits out of 43 trials for current or past practitioners (37%, exact $P = 0.051$).

In addition to individuals who meet those criteria, two studies have found that students in creative disciplines such as music and the arts perform better than unselected receivers. The participants in the first study (Schlitz & Honorton 1992) were students at New York's Julliard School, a prestigious institution for the performing arts. Ten of the 20 participants were successful (50%, exact $P = 0.014$). The participants in the second study (Dalton 1997) were artists, musicians, creative writers, and actors recruited at the University of Edinburgh in Scotland. Dalton conducted 128 sessions resulting in 60 hits, a hit rate of 46.9%, when 25% was expected by chance, and corresponding to a medium effect size of 0.46 (exact $P = 7 \times 10^{-8}$).

There are two possible confounding factors that should be considered in the interpretation of the results about creative participants. First, artists are accustomed to practicing good mental discipline outside the realm of normal intellectual endeavors. This practice may be similar to the practice of other mental disciplines, like meditation, which has been found to correlate with good performance in the ganzfeld studies. Second, Schlitz and Dalton have both been successful in obtaining results in other anomalous cognition experiments. Thus, there may be an 'experimenter effect,' rather than a participant effect, that explains the success of the studies with creative people.

Entropy and Contrast in Target Material

The next finding relates the quality of remote viewing output across sessions to a direct, intrinsic property of the target material (May et al 1994). The property is the change or 'gradient' in Shannon entropy, with respect to the intensity of color in the targets. Shannon entropy is unlikely to be familiar to most readers, so an explanation is in order. The concept will be explained using the example of photographs as displayed on a computer screen, but it can also be extended to more complex targets, such as video segments.

In general, entropy is a measure of order or disorder. High entropy values imply less order. In random systems, high entropy implies that the system is unpredictable while low entropy implies that it is more predictable. For instance, a series of coin tosses has high entropy if heads and tails occur equally often, and low entropy if either heads or tails occur most of the time. The latter situation makes it easier to predict the next toss, thus there is more order to it.

Entropy can be derived for small patches in a photograph by examining how much the intensity of color varies across the patch. This is done separately for the intensity of red, green and blue (which together define the picture), then summed. The entropy computation proceeds as follows:

1. On a standard computer screen, a photograph can be digitized into 640×480 pixels, each of which is represented by three strings of eight binary digits, one each for red, green and blue. These strings tell the computer the three intensities to display for the three colors, resulting in the image you see on your screen. Thus, there are $2^8 - 1 = 255$ possible intensities for each of the three colors. (A string of all 0s would be an absence of color so is excluded. A string of all 1s would be the most intense for that color.) In what follows, for simplicity we focus on a single color and use the letter m to designate the intensity for a pixel; thus m can range from 1 to 255.

2. A photograph is divided into $40 \times 40 = 1600$ small rectangles, which we call patches. Each patch contains $16 \times 12 = 192$ pixels. (Remember that a photograph is 640×480 pixels, so dividing 640 and 480 each into 40 segments results in little rectangles each with 16×12 pixels.)

3. Each of the 192 pixels has an intensity value m, ranging from 1 to 255. Within a patch, the relative frequency of each of the values of m is found; denote these by p_m. For instance, if 19 of the 192 pixels have intensity $m = 25$, then $p_{25} = 19/192 = 0.01$. Typically, within a patch the range of intensity values will be relatively small because color intensity does not tend to vary wildly in a small patch. Therefore, there will usually be a small number of non-zero p_m values.

4. The entropy is computed separately for each of the 1600 patches. It is also found separately

$$S = -\sum_{k=1}^{255} P_k \log_2 P_k$$

for each of the three colors, and then summed over them within a patch to create the entropy for that patch. For each color within a patch, the formula for Shannon entropy S is:

Note that small entropy values imply that there are only a few different intensity levels for that patch, while large entropy values imply that there is a wide range of intensity values for the patch. However, the measure of interest here is not the entropy itself, but how much it differs from that of neighboring patches.

May et al (1994) speculated that the quality of anomalous cognition would vary with the change in entropy across the patches in a target. They likened the reception of information in remote viewing sessions to the receipt of information detected by our known senses. Each of our five known senses is a 'change detector.' Our eyes detect changes in light, moving rapidly over what is being observed. Our ears detect changes in sound waves, and so on. Therefore, they speculated that however information is received in remote viewing, reception is likely to be enhanced if the target involves large changes of some sort.

The formula for measuring change in entropy is complex, but the idea is simple. The 'gradient' (change) of entropy across the patches is a summary of how the entropy changes when moving from one patch to all of its neighboring patches. Therefore, a photograph that has many adjacent patches with the same intensity will have a small entropy gradient. A photograph in which adjacent patches tend to differ in intensity will have a large entropy gradient.

Figure 6.3 displays the quality of each of 75 remote viewing trials, where quality is measured using the figure of merit described earlier. The triangles represent the entropy gradient of the target versus figure of merit, while the $\times$s represent the entropy of the target versus figure of merit. Notice that the correlation between the entropy gradient and figure of merit is statistically

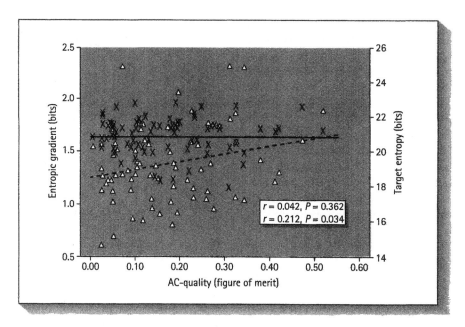

Figure 6.3 Correlation of anomalous cognition (AC) with the gradient of and with Shannon entropy.

significant ($r = 0.212$, $P = 0.034$) while the correlation between the entropy and figure of merit is not ($r = 0.042$, $P = 0.362$). The lines show the least squares fit to the data points.

The correlation between the entropy gradient and remote viewing quality has been replicated across five experiments. The combined correlation is $r = 0.294$ (95% CI is 0.127 to 0.363, $P = 5.2 \times 10^{-5}$). The fact that the gradient, or change, correlates with anomalous cognition, but that the entropy itself appears not to correlate is highly suggestive of a sensory system. All the familiar sensory systems act that way. For example, it is much easier to detect a weak flashing light than one that is steady with the same intensity. Perhaps Professor J. B. Rhine was right after all when he coined the term extrasensory perception.

Local Sidereal Time and Anomalous Cognition

One of the most intriguing patterns that has emerged in the study of anomalous cognition is that performance peaks and plummets at predictable times. However, these are not predictable clock times, they are predictable instances of local sidereal time (LST). The connection between performance and LST was discovered by Spottiswoode (1997a). Based on research showing that anomalous cognition may be enhanced when done in a Faraday cage, thus reducing electrical fields, Spottiswoode speculated that there might be some cosmic source of interference. If so, that source should vary based on the position of the earth relative to the cosmos. LST is one method for measuring that position.

One solar day is the length of time it takes for a fixed earth longitude to return to the same position with respect to the sun. Because the earth is moving around the sun, it must rotate almost 361° in one solar day. In contrast, a sidereal day is the length of time it takes for a fixed earth longitude to return to the same position with respect to distant stars. Because of the extreme distance, the earth does not move much in relation to distant stars, so one sidereal day corresponds to a rotation very close to 360°. A sidereal day is thus slightly shorter than a solar day; in fact it is 3 minutes and 56 seconds shorter.

Normal clock time can be thought of as the amount of time that has passed since a given longitude last went past a designated starting point (ignoring the discontinuity caused by rounding to the nearest hour to make convenient time zones). The reference starting point for clock time is directly away from the sun, thus at 3 a.m. it has been 3 hours since that midnight point was passed, and at noon it has been 12 hours.

Similarly, local sidereal time is the amount of time that has passed since a given longitude last went past a designated starting point. But in this case, the designated starting point is a distant location, called the vernal equinox. It is the position in the cosmos at which the celestial equator and the 'ecliptic' intersect. The celestial equator can be visualized as an expansion of the earth's equator stretched out into space, a constant distance from earth all around. The ecliptic is the ellipse that the sun seems to take as viewed from the earth. The vernal equinox is directly overhead at noon on the date in March that we call the vernal equinox. Thus, on that date, local sidereal time and clock time are off by 12 hours, because LST is 0 when clock time is 12 noon. At the date in September that we call the fall equinox, clock time and local sidereal time are the same (ignoring the discontinuity caused by rounding for time zones). After that date, the amount by which LST lags clock time accumulates at the rate of 3 minutes and 56 seconds a day, because it takes that much less time to complete a sidereal day than to complete a solar day.

Spottiswoode (1997a, p. 109) reported his findings as follows:

In this paper, an association between the local sidereal time (LST) at which a trial occurs and the resulting effect size is described. In an existing database of 1,468 free response trials, the effect size increased 340% for trials within 1 hour of 13.5 h LST ($P = 0.001$). An independent database of 1,015 similar trials was subsequently obtained in which trials within 1 hour of 13.5 h LST showed an effect size increase of 450% ($P = 0.05$) providing confirmation of the effect.

Further analyses ruled out potential explanations such as a relationship between LST and clock time for successful experiments. Further, a significant dip in effect size was observed at about 18 h LST. Curiously, each longitude is aligned with the galactic center of the Milky Way at 17 hours 46 seconds, close to the 18 h time of the observed dip in effect size, and each longitude is aligned with the galactic north pole of the Milky Way (pointed 90° away) at 12 hours 51 seconds, close to the observed peak in effect size at 13.5 LST. Therefore, it appears that anomalous cognition is enhanced when the longitude at which the session occurs is not aligned with the Milky Way, and is depressed when the longitude is aligned with the center of the Milky Way.

Geomagnetic Field Fluctuations, LST, and Anomalous Cognition

The geomagnetic field is the magnetic field that surrounds the earth. Its strength is constantly changing, mostly due to the influence of solar activity. There is some evidence that some biological systems are affected by the strength of the field. For instance, homing pigeons tend to get lost during magnetic storms.

There is a growing collection of evidence relating anomalous cognition to fluctuations in the geomagnetic field, with better performance corresponding to relatively quiet times (see Radin 1997a, p. 314, note 13, for a long list of references). However, results have been mixed, with some studies finding a connection and others failing to find one.

Following his discovery of the relationship between effect size and LST, Spottiswoode (1997b) examined the correlation between effect size and geomagnetic index for a large database of 2879 free-response trials. He found Spearman's $\rho = -0.029$ with a P value of 0.06. Although the correlation comes close to being statistically significant compared with zero correlation, the magnitude of it is unimpressive and the small P value is an artifact of having a very large sample size. Therefore, there did not appear to be a relationship between geomagnetic index and anomalous cognition effect size.

However, Spottiswoode (1997b) then calculated the correlation between effect size and geomagnetic index for 2-hour wide window of LST, sliding the starting point of the window by increments of 0.1 hours. He found that the correlation hovered around chance, except in a small segment of local sidereal time, centered at 12.9 h.

At that time, the correlation between effect size and geomagnetic index was $\rho = -0.33$ with a P value of 0.0001. The time of 12.9 h LST is very close to the peak found for anomalous cognition performance, at 13.5 h LST. Further, when he separated ganzfeld from remote viewing trials, the strong negative correlation occurred in both protocols.

In other words, there is a correlation between anomalous cognition effect size and geomagnetic index in a small region of local sidereal time. There is no appreciable correlation outside of this small window.

These results must be interpreted with caution because there are a number of interrelated variables involving solar activity, and other emissions from the galaxy. The results should be seen as a starting point for further investigation, rather than as a causal link between anomalous cognition and any specific physical variable.

Summary of Factors Associated with Anomalous Cognition

The seven factors associated with anomalous cognition (AC) discussed in this section can be summarized as follows:

1. Distance does not dampen AC performance.
2. AC experiments have been successful even when the target is generated after the response, suggesting that precognition is possible.
3. A sender is not a necessary component for successful AC, but when a sender is used, biologically related pairs perform exceptionally well.
4. There are certain characteristics of receivers that enhance AC performance, most notably practice of a mental discipline.
5. AC quality is correlated with the amount of change evidenced in the target.
6. AC performance peaks at about 13.5 hours local sidereal time, when the location of the experiment is orthogonal to the center of the galaxy, and dips at about 18 hours local sidereal time, when the location of the experiment is pointed toward the galactic center.

7. There is a moderate negative correlation between fluctuations in the earth's geomagnetic field and AC effect size in a 2-hour window surrounding 12.9 hours local sidereal time. Otherwise, there is very little correlation between them.

DISCUSSION

Let us revisit the classical model of information transfer, in which there was a source, a mode of transmission, and a receptor. Let us now add an additional concept used in information theory, that of a signal and noise. The signal is the information provided at the source that is supposed to be transmitted to the receptor. The strength of the signal is a combination of its original strength, and any signal-enhancing features that occur during transmission or at the receptor. For instance, the volume on a radio can be turned up to enhance the signal at the receiving end, and radio waves can be received and enhanced by intermittent transmitters.

Noise interferes with the transmission of information. Noise can be in the source, as when print on a page is smeared, it can be added during transmission, as when radio waves from two stations interfere with each other to create static, or it can be added at the receptor, as when one's eyesight begins to diminish, making it difficult to read a printed page.

We can speculate on how the seven factors presented in the previous session fit into this classical model of information transfer, hoping to find clues about how anomalous cognition works.

The fact that AC performance does not diminish with distance, and that precognition appears to be possible, suggest that the method of transmission may transcend our current understanding of space and time. For instance, perhaps the source is not the physical target material. Perhaps instead the source of the information is in the future, when the receiver eventually is given feedback and shown the target.

The third factor relates to the lack of sender, and to the enhanced performance with biologically close pairs. The fact that the sender is superfluous lends support to the idea that the source may be the future revelation of the target to the receiver. When there is no sender, the source is not clear, but it cannot be another human at a distant location. The source could be the existing target in real time, or it could be the target in the future, when it is revealed to the receiver. The biologically close pairing may lead to a reduction of noise, where the noise is caused when the receiver censors information he or she is not comfortable revealing to the listening sender.

The fourth factor is that receivers who practice mental disciplines have better success. This implies a reduction of noise in the receiver. Anecdotally, practices of mental discipline are supposed to 'quiet the mind.' Therefore, it is reasonable to assume that receivers who have had practice with eliminating sources of mental noise in the practice of their discipline would also be able to reduce mental noise when trying to perceive a remote target.

The fifth factor is the correlation between the quality of AC and the change in target entropy. This suggests that a stronger signal is sent from the source when a large amount of change is involved. This fits with anecdotal evidence for psi phenomena throughout history. It would be difficult to imagine a much bigger change for an individual than the transition from life to bodily death. There are frequent reports of people claiming to know when someone close to them has died, thus detecting a major change through anomalous means.

The sixth factor is the observation that AC performance peaks and dips at specific local sidereal times. This suggests one of three possibilities: there may be some cosmic source of noise that inhibits AC during specific times; or there may be some cosmic signal enhancement that occurs during specific times; or there may be some feature of those times that allows the transmission to occur more smoothly or less smoothly. In any case, related variables need to be explored further to try to identify something that could logically produce either a signal enhancement or noise reduction at differential local sidereal times.

The seventh factor is the realization that AC effect size is enhanced when the geomagnetic field is quiet, but that this relationship only holds

for a narrow band of local sidereal time. This finding implies that there is a complex interaction of signal enhancing and/or noise reducing cosmic forces that we have not yet uncovered.

In general, these findings tend to support a model of source, transmission, and receptor, but with features that are much different from what is traditionally envisioned. The transmission appears to occur at least partially from the future to the present. There appear to be steps that can be taken by receivers to reduce noise. There may be steps that can be taken to enhance the strength of the signal at the source, and there are clearly unknown variables lurking in the background that enhance the signal, reduce the noise, or both.

IMPLICATIONS FOR INTUITIVE MEDICAL DIAGNOSIS

Intuitive medical diagnosis occurs when a 'medical intuitive' appears to be able to provide information about the physical state of a distant patient. In these cases, the information must be somehow reaching the intuitive, much like target information reaches the receiver in free-response psi experiments.

There is one major difference between intuitive medical diagnosis and most free-response psi experiments. Using the classical transmission model for reference, the difference is that the assumed source of the information in medical diagnosis is the body of the patient. However, the results from AC experiments illustrate that caution should be used in making that assumption.

No matter what the source, the goal in medical diagnosis is clearly to enhance the signal and reduce the noise. The AC results may provide some clues, and research on intuitive diagnosis may provide some clues for understanding anomalous cognition.

Results from the anomalous cognition experiments point to the following implications for intuitive diagnosis:

- A large change from normal may be easier to diagnose than a small change, indicating that more serious diseases may be easier to diagnose.

- The mental state of the medical intuitive is important as a source of noise reduction. If the AC results generalize, then intuitives who practice mental disciplines may be more successful at reducing extraneous noise and thus receiving correct information.
- The source of information in anomalous cognition is poorly understood, so it is important to provide as much information to the intuitive as possible. Feedback should be given as soon as it is known whether or not the diagnosis was correct.
- Information does not seem to be transmitted through space as we know it, so distance between the patient and the intuitive is unlikely to matter unless there is a psychological enhancement from being in close proximity.
- The timing of diagnosis may not be as important as the timing of AC trials, with respect to LST, because the 'target' is not generated specifically for the medical diagnostic session. The source information is the state of the patient, and that remains nearly constant throughout a local sidereal 'day.' However, if the LST connection is a result of noise reduction in the receiver, then the timing of attempted diagnosis may be important.

The AC results and related factors raise interesting research questions for intuitive medical diagnosis. Some of these questions are:

- *Related to the source of information.* Does type of illness matter? Does feedback matter? Does intuitive diagnosis ever work in a precognitive mode?
- *Related to the method of transmission.* Does the distance between the patient and the intuitive matter?
- *Related to the receptor.* What are the characteristics of good diagnosticians? Does practice of mental disciplines seem to matter? Does relationship to the patient matter?
- *All three components.* Does timing of diagnosis matter, as it appears that it does for anomalous cognition? Does it matter what the relationship is between the patient and the intuitive? What information must be provided to the intuitive to focus her or his attention on the designated patient?

As a final note, the implications of the results of anomalous cognition and other psi studies for studies of distant healing are enormous, but are even more speculative than the implications for intuitive diagnosis, which more closely resembles anomalous cognition. For a discussion of the implications to studies of distant healing, see Chapter 15 in this volume.

REFERENCES

Alexander C H, Broughton R S 2001 Cerebral hemisphere dominance and ESP performance in the autoganzfeld. Journal of Parapsychology 65(4): 397–416

Bem D J, Palmer J, Broughton R S 2001 Updating the ganzfeld database: a victim of its own success? Journal of Parapsychology 65(3): 207–218

Dalton K 1997 Exploring the links: creativity and psi in the ganzfeld. Proceedings of the Parapsychological Association 40th Annual Convention. Parapsychological Association, Durham, NC, pp. 119–134

Dunne B J, Dobyns Y H, Intner S M 1989 Precognitive remote perception III: Complete binary database with analytical refinements. PEAR technical note 89002, Princeton University, Princeton NJ

Hansen G P, Utts J, Markwick B 1992 Critique of the PEAR remote viewing experiments. Journal of Parapsychology 56(2): 97–114

Honorton C 1997 The ganzfeld novice: four predictors of initial ESP performance. Journal of Parapsychology 61(2): 143–158

Honorton C, Ferrari D C 1989 Future telling: a meta-analysis of forced-choice precognition experiments, 1935–1987. Journal of Parapsychology 53: 281–308

Honorton C, Schechter E I 1987 Ganzfeld target retrieval with an automated testing system: a model for initial ganzfeld success [Abstract]. In: Weiner D H, Nelson R D (eds) Research in parapsychology 1986. Scarecrow Press, Metuchen, NJ, pp. 36–39

Jahn R G, Dunne B J 1987 Margins of reality. Harcourt Brace Jovanovich, New York

Lantz N D, Luke W L W, May E C 1994 Target and sender dependencies in anomalous cognition experiments. Journal of Parapsychology 58(3): 285–302

May E C 1996 American Institutes for Research review of the Stargate Program. Journal of Scientific Exploration 10(1): 89–107.

May E C, Utts J M, Trask V V, Luke W W, Frivold T J, Humphrey B S 1988 Review of the psychoenergetic research conducted at SRI International (1973–1988). SRI International Technical Report (March), Menlo Park, CA

May E C, Utts J M, Humphrey B S, Luke W L, Frivold T J, Trask V V 1990 Advances in remote viewing. Journal of Parapsychology 54: 193–228

May E C, Utts J M, Spottiswoode S J P 1995 Decision augmentation theory: application to the random number generator database. Journal of Scientific Exploration 9: 453–488

May E C, Spottiswoode S J P, James C L 1994 Shannon entropy: a possible intrinsic target property. Journal of Parapsychology 58(4): 384–401

Morris R L, Dalton K, Delanoy D, Watt C 1995 Comparison of the sender/no sender condition in the ganzfeld. Proceedings of the Parapsychological Association 38th Annual Convention. Parapsychological Association, Durham, NC, pp. 244–259

Radin D I 1997a The conscious universe. Harper Edge, San Francisco

Radin D I 1997b Unconscious perception of future emotions: an experiment in presentiment. Journal of Scientific Exploration 11(2): 163–180

Schlitz M J, Honorton C 1992 Ganzfeld psi performance within an artistically gifted population. Journal of the American Society for Psychical Research 86: 83–98

Spottiswoode S J P 1997a Apparent association between effect size in anomalous cognition experiments and local sidereal time. Journal of Scientific Exploration 11(2): 109–122

Spottiswoode S J P 1997b Geomagnetic fluctuations and free-response anomalous cognition: a new understanding. Journal of Parapsychology 61(1): 3–12

Puthoff H E, Targ R 1976 A perceptual channel for information transfer over kilometer distances: historical perspective and recent research. Proceedings of the IEEE 64(3): 329–354

Utts J M 1996 An assessment of the evidence for psychic functioning. Journal of Scientific Exploration 10(1): 3–30. Reprinted in: Journal of Parapsychology 59: 289–320

7

Non-sensory access to information: the ganzfeld studies

Marilyn Schlitz
Dean Radin

This chapter summarizes ongoing research on mechanisms of access to non-sensory information between untrained individuals.

In many cultures, alteration of consciousness, such as through hypnosis or trance, is used to access information not otherwise available to the conscious mind. In Western science, it is assumed that such techniques allow access only to intrapersonal unconscious information – that is, information within the mind of the person in the trance. Most non-Western cultures (and some Western thinkers such as C. G. Jung), however, believe that some unconscious information is 'collective' or interpersonal, and so can be shared by more than one individual. In some cases, access to this collective state is made by blocking out normal sensory cues through special meditative techniques. In other situations, sensory masking is used as with drums or in dim enclosures.

Over several decades of research by a number of investigators, a standardized way of masking sensory cues (called the ganzfeld) in order to study access to non-sensory information has been developed. Detailed methodological protocols for acceptable evidence were established in the 1980s with input from both believers and skeptics of this ability. In this chapter, Marilyn Schlitz and Dean Radin summarize past and current research using these high-quality methods. The history of how these standard methods were developed is a model for quality science in the investigation of intuitive diagnosis. **WBJ**

INTRODUCTION

The experience of direct communication between two minds has been reported so frequently throughout history that it eventually gained its own name: telepathy. Coined in 1882 by the British scholar Frederic W. H. Myers (1963), the word telepathy literally means 'feeling at a distance.' More recently, telepathy has been considered a subset of a broader set of experiences known as psi phenomena. In most cases, the reason such communications are reported is because they are especially meaningful to the experiencer. We often place telephone calls to each other, we often receive letters from old friends, we sometimes *seem* to know what others are thinking, and some alternative healers report knowing something about the state of a distant patient without the aid of any conventional sensory means (known as 'intuitive diagnosis'). But when we have strong feelings about such events and we know we did not use the ordinary senses to get this information, and the information was objectively verified in due course, this may be a reflection of genuine psi abilities.

EXPERIMENTAL TECHNIQUES

Because psi experiences have been reported frequently, there is a long legacy of academic psychologists who have applied the best experimental techniques of the day to investigate these phenomena under controlled conditions. Figure 7.1 provides an overview of some of the university and private laboratories that have studied mind-to-mind information transfer. As the list indicates, the primary experimental focuses have evolved over the years, starting with tests of 'thought transference,' to experiments in the dream state, to the present *ganzfeld* method.

There are two general categories of psi experiments involving the apparent transfer of information. The first, forced-choice tests, constrain the research participant to select one among a small number of target possibilities. The second, free-response tests, allow the participant to respond freely about his or her impressions of a target. The protocols for obtaining data within these methodologies are similar for each experimental trial:

- A target – typically a symbol, photograph, or video clip – is chosen randomly from a pre-defined set of possibilities.
- A 'sender' attempts to send information about this target to a 'receiver' who is isolated from all conventional sensory cues.
- The receiver, who is, of course, blind to the target choice, is asked to register or otherwise announce his or her impressions of the target.
- An objective method is used to judge whether those impressions match the target. This is done either by directly matching symbols, or by asking the receiver to select which one of several possible targets best matches his or her subjective impressions.
- A statistical assessment determines whether the number of matches obtained over a series of trials was within or above chance expectation.

There has been considerable variation on this theme, and significant care is usually taken to assure that there is no chance of leakage of information from the target to the participant via the recognized senses. Complete protocols include such details as the precise randomization procedure, methods of ensuring target and data security, the planned methods of analysis, and specifics such as the number of trials and participants.

Historically, free-response experiments have resulted in larger effect sizes than the forced-choice, and free-response tests have also proven to be easier to replicate. This is probably because free-response techniques engage participants more deeply than the highly repetitive and ultimately boring free-response tasks. Among free-response methods, the ganzfeld technique for studying psi phenomena has proven to be one of the most successful.

THE GANZFELD TECHNIQUE

Ganzfeld is a German word meaning 'whole field.' The ganzfeld technique was developed at the turn of the 20th century by psychologists investigating the nature of mental imagery. In a ganzfeld trial, the information receiver (R) is sequestered in a soundproof room. A uniform visual field is created

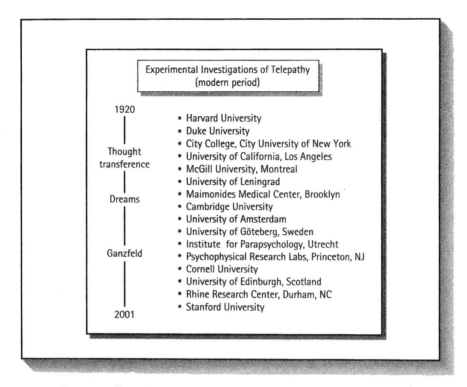

Figure 7.1 Sites where scientific investigations of telepathy have taken place.

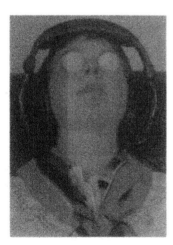

Figure 7.2 A participant in a ganzfeld telepathy test.

for R by placing translucent ping-pong ball halves over each eye, and then illuminating the face with a soft red light. The audio equivalent of this unpatterned stimulus is accomplished by providing near-white noise over headphones. While relaxing in this state on a reclining chair, within a few minutes most Rs report that the red glow and static noise vanish from conscious awareness, and are replaced by mild visual and auditory hallucinations. A receiver in the ganzfeld is illustrated in Figure 7.2.

Psi researchers rediscovered the ganzfeld stimulation method in the 1970s while in the process of searching for a way to test a 'noise reduction' model of psi. This model proposed that psi effects in the laboratory were variable and weak primarily because internal somatic and external sensory information mask our perception of subtle psi-mediated signals. The ganzfeld technique looked especially promising because it provided a fast, inexpensive, and non-intrusive way to provide a sensory reduction environment, which could then be used to test the noise reduction model (Honorton et al 1990, Bem & Honorton 1994).

In the standard ganzfeld test, while R is isolated in the ganzfeld condition, the information sender (S) views a short video clip, as illustrated in

Figure 7.3. R is encouraged to speak aloud his or her subjective impressions, and in some experimental setups this mentation can be heard by S to help guide him or her in 'sending' the target information. Many researchers today doubt that a sender is necessary for a receiver to gain distant target information, because evidence from remote viewing experiments indicates that information about distant objects and events can be received directly without a distant sender (Targ & Katra 1999). Nevertheless, senders are still commonly used in telepathy tests because the phenomenon seems to involve direct mind-to-mind connection, and because of the prospect that the sender's intention may assist the receiver in some way.

Analysis of the results of each trial is typically carried out by R, who at the time of the evaluation is, of course, blind to the target picture. After R's impressions are recorded, R is presented with a predefined target pack that contains the actual target and three decoys, as illustrated in Figure 7.4. These packs are designed so that all four targets are as different as possible from one another. Under the null hypothesis of no telepathy, the probability of guessing the correct answer is 1 in 4, or 25%.

META-ANALYSES OF GANZFELD TESTS

Systematic reviews of experimental outcomes in carefully circumscribed domains are called meta-analyses (Utts 1991, Rosenthal 1986, Rosenthal 1991). In 1985, psi researcher Charles Honorton (1985) and skeptical psychologist Ray Hyman (1985) independently published meta-analyses of ganzfeld telepathy tests. While 42 experiments had been published at that time, only 28 studies reported the hit rates, and thus those were the studies subjected to the meta-analyses. The combined hit rates for all 28 studies was an impressive 37% instead of the 25% expected by chance. This corresponds to odds against chance of about a trillion to one. Figure 7.5 shows the point estimates and 95% confidence intervals for these 28 studies, involving a total of 762 sessions. The overall estimate is shown at the right of the graph.

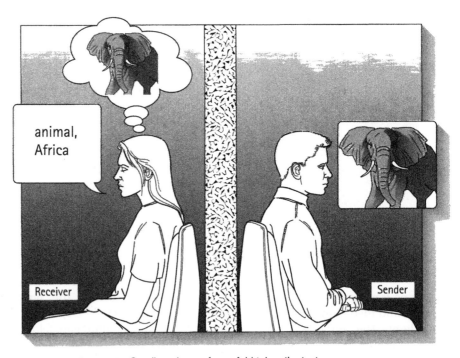

Figure 7.3 Sending phase of ganzfeld telepathy test.

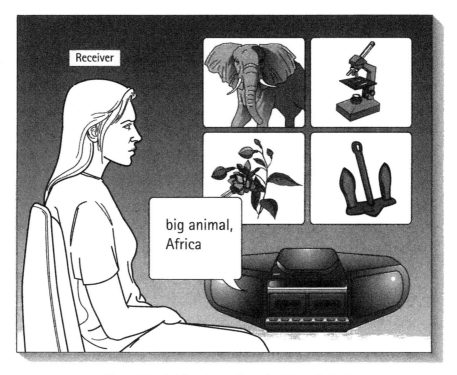

Figure 7.4 Judging phase of ganzfeld telepathy test.

As a result of their 1985 meta-analyses, Honorton and Hyman (1986) agreed on the design criteria required to conduct a prospective test of the telepathy hypothesis in the ganzfeld. Later, they wrote in a joint publication:

We agree that there is an overall significant effect in this database that cannot reasonably be explained by selective reporting or multiple analysis. We continue to differ over the degree to which the effect constitutes evidence for psi, but we agree that the final verdict awaits the outcome of future experiments conducted by a broader range of investigators and according to more stringent standards. (Hyman & Honorton 1986, p. 351)

After nearly a decade of research, Honorton and colleagues published a grand replication experiment that had been conducted according to a design that eliminated all of the skeptical objections that had arisen in criticisms of the previously reported studies (Honorton et al 1990, Bem & Honorton 1994). Out of 354 sessions in an automated ganzfeld experiment, Honorton's team obtained 122 direct hits, for a 34% hit rate.

This was associated with odds against chance of 45 000 to 1.

Later, Milton & Wiseman (1999) published a meta-analysis of 30 additional ganzfeld studies that had been reported after Honorton's study. They concluded that the new studies provided a positive but statistically not significant outcome. This raised questions about the repeatability of the ganzfeld technique. However, when we recently reviewed Milton & Wiseman's article to determine the overall hit rate in those 30 studies, we found 330 hits in 1198 trials, for a hit rate of 28%. While smaller than the previous meta-analytic estimates, this hit rate is significantly above chance expectation, $z = 2.04$, $P < 0.03$. The reason for the discrepancy in our results *vs.* Milton & Wiseman's is that the latter used a method of combining studies outcomes that introduced a small, negative bias.

In any case, Milton & Wiseman's (1999) pessimistic conclusion seems especially unwarranted in light of a more recent meta-analytic review by

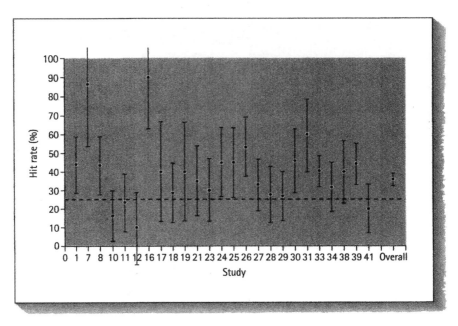

Figure 7.5 Ganzfeld telepathy meta-analysis to 1985, involving 762 sessions. The dotted line shows chance expectation.

Bem et al (2001). The authors found 10 new experiments published after Milton & Wiseman's (1999) review. Those new studies consisted of 170 hits in 463 trials, for a hit rate of 37%, $z = 5.82$, $P < 10^{-8}$.

Bem et al (2001) also discovered why Milton & Wiseman's meta-analysis resulted in a lower average hit rate than previous meta-analyses. They noticed that studies that were similar to the simple, proof-oriented designs conducted by Honorton et al (1990) showed larger effect sizes than 'non-standard' studies that were conducted to explore process-oriented questions. To test their observation, they asked three independent judges to blindly rate each of the studies considered by Milton & Wiseman according to a written criterion of ganzfeld study 'methodological standardness.' They predicted and found a significant correlation between the degree to which each study corresponded to the measure of standardness, and its effect size. Using a median split to partition standard from non-standard studies, we illustrate the findings of Bem et al (2001) in Figure 7.6.

We know now that Milton & Wiseman's (1999) review was ill-timed in the sense that had they

waited a year before conducting their meta-analytic update, they would have confirmed Honorton et al (1990) findings. Indeed, as of late 2001, when we compiled this chapter, all known ganzfeld experiments resulted in 929 hits out of 2878 trials, for an overall hit rate of 32%, associated with $z = 8.75$, $P << 10^{-15}$.

CONCLUSION

Based on meta-analyses of ganzfeld telepathy experiments published in 1985, 1994, 1999, 2001, and the present review, it is clear that the statistical results in these experiments are far beyond what is expected by chance expectation. These tests continue successfully to demonstrate an approximately 32% hit rate with unselected volunteers, where chance expectation is 25%, at least when 'standard' ganzfeld designs are employed. With this high level of consistency reported by at least 10 independent laboratories around the world, and for over three decades, it is unlikely that such results are due to systematic methodological flaws. Because these results continue to be demonstrated repeatedly, most researchers actively involved in this line of research have moved

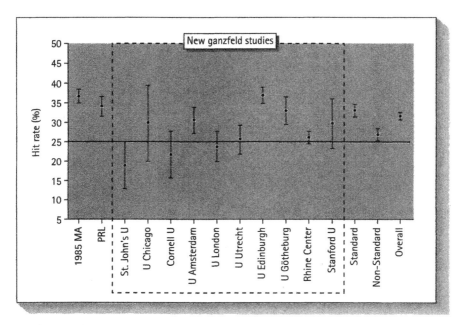

Figure 7.6 All ganzfeld experiments to 2001, with point estimates and one standard error bars. The two points at the far left show the meta-analytic estimates for the 1985 and 1990 meta-analyses. The studies in the dotted area were published after the 1990 meta-analysis. The 'standard' and 'non-standard' estimates to the right of the dotted area show hit rates for studies that followed and did not follow the standard ganzfeld method used in the earlier studies. The overall hit rate estimate is shown at the far right.

beyond the question of proof, and they are now involved in process-oriented questions designed to elucidate the underlying mechanisms.

The five meta-analyses of the ganzfeld experiment now also indicate that frequently voiced skeptical opinions about psi phenomena are often based on prejudice, and not upon a careful consideration of the available data. For example, in the September 30, 2001 issue of the *Observer* (McKie 2001), a major British newspaper, a well-known physicist at Oxford University named David Deutsch was asked for his opinion that quantum physics might one day explain telepathy. Deutsch replied: 'It is utter rubbish. Telepathy simply does not exist.' With all due respect to Dr Deutsch, it is now quite clear that such unequivocal statements are merely embarrassing displays of ignorance.

How these data relate to healing and intuitive medical diagnosis remains unclear. To date, little attention in telepathy research has been directed towards medically relevant outcomes (Schlitz 1996). Until such research is conducted under rigorously controlled conditions, we can only speculate that some forms of intuitive medical diagnosis may have a telepathic component. Because of widespread use, however, such research deserves to be given high priority as we develop an agenda for serious investigation of biofields and distant healing.

REFERENCES

Bem D, Honorton C 1994 Does psi exist? Replicable evidence for an anomalous process of information transfer. Psychological Bulletin 115: 4–18

Bem D, Palmer J, Broughton R 2001 Updating the ganzfeld database: a victim of its own success? Journal of Parapsychology 65: 207–218

Honorton C 1985 Meta-analysis of psi ganzfeld research: a response to Hyman. Journal of Parapsychology 49: 51–91

Honorton C, Berger R E, Varvoglis M P et al 1990 Psi communication in the ganzfeld: experiments with an automated testing system and a comparison with a meta-analysis of earlier studies. Journal of Parapsychology 54: 99–139

Hyman R 1985 A critical overview of parapsychology. In: Kurtz P (ed) A Skeptic's Handbook of Parapsychology. Prometheus Books, Buffalo, NY, pp. 1–96

Hyman R, Honorton C 1986 A joint communique: the psi ganzfeld controversy. Journal of Parapsychology 50: 351–364

McKie R 2001 Royal Mail's Nobel guru in telepathy row. Observer, September 30, 2001

Milton J, Wiseman R 1999 Does psi exist? Lack of replication of an anomalous process of information transfer. Psychological Bulletin 125: 387–391

Myers F W H 1963 Human personality and its survival of bodily death, 2 vols. Longmans, Green, New York [(Original work published in 1903)]

Rosenthal R 1986 Meta-analytic procedures and the nature of replication: the ganzfeld debate. Journal of Parapsychology 50: 315–336

Rosenthal R 1991 Meta-analytic procedures for social research. Sage Publications, Newbury Park, London

Schlitz M 1996 Intentionality and intuition and their clinical implications: a challenge for science and medicine. Advances 12(2): 58–66

Targ R, Katra J 1999 Miracles of mind: exploring nonlocal consciousness and spiritual healing. New World Library, Novato, CA

Utts J 1991 Replication and meta-analysis in parapsychology. Statistical Science 6(4): 363–403

8

'Energy' healing research

Sara L Warber, Gaia LM Kile, Brenda W Gillespie

This chapter summarizes randomized controlled trials on so-called 'energy' healing systems developed in the West such as therapeutic touch.

While all healing systems involve the use of consciousness such as focused attention or healing intention to direct therapy, some also visualize an 'energy' or healing force that contains therapeutic power. Terms such as chi, prana, huna, and ki encompass the idea of an energy that emanates off the body and produces biological effects. Modern Western medicine sees most energy emanating off the body as an epiphenomenon of biochemical activity in cells and of no therapeutic value in itself. Spiritual, psychic, and bioenergy healers imagine this energy as directly interacting with the person to facilitate healing.

In this chapter, Sara Warber systematically reviews the literature of controlled trials on studies that use energy methods such as therapeutic touch, healing touch, and other methods. As with the research on prayer reviewed in a previous chapter, the quantity and quality of research is too limited to draw definitive conclusions. Yet some high-quality studies have reported positive effects. A major problem is there are no accepted standards for how to conduct quality energy healing studies or what to measure – two concerns taken up by later chapters in this book.

The definition of 'energy' is also not clear. The concept is ambiguous, holding itself at a midpoint between mind and matter. Conventional Western science uses energy to refer to a spectrum of electromagnetic waves or other static forces such as gravity. The concept of energy in Eastern systems of medicine often has characteristics similar to consciousness or spirit, yet is also treated like a physical substance that can be stored, enhanced, projected, and withdrawn. Some researchers call this 'bioenergy' and treat it in a manner similar to extremely low frequency and treat it (ELF) electromagnetic fields. Measurement of fields that come off the body has rarely been accomplished and the relationship with 'bioenergy', spiritual power and non-locality has not been clarified in more recent studies.   **WBJ**

USING TOUCH TO HEAL

Many ancient cultures appear to use touch for healing (Older 1984), and written accounts of off-body healing date back at least 2500 years (Miller 1979). A number of contemporary analogous techniques use the hands in an attempt to affect the patient's bio-energy field for the purpose of healing. These related energy healing modalities include: therapeutic touch, laying-on of hands, healing touch, polarity therapy, Reiki, pranic healing, and external Qigong. This chapter is a critical review evaluating the literature on these energy therapies (excluding external Qigong). Among contemporary healing modalities, therapeutic touch dominates the literature with a wealth of research available including several randomized controlled trials (RCTs).

Therapeutic Touch (TT)

Therapeutic touch (TT) is currently used by between 20 000 and 30 000 health care practitioners to reduce patients' anxiety or pain in many clinical settings (Mulloney & Wells-Federman 1996). A broad description of TT includes a practitioner placing his or her hands on or near the body of a patient with an intent to help, heal, or convey caring (Krieger 1975). The formal practice of TT, as originally conceived, involves four steps:

1. meditative 'centering' by the practitioner
2. the practitioner then passes her or his hands near the body of the patient to assess for qualitative differences in the patient's energy field
3. using long strokes with the hands, the practitioner mobilizes the patient's energy field

4. the practitioner directs his or her own energy through the hands to modulate areas of imbalance in the patient's energy field (Krieger et al 1979).

A fifth step of reassessing the patient's energy field is sometimes added to the original four steps (Steckel & King 1996). The fourth step of TT energy modulation may involve physical touch or it may only involve simply placing the hands close to the body; this is called non-contact TT (NCTT).

CRITICAL REVIEW

This chapter examines published randomized controlled trials of energy healing applied to humans. At this time, all available non-Qigong RCTs except one evaluate TT as the intervention, the single exception being an RCT of laying-on of hands (LOOH) (Beutler et al 1988). Whether the designs and outcomes of this body of research are applicable to the other analogous techniques is open to discussion. Qualitative analysis of energy healers' utterances about the nature of energy for healing indicate that they do indeed speak of energy and the process of healing facilitation in similar ways (Warber et al 2000b, Warber et al 2000c). This qualitative groundwork suggests that energy healing techniques may be studied using similar methodology and that the results may be extrapolated from one technique to the others.

Methods

Literature search

The literature search was carried out in two phases, the first in preparation for our group's meta-analysis of TT (Warber et al 2000a) and the second in preparation for the current critical review (Fig. 8.1).

In the first phase, we searched the medical literature from 1966 to March 1998 using the terms 'therapeutic touch,' 'healing touch,' and 'laying-on of hands' via Medline, CINAHL, Scientific Citations Index, Social Science Index, and Dissertation Abstracts. We retained experiments and reviews from this search. We then hand-searched references of the retained articles for

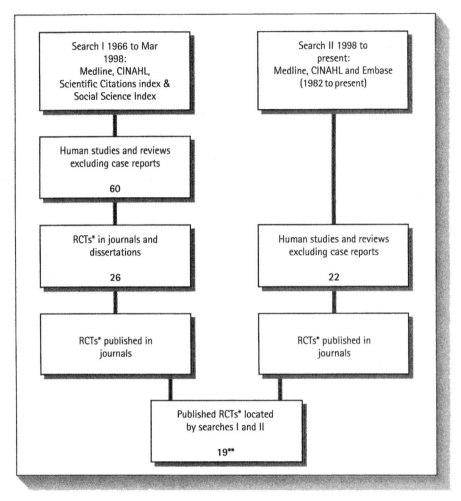

Figure 8.1 Path to entry into the critical review.

* RCT = randomized controlled trial.

** Two separate reports of the same study were counted as a single study for the purposes of this review.

experimental reports not found in databases. Additionally, we contacted researchers in the field to locate possible unpublished material.

In the second phase, to update our records, we searched Medline and CINAHL from 1998 to the present and Embase from its inception (1982) to the present, for the following terms: 'therapeutic touch,' 'Reiki,' 'polarity therapy,' 'healing touch,' and 'laying-on of hands,' 'pranic,' and 'biofield.' We reviewed titles and abstracts for likely research studies or scientific reviews. A search by hand for citation of other pertinent articles was also conducted.

We prospectively determined the following inclusion/exclusion criteria. Only published studies that reported the effects of energy healing in humans with or without disease were included. We required each study included in the review to be randomized and controlled with a comparison group. Outcomes needed to be measured quantitatively and reported such that an effect size could be calculated. We excluded: single case reports, qualitative studies of the narrative type, quasi-experiments of a pre-post design without a comparison group, studies of effects or educational outcomes in people performing energy healing, and studies of energy healing effects in animals or plants. Studies were examined for inclusion/ exclusion by one of our group. Data extractors in the group confirmed that studies met the inclusion criteria. Discrepancies were resolved in consultation with our biostatistician. Studies that met the criteria are included in this critical review.

Data extraction

Elements extracted from the study descriptions included patient condition, experimental setting, type, duration, and frequency of TT, type of control(s), who performed experimental and control interventions, outcome measures, sample sizes, means and standard deviations, type of analysis performed, and significance of differences.

Quality assessment

The quality of the studies was rated using the previously validated five-point Jadad scale (Jadad et al 1996). This scale assigns one point for randomization, an additional point for describing appropriate randomization, one point for double blinding, an additional point for describing appropriate double blinding, and one point for describing withdrawals. All included articles were rated by at least two independent reviewers and differences were resolved by consensus in consultation with the biostatistician. The Jadad scores of the entire group of studies were reviewed again to assure uniform application of criteria.

The articles were further assessed according to the CONSORT (consorted standards of reporting trials) criteria for reporting RCTs (Begg et al 1996). These criteria consist of 21 elements that should be included in the following specific portions of a scientific report: title, abstract, introduction, methods, results, and comment. Further assessment was based on criteria suggested by the conference organizer, Wayne Jonas, and focused on therapeutic interference and clinical significance of outcomes (personal communication, September 1, 2000).

Effect sizes, using Cohen's d, were calculated for all studies to compare the effect between intervention and control group. An effect size of 0.2 is considered small, 0.5 is moderate, and 0.8 is large (Cohen 1977). This statistic is calculated using the difference between the outcome means of the treatment group and the control group divided by the standard deviation of the control group (McGaw & Glass 1980). Because not all studies reported standard deviations, some standard deviations were estimated based on reported t and F statistics in addition to outcome means. The outcome used from each study was based on the identified main outcome following the full course of treatment. When more than one control group was used in the study design, effect size comparison was made with the placebo group that consisted of a mimic intervention. Studies were grouped by type of outcome (global, psychological, pain, physiological, wound healing) and mean effect size was calculated for each group and for the entire group of studies. We tested the sensitivity of effect size by removing the lowest quality studies and recalculating the mean effect for the remaining studies. Effect size versus sample size was plotted for all studies to determine whether overall effect was driven by smaller, less reliable studies.

Synthesis of the overall quality of the research in the field and development of recommendations was made by one of our group in consultation with the biostatistician.

Results

Literature search

Eighty-two energy healing research reports were identified through our two phases of literature searching. They were as follows: Alandydy & Alandydy (1999), Beutler et al (1988), Bowers (1992), Brown (1981), Bush & Geist (1992), Cooper (1997), Cox & Hayes (1998), Dollar (1993), Donohue (1998), Dowling & Bright (1999), Eliopoulos (1998), Evanoff & Newton (1999), Faughnan & Lagace (1998), Fedoruk (1984), Gagne & Toye (1994), Garrad (1998), Giasson & Bouchard (1998), Gordon et al (1998), Grad (1963), Grad (1964), Grad (1965), Grad et al (1961), Green (1998a), Green (1998b), Griffin & Vitro (1998), Guerrero (1985), Hale (1986), Hayes & Cox (1999), Heidt (1981), Huebscher

(1999), Hughes et al (1996), Ireland (1998), Keller & Bzdek (1986), Kemp (1994), Kramer (1990), Krieger (1975), Krieger (1976), Krieger (1979), Lafreniere et al (1999), Ledwith (1995), Leskowitz (2000), Lewis (1999), MacNeil (1995), Markides (1996), Meehan (1993), Mersmann (1993), Misra (1993), Mueller Hinze (1988), Nodine (1987), Olson et al (1992), Olson & Sneed (1995), Papantonio (1998), Parkes (1985), Peck (1997), Peck (1998), Pomerhn (1987), Post (1990), Quinn (1984), Quinn (1989), Quinn & Strelkand (1993), Randolph (1984), Robinson (1995), Rosa et al (1998), Samarel et al (1998), Simington & Laing (1993), Smith (1973), Sneed et al (1997), Snyder et al (1995), Sodergen (1990), Tharnstrom (1993), Turner et al (1998), Villaire (1999), Wilkinson (1997), Wirth (1990), Wirth (1993), Wirth (1994), Wirth & Cram (1993), Wirth et al (1992), Wirth et al (1993), Wirth et al (1996), Yamashita et al (1998). Of these, 20 were published randomized controlled trials in humans and met the overall inclusion criteria. These were Beutler et al (1988), Gagne & Toye (1994), Giasson & Bouchard (1998), Gordon et al (1998), Ireland (1998), Keller & Bzdek (1986), Lafreniere et al (1999), Meehan (1993), Peck (1997), Peck (1998), Quinn (1984), Quinn (1989), Randolph (1984), Samarel et al (1998), Simington & Laing (1993), Turner et al (1998), Wirth (1990), Wirth & Cram (1993), Wirth et al (1993), Wirth et al (1996) (see Fig. 8.1). Two articles by Peck (Peck 1997, 1998), were reports of different outcomes based on the same data set and were considered as one study for purposes of this review, thus bringing the total number of studies in the critical review to 19, of which 18 examined the effects of TT, while one looked at LOOH.

Quality scoring

Using the five-point Jadad score, quality scores of the TT studies ranged from 1 to 4 with a median and mode value of 3 (Table 8.1). Eleven of 19 studies received the full two points for randomization. Eight studies were identified as randomized but failed to describe the process of randomization, therefore scoring only one point in this category. Six of 19 studies received two points for double blinding, indicating the use of an appropriate

Table 8.1 A summary showing study author(s), date of publication, comments on blinding, and Jadad scores.

Study author(s)	Year	Comments on blinding	R	B	W	T
Giasson & Bouchard	1998	Not enough information	1	0	1	2
Lafreniere et al	1999	Open trial	1	0	0	1
Samarel et al	1998	Subjects blinded	2	0	1	3
Ireland	1998	Subjects blinded, evaluators not blinded	2	0	1	3
Gagne & Toye	1994	Subjects blinded, evaluator not blinded	2	0	1	3
Simington & Laing	1993	Double blinded	2	2	0	4
Quinn	1989	Standard care subjects unblinded, evaluator blinded	2	0	0	2
Quinn	1984	Subjects blinded	1	0	0	1
Turner et al	1998	Double blinded	2	2	0	4
Gordon et al	1998	Evaluator blinded	1	0	1	2
Peck	1997/8	Not blinded	2	0	1	3
Meehan	1993	Evaluator blinded	2	0	1	3
Keller & Bzdek	1986	Subjects blinded	2	0	1	3
Wirth & Cram	1993	Subjects blinded	1	0	0	1
Beutler et al	1988	Treatment group unblinded, two control arms double blinded	2	0	1	3
Randolph	1984	Double blinded	1	2	0	3
Wirth et al	1996	Double blinded	1	2	0	3
Wirth et al	1993	Double blinded	1	2	0	3
Wirth	1990	Double blinded	1	2	1	4

R = randomization score (0–2); B = blinding score (0–2); W = withdrawal score (0–1); T = total Jadad score (0–5).

placebo control with all study participants blinded and either instruction in performing a subject self-administered questionnaire or actual outcome measurement by a blinded assistant. According to the Jadad criteria, those performing the intervention or statistical analysis do not necessarily need to be blinded in order to receive full points in this category (Jadad et al 1996). In the 13 studies in which no points were earned for double blinding, six were single blinded with respect to the participants and four were single blinded with respect to those administering the outcome measures. In two studies, no one was blinded (Lafreniere et al 1999; Peck 1997, 1998), and in one report there was insufficient information to assess blinding (Giasson & Bouchard 1998). Ten of 19 studies described withdrawals and dropouts or indicated that there were none, thus receiving an additional point. The remainder either did not report the existence of dropouts or withdrawals or did not describe their characteristics.

THE STUDIES

Methods

Populations and setting

Six studies were conducted on healthy adult volunteers (Lafreniere et al 1999, Randolph 1984, Wirth 1990, Wirth & Cram 1993, Wirth et al 1993, Wirth et al 1996), one on adult volunteers with tension headache (Keller & Bzdek 1986), and one on adult volunteers with hypertension (Beutler et al 1988) (see Table 8.3). Three studies involved elders, either institutionalized with a variety of conditions or outpatient volunteers with arthritis (Gordon et al 1998; Peck 1997, 1998; Simington & Laing 1993). Three studies were performed on volunteers in the pre- or post-surgical (cardiac, breast, and abdominal or pelvic surgery) period (Meehan 1993, Quinn 1989, Samarel et al 1998). Four studies used inpatient volunteers from various units: terminal cancer patients on a palliative care unit (Giasson & Bouchard 1998); psychiatric patients (Gagne & Toye 1994); cardiovascular patients (Quinn 1984); and burn patients (Turner et al 1998). A single study examined the effects in outpatient children with HIV (Ireland 1998).

Although the subject sample was generally clearly described in all studies, few authors explicitly stated their inclusion or exclusion criteria.

These 19 studies took place in a variety of locations including: five in laboratory settings, six in conventional institutional settings, four in conventional outpatient settings, two in either subject homes or TT practitioner offices, one at a yoga retreat center, and one in an unspecified location (although probably an outpatient clinic). Of these, a single study is notable for being conducted in five different extended care settings (Simington & Laing 1993).

Intervention

The experimental intervention employed was non-contact TT in 16 of 19 studies (see Table 8.2). A single study, the earliest reported in this data set, used contact TT (Randolph 1984) and another study used LOOH with contact (Beutler et al 1988). In one other study, the most recently reported, the description of TT was inadequate to determine if NCTT or CTT was used (Lafreniere et al 1999). The predetermined duration of a single treatment ranged from 3 to 20 minutes in 14 of the studies. Four of the more recent studies allowed the practitioner to determine the length of treatment (Giasson & Bouchard 1998; Gordon et al 1998; Peck 1997, 1998; Turner et al 1998). Lafreniere and colleagues failed to report the duration of therapy sessions (Lafreniere et al 1999). Ten studies, generally the earlier ones, used a single session as the intervention. The remaining nine studies used multiple treatments such as daily treatment over 2–16 days, weekly treatment for 6–15 weeks, or monthly treatments for 3 months.

Blinding/masking/control procedures

Several schemas were attempted for establishing a blinded control group (see Table 8.2). Two treatment arms were used in 13 studies and three treatment groups were employed in six studies. In Randolph's early study employing contact TT, she used physical touch as a control (Randolph 1984). Beutler et al compared physical contact LOOH to distant healing with a hidden healer (Beutler et al 1988).

Table 8.2 Study authors, factors related to the intervention, and control states.

Study author	Therapy	Control groups				Session length (min)	Number of sessions
		Mimic	Physical touch	Other therapy/ human	No treatment		
Giasson & Bouchard	NCTT			Rest period		15–20	×3 (3 days)
Lafreniere et al	? CTT, music and rest				No Tx	Unknown + 5–10 rest	×3 (1 ×/mo)
Samarel et al	NCTT, music and talk			Quiet time music and talk		10 + 20 talk	×2 (preop, postop)
Ireland	NCTT	Mimic				5–7	×1
Gagne & Toye	NCTT	Mimic		Relaxation (20–30 min)		15	×2 (2 days)
Simington & Laing	NCTT and massage			Massage, two groups		3	×1
Quinn (1989)	NCTT	Mimic			Standard care, no Tx	5	×1 (preop)
Quinn (1984)	NCTT	Mimic				5	×1
Turner et al	NCTT, music and rest	Mimic, music and rest				5–20 + 5–10 rest	×5 (5 days)
Gordon et al	NCTT	Mimic			Standard care, no Tx	Variable	×6 (6 wks)
Peck (1997/8)	NCTT	Mimic		Progressive muscle relaxation		10–33	×6 (6 wks)
Meehan	NCTT	Mimic			Standard care (narcotics)	5	×1 (postop)
Keller & Bzdek	NCTT and deep breathing	Mimic and deep breathing				5 + 5 rest	×1
Wirth & Cram	NCTT and meditation	Mimic and meditation				5–7	×1
Beutler et al	LOOH and music			Distance healing and music	No healing, just music	20	×15 (15 wks)
Randolph	CTT					15	×1
Wirth et al (1996)	NCTT				No Tx vacant room	5	×10 (10 days)
Wirth et al 1993	NCTT				No Tx vacant room	5	×10 (10 days)
Wirth 1990	NCTT				No Tx vacant room	5	×10 (10 days)

NCTT = non-contact therapeutic touch; CTT = contact therapeutic touch; LOOH = laying-on-of-hands; Tx = treatment.

Nine of the 16 non-contact TT studies used a mimic TT procedure, developed and validated by Quinn in a study in which 15 blinded observers could not distinguish between TT and mimic TT (Quinn 1984). In this procedure, the motions of TT are imitated but the mind of the practitioner is occupied with a mundane task, thus removing the element of focused intention to help or heal. In three of these nine studies, experienced TT practitioners performed the mimic procedure (Keller & Bzdek 1986, Quinn 1989, Wirth & Cram 1993). When Quinn's large study showed no effect using this type of control it was postulated that a trained TT practitioner may not be able to block the putative therapeutic effects. The other six studies employing a mimic TT control group used naïve people who were taught the hand motions of TT (Gagne & Toye 1994, Gordon et al 1998, Ireland 1998, Meehan 1993, Quinn 1984, Turner et al 1998).

Five of the 16 NCTT trials used another therapy as a comparison or camouflage for the TT therapy. Peck (1997, 1998) used relaxation training as the comparison. Gagne & Toye (1994) used a relaxation group in addition to a mimic TT group. Samarel et al compared music, dialogue, and TT to music, dialogue, and quiet time (Samarel et al 1998). Simington & Laing compared massage plus TT vs. massage alone done by a TT practitioner vs. massage alone done by a naïve person (Simington & Laing 1993). Giasson & Bouchard used a rest period with a TT practitioner in the room as the control state (Giasson & Bouchard 1998).

Standard care or no treatment was employed in eight of the 19 studies as a comparison group. Depending on execution, this may or may not have been done in a blinded manner. Wirth, in his three studies of wound healing, effectively blinded a no treatment control by having the intervention performed in a room adjacent to the one occupied by the subject. For the control state the room was unoccupied, but this could not be detected by the subject or evaluator of outcomes (Wirth 1990; Wirth et al 1993; 1996). Beutler and colleagues' LOOH study also employed a no treatment arm without a healer present in the designated space vs. the arm with a hidden healer

present. Beutler et al describe these two groups as double-blinded; however, the intervention LOOH group was unblinded (Beutler et al 1988). In three other studies, investigators used a standard care arm in addition to a mimic TT arm (Gordon et al 1998, Meehan 1993, Quinn 1989). These studies might be termed semi-double blinded. Evaluators of outcomes were blinded for all three groups; however, approximately one-third of the subjects in the standard care arm were unblinded. In the study by Lafreniere et al (1999), no one was effectively blinded by the untreated control state.

Outcomes

Most studies measured multiple outcomes (Table 8.3). Global well-being and quality of life were measured in four studies. Giasson & Bouchard used global well-being as the primary outcome in their study that included validation of Giasson's Well-being Scale (Giasson & Bouchard 1998). Other studies included quality of life with a single question (Beutler et al 1988), the validated Stanford Health Assessment Questionnaire (Gordon et al 1998), or a disease-specific Arthritis Impact Scale (Peck 1998).

Psychological outcomes were the main interest in seven studies. These measured transient anxiety using the validated anxiety state index (X-1 or Y-1) from Spielberger's State-Trait Anxiety Index (STAI) or the children's version (Gagne & Toye 1994; Ireland 1998; Lafreniere et al 1999; Quinn 1984, 1989; Samarel et al 1998; Simington & Laing 1993). Two of these studies also had mood as an outcome as measured by the validated Profile of Mood States (Lafreniere et al 1999) or the Affects Balance Scale (Samarel et al 1998). A single study used a visual analog scale (VAS) to measure anxiety as a secondary end-point (Turner et al 1998).

Pain was a primary outcome in five studies (Gordon et al 1998; Keller & Bzdek 1986; Meehan 1993; Peck 1997, 1998; Turner et al 1998) and was measured in two additional studies (Giasson & Bouchard 1998, Samarel et al 1998). Two studies used the validated Magill–Melzak Pain Questionnaire (Keller & Bzdek 1986, Turner et al 1998) and one used the validated

Multidimensional Pain Inventory (Gordon et al 1998). Turner and Gordon both added a pain visual analog scale (VAS) as a check to the validated tool (Gordon et al 1998, Turner et al 1998). Three other studies measured pain only with the VAS (Meehan 1993, Peck 1998, Samarel et al 1998). Peck differentiated two aspects of pain by using a VAS for pain intensity and one for distress from pain (Peck 1997). Giasson's Wellbeing Scale also included a VAS for pain (Giasson & Bouchard 1998).

Several studies used some form of objective measurement of the physical status of the study participants. Three studies measured physiological states thought to correlate with decreased anxiety or increased relaxation. The measures included: systolic blood pressure, heart rate, skin conductance, EMG, or skin temperature (Quinn 1989, Randolph 1984, Wirth & Cram 1993). The LOOH study looked at the effects on blood pressure in subjects with hypertension (Beutler et al 1988). Another study assessed spontaneous body movements in a specified time interval (Gagne & Toye 1994). Only two studies examined body fluids for signs of TT effects. Turner measured CD4 counts as an indicator of immune function and Lafreniere measured cortisol, dopamine, and nitric oxide in urine which are indirectly related to emesis (Lafreniere et al 1999, Turner et al 1998). Another physical outcome, wound healing, was measured by two common methodologies, direct tracing and digitization or observation of the wound or a photograph (Wirth 1990; Wirth et al 1993, 1996).

Outcomes were frequently assessed both pre- and post-experimental intervention. When multiple applications of the interventions were performed over days, weeks, or months, the outcome measure was generally taken on multiple occasions both before and after treatment. Long-term effects were examined by looking at pre-treatment measures over time.

Outcomes were checked for clinical significance with the subjects in an open-ended fashion for 10 out of 19 studies. However, the process of the qualitative analyses was rarely specified in the methods section, so the validity of the findings is unknown. They may merely represent the most favorable comments made by subjects.

Analyses

Sample sizes ranged from 12 to 153, with a total of 1122 subjects in all 19 studies (see Table 8.3). Thirteen studies might be termed pilot studies as they each had 60 subjects or fewer. Six studies ranged from 80 to 153 subjects. Only two authors (Peck 1997, 1998; Quinn 1989), gave a sample size calculation. No study indicated using an intent-to-treat analysis. Only five gave a rationale for the statistics chosen (Gordon et al 1998, Ireland 1998, Keller & Bzdek 1986, Meehan 1993, Turner et al 1998).

All studies commented on or evaluated the baseline comparability of groups. Most looked at some aspect of demographics, many also assessed co-morbidities or variables related the clinical condition of the subjects. Three studies are notable for also examining beliefs or expectancy related to the treatment or experience with meditation (Gagne & Toye 1994, Keller & Bzdek 1986, Quinn 1984).

Statistical analysis methods varied widely across the studies, partly depending on whether a continuous or dichotomous outcome measure was employed, and whether normality could be assumed for continuous outcomes (see Table 8.3). For continuous measures, between group analyses included ANOVA (analysis of variance) or MANOVA (multivariate analysis of variance), ANCOVA (analysis of covariance) or MANCOVA (multivariate analysis of covariance) with pre-treatment measures as covariates, and multiple or stepwise regression. Student's t test was used for two-group comparisons, either as a main or pairwise post hoc analysis. Other post hoc multiple comparison procedures included Tukey's honestly significant difference and Sheffe's method. Mann–Whitney U or Wilcoxon rank sum tests were used for between group analyses of non-normal data. Fisher's exact test was used to test for independence in a 2×2 table.

Within group analyses were made with ANOVA for comparison of multiple time points (Gagne & Toye 1994, Giasson & Bouchard 1998)

Table 8.3 Study authors, patient population, outcome, and statistical analysis.

Study author(s)	Patient population	N	Outcome	Outcome measures	Statistical analysis
Giasson & Bouchard	Terminal CA	20	Well-being (incl. pain)	Giasson well-being scale, VAS-pain	Student's t on pre–post differences between groups, ANOVA within group
Lafreniere et al	Healthy women	41	Mood, anxiety	POMS, STAI, urine: cortisol, dopamine, NO	ANOVA over time
Samarel et al	Women with breast CA	31	Anxiety, mood, pain	STAI, affects balance scale, VAS-pain	MANCOVA with baseline trait anxiety as covariate, univariate controlled for trait anxiety
Ireland	Children with HIV	20	Anxiety	STAI for children	ANCOVA with baseline scores as covariate, pre–post change within group
Gagne & Toye	Psych inpt with anxiety	31	Anxiety	STAI, movement score	MANOVA between groups, ANOVA within group
Simington & Laing	Elderly	105	Anxiety	STAI	ANCOVA on post-test scores, *post hoc* Scheffe
Quinn 1989	Cardiac preop	153	Anxiety	STAI, SBP, HR	ANCOVA with baseline scores as covariates
Quinn 1984	Cardiovascular	60	Anxiety	STAI	t test on between group partial correlation, paired t within group (pre–post)
Turner et al	Burn	99	Pain, anxiety, immune function	MMPQ, VAS, CD4 cts	Stepwise regression: outcome on treatment group and baseline scores
Gordon et al	Osteoarthritis	25	Pain, well-being, health status	MPI, VAS, HAQ	ANOVA between groups, ANOVA over time, paired t within group (pre-post), χ^2 for categorical data
Peck 1997/8	Arthritis; OA and RA	82	Arthritis impact, including pain	AIMS incl. 11 subscales + pain, satisfaction, mood, tension, VAS	ANOVA between groups on subscales, MANOVA between groups adj. for baseline measures, paired t within group (pre–post)
Meehan	Postop pain (abd/pelvic surg)	108	Pain	VAS	Hierarchical multiple regression adjusted for baseline, Tukey HSD *post hoc*

Study	Condition	N		Measure	Analysis
Keller & Bzdek	Tension headache	60	Pain	MMPQ	Wilcoxon rank sum test between groups, Wilcoxon signed rank test within groups
Wirth & Cram	Healthy	12	Relaxation	EMG, skin temp., HR, CO_2, PR	ANOVA on diff. between groups, Student's t with Bonferroni correction, ANOVA within group
Beutler et al	Essential HTN	115	Blood pressure and well-being	SBP, DBP, single question	Between group MANOVA ± covariates, Kruskal-Wallis (non-parametric) with Bonferroni correction, within group ANOVA ± covariates, Wilcoxon rank sum test (non-parametric)
Randolph	Healthy college women	60	Anxiety or relaxation	Skin conductance, EMG, skin temp.	ANCOVA with baseline scores as covariate
Wirth et al 1996	Healthy, punch biopsy	32	Number of wounds healed	Observer + photo, three individual observers	2×2 Fisher's exact test on day 10 only
Wirth et al 1993	Healthy, punch biopsy	24	Number of wounds healed	Observer + photo, four individual observers	2×2 Fisher's exact test on day 5 and day 10
Wirth 1990	Healthy, punch biopsy, men	44	Wound surface area, number of wounds healed	Direct tracing and digitalization	Mann–Whitney U between groups day 8, χ^2 on 2×2 table of number of healed wounds day 16

CA = cancer; HIV = human immunodeficiency virus; OA = osteoarthritis; RA = rheumatoid arthritis; HTN = hypertension; VAS = visual analogue scale; POMS = profile of mood states; STAI = state-trait anxiety inventory; NO = nitric oxide; SBP = systolic blood pressure; HR = heart rate; MMPQ = McGill-Melzak pain questionnaire; MPI = West Haven–Yale multidimensional pain inventory; HAQ = Stanford health assessment questionnaire; AIMS = arthritis impact measurement scale; EMG = electromyography; CO_2 = carbon dioxide; RR = respiratory rate; DBP = diastolic blood pressure; ANOVA = analysis of variance; MANCOVA = multivariate analysis of covariance; ANCOVA = analysis of covariance; MANOVA = multivariate analysis of variance; HSD = honestly significant difference.

or comparison of treatment sequence and subject (Wirth & Cram 1993). The paired t test on pre–post treatment data was also frequently used for continuous outcomes and non-normal data were analyzed within group by the Wilcoxon signed rank test.

Effect sizes were not reported by any study, but could be calculated or reasonably estimated for all studies (Table 8.4). Because not all studies reported the needed standard deviations (SD), several assumptions were necessary in order to calculate Cohen's d. For Gagne & Toye's study (1994), the SD of the STAI was estimated from the SDs reported in four other studies using the same outcome measure. For Lafreniere et al's study (1999), the SD was calculated based on the reported F statistic, cell means read from a graph, and the reported mean squared error of the interaction of groups over time. In the study by Turner et al (1998), the SD was estimated assuming that the loss to follow-up was evenly distributed across the groups and that SDs were equal in each group. For the work of Keller & Bzdek (1986), we used the reported pre-test SD, since the post-test SD was described as 'within one point' of the pre-test. Two of the studies by Wirth et al (1993, 1996) reported the number of wounds healed as recorded by multiple observers. We calculated the percentage of wounds healed in both treatment groups. To calculate a SD, we used the percentage of observers rating the wound as healed for each subject and calculated the SD of those values.

Effect sizes across all studies ranged from – 0.56 to + 1.97, with an average of 0.60 which is a moderate effect (see Table 8.4). When we looked at average effect size in each type of outcome, the strongest effects were seen in the wound healing (0.78) and pain studies (0.72). Moderate effects were seen in physiological outcomes (0.45) and in emotional outcomes (0.55). We tested the sensitivity of the average effect for all studies by removing the six studies with the lowest quality scores (Jadad ≤ 2). The resulting range was – 0.56 to + 1.84 and the average effect was lowered to 0.54, still reflective of a moderate effect. The effect sizes of all studies were plotted versus sample sizes which produced a classic funnel plot with the effect sizes of largest quality studies nearly approximating the mean effect (Fig. 8.2).

To further understand the effect of energy healing, it is useful to look at those studies with the best designs. Three studies scored 4s on the Jadad scale and all were successfully double blinded, thus removing a major potential for systematic bias (Simington & Laing 1993, Turner et al 1998, Wirth 1990).

Simington & Laing studied an elderly population in five different extended care facilities, measuring the effects of a 3-minute application of massage with or without NCTT on the STAI Y-1 as a measure of anxiety (Simington & Laing 1993). Analysis of variance among 105 subjects on post-test scores showed that massage plus TT was more effective ($P = 0.001$). This study evaluated a brief intervention in an important population, was well controlled, and had a substantial number of subjects, with only three dropouts unaccounted for across the whole study. The outcome measure and analysis were appropriate, thus making the result meaningful. The calculated effect size was 0.70, a moderate to large effect.

Turner et al looked at patients in a hospital burns unit and compared the effects of music and a rest period plus NCTT or mimic TT on pain, anxiety, and immune cell counts (Turner et al 1998). The treatment was allowed to vary and took place daily over 5 days. Outcomes in 99 subjects were measured using validated scales and VASs at baseline and on the day following conclusion of treatment. A stepwise regression of outcome on treatment group with baseline scores, demographic variables, beliefs about treatment, and pain medications as covariates showed that the NCTT group experienced less pain ($P = 0.005$) and less anxiety ($P = 0.031$). The calculated effect size for pain as measured by the McGill–Melzak Pain Rating Index was 0.71, indicating a moderate to large effect. Criticism of this trial includes the significant number of dropouts or withdrawals (16), and the inadequate reporting of their characteristics or group assignment. A flow diagram of numbers of subjects through different phases of the study would have been useful. It is unfortunate that the deviations from protocol resulted in too few blood samples for

Table 8.4 Effect size (Cohen's d) calculated for primary outcomes ((control mean–treatment mean) / control standard deviation).

Study author(s)	Outcome measure	Direction of positive outcome	Treatment group mean	Control group mean	Standard deviation (SD)	Effect size (Cohen's d)	Average effect	Type of outcome
Giasson & Bouchard[a]	Well-being	Higher[o]	−6.3	−5.6	1.9	0.37	0.37	Global
Lafreniere et al[b]	POMS[i]	Lower	−6	14	11.67	1.71		
Samarel et al	STAI[j]	Lower	31	36.4	12	0.45		
Ireland	STAI	Lower	26.7	29.5	3.37	0.83		
Gagne & Toye[c]	STAI	Lower	40.1	43	24.34	0.12		
Simington & Laing	STAI	Lower	27.09	36.53	13.4	0.70		
Quinn 1989	STAI	Lower	37.62	35.19	11.84	−0.21		
Quinn 1984	STAI	Lower	31.79	34.3	11.34	0.22	0.55	Psychological
Turner et al[d]	McGill PRI[k]	Lower	27.9	36.3	11.8	0.71		
Gordon et al[e]	Pain severity	Lower	2.14	3.27	0.574	1.97		
Peck 1997/8	Pain subscale	Lower	4.88	4.42	1.86	−0.25		
Meehan	Pain VAS[l]	Lower	50.25	61.72	22.15	0.52		
Keller & Bzdek[f]	McGill PRI	Lower	4.57	10.4	8.8	0.66	0.72	Pain
Wirth & Cram	Neck EMG[m]	Lower	3.2	5	4.1	0.44		
Beutler et al[g]	SBP[n] reduction	Higher[o]	−19.3	−14.2	5.9	0.86		
Randolph	Skin conductance	Lower	21.77	22.43	14.84	0.04	0.45	Physiological
Wirth et al 1996[h]	% healed	Higher[o]	0	−0.25	0.45	−0.56		
Wirth et al 1993[h]	% healed	Higher[o]	−0.84	−0.34	0.48	1.04		
Wirth 1990	Wound size	Lower	0.418	5.855	2.952	1.84	0.78	Wound healing

[a]Mean and SD calculated from reported individual scores; [b]SD estimated based on mean squared error (mean squared interaction/F statistic); outcome values read from graph; [c]SD estimated by averaging SDs for STAI reported by other authors; [d]means adjusted for baseline score and use of pain medication; SD estimated assuming loss of n evenly distributed on day 6 and SD equal for treatment and control group; [e]Article reports standard errors labeled as standard deviation; appropriate SDs calculated based on P values of between group post hoc analysis; [f]used pre-test SD since post-test SD only reported as 'within one point' of pretest; [g]SD calculated from reported confidence intervals; [h]Percent healed calculated from reported number healed; SD calculated assuming least interobserver variability; [i]profile of mood states; [j]state-trait anxiety inventory; [k]pain rating index; [l]visual analogue scale; [m]electromyography; [n]systolic blood pressure; [o]higher score reflects positive effect therefore the sign was reversed on outcomes prior to calculation of effect size.

meaningful statistical analysis of the effect on immune cell counts. More data on objective physiological outcomes is needed in this field of healing energy research.

Wirth did examine a physiological process, wound healing, in healthy volunteers who received a uniform punch biopsy in the arm (Wirth 1990). In his original study, Wirth compared a 5-minute NCTT treatment to an effectively blinded no treatment control administered daily for 16 days, measuring wound surface area quantitatively with direct tracing and digitization in 44 subjects. On day 8 after wounding, the TT group had significantly smaller wounds ($P <0.001$) using a Mann–Whitney U test between groups. At day 16 the number of wounds healed was significantly different between groups. The χ^2 test for independence on a 2×2 table showed TT to be significantly more effective ($P < 0.001$). The effect size on day 16 was calculated to be 1.84, a very large effect. Criticism of this study includes failure adequately to describe the randomization process and the questionable feasibility of implementing this type of treatment in the outpatient setting. It may be most useful in the inpatient postoperative set-

ting. Wirth has published two replications of this work, one with positive results (effect size = 1.04) (Wirth et al 1993) and one with negative results (effect size = −0.56) (Wirth et al 1996). The 1996 study with negative results is important for suggesting that the health of the TT practitioner may significantly affect the direction of TT effects; however, that study had several dropouts who were not well characterized and could have changed the outcome to one of overall non-significance. Replication by other investigators in meaningful clinical settings would be useful.

Reporting

When examined as a group on aspects of reporting via the CONSORT criteria, this body of literature has several strengths and several weaknesses. Looking at the initial CONSORT requirements, no articles included in this review used the word 'randomized' in the title and only two used a structured abstract (Gordon et al 1998, Samarel et al 1998). Eighteen of 19 studies clearly stated the clinical objectives of the research, with 16 authors further stating clear hypotheses to be tested.

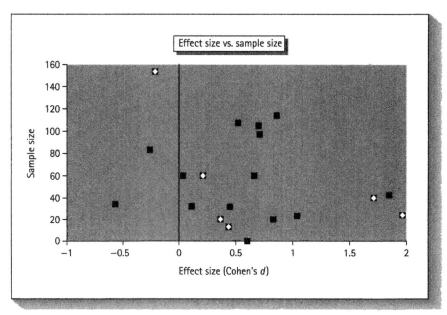

Figure 8.2 Effect size *vs.* sample size for all studies. White diamonds on black squares equal the poor quality studies (Jadad score ≤ 2); black squares equal the good quality studies (Jadad score ≥ 3). The effect size positioned on y = 0 is the overall effect size for this group of studies.

Methods of intervention and outcome measures were generally well described. Often, inclusion/exclusion criteria, sample size calculation, and allocation of dropouts were not reported. Frequently randomization was not fully described, and blinding with respect to subjects, outcome assessors, practitioners, and analysts was variously reported. No authors provided a participant flow diagram and few identified whether or not there were protocol deviations. Results were provided with means and standard deviations in most cases and groups were examined for comparability at baseline, with important variables often used as covariates or adjustments in the analyses. Most authors were insightful in their handling of the discussion section of their reports, but a strong assumption permeating the work is the existence of human energy fields or transferable energy for healing.

DISCUSSION

This critical review brings several important observations to light about the state of healing energy research. First, there is a relatively large body of experimental literature available between published works and unpublished dissertations. Further, the literature includes 19 randomized controlled clinical trials – a substantial number, particularly for a complementary medicine technique. Therapeutic touch clearly dominates this research with only a single RCT of another modality, laying-on of hands. The overall quality of these trials, as assessed by the Jadad score, is comparable to the general medical literature with the majority of trials scoring 3 or 4 out of a possible 5. In general, the studies cover a wide variety of subject populations and settings. Energy healing is assessed for its effects on a number of important subjective outcomes including general well-being, anxiety, mood, and pain. Certain objective physiological states, such as muscle contraction, blood pressure, heart rate, serum immune cell counts, and urinary neuropeptides are also measured. The outcome measures are carefully selected with previously validated scales predominating for subjective data and standard physiologic testing for objec-

tive data. Uniformly, the statistical methods chosen are appropriate to the data and hypotheses. A flaw in reporting or design is the general inattention to identification of clinically important differences in the outcome measures. However, many studies use some kind of qualitative check on the perceptions of the subjects about the importance of the effects. Examination of the three best-designed and reported experiments demonstrated statistically significant positive effects of NCTT on anxiety, pain control, and wound healing. Effect sizes were not reported, but could be calculated or estimated after making reasonable assumptions. Overall, there was a moderate positive effect of healing energy across all primary outcomes. Reporting of the experiments could be significantly improved by careful attention to the CONSORT criteria.

Adequate blinding is the most important threat to the internal validity of these studies. Several strategies for double blinding were employed, with two standing out as adequate: the first was non-contact TT *vs.* mimic TT, and the second non-contact TT with the healer in a visually separated space adjacent to the subject *vs.* no healer in that separate space. Two caveats are important here. First, mimic TT is best performed by TT naïve individuals, and second, where healers are operating from a different space, an even better control may be a TT naïve individual present in that space. Another issue in blinding is maintaining the blinding of the administrator of measures, even those who give instructions or initiate so-called subject self-evaluations. This is a logistical problem that can be solved with careful forethought. A more perplexing question is whether the practitioners administering the healing energy must be blinded. The concern here is that there may be subtle cues that the subject will detect that will unblind the subject. Quinn's creation of the mimic procedure was tested and a recent report of a similar approach to sham Reiki also demonstrated that it was an effective blinding procedure (Mansour et al 1999). Lastly, good practice would dictate that even the statistical analyst should keep their blinders on until the pre-stated hypotheses have been tested. Even biostatisticians may have opinions on the outcome of studies.

The most important threat to external validity among this body of work is the selection of outcomes. While the selected measures are good approximations of the subjective concepts identified as clinically important, that is, anxiety or pain perception, little evidence here substantiates an effect of energy healing on physiological processes. For example, the arthritis studies would benefit from objective measures of arthritis, and tension headache might be assessed with EMG. Wounds might be assessed as to time to full healing or wound strength. Measures of physiological processes that might elucidate mechanism of action of healing energy should be included in future clinical trials. Other important aspects of efficacy that have not been fully explored, but could be designed into trials, include dose effect and residual effect.

One difficulty with this research is that the underlying theory, that in some way humans can interact on an energetic level to heal each other, is only indirectly assessed by this body of literature. However, there are many mysteries about the underlying mode of action of even our most well-studied therapeutic interventions and this has not caused medical professionals to abandon them. Thus the examination of theory, including the measurement of so-called energy fields, is an important area of further study.

This critical review has its own limitations that should be considered when evaluating the conclusions expressed therein. First, only published reports of randomized controlled trials were included. The first phase of our search included unpublished dissertations, and arguments can be made that unpublished negative studies would sway our overall evaluation of the literature. This is most important in meta-analyses where the major objective is to calculate overall effects. The major objective here was focused on evaluation of research process and reporting, so that limitation to previously peer-reviewed reports seemed justified. Second, no matter what criteria one uses to objectively 'score' a research report, there is still a great deal of interpretation that enters into the process. We attempted to overcome this problem by using more than one reviewer and a

process of coming to consensus in consultation with a biostatistician. Finally, synthesis of the extracted data and scorings was done primarily by only one of our group using a simple method of counting numbers of studies with or without the characteristics of interest. While this gives an overall gestalt of the status of this literature, it is necessarily subject to the investigator's biases, knowledge base, attention to detail, and perseverance. However, other reviewers and meta-analysts have looked at similar groupings of the literature and obtained similar results. Our group (Warber et al 2000a) has made a preliminary report of a meta-analysis of the TT anxiety studies, finding an overall positive effect of TT on pre–post difference scores between experimental groups. Both published and unpublished studies prior to 1998 were included in that meta-analysis. Peters (1999) has published a recent meta-analysis in which she calculated effect sizes using Cohen's d as was done in this review. She found an average effect of 1.20 for physiological studies and 0.48 for psychological outcomes. She limited the group to studies published between 1986 and 1996. Astin et al (2000) included eleven TT studies in a systematic review of 'distant healing' trials published before the end of 1999. This group reported Jadad scores and Cohen's d weighted by sample size. They found a moderate effect of 0.63 for 10 of the TT studies, a similar finding to our own of 0.60 for the overall effect among our 19 studies.

Overall, the clinical research on healing energy as exemplified by these randomized controlled trials of, primarily, therapeutic touch has important strengths and weaknesses. Careful attention to blinding procedures, expansion of outcome measures, and investigation of theoretical underpinnings will improve the credibility of the research. Future authors can easily enhance the value of their contributions by applying the CONSORT criteria to their manuscripts. Given the current body of published reports, including two recent meta-analyses and a systematic review, the overall quality of evidence for this topic area, as specified by the Guidelines for Quality of Evidence, is of the highest level.

REFERENCES

Alandydy P, Alandydy K 1999 Using Reiki to support surgical patients. Journal of Nursing Care Quality 13(4): 89–91

Astin J A, Harkness E, Ernst E 2000 The efficacy of 'distant healing': a systematic review of randomized trials. Annals of Internal Medicine 132(11): 903–910

Begg C, Cho M, Eastwood S et al 1996 Improving the quality of reporting of randomized controlled trials: the CONSORT statement. Journal of the American Medical Association 276(9): 637–639

Beutler J, Attevelt J T M, Schouten S A, Faber J A, Mees E J D, Geijskes G G 1988 Paranormal healing and hypertension. British Medical Journal 296: 1491–1494

Bowers D P 1992 The effect of TT in state anxiety and physiological measurements in preoperative clients. San Jose State University, San Jose

Brown P R 1981 The effects of therapeutic touch on chemotherapy-induced nausea and vomiting. University of Nevada, Las Vegas, Nevada

Bush A M, Geist C R 1992 Geophysical variables and behavior: LXX. Testing electromagnetic explanations for a possible psychokinetic effect of therapeutic touch on germinating corn seed. Psychological Reports 70(3/1): 891–896

Cohen J 1977 Statistical power analysis for the behavioral science. Academic Press, New York

Cooper R E 1997 The effect of TT on irritable bowel syndome. Clarkson College, Potsman, New York

Cox C, Hayes J 1998 Experiences of administering and receiving therapeutic touch in intensive care. Complementary Therapies in Nursing and Midwifery 4(5): 128–132

Dollar C E 1993 Effects of TT on perception of pain and physiology measurements tension headaches in adults: a pilot study. University of Mississippi, Oxford, Mississippi

Donohue M 1998 What is energy work? Nursing Spectrum 8(7): 11

Dowling J S, Bright M A 1999 A collaborative research project on therapeutic touch. Journal of Holistic Nursing 17(3): 296–307

Eliopoulos C 1998 Therapeutic touch. Director 6(4): 150–151

Evanoff A, Newton W P 1999 Therapeutic touch and osteoarthritis of the knee. Journal of Family Practice 48(1): 11–12

Faughnan J G, Lagace E A 1998 Science and the alternative. Journal of Family Practice 47(4): 262–263

Fedoruk R B 1984 Transfer of the relaxation response: therapeutic touch as a method for reduction of stress in premature neonates. University of Maryland, Baltimore, Maryland

Gagne D, Toye R C 1994 The effects of therapeutic touch and relaxation therapy in reducing anxiety. Archives of Psychiatric Nursing 8(3): 184–189

Garrad C T 1998 The effect of therapeutic touch on stress reduction and immune function in persons with AIDS. University of Alabama at Birmingham, Birmingham, Alabama

Giasson M, Bouchard L 1998 Effect of therapeutic touch on the well-being of persons with terminal cancer. Journal of Holistic Nursing 16(3): 383–398

Gordon A, Merenstein J H, D'Amico F, Hudgens D 1998 The effects of therapeutic touch on patients with osteoarthritis of the knee. Journal of Family Practice 47(4): 271–277

Grad B 1963 A telekinetic effect on plant growth. International Journal of Parapsychology 5(2): 117–133

Grad B 1964 A telekinetic effect on plant growth: II. Experiments involving treatment of saline in stoppered bottles. International Journal of Parapsychology 6: 473–498

Grad B 1965 Some biological effects of the 'laying on of hands': a review of experiments on animals and plants. Journal of American Society for Psychical Research 59: 95–127

Grad B, Cadoret R J, Paul G I 1961 An unorthodox method of treatment on wound healing in mice. International Journal of Parapsychology 3(2): 5–24

Green C A 1998a Critically exploring the use of Rogers' nursing theory of unitary human beings as a framework to underpin therapeutic touch practice. European Nurse 3(3): 158–169

Green C A 1998b Reflections of a therapeutic touch experience: case study 2. Complementary Therapies in Nursing and Midwifery 4(1): 17–21

Griffin R L, Vitro E 1998 An overview of therapeutic touch and its application to patients with Alzheimer's disease. American Journal of Alzheimers Disease 13(4): 211–216

Guerrero M A 1985 The effects of therapeutic touch on state-trait anxiety level of oncology patients. University of Texas Medical Branch at Galveston, Galveston, Texas

Hale E H 1986 A study of the relationship between therapeutic touch and the anxiety levels of hospitalized adults. Texas Woman's University, Denton, Texas

Hayes J, Cox C 1999 Clinical. The experience of therapeutic touch from a nursing perspective. British Journal of Nursing 8(18): 1249–1250

Heidt P 1981 Effect of therapeutic touch on anxiety level of hospitalized patients. Nursing Research 30(1): 32–37

Huebscher R 1999 Therapeutic touch – what is the controversy and why does controversy exist? Nurse Practitioner Forum 10(2): 43–46

Hughes P P, Meize-Grochowski R, Harris C 1996 Therapeutic touch with adolescent psychiatric patients. Journal of Holistic Nursing 14(1): 6–23

Ireland M 1998 Therapeutic touch with HIV-infected children: a pilot study. Journal of the Association of Nurses in AIDS Care 9(4): 68–77

Jadad A R, Moore R A, Carroll D et al 1996 Assessing the quality of reports of randomized clinical trials: is blinding necessary? Controlled Clinical Trials 17(1): 1–12

Keller E, Bzdek V M 1986 Effects of therapeutic touch on tension headache pain. Nursing Research 35(2): 101–106

Kemp L 1994 The effect of therapeutic touch on the anxiety levels of patients with cancer receiving palliative care. Dalhousie University, Halifax, Nova Scotia, Canada

Kramer N A 1990 Comparison of therapeutic touch and casual touch in stress reduction of hospitalized children. Pediatric Nursing 16(5): 483–485

Krieger D 1975 Therapeutic touch: the imprimatur of nursing. American Journal of Nursing 75(5): 784–787

Krieger D 1976 Healing by the 'laying-on' of hands as a facilitator of bioenergetic change: the response of in-vivo human hemoglobin. Psychoenergetic Systems 1: 121–129

Krieger D 1979 The therapeutic touch: how to use your hands to help or to heal. Prentice-Hall, Englewood Cliffs, NJ

Krieger D, Peper E, Ancoli S 1979 Therapeutic touch: searching for evidence of physiological change. American Journal of Nursing 79(4): 660–662

Lafreniere K D, Mutus B, Cameron S et al 1999 Effects of therapeutic touch on biochemical and mood indicators in women. Journal of Alternative and Complementary Medicine 5(4): 367–370

Ledwith S P 1995 Therapeutic touch and mastectomy: a case study. RN 58(7): 51–53

Leskowitz E D 2000 Phantom limb pain treated with therapeutic touch: a case report. Archives of Physical Medicine and Rehabilitation 81(4): 522–524

Lewis D 1999 A survey of therapeutic touch practitioners. Nursing Standard 13(30): 33–37

McGaw G, Glass G 1980 Choice of the metric for effect size in meta-analysis. American Educational Research Journal 7(2): 325–337

MacNeil MS 1995 Therapeutic touch and tension headaches: a Rogerian study. D'Youville College, Buffalo, NY

Mansour A A, Beuche M, Laing G, Leis A, Nurse J 1999 A study to test the effectiveness of placebo Reiki standardization procedures developed for a planned Reiki efficacy study. Journal of Alternative and Complementary Medicine 5(2): 153–164

Markides E J 1996 Complementary energetic practices: an exploration into the world of Maine women healers. University of Maine, Orono, ME

Meehan T C 1993 Therapeutic touch and postoperative pain: a Rogerian research study. Nursing Science Quarterly 6(2): 69–78

Mersmann C A 1993 Therapeutic touch and milk letdown in mothers of non-nursing preterm infants. New York University, New York

Miller L A 1979 An explanation of therapeutic touch using the science of unitary man. Nursing Forum 18(3): 278–287

Misra M M 1993 The effects of TT on menstruation. California State University at Long Beach, Long Beach, California

Mueller Hinze M 1988 The effects of therapeutic touch and acupressure on experimentally-induced pain. University of Texas at Austin, Austin, Texas

Mulloney S S, Wells-Federman C 1996 Therapeutic touch: a healing modality. Journal of Cardiovascular Nursing 10(3): 27–49

Nodine J 1987 The effect of therapeutic touch on anxiety and well-being in pregnancy. University of Arizona, Tuscou, Arizona

Older J 1984 Teaching touch at medical school. Journal of the American Medical Association 252(7): 931–933

Olson M, Sneed N 1995 Anxiety and therapeutic touch. Issues in Mental Health Nursing 16(2): 97–108

Olson M, Sneed N, Bonadonna R, Ro J, Dias J 1992 Therapeutic touch and post-hurricane Hugo stress. Journal of Holistic Nursing 10(2): 120–136

Papantonio C 1998 Alternative medicine and wound healing. Ostomy Wound Management 44(4): 44–46

Parkes B 1985 Therapeutic touch as an intervention to reduce anxiety in elderly hospitalized patients. University of Texas at Austin, Austin, Texas

Peck S D 1997 The effectiveness of therapeutic touch for decreasing pain in elders with degenerative arthritis. Journal of Holistic Nursing 15(2): 176–198

Peck S D 1998 The efficacy of therapeutic touch for improving functional ability in elders with degenerative arthritis. Nursing Science Quarterly 11(3): 123–132

Peters R M 1999 The effectiveness of therapeutic touch: a meta-analytic review. Nursing Science Quarterly 12(1): 52–61

Pomerhn A 1987 The effect of therapeutic touch on nursing students' perceptions of stress during clinical experiences. D'Youville College. Buffalo, New York, USA

Post N W 1990 The effects of therapeutic touch on muscle tone. Dissertation written at San Jose State University, San Jose, CA

Quinn J F 1984 Therapeutic touch as energy exchange: testing the theory. Advances in Nursing Science 6(2): 42–49

Quinn J F 1989 Therapeutic touch as energy exchange: replication and extension. Nursing Science Quarterly 2(2): 79–87

Quinn J F, Strelkand A J 1993 Psychoimmunologic effects of TT on practitioners and recently bereaved recipients: a pilot study. Advanced Nursing Science 15(4): 13–26

Randolph G L 1984 Therapeutic and physical touch: physiological response to stressful stimuli. Nursing Research 33(1): 33–36

Robinson L S 1995 The effects of therapeutic touch on the grief experience. University of Alabama at Birmingham, Birmingham, Alabama

Rosa L, Rosa E, Sumer L, Barett S 1998 A close look at therapeutic touch. Journal of the American Medical Association 279(13): 1005–1010

Samarel N, Fawcett J, Davis M M, Ryan F M 1998 Effects of dialogue and therapeutic touch on preoperative and postoperative experiences of breast cancer surgery: an exploratory study. Oncology Nursing Forum 25(8): 1369–1376

Simington J A, Laing G P 1993 Effects of therapeutic touch on anxiety in the institutionalized elderly. Clinical Nursing Research 2(4): 438–450

Smith M J 1973 Paranormal effects on ezyme activity. Human Dimensions 1: 15–19

Sneed N V, Olson M, Bonadonna R 1997 The experience of therapeutic touch for novice recipients. Journal of Holistic Nursing 15(3): 243–253

Snyder M, Egan E C, Burns K R 1995 Interventions for decreasing agitation behaviors in persons with dementia. Journal of Gerontological Nursing 21(7): 34–40

Sodergen K A 1990 The effects of absorption and social closeness on responses to educational and relaxation therapies in patients with anticipatory nausea and vomiting secondary to cancer chemotherapy. University of Minnesota, Minneapolis, MN

Steckel C M, King R P 1996 Therapeutic touch in the coronary care unit. Journal of Cardiovascular Nursing 10(3): 50–54

Tharnstrom C 1993 The effects of non-contact therapeutic touch on the parasympathetic nervous system as evidenced by skin temperature and perceived stress. San Jose State University, San Jose

Turner J G, Clark A J, Gauthier D K, Williams M 1998 The effect of therapeutic touch on pain and anxiety in burn patients. Journal of Advanced Nursing 28(1): 10–20

Villaire M 1999 Healing touch therapy makes a difference in surgery unit. Critical Care Nurse 19(1): 104

Warber S, Kile G, Gillespie B, Gorenflo D, Bolling S 2000a Meta-analysis of the effects of therapeutic touch on anxiety symptoms [abstract]. FACT: Focus on Alternative and Complementary Therapies 5(1): 106

Warber S, Kile G, Straughn J 2000b The nature of biofield energy for healing: a qualitative study [abstract]. Forschende Komplementarmedizin und Klassische Naturheikunde [Research in Complementary and Natural Classical Medicine] 7: 55

Warber S, Straughn J, Kile G 2000c The complementary medicine healer-client relationship. North American Primary Care Research Group 28th Annual Meeting, Amelia Island, Fla, Nov 4–7, 2000

Wilkinson T 1997 The effects of therapeutic touch on the experience of acute pain in postoperative laminectomy patients. Bellarmine College, Louisville, NY

Wirth D P 1990 The effect of non-contact therapeutic touch on the healing rate of full thickness dermal wounds. Subtle Energy 1(1): 1–20

Wirth D P 1993 Non-contact therapeutic touch and wound re-epithelialization: an extension of previous research. Complementary Therapies in Medicine 3: 187–192

Wirth D P 1994 Complementary healing therapies. International Journal of Psychosomatics 41(1–4): 61–67

Wirth D P, Cram J R 1993 Multi-site electromyographic analysis of non-contact therapeutic touch. International Journal of Psychosomatics 40: 47–55

Wirth D P, Johnson C A, Horvath J S, MacGregor J D 1992 The effect of alternative healing therapy in the regeneration rate of salamander forelimbs. Journal of Scientific Exploration 6(4): 375–390

Wirth D P, Richardson J T, Eidelman W S, O'Malley A C 1993 Full thickness dermal wounds treated with non-contact therapeutic touch: a replication and extension. Complementary Therapies in Medicine 1(3): 127–132

Wirth D P, Richardson J T, Martinez R D, Eidelman W S, Lopez M E 1996 Non-contact therapeutic touch intervention and full-thickness cutaneous wounds: a replication. Complementary Therapies in Medicine 4(4): 237–240

Yamashita M, Jensen E, Tall F 1998 Therapeutic touch: applying Newman's theoretic approach. Nursing Science Quarterly 11(2): 49–50

9

Qigong: basic science studies in biology

Xin Yan, Ping Y Lu,
Juliann G Kiang

The concept of qi is the main theoretical basis for traditional Chinese medicine (TCM), physical exercise, philosophy, culture and natural science. Qi is also used to describe the universal life force. Interaction of qi to produce balance and order of energy flow in the body with needles (acupuncture) or mind-body adjustment (qigong) contributes to the foundation of TCM therapy. Qigong is therefore sometimes called Chinese energy medicine in the West. While it has characteristics of energy such as the ability to do work, to be accumulated, stored, discharged and projected from the body, qi also has characteristics of intelligence and information in that it can be directed by the mind. Therefore, qi is not identical to energy or consciousness as understood in the West.

The therapeutic claims of Qigong are vast, and there are extensive reports of research both clinical and in the laboratory of its effects. However, this literature is mostly in Chinese and not easily accessible in the West. In addition, the research methodology of many studies in Qigong is often not of the type or quality accepted in the West. Most Chinese research on qigong accepts qi as a given and is done to explore its mechanisms and use rather than to prove that it exists as is usually desired in the West where qi is not accepted. In addition, negative studies of qigong are not generally published in the Chinese literature so the parameters for its generalizability are not available. There has been debate in China lasting several decades about the value of research focused on proof of the existence of qi. No consensus has emerged and further research to advance qigong will likely require improved methods and measurement techniques. These issues are discussed in more detail in Chapter 20 on methods in laboratory research.

In this chapter, Xin Yan, Ping Y Lu and Juliann G Kiang have analyzed a sample of qigong research done in laboratory models. These types of studies are thought not to be subject to expectation and placebo effects and so are more useful for further exploring the mechanisms of qigong and for proof of concept research. Although some renowned scientists, such as Dr. Hsue-Shen Tsien have lauded qigong research as "a scientific revolution", the quality of the research has not been convincing by Western criteria. However, a number of technologically sophisticated studies have been done and can serve as a basis for improved study design and replication in future research. ***WBJ***

INTRODUCTION

'Qi', in ancient Chinese texts, implies a fundamental dynamic of existence at the microscopic level, somewhat similar to the concept in modern science of energy and information. The concept is not entirely translatable into Western terminology. Qi is capable of doing work, and can exist in the state of radiation, propagation, and of concentration or distribution. Some modern concepts associate qi with a 'qi field', which is roughly characterized as a form of life-information-energy field. Qi is believed to connect energy and information through special meridian points such as one's Baihui point (the λ position of the skull, facing the sky), thereby improving health through "correspondence and harmony between man and universe" (Yan 2000). Any partial or full blockage of the qi flow within the body may result in symptoms ranging from subjective feelings of discomfort to symptomatic expression of disease, while a fluent and ordered cycling of internal and external qi in good quality is believed to be vital for an overall feeling of happiness and physical well-being.

'Qigong' is the practice of control and manipulation of qi. It consists of four elements: training in consciousness (including intention), breathing, physical movement, and the excitation and adjustment of one's potential energy. Qigong and its practice includes methods for strengthening the body, preventing and curing diseases, prolonging lifespan, developing wisdom, exploring potentiality, and healing and self-healing. General traditional Chinese qigong (TCQ) has been known for more than 7000 years according to archeologically discovered pictorial depictions, and was documented in literature between 3500 and 5000 years ago (Yan 2000). General TCQ is arguably one of the most ancient technologies of healing and mind-body fitness known to man.

In its long history, Chinese qigong has evolved various schools. Advanced TCQ is the result of many thousand years of development and experimentation by various qigong schools and individuals such as medical doctors, martial artists, scholars, masters and adepts, and includes those of many faiths including Daoism, Buddhism, and Confucianism. Advanced TCQ emphasizes the simultaneous training of mind and body, and cultivation in one's disposition and fortune. Seeking *De* (roughly, 'virtue') as general guidance, it develops one's potentiality and aims towards a high quality of health and longevity of both mind and body. Today, the application of general TCQ can be found in acupuncture, traditional herbal medicine, the martial arts, feng shui (i.e. 'wind-water'), and generic health care systems. Methods of general TCQ cover many of the methods similar to those under the category of complementary and alternative medicine (CAM), such as relaxation and meditation, imagery, dietary supplements and nutrition treatment, aromatherapy and music therapy (Kiang 2000).

However, it was not until about two decades ago that TCQ technology became more available to the vast majority of Chinese society as well as to the rest of the world. There were important historical reasons. TCQ has been a highly specialized technology done by traditional 'masters', who were extremely strict and secretive in selecting their students. It was often misconstrued by conventional wisdom to be a religious, feudalistic, and occult mystery. Making TCQ available to the public meant transforming both of these traditional views. There were three fundamental difficulties in achieving this transformation. The first was the need for a large enough number of general or even advanced TCQ specialists who had mastery of both traditional and modern technology; the second was finding a way to adapt traditional techniques to a wider population; last, and most critically, was a need for scientific study. During the economic and cultural renaissance of contemporary China, the Chinese government has made tremendous effort to preserve and promote the nation's traditional treasure of TCQ. Qigong was given official state status to become legalized in medical practice and physical excise. Thanks to the pioneering collaboration of reputable scientists at Tsinghua University, together with qigong specialists and medical doctors such as Xin Yan (Lu 1997), there was a modern upsurge of interest and research in TCQ (Yan, 1999 & 2001).

The needs and preferences of health have changed and people now seek new ways to improve both the quantity and quality of life. TCQ is felt by its promoters to offer a powerful approach to improving health. In this chapter we systematically review a selection of 58 studies on the effects of qigong in biology, physics and chemistry. We will first describe some of the research reported in laboratory studies of qigong, the parameters that seem to influence the consistency of results and then evaluate the quality of the research using scientific criteria for causation and internal validity including criteria on experimental design, data analysis, outcomes, clinical importance, and independent replication.

BIOLOGICAL EFFECTS OF QIGONG

External qi experiments on humans cannot completely exclude psychological factors such as the placebo effect. To better control these factors, basic scientific studies were conducted on *in vivo* animal models, *in vitro* models, and non-living substances.

In Vivo Studies

External qi treatment

Due to the inconsistent effectiveness of qi emitted by each specialist, and among qigong specialists (see the section on Inconsistent Effectiveness of Qi, below), results generated from studies are varied and sometimes inconclusive. Both positive and negative results have been reported.

Positive results. The application of external qi emitted from qigong specialists has been reported to protect normal cells from harmful assaults, increase anti-tumor immunity, reduce tumor metastases, promote cell death of tumor cells, and increase survival time of tumor-embedded animals. In mice treated with qi, a reduced level of interleukin 2 and an increased activity of interferon-γ in Con A-treated spleen cells were observed (Cao et al 1988b, Guan & Yang 1989). In peritoneal macrophages, qi treatment increased their phagocytotic function, the activity of acid phosphatase, and the amount of IgM antibodies (Feng et al 1988b). Numbers of lymphocytes, leukocytes, and neutrophils were also elevated (Lin et al 1990). When C57BL/6 mice were inoculated with B16 melanoma tumor cells via the tail veins, treatment with qi markedly reduced the number of B16 melanoma pulmonary metastases nodules in the lungs and the survival time of these animals was longer than that of those without the treatment (Cao et al 1988a). Similar results were found with mice injected with M04 cells (Qian & Shen 1993, Qian et al 1993) or U27 cancer cells (Qian et al 1993). Mice injected with ascitic cancer fluid followed by treatment with qi displayed increases in hemoglobin level, numbers of red blood cells and white blood cells, and a smaller tumor compared to untreated control mice (Zhao et al 1988). Other studies showed that reduced tumor formation in NC-Z strain mice inoculated with nasopharyngeal squamous carcinoma CNE-2 cells (Chen et al 1993) or human hepatocarcinoma BEL-7420 cells (Chen 1993) and weight reduction of sarcoma 180 tissue (Liu et al 1988a, Xu et al 1990). External qi has also been reported to have reduced the size of G422 cell neuroglioma implanted into mice (Li 1992). In external qi-treated human patients, natural killer cell activity increased while the CD4/CD8 ratio remained unchanged (Higuchi et al 1999). Guan & Yang (1990) reported that qi treatment increased interleukin activity and spleen cell numbers in mice, and this is in disagreement with findings reported by Cao et al (1988b).

In a rat diabetic model, qi treatment increased weight, reduced blood glucose levels, increased insulin activity (Feng et al 1995), and decreased MDA and lipid peroxides (Liu et al 1996). In a rabbit model with bone fracture, treatment with qi after the fracture prevented the pathological changes such as muscle fiber edema and breaking and disappearance of myofibrils as well as Z lines (Jia & Jia 1988). Histological examination indicated that qigong transformed fibroblasts into osteocytes, and induced both chondrocytes and fibroblasts to generate bone tissue (Jia et al 1988).

There are reports of qi treatment resulting in sedative and analgesic effects (Lin 1988), probably by increasing the pain threshold (Yang et al 1988b). This analgesic effect of qi was blocked partially by bilateral ventral lesions at periaqueductal gray (PAG) or by the injection of naloxone, an opiate receptor antagonist (Yang et al 1988a).

In rabbits, qi increased the volume of blood flow in important visceral organs under normal and hemorrhagic shock conditions by decreasing the tension of smooth muscles of blood vessels so as to cause the increase in blood volume of the organs (Zhang 1990).

In an immunosuppressive mouse model induced by cyclophosphamide, qi treatment resumed T cell proliferation and the activity of interleukin 2 (Zhang et al 1988).

Tobacco cell tissues (Li & Li 1995) responded to external qi by accelerating cell fission and differentiation.

Negative or inconclusive results. A few studies have reported "negative", "inconclusive", or "questionable" results. Li (1992) reported that 13 qigong specialists were invited to exert external qi on experimental mice implanted with G422 cells of neuroglioma. Only four out of thirteen qigong specialists were able to reduce the glioma size and increase the activities of Tu cells, NK cells and K cells in spleens. The other nine qigong specialists failed to achieve a result.

Another report was of experiments on cats studying the external qi effects on the auditory brainstem evoked responses (ABER) and auditory middle latency evoked responses (MLR) after application of external qi. For ABER, two cats showed facilitation and two displayed inhibition, whereas for MLR, six cats exhibited facilitation and another six elicited inhibition (Liu et al 1988b). The conflicting results were not explained, but may imply the presence of bidirectional effects.

A similar outcome was observed with mice injected with M04 cells (Qian & Shen 1993). Tumors induced by intraperitoneal injection of M04 cells were small in size in mice treated with external qi, but these mice did not survive longer compared with those not treated with external qi. In contrast, the size of tumors induced by subcutaneous injection of M04 cells in qi-treated mice was not different from that in controls. However, the qi-treated mice lived longer than the control mice. It was difficult to distinguish whether the discrepancy in results was due to the different routes of injections, stress generated by the handling, or inconsistent effectiveness of qi (see section on Inconsistent Effectiveness of Qi, below).

Another report (Lu et al 1990a) indicates that more than 10 experiments were conducted with the same qigong specialist, but only four of them worked to reduce the temperature of growing an obligate thermophile A sub 4-3 that normally has optimal growth between 50 and 60°C. Although the purpose of the experiment indicated in the report was to screen and pick the mutants that could grow at a lower temperature, such as 30°C, the fact that some of the successful four experiments succeeded showed that changes occurred in both qi-treated and untreated samples. This weakens the argument for drawing the conclusion that external qi causes the temperature shift.

Internal qi treatment

Internal qi is generated in the body by exercising qigong techniques. This internal qi has been reported to produce anti-tumor immunity, reduce free radicals, and increase blood flow. Wang & Xu (1991) reported that after practicing qigong for 1 year, cardiac output was increased, total peripheral resistance was decreased, and ejection fraction mitral valve diastolic closing velocity and mean velocity of circumferential fiber shortening tended to be increased. Other laboratories showed reduction of lipid peroxide in the serum (Wang et al 1989), a decreased ATP content in the blood (Wang et al 1988), reduced cerebral blood flow and respiration rate (Zhao 1988), and increased excretion of urinary catecholamines (Tang et al 1988). IgG, a-naphthyl-acetate esterase staining assar, leukocytes, and active E rosette formation increased as well (Xu & Qi 1989).

There are numerous reports of prolonged qigong practice improving function, well-being and reducing disease severity and incidence. It is not the purpose of this chapter to review this research, which is vast. Chapter 10 reports a systematic evaluation of all controlled research on the effects of internal qigong practice on hypertension.

In Vitro Studies

Studies at cellular level

Similar reports are in the literature on the study of cultured cells after external qi treatment. Hale cells and SGC-7901 human gastro-adenocarcinoma cells treated with external qi exhibited poor growth rate (Feng et al 1988a). The optimal growth temperature for growing thermophile A sub 4–3 bacteria was inconsistent altered after qi (Lu et al 1990a). Serum cAMP, hemoglobin, white blood cells, and platelets were increased after the blood was exposed to external qi (Luo et al 1988). Qi promoted the growth of normal human lymphocytes, but inhibited the growth of human erythroleukemia K sub 562 cells (Yang & Guan 1990). Chen et al (1990) reported that emitted qi could inhibit the cell growth and DNA synthesis of CNE-2 cells. The colony formation of *Escherichia coli* and *Shigella* was also altered by qi (Tables 9.1 and 9.2, Lu 1997). Recently, our laboratory has shown that external qi significantly increased cytosolic free calcium, which is indicative about the biological effects produced by application of external qi (Kiang et al 2002).

Studies at molecular level

There are reports that external qi enables change in the intrinsic property of molecules. For example, exposure of yeast RNA (Sun et al 1988a, Yan et al 1988c), fish sperm DNA (Sun et al 1988b), and calf thymus deoxyribonucleic acid displayed significant increases in relative absorption intensity at 256 nm after treatment with external qi. Other chemicals or molecules exposed to external qi were samples of lithium fluoride crystal luminescence (Wang et al 1988), tap water, saline, glucose, medemycine solution (Yan et al 1988a, Yan et al 1999), dipalmitoyl phosphatidyl choline liposome (Yan et al 1988b), synthesis gas system (Yan et al 1988d), n-hexane and bromine (Yan et al 1988e). Thyme quinguecostatus oil, lemon oil, jasmine tea vapor, and michelia alba vapor (Lu 1997) demonstrated changes in the profile of

Table 9.1 Effect of external qi with different intentions on the number of colonies of *E. coli* formed (Lu 1997)

Sample no.	Numbers of colonies		% change
	Without qi	With qi	
With 'kill' intention			
1	611	312	59.0
2	295	164	56.0
3	403	41	10.2
4	403	50	12.4
With 'growth' intention			
1	295	>700	237
2	66	456	690

Table 9.2 Effect of external qi with different intentions on the number of colonies of *Shigella* formed (Lu 1997)

Sample no.	Numbers of colonies		% change
	Without qi	With qi	
With 'kill' intentions			
1	182	2	1.1
2	182	8	4.4
3	63	21	33.3
4	6	1	16.7
With 'growth' intentions			
1	63	196	310
2	6	42	700
3	71	103	131
4	16	21	131

their gas chromatograms. Furthermore, the half-life of americium isotope 241 (^{241}Am) was altered by qi (Yan et al 1988f, Lu 1990, Lu et al 1993).

Figure 9.1 gives an example with a profile of DNA absorbance before and after qi application. Treatment with external qi increased the peak absorbance of DNA at 256 nm from 0.428 to 0.579. Figure 9.2 shows changes in the property of jasmine tea vapor by qi treatment that significantly reduced the peaks B and C.

ANALYSIS ON SPECIFIC CHARACTERISTICS OF QIGONG

Inconsistent Effectiveness of Qi

It is possible that the effectiveness of the external qi from a qigong specialist becomes inconsistent due to changes in time, location, environment, and psychological and pathological factors during the generation of qi. Certain experiments involving external qi treatment have been made either directly or indirectly through qi emission by qigong specialists. Qi emission consumes qigong specialists' vital energy (Wang et al 1988) and its quality is subject to their physical and mental condition.

Figure 9.3 shows different output voltage profiles of a qigong practitioner and a non-qigong practitioner. Figures 9.4 and 9.5 depict the infrared temporal radiation spectrum of a specialist in good health (tracing A) and in poor health (tracing B). Furthermore, the magnetic signals given by different specialists are very different (Fig. 9.4A vs. Fig. 9.6). As a result, qi emitted at different times by the same specialist may not have the same quality and, therefore, may not reproduce the same result. For example, external qi is capable of increasing resting cytosolic free calcium concentration ($[Ca^{2+}]_i$) in human Jurkat T cells. Since the experiment was conducted on two different days, the specialist, in this case a bioenergy expert, was under two different physical conditions. The tracings collected from two different days were different (Fig. 9.7), although increases in $[Ca^{2+}]_i$ were clearly evident. Furthermore, the responses varied even on tracings collected on the same day. Figure 9.8 shows that tracing A was done when the bioenergy expert was fresh and rested. The $[Ca^{2+}]_i$ increased from 61 nM to 79 nM after 15 minutes of qi treatment. Tracing B shows a tiny $[Ca^{2+}]_i$ response to external qi or indirectly through the qi emission by qigong specialists. Qi emission consumes qigong specialists' vital energy (Wang et al 1988), and its quality is subject to their physical and mental condition.

Likewise, the qi emitted by different qigong specialists never falls into the same pattern. Therefore, specialists cannot be asked to behave like a mechanical device emitting the same quantity and quality of qi many times within a given period of time. Thus, only similar but not identical results are expected from either repeated qi emissions from the same specialist or simulated emissions among different specialists.

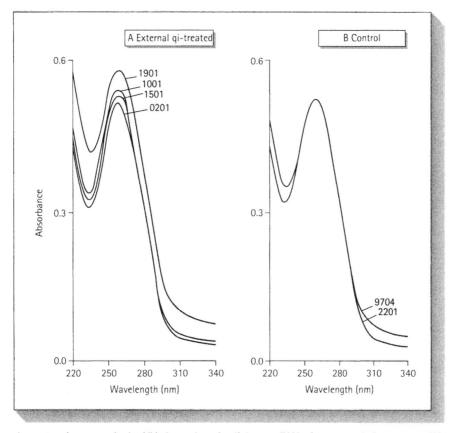

Figure 9.1   Increases in the UV absorption of calf thymus DNA after external qi treatment. (A) Qi was applied to calf thymus DNA for 10 minutes. Line 0201 was the background reading of the sample before qi treatment. Lines 0501 and 1001 were readings at 5 minutes and 55 minutes, respectively. Line 1901 was from a sample that received three qi applications (10 minutes each, 1 h interval) read 9 h after the third treatment. (B) Line 9704 was a reading from a sample sham-treated as line 0201. Line 2201 was the reading from a sample sham-treated as line 1901. Both samples received no qi treatment. (Modified from data in Lu 1997.)

Traditional physiology and pharmacology teach us that in order to study the effects of chemical or physical stimuli, a dose–response relationship and time course should be established to determine their median effective dose or concentration before further investigation. It is not apparent how, without qualitative and quantitative measuring methodology and equipment from modern medicine and science, to establish such relations for qi as indicated above.

Traditional approaches also indicate that in order to determine the specificity of the effect of the stimuli, various antagonists are used. If qi exhibits properties such as bi-directionality, no antagonist is apparent suggesting the need for a different methodology.

Distant Effects of External Qi

External qi emission is said to produce local effects and in that sense is similar to electromagnetic and gravitational interactions. However, unlike research conducted in the conventional fields of life sciences, external qi is reported to induce remote effects on tested subjects at a distance. This distance ranges from several to thousands of kilometers. An example experiment was conducted remotely on [241]Am (Lu 1990, Lu 1997).

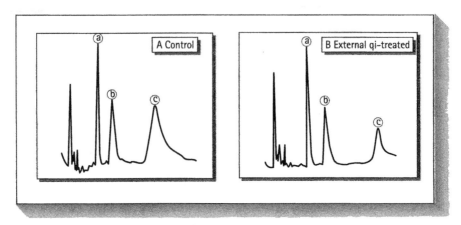

Figure 9.2 Changes in relative abundance of peaks of jasmine tea vapor after external qi treatment. (A) A representative gas chromatogram from a sample before external qi treatment. (B) A representative gas chromatogram from a sample after external qi treatment. Peaks b and c were reduced. (Modified from data in Lu 1997.)

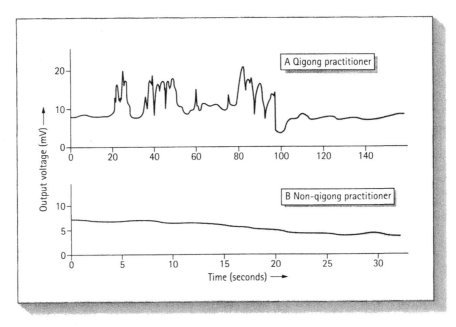

Figure 9.3 Different magnetic signals detected from a qigong practitioner and a non-qigong practitioner. Voltage output of magnetic signals was taken 2 cm from the Laogong acupuncture point in the right hand of a qigong practitioner (A) and a non-qigong practitioner (B). (Modified from data in Lu 1997.)

Ultra long-distance effects are characteristic of the experiments done with Yan (Lu 1997, Kiang 2000). Among other unknowns, it is often asked how a qigong specialist is able to work with experimental samples from such distances as in experiments with yeast RNA (Sun et al 1999, Lu et al 1993). Experimentations with [241]Am were also conducted from the United States to Beijing over 10 000 km apart (Lu 1997). Qi emission is sometimes thought to be like thrusting out one's arm: the force will be stronger if the arm is first drawn back and then thrust forward; as a result,

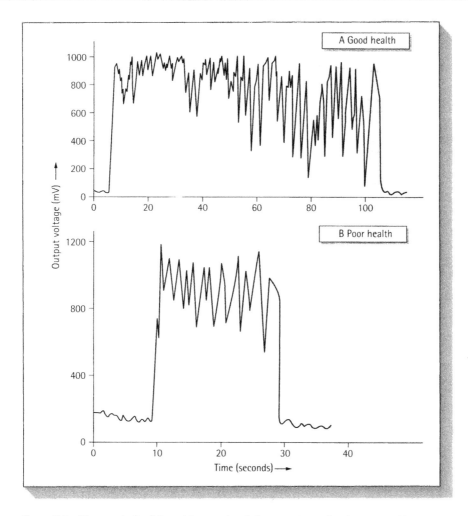

Figure 9.4 Changes in the infrared temporal radiation spectrum of a qigong practitioner under different health conditions. The external qi was measured with a model HD-I infrared low temperature thermometer, a remote sensing apparatus for distant objects with a focal length of 1 meter and detector window of 7–20 microns. Output voltage was detected from a qigong practitioner in good health (A) and in poor health (B). (Modified from data in Lu 1997.)

the longer the distance, the stronger the effect of external qi (Lu, 1997). However, this action-at-a-distance does not seem to fit with the concept of qi as an energy and so various theories of qi as having informational characteristics have arisen. This is the most controversial claim of qigong and is often dismissed by scientists as impossible.

Bi-directional Effects of External Qi

It is thought that practicing qigong can lower the blood pressure of a person with hyperten-sion. On the other hand, it also can raise the blood pressure to a normal level for a person with hypotension (see review by Mayer 1999). This bi-directional effect on adjusting blood pressure is very distinct from the modern drug therapeutic remedy in which the treatment can either raise or lower the blood pressure, working in only one direction. The bi-direction-al phenomenon is explained in TCM theories as a result of adjusting the body from a state of non-equilibrium to one of equilibrium of Yin-Yang.

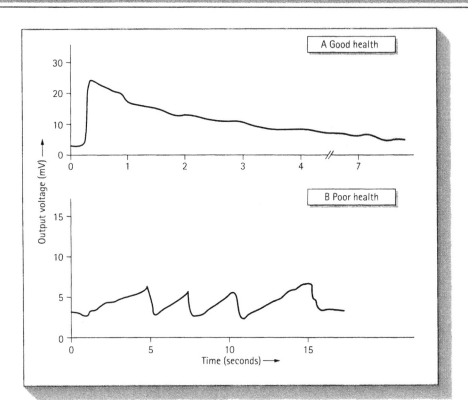

Figure 9.5 Changes in the magnetic signal of a qigong practitioner under different health conditions. Voltage output of magnetic signals was taken 6 cm from the Baihui acupuncture point at the top of the head of a qigong practitioner in good health (A) and in poor health (B). (Modified from data in Lu 1997.)

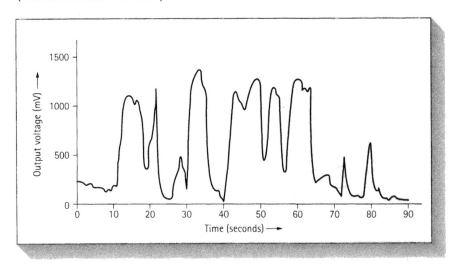

Figure 9.6 Infrared temporal radiation spectrum of a qigong practitioner. The external qi was measured with a model HD-I infrared low temperature thermometer, a remote sensing apparatus for distant objects with a focal length of 1 meter and detector window of 7–20 microns. Output voltage was detected from a qigong practitioner in good health. (Modified from data in Lu 1997.)

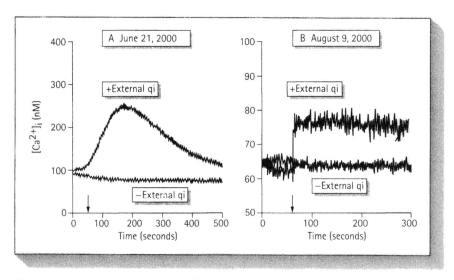

Figure 9.7 Increases in cytosolic free Ca^{2+} concentrations in human Jurkat T cells by external qi treatment. Jurkat T cells were treated with external qi for 15 minutes by a bioenergy expert. Then, cytosolic free Ca^{2+} concentrations ($[Ca^{2+}]_i$ were measured using fluorescent probe Indo-1. The initial portion of the tracing is the resting $[Ca^{2+}]_i$. The arrow indicates the qi treatment. (A) A representative tracing obtained on June 21, 2000. (B) A representative tracing obtained on August 9, 2000.

But do such effects occur in the laboratory? Feng & Bao (Lu 1997) were the first to report that qi emitted for 1 minute to test tubes containing cultures of *Escherichia coli* or *Shigella* was able to either reduce or in another experiment to increase the numbers of colonies by wishing for kill or growth, respectively. Tables 9.1 and 9.2 show in the "kill" experiment, qi decreases *E. coli* by 44–89.8% and *Shigella* by 66.7–98.9%. While in a "growth" experiment, *E. coli* is increased 237–690% and *Shigella* 131–700%. Similar results were obtained from experiments in other systems including with a mixture of bromocarbon tetrachloride and n-hexane (Lu 1997), the electrogastric activity in humans (Feng et al 1988c, Feng et al 1989), adherence of tumor cells to red blood cells in mice and humans (Lu et al 1990b), and emanation of tobacco cell tissues (Li & Li 1995). Apparent bi-directionality was observed in a nucleic acid experiment (Yan et al 1988c), the bromine and n-hexane reaction (Lu 1997), and the radioactive decay rate of ^{241}Am (Yan et al 1988f). Thus, the intent of the practitioner is reported to have an effect on the direction of the results. How both bi-directionality and directional intention interact has got to be adequately studied.

CRITERIA-BASED ANALYSIS OF QIGONG STUDIES ON BASIC SCIENCE

Since the biological effects of external qi are new to most Western scientific communities, conventional scientific approaches are needed before they gain acceptance. We analyzed 56 laboratory studies for their incorporation of several quality areas including experimental design, data analysis, outcomes, clinical importance, and independent replicability.

Experimental Design

Randomization

Many *in vivo* studies with external qi have used mice or rabbits, and the question of whether animals were randomly assigned to control or treated groups is not indicated. Of the 34 reports with *in vivo* models listed in the references, only eight (Feng et al 1995, Kuang et al 1991, Qian & Shen 1993, Qian et al 1993, Qian 1994, Wang et al 1993, 1995, Xu & Qi 1989, Zhang 1990, Zhang et al

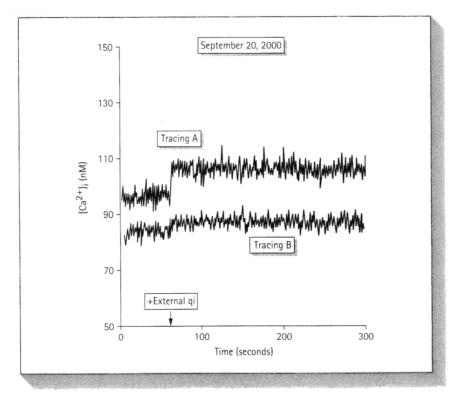

Figure 9.8 Variation of increases in cytosolic free Ca2 + concentrations in human *Jurkat T cells* by external qi treatment. *Jurkat T cells* were treated with external qi for 15 minutes by a bioenergy expert. Then, cytosolic free Ca2+ concentrations ([Ca2+li) were measured using fluorescent probe Indo-1. The initial portion of the tracing is the resting [Ca2+li. The arrow indicates the qi treatment. Tracing A was obtained when the expert was in good spirit; tracing B was obtained when the same expert felt tired and bored. Both tracings were collected on September 20, 2000.

1988, Zhao et al 1988) clearly indicated that there was randomization of tested animals before the study was conducted.

Baseline comparability

Control groups or sham-operated groups were usually used in these articles. However, the gender in animal studies was mentioned in only a few reports (Chen 1993, Feng et al 1995, Jia & Jia 1988, Jia et al 1988, Lin et al 1990, Qian & Shen 1993). In *in vitro* studies, cultured cells or non-living tested subjects were used for qi treatment and a matched baseline comparability was present.

Duration of effects

This area is rarely studied. Qigong specialists report that the qi effect can be long-lasting (up to 120 days in human patients). Some reports on the effect of external qi on a gas chromatogram of michelia alba vapor also suggest that the effect of external qi is long-lasting. Lu (1997) indicated that the profile of a gas chromatogram of michelia alba vapor treated with external qi remained different from the untreated one for up to 163 days after qi treatment. Lu also reported similar results with qi-treated calf thymus DNA solution absorbing UV. Untreated control samples did not show any alteration with time.

Blinding

Studies conducted blindly can better control for a number of potential biases. Therefore, double-blindness or single-blindness is desirable in both *in vivo* and *in vitro* studies. Only two reports explicitly indicated they were conducted blindly in *in vivo* models (Yang et al 1988a, Yang et al 1990). Others do not mention blinding though some distant healing qigong studies are said by their authors to have been conducted blind (Lu 1997, personal communication).

Data Analysis

Sample size

One major criticism of qigong experiments is that the number of samples used in the experiments was too small to draw significant conclusions. The ability to achieve a satisfactory sample size may rely on the subjects' qigong ability and willingness of the qigong specialist.

Difficulty with the consistency of qi suggests that we need to look for ways to improve the quality and quantity of the emitted qi. New protocols should be tailored for the particular characteristics of qigong studies so that proper subject screening and practitioner training and entry criteria can be established.

Some of the variability can be reduced if a mechanical device could be devised to emit the same type of qi as humans. Indeed, Yamauchi et al (1996) attempted to develop an *in vitro* experimental system, the effect of stimulant emission (ESE), to replace external qi application. Their results with cultured human cells exposed to G418 or X-ray irradiation showed no cytoprotection by ESE against cytotoxicity produced by G418 or X-ray irradiation. Thus, no successful attempt in developing a mechanical device to emit qi has yet been documented.

Statistical analysis

Statistical analysis is necessary in order to detect significant changes caused by experimental treatments. Many *in vivo* and *in vitro* studies of qigong reports have conducted statistical analyses and stated P values. In the studies at a molecular level, the change caused by external qi treatment was clearly evident even without any statistical analysis. In all of these studies, however, the type of statistics used to carry out the analysis was not stated.

Generalizability and independent reproducibility

Before acceptance in conventional scientific practice, qigong research results should be subject to repeated experiments in different laboratories. In this way, the generalizability and independent reproducibility of external qi effects can be examined. Some findings of similar *in vivo* and *in vitro* models by different qigong specialists in different laboratories have been reported. For example, the study of tumor weight after sarcoma 180 tissue implanted into mice was reported to be reduced by qi treatment conducted in two different laboratories (Liu et al 1988a, Xu et al 1990).

We found no experimental sets of high quality that were independently reproduced. The results from experiments with ^{241}Am done in several labs were said to have led to the modern upsurge of interest in qigong in China (Lu 1997). Studies with negative controls done by non-qigong practitioners are essential in such studies. Only four experiments included such negative controls (Lu et al 1990a, Qin et al 1989, Wang et al 1988, Yang et al 1990).

Clinical Significance and Therapeutic Potential

Most of the qigong studies cited here show limitations in the randomization of tested animals or samples, a lack of good controls and blindness in conducting experiments, and incomplete data analysis. Nevertheless, they do provide examples of how studies on qi can be conducted and point in the direction of future research of better quality.

Since currently qi-treatment can only be performed by human qigong specialists, the quality and strength of qi depend on the mind-body status of the specialist and the environmental setup, and also are equally influenced by the state of the qi recipient. Thus, verification of therapeutic qi-treatment is not easily obtained. It appears that qigong's clinical potential lies both in treatment and in self-healing practice for the enhancement of qi directly from within.

PERSPECTIVES

Straus (2000) and others suggest guidelines for a systematic review of evidence using the evidence hierarchy which are in sequence: anecdotes, case studies, observational studies, uncontrolled trials, small randomized clinical trials, and large randomized clinical trials and meta-analyses. Qigong has been embedded in traditional Chinese culture from its infancy and has been associated with an increase in clinical study for a decade. However, modern studies of qigong were not conducted until the 1980s. Currently, the study of qigong has not proceeded beyond the stage of small randomized clinical trials in the West.

It may take many years of training and a determined mind to become a good ballerina, a great musician, or an outstanding athlete. Likewise, it takes a long technical training, cultivation of culture, science, virtue and merit, plus body alignment to reach the level of a qigong master. If the optimal result produced by a qi specialist is mediated by organic pathways as well as through mind and virtuous alignment, then the mind-virtuous merit-body axis needs to be explored. Biological exploration of qi may unfold the organic pathways of qi action. Efforts from areas other than life sciences should be recruited for a comprehensive investigation and appreciation of the healing potential of qigong.

The current data in qi research provide a beginning towards establishment of research standards for the study of qigong. A creative yet conventional experimental design will be needed to set-up standard qi protocols. Ultimately, innovations in the development of qi measurement and quantification, bionic qi-devices, or qi-empowered medicines might be developed.

CONCLUSION

Qigong has been reported in numerous *in vivo* and *in vitro* studies to increase anti-tumor immu-nity, reduce tumor metastases, promote tumor cell death, increase survival time of tumor-bearing subjects, produce analgesic effects, and increase blood flow to vital organs. Research is needed to correlate the basic science of qigong with clinical observation of qigong treatment but better quality research should be the initial goal.

We believe that qigong research is one of the most exciting subjects in science today. We hope that Western researchers will work together with those in Asian countries since much benefit may be achieved from further collaboration done with established standards. At first, a multi-directional in-depth study is needed on the originally reported qigong effects. Once quality research standards are developed, exploring qigong mechanisms and inventing qi-interactive devices will further qigong research in the direction of improving public health.

ACKNOWLEDGEMENTS

We thank Dr Wayne B Jonas for his invitation to write the original review and Ms Cindy Crawford for assistance. Author JGK is also grateful to Mr Mietek Wirkus, Ms Margaret Wirkus and Dr Diane Marotta for the $[Ca^{2+}]_i$ experiments. As authors of this review article, we are greatly indebted to all the original authors, and especially to scholars Prof Zuyin Lu, Prof Shengping Li and Dr Y T Fong, who pioneered the breakthrough scientific collaboration with author XY. Thanks also go to the International Yan Xin Qigong Association and to the contributions to world qigong made by the originators, supporters, leaders and participants of the modern Chinese qigong upsurge. Finally, and most gratefully, authors PYL and JGK thank Dr Xin Yan for his long-time teaching about Traditional Chinese Qigong, as well as his general guidance in academic and technical matters. This work is supported in part by the Laurance S. Rockefeller Fund. This article was written in the authors' private capacity. No official support or endorsement by U.S. Department of the Army and Uniformed Services University of the Health Sciences should be inferred.

REFERENCES

Cao X, Ye T, Gao Y 1988a Antitumor metastases activity of emitted qi in tumor bearing mice. 1st World Conference of Academic Exchange of Medicine and Qigong, Beijing, China, p. 50

Cao X, Ye T, Gao Y 1988b Effect of emitted qi in enhancing the induction in vitro of lymphokines in relation to antitumor mechanisms. 1st World Conference of Academic Exchange of Medicine and Qigong, Beijing, China, p. 51

Chen Y 1993 Analysis of effect of emitted qi on human hepatocarcinoma cell (BEL-7402) by using flow cytometry. 2nd World Conference of Academic Exchange of Medicine and Qigong, Beijing, China, p. 102

Chen X, Gao Q, Jao X, Zhang J, Huang C, Fan X 1990 Effects of emitted qi on inhibition of human NPC cell line and DNA synthesis. 3rd National Academic Conference on Qigong Science, Guangzhou, China, p. 79

Chen X, Yi Q, Liu K, Zhang J, Chen Y 1993 Double-blind test of emitted qi on tumor formation of a nasopharyngeal carcinoma cell line in nude mice. 2nd World Conference of Academic Exchange of Medicine and Qigong, Beijing, China, p. 105

Clifford L 2000 Getting over the hump before you're over the hill. Fortune 142: 145–152

Feng L, Qian J, Chen S 1988a Effect of emitted qi on human carcinoma cells. 1st World Conference of Academic Exchange of Medicine and Qigong, Beijing, China, p. 1

Feng L, Wang Y, Chen S, Chen H 1988b Effect of emitted qi on the immune functions of mice. 1st World Conference of Academic Exchange of Medicine and Qigong, Beijing, China, p. 4

Feng Y, Qing C, Yu Y, Xie S, Gann S 1988c Bidirectional influence on the electrogastric activity in man. 1st World Conference of Academic Exchange of Medicine and Qigong, Beijing, China, p. 105

Feng Y, Qin C, Yu Y, Wang R 1989 The intention control effect of qigong imagery on electrogastric activity in man. 2nd International Conference on Qigong, Xian, China, p. 90

Feng L, Peng L, Qian J, Cheng S 1995 Effect of qigong information energy on diabetes mellitus. 4th International Conference on Qigong, Vancouver, British Columbia, Canada, pp. 17–19

Guan H, Yang J 1989 Effect of external qi on IL-2 activity and multiplication action of spleen cells in mice. 2nd International Conference on Qigong, Man, China, p. 92

Guan H, Yang J 1990 Effect of qigong waiqi (emitted qi) on IL-2 activity and multiplication action of spleen cells in mice. 3rd National Academic Conference on Qigong Science, Guangzhou, China, p. 84

Higuchi Y, Kotani Y, Higuuchi H, Yu Y, Chang Y U 1999 Immune changes during qigong therapy. Journal of International Society of Life Informational Science 17: 297–300

Jia L, Jia J 1988 Effects of the emitted qi on healing of experimental fracture. 1st World Conference of Academic Exchange of Medicine and Qigong, Beijing, China, p. 13

Jia L, Jia J, Lu D 1988 Effects of emitted qi on ultrastructural changes of the overstrained muscle of rabbits. 1st World

Conference of Academic Exchange of Medicine and Qigong, Beijing, China, p. 14

Kiang J G 2000 Introduction to alternative medicine. NEWSDOM 2441: 39–42

Kiang J G, Marotta D, Wirkus M, Wirkus M, Jonas W B 2002 External bioenergy increases intracellular free calcium concentration and reduces cellular response to heat stress. Journal of Investigative Medicine, 50: 38–45

Kuang A, Wang C, Xu D, Qian Y 1991 Research on anti-aging effects of qigong. Journal of Traditional Chinese Medicine 11:153–158, 224–227

Li C 1992 Effect of qigong-waiqi on immune function of mice. Chinese Journal of Somatic Science 2: 67–72

Li C, Li J 1995 Preliminary study on the research of the effect of qigong emanation on plant cell tissue concrescence. 4th International Conference on Qigong, Vancouver, British Columbia, Canada, pp. 1–2

Li S, Su M, Meng G, Cui Y, Xin Y 1988 Effect of emitted qi on bovine serum albumen by the ultraviolet and fluorescence spectrophotometer. 1st World Conference of Academic Exchange of Medicine and Qigong, Beijing, China, p. 176

Lin H 1988 Clinical and laboratory study of the effect of qigong anaesthesia on thyroidectomy. 1st World Conference of Academic Exchange Medicine and Qigong, Beijing, China, p. 84

Lin M, Zhang J, Hu D, Ye Z 1990 Effect of qigong waiqi (emitted qi) on blood chemistry of mice radiated with X-rays. 3rd National Academic Conference on Qigong Science, Guangzhou, China, p. 58

Liu T, Wan M, Lu O 1988a Experiment of the emitted qi on animals. 1st World Conference of Academic Exchange of Medicine and Qigong, Beijing, China, p. 60

Liu G, Wan P, Peng X, Zhong X 1988b Influence of emitted qi on the auditory brainstem evoked responses (ABER) and auditory middle latency evoked responses (MLR) in cats. 1st World Conference of Academic Exchange of Medicine and Qigong, Beijing, China, p. 31

Liu C, Sun C, Dong X 1996 Study of the mechanism of the effect of qigong for diabetes. 3rd World Conference of Academic Exchange of Medicine and Qigong, Beijing, China, p. 107

Lu Z 1990 Effect of qi on the half-life of radioactive isotope Am-241. 1st International Congress of Qigong, University of California at Berkeley, California, USA, p. 108

Lu, Z 1997 Scientific qigong exploration: the wonders and mysteries of qi. Amber Leaf Press, Malvern, Pennsylvania

Lu G, Ye Y, Ye S, We H, Li X, Qin W, Deng B 1990a Preliminary study of the variation of growth temperature of bacteria by qigong external qi treatment. 3rd National Academic Conference on Qigong Science, Guangzhou, China, p. 61

Lu H, Wang L, Zhen J, Chang J, Xie C, Xiao L, Luo J, Lin Z 1990b Qigong's effect on the adhesive capacity of erythrocytes to tumor cells. 3rd National Academic Conference on Qigong Science, Guangzhou, China, p. 89

Lu Z, Zhu R, Ren G 1993 External qi experiments from the United States to Beijing (China) by Yan Xin. China Qigong 1: 4–6

Luo S, Chai S, Yi W, Ren H, Cao B 1988 Molecular biological effects of emitted qi on man. 1st World Conference of Academic Exchange of Medicine and Qigong, Beijing, China, p. 42

Mayer M 1999 Qigong and hypertension: a critique of research. Journal of Alternative and Complementary Medicine 4: 371–382

Qian Z 1994 Experimental research of influence of qigong waiqi on the cancer growth metastasis and survival time of host. Chinese Journal of Somatic Science 4: 117–118

Qian S, Shen H 1993 Curative effect of emitted qi on mice with M04 tumors. 2nd World Conference of Academic Exchange of Medicine and Qigong, Beijing, China, p. 107

Qian S, Sun W, Liu Q, Wan Y, Shi X 1993 Influence of emitted qi on cancer growth, metastasis and survival time of the host. 2nd World Conference of Academic Exchange of Medicine and Qigong, Beijing, China, p. 106

Qin C, Feng Y, Yu Y, Wang R, Shu K 1989 A primary study of the influence of qigong waiqi on electrogastric activity in man. 2nd International Conference on Qigong, Xian, China, p. 92

Straus S 2000 Complementary and alternative medicine: challenges and opportunities for pharmacology and therapeutic research. Pharmacologist 42: 74–76

Sun M, Li S, Meng G, Cui Y, Xin Y 1988a Effect of emitted qi on ultraviolet spectrum of a yeast RNA solution. 1st World Conference of Academic Exchange of Medicine and Qigong, Beijing, China, p. 178

Sun M, Li S, Meng G, Cui Y, Xin Y 1988b Effect of emitted qi on trace examination of UV spectroscopy on the DNA solution of fish sperm. 1st World Conference of Academic Exchange of Medicine and Qigong, Beijing, China, p. 172

Tang C, Sun L, Aheng L, Xiang X 1988 Preliminary study of the biological effects of qigong. 1st World Conference of Academic Exchange of Medicine and Qigong, Beijing, China, p. 20

Wang Z, Huang J, Wu Z 1988 Preliminary study of the relationship between qigong and energy metabolism; the changes in blood ATP content. 1st World Conference of Academic Exchange of Medicine and Qigong, Beijing, China, p. 58

Wang Y, Zhang G, Zhang Y, Wang X 1989 Effects of qigong on lipid peroxides (LPO) of human serum. 2nd International Conference on Qigong, Xian, China, P. 78

Wang C X, Xu D H 1991 The beneficial effect of qigong on the ventricular function and microcirculation in deficiency of heart-energy hypertensive patients. Chung Hsi I Chieh Ho Tsa Chih 11: 659–660

Wang C, Xu D, Qian Y, Shi W 1993 Effects of qigong on preventing stroke and alleviating the multiple cerebrocardiovascular risk factors: a follow-up report on 242 hypertensive cases over 30 years. 2nd World Conference of Academic Exchange of Medicine and Qigong, Beijing, China, p. 123–124

Wang C, Xu D, Qian Y, Shi W, Bao Y, Kuang A 1995 The beneficial effects of qigong on the ventricular function and microcirculation of deficiency inherit energy hypertensive patients. Chinese Journal of Internal Medicine 1: 21–23

Xu H, Qi Y 1989 Preliminary study on qigong and immunity. 2nd international Conference on Qigong, Xian, China, p. 99

Xu H, Xue H, Zhang C, Shao X, Liu G, Zhou Q, Yu F, Wu K 1990 Study of the effects and mechanism of qigong waiqi (emitted qi) on implanted tumors in mice. 3rd National Academic Conference on Qigong Science, Guangzhou, China, p. 82

Yamauchi M, Saito T, Yamamoto M, Hirasawa M 1996 Attempts to develop an in vitro experimental system for detecting the effect of stimulant emission using cultured human cells. Journal of International Society of Life Informational Science 14: 266–271

Yan X 2000 The practice and principles of qigong. In: Ai R, Jing W (eds) The philosophy and practice of Yan Xin qigong. Ru-Lin, Taipei, Taiwan

Yan X, Li S, Yu J, Li B, Lu Z 1988a Laser Raman observation on tap water, saline, glucose and medemycine solutions under the influence of external qi. Nature Journal 11:567–571

Yan X, Zhao N, Yin C, Lu Z 1988b The effect of external qi on liposome phase behavior. Nature Journal 11: 572–573

Yan X, Zheng C, Zhou G, Lu Z 1988c Observations of the effect of external qi on the ultraviolet absorption of nucleic acids. Nature Journal 11: 647–649

Yan X, Li S, Liu C, Hu J, Mao S, Lu Z 1988d The observation of the effect of external qi on synthesis gas system. Nature Journal 11: 650–652

Yan X, Li S, Yang Z, Lu Z 1988e Observations on the bromination reaction in solution of n-hexane and bromine under the influence of external qi. Nature Journal 11: 653–655

Yan X, Lu Z, Zhang T, Wang H, Zhu R 1988f The influence of external qi on the radioactive decay rate of 241 Am. Nature Journal 11: 809–812

Yan X, Lin H, Li H, Traynor-Kaplan A, Xia Z Q, Lu F, Fang Y, Dao M 1999 Structure and property changes in certain materials influenced by the external qi of qigong. Material Research and Innovation 2: 349–359

Yan X, Fong Y T, Wolf G, Wolf D, Cao W 2001 Protective effect of XY99-5038 on hydrogen peroxide induced cell death in cultured retinal neurons. Life Science 69: 289–299

Yang J, Guan H 1990 Effect of emitted qi on human lymphocytes and tumor cells in vitro. 3rd National Academic Conference on Qigong Science, Guangzhou, China, p. 81

Yang K, Guo Z, Xu H, Lin H 1988a Influence of electrical lesion of the periaqueductal gray (PAG) on the analgesic effect of emitted qi in rats. 1st World Conference of Academic Exchange of Medicine and Qigong, Beijing, China, p. 43

Yang K, Xu H, Guo Z, Zhao B, Li Z 1988b Analgesic effect of emitted qi on white rats. 1st World Conference of Academic Exchange of Medicine and Qigong, Beijing, China, p. 45

Yang S, Shi J, Yang Q, Zheng Z 1990 Experimental research on the braking phenomenon of the upper limbs evoked by qigong waiqi (emitted qi). 3rd National Academic Conference on Qigong Science, Guangzhou, China, p. 44

Zhang J 1990 Influence of qigong waiqi (emitted qi) on volume of blood flow to visceral organs in rabbits under normal and hemorrhagic shock conditions. 3rd National Academic Conference on Qigong Science, Guangzhou, China, p. 47

Zhang L, Yan X, Wang S, Tao J, Gu L, Xu Y, Zhou Y, Liu D 1988 Immune regulation effect of emitted qi on immunosuppressed animal model. 1st World Conference of Academic Exchange of Medicine and Qigong, Beijing, China, p. 27

Zhao B 1988 Effects of qigong on cerebral blood flow and extremitic blood flow. 1st World Conference of Academic Exchange of Medicine and Qigong, Beijing, China, p. 83

Zhao S, Mao X, Zhao B, Li Z, Zhou D 1988 Preliminary observation of the inhibitory effect of emitted qi on transplanted tumors in mice. 1st World Conference of Academic Exchange of Medicine and Qigong, Beijing, China, p. 46

Qigong clinical studies

Michael Mayer

Drs Yan, Kiang and Lu summarized the laboratory research on qigong in Chapter 9. In this chapter Dr Mayer summarizes the clinical research on qigong with a focus on the studies of hypertension.

There are two primary forms of qigong – internal and external. Internal qigong involves using the mind, breath and physical exercises to circulate qi within the body. It is similar in execution to meditative and exercise techniques known to be healthful in the West. External qigong involves projection of qi outside the body to influence another. While the laboratory studies evaluated in the last chapter involve external qi, clinical qigong often involves cultivation of internal qi through daily practice. Internal qigong is not conceptually difficult, but external qigong is conceptually very difficult for most conventional scientists.

The clinical research conducted on therapeutic effects of qigong is extensive. The vast majority of this research is done in China and reported in Chinese journals not accessible to the West. Michael Mayer selected a sample of qigong research on hypertension in order to assess the quantity and quality of research on this condition. While over 70 studies on the effects of qigong on hypertension were found, only 33 could be evaluated for quality. Of these, none was considered of adequate quality to say definitively that qigong improves hypertension. While it is likely that the combination of meditation and exercise involved in qigong can be beneficial for those with high blood pressure, this effect has not yet been adequately demonstrated. **WBJ**

INTRODUCTION

We are in the midst of a revolution in health care where age-old healing methods from other cultures are now being integrated into the Western health care system (Eisenberg et al 1998, Ornish 1990, Zinn 1990). Among the treatment methods being researched is qigong, a practice that has existed for several thousand years and that invokes awareness, intention, breath, posture, movement, touch, and sound to cultivate *qi*, understood as the vital energy of life.

This chapter first briefly reviews selected research on hypertension and the practice of qigong to evaluate its potential efficacy as a treatment for hypertension. Second, methodological issues are discussed to guide future researchers in the field.

Hypertension affects 20% or more of the adult population in Western societies and is a significant risk factor for stroke, myocardial infarction, and congestive heart failure. Together, these account for more than 50% of deaths in the United States (Wollam et al 1988). It is estimated that about 50 million Americans have elevated blood pressure (BP) which is defined as systolic BP of 140 mmHg or greater, or diastolic BP of 90 mmHg or greater (Joint National Committee on Detection, Evaluation and Treatment of High BP (JNC-V) 1993).

The disadvantages of conventional treatments that use medication include high costs and negative side-effects in mood state, cognitive functioning, and sexual performance (Polare et al 1989, Medical Research Council Working Party 1985, Kostis et al 1990). Therefore, a growing body of research in the West has focused upon lifestyle modification as an alternative to hypotensive drugs. According to the Joint National Committee report (JNC-V 1993), lifestyle modification can provide multiple benefits at little cost and minimal risk and may be used as a first step therapy for hypertension or as a means of reducing the number and doses of hypotensive medications required (Little et al 1991).

REVIEW OF LITERATURE ON QIGONG AND HYPERTENSION

To survey the field, the Qigong Institute of San Francisco's computer database was searched (Sancier 1997). Seventy-three studies on hypertension were reviewed. These came mostly from conference proceedings. It should be emphasized that even though this is one of the best sources of data available in the West, making judgements about the efficacy of qigong from this source may create a bias against qigong. Since these conference reports are often in the form of abstracts, the limited information may be incomplete, so that one cannot determine whether the original studies addressed significant research methodology issues.

Other reviewed sources include various journal articles (Shih et al 1998, Kuang et al 1991, Wang et al 1995, Sukuki et al 1993), books (Cai 1986, Chia 1990, Chuen 1991, McGee & Chow 1994, Cohen 1997, Johnson 2000, Sha 2000), write-ups from qigong institutes (Xu & Wang 1993), journals (Kuang et al 1991, Wang et al 1995) and reports from peer-reviewed scientific journals (Sancier 1996a, 1996b; Yasutami 1999). Of the 73 studies, 33 representative studies were selected for review. The selection process was based upon first choosing the best designed studies, i.e. studies which were randomly assigned, or appeared in journals preferably which were peer reviewed. Since the purpose of our review was to illustrate and discuss methodological problems in the literature in the field, other representative studies were chosen to meet this heuristic goal. Presenting the studies in a table was considered, along the lines of a meta-analytic design, but rejected on the grounds that it would tend to concretize and reify potentially unreliable data.

In total, approximately 3409 subjects were represented by our original research of 33 studies (Mayer 1999). In this follow-up report, Wen (1998) adds a reported 2114 subjects, Yasutami et al (1999) add four, and Zdravkovic and colleagues (1998) 18 subjects. Thus, a grand total of approximately 5545 subjects are represented.

Blood Pressure

Almost all of the studies suggest that qigong lowers BP to various degrees over various time periods (Bornoroni et al 1993; Huang 1990; Jing 1988; Kuang et al 1989, 1991; Li et al 1988; Pan & Zhang 1990; Qu 1990; Shih et al 1998; Tainjin Research Institute 1988; Wang et al 1994, 1995; Wu & Liu 1993; Xu & Wang 1994; Young et al 1998; Yuan et al 1996). The most in-depth of these studies is the Kuang study (Kuang et al 1991, updated by Wang et al 1994), which took place over 20 years. The basic design involved 204 patients with hypertension, randomly assigned to qigong practice and control groups. Age of subjects was not mentioned. Both groups were given antihypertensive drugs. The qigong group of 104 patients reportedly practiced 30 minutes twice per day, over 20 years.

During the first 2 months, the BP of all patients dropped in response to the hypotensive drug. Subsequently, and consistently over the period of 20 years, the BP of the group practicing qigong stabilized while that of the control group increased ($P < 0.01$). Due to the stabilized BP, 48% of those in the qigong practice group reduced the hypotensive dosage, and for 30% in this group, the BP medication was eliminated. In contrast, 31% in the control group increased the hypotensive dosage (Kuang et al 1991).

Other studies report that patients suffering from various degrees of hypertension can withdraw from their medication, and that BP reduced over various time periods: after one session (Li et al 1988, Tianjin Research Institute 1988), 14 days (Wu & Liu 1993), 2 months (Jing 1988, Tainjin Research Institute 1988, Shih et al 1998, Yuan et al 1996), and 1 year (Huang 1990). In a group of 18 borderline hypertensive males with a group mean value of 142/92 mmHg who practiced Chow qigong bi-weekly there was no significant change of blood pressure over the course of each session or after 2 months of training. However, after 2 months of training there was a slight reduction (139/90) of BP in 70% of the subjects. This slight reduction was noted in 78% of the 18 subjects (Zdravkovic et al 1998). Jing (1988) reports that for patients with a long history of hypertension and no satisfactory results with medication, BP stabilized within 2 months and was maintained in a follow-up study 3 years after starting to practice qigong.

Other Blood Measures

In studies that were not specifically described as randomly assigned control group studies, significant differences were reported between qigong and control groups on eight blood flow measures (Chu et al 1988), in 10 indices of microcirculation ($P < 0.05–0.01$) (Wang C et al 1995). At three major laboratories in China, Wang and colleagues (Wang B et al 1990), using a photoelectric earlobe sphygmograph that measures blood volume, reported a 30% increase in the group practicing qigong versus ordinary state ($P < 0.01$). Chai & Wang (1990) used a laser microcirculation blood flow meter to measure blood flow, and found an increase in experimental versus control group ($P < 0.001$). Qu et al (1998) found blood flow resistance and vascular tension reduced in the group practicing qigong versus the control group ($P < 0.001$) even after an hour and a half of rest.

In randomly assigned controlled group studies, Kuang reports, in his 20 year study, fewer cardiovascular lesions ($P < 0.05$), decreased blood viscosity, improved platelet aggregation, decreased triglycerides, and increased high density lipoprotein cholesterol (HDL-C, good cholesterol) in the groups practicing qigong. Beneficial changes were reported in total peripheral vascular resistance, plasma cholesterol, and in two messenger cyclic nucleotides (cAMP and cGMP) in the qigong compared to the control group (Kuang et al 1991). Xian (1990) reports that after 6 months of practice, the blood of the group practicing qigong, compared to the control group, showed less tendency to form abnormal blood clots and contained significantly higher levels of high density lipoprotein cholesterol (HDL-C).

Wen (1998), in a conference proceeding, reported that during a 4 year research project, the Shanghai Institute of Hypertension repeatedly tested 2114 cases. Qigong increased the volume of blood flow in the limbs and the cardiac index of the heart. The capacity of blood vessels in the fingertips was raised 20%, and improved blood circulation was measured in the brain.

Other Cardiovascular Outcome Measures

A wide variety of other cardiovascular measures are reportedly improved by practicing qigong. Less congestive heart failure and acute myocardial infarction was reported ($P < 0.001$) by Xing & Li (1991), but the existence of control groups was not mentioned. A shorter comparative study (Kuang et al 1991, p. 157) was done on a randomly divided subgrouping of 98 cases of hypertension accompanied by coronary heart disease. There was a comparable control group based upon age, gender, and course of disease. Significant improvement was reported in the group practicing qigong compared to the control group in retinopathy ($P < 0.05$) and fewer cardiovascular lesions were found ($P < 0.05$).

In the latest update of the research of Kuang by Wang et al (1995), significant differences were reported in subjects who reportedly practiced qigong for 30 years, with sessions of 30 minutes twice a day. The accumulated mortality rate was 25.41% in the qigong group and 40.8% in the control group. The incidence of strokes was also significantly different in the qigong practice groups as compared to the control group, with 20.5% and 40.7%, respectively. The death rate due to strokes was 15.6% and 32.5% respectively ($P < 0.01$) (Wang 1993, cited in Sancier 1996a).

Wang et al (1995, in Sancier 1996a, p. 41) reported that after 1 year, many significant changes took place in a subset of 80 elderly hypertensive patients with Heart Energy Deficiency (a Chinese medical diagnosis), which often presents as a weakened function of the left ventricle and a disturbance of microcirculation. Researchers evaluated the results of qigong exercises on patients through measurements done by ultrasonic cardiography and indices of microcirculation. Subjects were divided into three groups: hypertensive patients with Heart Energy Deficiency, without Heart Energy Deficiency, and with normal BP. Left ventricular function (LVF) improved in the group practicing qigong compared to the normal BP group ($P < 0.05$–0.01), and other cardiac measures increased including 10 indices of abnormal clinical blood conditions, for example

blood flow and petechiae (fragile capillaries creating red dots on the skin) ($P < 0.05$). This study exemplifies problems related to regression to the mean, discussed in a later section.

Other Symptoms Reduced

Reports suggest qigong practice affects other chronic diseases and physical complaints associated with hypertensive states. Aching, distention, dizziness, and insomnia were reduced in a hypertensive group practicing qigong compared to a control group (Jing 1988). In a group of chronic renal failure patients, swelling disappeared, and fatigue was reduced (Suzuki et al 1993), attributed to qigong exercises. In the Kuang et al (1991) study, a subgrouping of 16 male patients with hypertension associated with diabetes reportedly had, after 6 months of practice, significant reduction ($P < 0.01$) in symptoms of polydipsia (excessive thirst), polyphagia (overeating), polyuria (excessive urination), fatigue, weakness, blurred vision, and hyperesthesia (skin sensitivity); and when 40 patients from the qigong group were examined by ultrasound, they were found to have better left ventricular function (Wang et al 1995; Cohen 1997, p. 58).

RESEARCH CRITIQUE: METHODOLOGICAL ISSUES AND PROBLEMS

Inadequate design makes the scientific validity of these studies difficult to determine. However, faulty methodology does not mean that the phenomenon under study is not worthy of further research. The methodological inadequacies of each individual study above will not be analyzed but rather, the focus of the next section is general themes, for illustrative purposes. The Kuang study (Kuang et al 1991) has been selected as an example since it is one of the longest qigong studies and the methodology has been clearly described.

Source of Studies

The bulk of the studies reviewed have been collected from the San Francisco Computerized

Database and, for the most part, come from proceedings from various qigong conferences. Some relevant data is missing, particularly from secondary reports. Many of the journal articles, reports from various qigong institutes, and books reviewed are difficult to assess methodologically, since these reports generally have not appeared in peer reviewed journals that adhere to accepted scientific standards of reporting.

Random Assignment

Of the many studies surveyed, only five authors (Huang 1990, Kuang et al 1991, Li et al 1990, Wang et al 1994, Yuan et al 1996) explicitly state in the source material that they used randomly assigned control groups. These studies contain a total of 778 subjects. All of these studies to one degree or another report positive effects of qigong on hypertension in the area of blood pressure, various other blood measurements, other cardiovascular measurements and other health related measures. Without such random assignment, outcome measures are open to other interpretations, including habituation, seasonal effects, placebo response and changes in instrumentation.

Even in the randomly assigned control group studies, there can be other potential explanations for the reported results, for example not including all subjects who were assigned in follow-up measures, isolating causes of reported treatment effects, patient's biases that arise because of expectancy of treatment effect, and lack of blinded outcome assessment.

Selection Biases

Even in studies where there was a randomly assigned control group, methodology of the selection process may be problematic. In the Kuang study, for example, although it is reported that patients with hypertension were randomly divided into qigong and control groups, specific relevant factors of the recruitment process were not mentioned. For example, we do not know how many people refused to participate, nor do we know

when or how the random assignment was made. This makes it difficult to determine whether the two groups were similar at baseline.

These questions may affect the ability to generalize to the larger population and the external validity of the study. This problem may reflect a population selection bias. If some people selected for the qigong group refused to enter into the 30-minute twice a day practice, and were eliminated from the study, this could be because they were too sick, busy, or tense. This could bias the results by eliminating the most unhealthy people from the treated group, and falsely increase the qigong practice group's health outcomes. Likewise, if some of the subjects initially selected for the control group wanted to practice qigong and were eliminated, this could eliminate the healthier controls.

Treatment Effects

What are the results of the various studies actually measuring? In virtually all of the studies reviewed, including the Kuang et al (1991) study, we do not know whether the improved health of the qigong practice group was a function of qigong exercises, or some epiphenomenon associated with qigong practice, such as general physical exercise. In most of the studies (e.g. Huang 1990, Kuang 1991) there is not sufficient information to determine whether measurements took place shortly after qigong practice, and therefore whether improvements in BP or other blood flow measurements were lasting effects of qigong or a temporary result of movement and exercise.

Physical exercise is a possible source of explanation in the Wang B et al (1990) sphygmograph blood volume study, which showed a 30% increase in qigong *versus* ordinary state ($P < 0.01$), and Chai & Wang's (1990) finding of a significant increase in blood flow in experimental versus control group ($P < 0.001$). Other studies state that BP reductions and other blood flow measures were maintained between 2 months and 3 years (Jing 1988), and 1 to 3 years (Li & Zhang 1988) of practice. However, reports do not specifically mention how long after qigong practice measures were taken. In the Shih et al (1998) study it is stated that BP measures were taken after the study; but it was not stated how long after or whether qigong was practiced before measures were taken. A study that did take this variable into account was that conducted by Qu et al (1998), who found that blood flow resistance and vascular tension were reduced in qigong versus control ($P < 0.001$) groups, even after an hour and a half of rest.

In future research, it would be useful to add a control group who exercise but do not practice qigong. If this exercise group has fewer beneficial health results, a useful step would be made in ruling out exercise as a confounding variable. Also, it should be more clearly stated how long after qigong practice measures are taken to determine how long lasting the results are.

Two studies are of interest in this regard. First, the Journal of the American Medical Association recently reported on a study that Taiji, the most popular form of qigong, helped to reduce falls among the elderly more than seven other different forms of physical exercise measured at eight different medical facilities (Province et al 1995). Second, Johns Hopkins University researchers exploring whether exercise lowers BP needed a control group that did not exercise. They picked Taiji because they thought it was so slow that it would not affect BP (Young et al 1998, unpublished). To their surprise, by the end of the 12 week study, BP of both groups dropped nearly the same amount. This latter study is important in factoring out certain expectancy biases inherent in studies done by Taiji advocates.

Finally, in terms of other alternative explanations for results, even in controlled studies the validity of qigong could be better determined by giving both groups a questionnaire addressing diet, exercise regimens, possible differences in setting between the qigong and the control group, occupation, adherence to treatment (taking medication and practicing qigong), personality measurements, or other significant variables. The authors in the Kuang study did not report measuring differences with regard to such possible confounding variables between the two groups at the beginning, middle, or end of treatment. Since there was reportedly a random division into experimental and control groups at the beginning of the study, this might mean that such variables were controlled; however, a questionnaire could help determine the extent to which differences in health were related to qigong.

Placebo Response: Expectancy Biases and Double Blind Issues

In behavioral research with humans, unlike in animal or drug research, it is difficult to have a double blind study since the subjects usually know the group to which they belong and the therapist knows which group is receiving treatment. With qigong research, qigong practitioners are aware that they are practicing a specific healing technique, and the qigong teacher/therapist knows that the qigong students are being treated. Thus, results of many of the studies cited could be based on placebo response rather than upon qigong *per se*.

A placebo response is a type of expectancy bias based upon the belief of the patient, the belief of the therapist, and the interaction between the two. A well designed study attempts to tease out how much expectancy biases and the treatment effects cause reported differences between the treatment and control groups. For example, if the qigong students had a teacher who showed them positive regard, or if students had a sense of mission and purpose to prove the efficacy of qigong as compared to a control group, these factors rather than qigong itself could have caused the reported differences. The Kuang study and others in the review of the literature (e.g. Chai & Wang 1990, Huang 1990, Jing 1988, Qu et al 1998) did not address this in the discussion section, nor did they attempt to control for these potential sources of bias.

Blinded Outcome Assessment

It was not reported in the Kuang study, nor in other studies reviewed, whether the data collectors were blinded to group assignment. This source of potential bias could be a source of conscious or unconscious skewing of measurements. In subsequent research, it should be reported whether the data collectors were blinded to group assignment.

The one study in our review which did address this issue was a Master's degree thesis from Columbia University's Program in Physical Therapy (Shih et al 1998). To the credit of this study, the investigators taking measurements were blind to group affiliation, and baseline measurements were taken on each subject before treatment establishing a greater chance of validity of BP measurements. This study involved subjects who practiced qigong twice a week during an 8 week period. Subjects reportedly showed significant decreases in systolic and diastolic BP, mean arterial pressure, and respiratory rate. In this study a quality-of-life questionnaire and a subjective self-report questionnaire indicated improvements in many areas such as relief of chronic back pain, migraine headaches, and insomnia, better ability to cope with life stresses, decreased anxiety, and increased peace and contentment. However, since the control group was taken from drop-outs of the study, the positive results could be explained by differences between groups in such variables as personality characteristics or health rather than qigong. Also, it cannot be determined whether the treatment group's positive results are due to other variables such as exercise in general, group support, or general expectancy biases.

Adherence and the Dose–Response Effect

The dose–response effect – i.e. that a greater dose of the experimental variable increases positive outcome – is important to consider in therapeutic studies. If we knew that people who practiced qigong for longer periods of time, or were more skilled, had increased health, this could increase our confidence in the effects of qigong.

In the Kuang et al (1991) study, how many in the qigong group actually practiced 30 minutes per day twice a day? The original research by Kuang did not specifically report how long the qigong practitioners practiced per day; however,

Wang et al (1993; reported in Sancier 1996a, p. 41) report that the qigong group practiced 30 minutes twice a day. Still, from this report we cannot be certain specifically how many subjects practiced this long. Among the people who died in the qigong group, did they practice more or less, or were they more or less skilled than those who lived longer? Were members of the qigong group eliminated from the analysis if they did not practice? How was adherence to the practice regimen assured? Since qigong in China is practiced by many millions of people, and is as common as aerobics in our culture, how did the researcher ensure that the control group did not practice any qigong over a 20 year period?

An important part of an analysis of a clinical trial is called the intention to treat principle, which means that to maximize validity, every patient assigned to a group must be analyzed, including those who dropped out at the beginning or during the course of the study. To the authors' credit, and adding to the study's validity, they did address the issue of drop-outs during treatment. It was reported that 204 of the 218 cases (93.58%) were included in the study over the 20 year time line, and were continuously monitored and analyzed. The inclusion of this impressive percentage in the analysis lessens the potential of this selection bias.

Most of the studies reviewed do not mention how many subjects actually adhered to the practice regimen, and therefore it cannot be determined whether there was a dose–response effect. If we knew this then it would be more likely that the qigong practice contributed to the treatment effects, rather than expectancy effects from being involved in a qigong group.

Chai & Wang (1990) did report a direct relationship between blood flow and the subjects' length and level of qigong training ($P < 0.001$), which is a dose sensitive relationship, but these researchers did not randomly assign a control group. Likewise Shih et al (1998) report a dose–response effect, but due to the problems with the selection of control group from drop-outs described earlier, alternative explanations could be posited for reported treatment effects.

Problems with Reliability of Blood Pressure Measurements

There are general difficulties in establishing reliable BP measurements in terms of establishing a stable baseline for any researcher. A subject's BP may fluctuate for a variety of reasons at different times, making analysis difficult. Many studies in our review do not adequately address this problem, though some studies have given attention to establishing stable baseline BP measures, and monitoring BP continuously over the course of the study, for example Shih et al (1998). However, even in this study, it was not reported whether such measures were taken at times other than directly after the qigong meditation period. Such measures would help to determine whether meditative exercise itself is a confounding variable (i.e. whether qigong versus control groups temporarily reduces BP after exercise) or if qigong produces longer lasting effects.

Regression to the Mean

Studies which select subjects by extremely high or low levels of any variable have the methodological problem of follow-up measures having a general tendency to move toward the center. In the earlier cited Wang study (Wang et al 1995; Wang et al 1993, in Sancier 1996a, p. 41), 80 elderly hypertensive patients were divided into three groups: hypertensive patients with Heart Energy Deficiency (HED), without Heart Energy Deficiency, and with normal BP, and were given treatment targeted to decrease Heart Energy Deficiency. Left ventricular function (LVF), other cardiac measures, and 10 indices of abnormal clinical blood conditions improved ($P < 0.05$) in the qigong group versus both control groups. However, the non-random division into groups of greater and lesser heart deficiency at the outset allows for regression to the mean to explain the positive results.

Regression to the mean could be a confounding variable in Xu & Wang's (1993) use of a pre- and post-test design in reports regarding patients with degeneration of the heart, brain and kidney functions, and senility, and their improvements in these functions.

Publication Bias

Any field of research is subject to publication biases. Studies that support a given treatment are published, while those that do not lend support tend not to be published. Studies coming from China are suspect in the West for being influenced by political and cultural factors which could bias scientific methods and data. Thus there is a need for replication of the work in the West.

All the sources reviewed on hypertensive patients (except Zhang & Hou 1993) report that the practice of qigong positively affects BP, other blood flow measures, cardiovascular outcome measures, and other aspects of health to varying degrees.

Zhang & Hou (1993), in a study that addresses qigong practice problems, report that a qigong group that thought they could open their 'third eye,' 'emit qi' and develop natural gifts had worse systolic and diastolic BP and heart rates after treatment. The article warns that patients with hypertension must be careful when practicing qigong to concentrate their minds on the lower abdomen ('*tan tien*'). Regarding the believability of the studies on the reduction of BP, the various studies cited report different rates of reduction over time from one session to 1 year. In the Zdravkovic (1998) study it was reported that there was no significant change of BP in up to 2 months of training. If there was extreme publication bias, the varied reports of time to decrease hypertension and studies reporting limited effects would be absent.

LACK OF CONSISTENCY OF MEASUREMENT

Many Types of Hypertension and Many Styles of Qigong

Further research needs to be conducted on the varied qigong traditions to determine which particular type or sequence of qigong movements may be most beneficial to a given patient at a given time. In any sample of the many qigong traditions (Cohen 1997, Johnson 2000), each may focus upon various combinations or types of self-healing qigong exercises (SHQE) such as qigong healing internal organs, stretching muscles, dispersing stagnant qi, tapping, breathing, making sounds, using pulsing movements, animal like movements, self-massaging, visualization techniques, and spiritual awareness exercises. Qigong also uses non-movement, called static qigong, such as standing meditation, to activate qi (Cai 1986, Chuen 1991, Diepersloot 1995, Ha & Olsen 1996, Johnson 2000, Mayer 1997c, Wen 1998). As well, external qigong (EQ) is used where the practitioner does not touch the patient, or the practitioner may touch specific points on the patient's body such as acupressure points or vital zones.

We should also be aware that qigong practices are not so easily oriented towards Western notions of prescribing a single pill or movement. Such an approach provides ease of scientific measurement, but does not fit into holistic Chinese medical philosophy which includes disease categories that do not conform to nomothetic categories.

For example, the Western diagnostic category of hypertension in Chinese medicine may be due to a wide variety of energetic imbalances such as 'an imbalance of the Yin and Yang functional aspects of Deficient Kidney Yin and Excess Liver Yang, and/or an overabundance of phlegm and dampness within the body' (Johnson 2000). Two different people with the same Western diagnosis of 'hypertension' are treated differently depending upon specific diagnostic considerations that come from such general categories and from tongue and pulse analysis. Ideographic factors related to the unique patient and the background of the particular qigong healer/Chinese doctor are also part of the decision about what treatment or combination of treatments is chosen. Unique combinations of herbs, acupuncture, and a wide variety of qigong movements are prescribed based upon what is suited to the individual whole person.

OVERVIEW OF QIGONG TREATMENT FOR HYPERTENSION

Each different system of qigong has its own self-healing qigong exercises for disorders of the heart, including hypertension. Sometimes these treatments use the same or similar methods; at other times they use different ones. The recently published 'comprehensive clinical text' on qigong (Johnson 2000) is an English translated source that gives a compendium of the variety of qigong treatments used for different types of hypertension in China today. We will use this text to exemplify the depth and breadth of the tradition of 'medical Qigong therapy.' This text describes a variety of qigong techniques including breathing exercises, self-healing qigong exercises (SHQE), healing sounds, acupressure, self-rubbing techniques, static qigong, visualizations, and external emission qigong (EQ) where the practitioner does not touch the patient. The techniques may be used in particular combinations in clinical practice with different patients.

Johnson states that 'scientific studies confirm that 90% of hypertensive patients practice *Reverse Breathing* chronically.' However, no reference is given for the research behind this claim. Reverse breathing involves contracting the abdomen when inhaling and expanding the abdomen upon exhaling. Various breathing techniques are given to the patient to restore normal abdominal breathing such as Abdominal Breathing where the patient's stomach expands on the in-breath and expands on the out-breath. A wide variety of other breathing techniques are used, for example Deep Exhalation Method, Abdominal Breath Holding Method, and Microcosmic Orbit Breathing.

SHQE exercises may be prescribed. For example, the patient may be instructed to move his or her hands with palms downward along the front and side of the body to purge and guide toxic qi so that it descends down the liver and gall bladder channels, or down the torso to the hips. Specific points such as acupuncture point GB30 may be focused upon. Self-rubbing techniques are prescribed and sometimes combined with vocalization of healing sounds suited to a specific type of hypertension. Other SHQE are used for different situations including static postures where the patient lies, sits or practices standing meditation. The text advises first practicing sitting, and later both sitting and standing meditations to direct qi downward. Intricate imaginal techniques, including the visualization of colors, may be practiced in conjunction with assuming such postures. For example, the patient may be instructed to imagine and feel warm water pouring down over the head. Beating a bag filled with rice to expel excess anger may be practiced, similar to cathartic methods of Western psychotherapy.

Regarding EQ versus SHQE exercises, Johnson states that EQ techniques are employed if the person is 'sensitive to energy.' For example, the EQ technique called the Extended Fan Palm Technique (EFPT) may be used; the practitioner moves his hands up and down over the center line in the back and front of the body with fingers extended like a fan for 'Cleaning the Conception and Governing Vessels (*Ren Mai and Du Mai*).' While working with a patient the practitioner may also use intentionality techniques such as visualizing two streams joining. In cases with Excess Liver Fire, acupressure points such as Lv 13–14 may be touched to direct the energy to the earth leading the qi down the right gall bladder meridian. When treating hypertensive patients with Kidney Yin or Yang deficiency, the qigong therapist may focus the treatment differently, using EFPT and moving the hands to direct energy to the belly (*Tan Tien*) or the lower back (*Ming Men*). Johnson says that for patients 'not sensitive to energy,' a 'Sword Finger Technique (the thumb holds the ring and small fingers while the middle and pointer fingers are outstretched)' is used touching the patient on the crown of his head (*Bai Hui*), while the practitioner's other hand is on the patient's lower back. Different acupressure points are used; these patients are touched on both sides of the body using points such as Li 11, St 26, Lv 2 and Sp 6. Some EQ techniques and Energy Point Therapy such as the Invisible Needle Technique are reportedly contraindicated for hypertensive patients in acute stages.

In this clinical text (Johnson 2000), scientific studies that lie behind the assumptions of clinical efficacy with the various techniques are not stated, nor is the reliability and validity of the diagnostic categories. The evidence for the specific treatments cited in the text presumably comes from

centuries of empirical evidence and on acupuncture and qigong theory and practice, not scientific evidence *per se*. It is difficult to determine how much placebo and other factors discussed in our critique of the research relate to the success of treatment. How 'sensitive' patients are differentiated from 'non-sensitive' ones is not made clear. Further research could investigate if they correlate with 'highly hypnotizable subjects' (Wickramasekera 1998), or examine what other criteria could be used to measure those 'sensitive to energy.'

From a Western viewpoint, once diagnostic criteria are reliably established for sensitive/insensitive, Excess Liver Yang and Kidney Yin and Yang Deficiency, groundwork is laid for research designs using mock treatments on the subjects who are controls, and comparing it to the qigong treatment group to determine efficacy of treatment. However, as will be discussed further below, the attempt to isolate a specific treatment and separate it from ideographic dimensions of a patient, and holistic dimensions of Chinese medicine, is itself problematic. Finding a general prescription is difficult due to unique clinical situations. For example, a subject in a group of Excess Liver Yang who normally might be given a visualization SHQE of imagining a river flowing down the body to lower qi to the feet might have a water phobia, and the treatment might be detrimental or not work. Likewise, as can be seen from the discussion above, a researcher who wanted to investigate EQ might choose a method of EQ that could be detrimental to a patient, or not work, due to the particularities of the patient's situation.

Another example of treatment application of qigong to hypertension is the work of Dr Zhi Gang Sha (Sha 2000). His system of healing combines standing meditation, hand postures, sound and visualizations. The theoretical basis for his method is based upon energy in the body naturally moving from high to low intensity fields, and using the aforementioned elements to facilitate such movement of energy. In a case of excess, the patient puts one hand closer to the area of excess and their other hand further away from another body part to move the excess away from the area of high intensity. In cases of deficiency, the patient places one hand further away from the deficient area of the body and the other hand closer to another body part to bring the energy from the high intensity, strong area to low intensity, deficient area. For high systolic and high diastolic hypertension the near hand is placed over the crown of the head or facing the forehead; the far away hand is by the lower adbomen. The patient visualizes light flowing from the head to the lower adomen as he or she repeats the sound *yi* (for the head) and *jiu* (for the abdomen). He has other hand postures and sounds for normal systolic and high diastolic blood pressure, and for hypotension. Group ritual, where the whole group chants sounds together, amplifies the placebo effect, and perhaps increases the healing dimensions of the 'energy field' itself. Many anecodotal reports exist of the healing effects of his method. Dr Sha does many large demonstrations in the United States; however, to my knowledge, there have not been any scientific studies documenting the efficacy of his methods along the lines suggested in this chapter.

INTERNAL VERSUS EXTERNAL QIGONG

In terms of scientific studies on external emission techniques of qigong (EQ) and internal qigong, also called self-healing qigong movement exercises (SHQE), of the studies reviewed, two involved external emission (Huang 1993, and Pan & Zhang 1990). Huang's study was not stated as being with hypertensive patients, but with 'male intelligensia.' For the first 3 months of his study, Huang's subjects received emitted qi twice a week in addition to SHQE twice a day. In the next 9 months the trainees practiced by themselves without emitted qi. After 3 months, various heart measurements showed no significant difference. However, after 1 year of practice many heart measures improved including electrocardiogram, carotid artery pulse, systolic and diastolic pressure. Due to design problems, no determination can be made about the efficacy of internal versus external qigong from this study. Positive changes in heart measures in the longer

term internal practice qigong group could be due to time itself and its concomitant attributes such as the amount of time of doing exercise in general, group cohesion, expectancy biases, etc.

Pan & Zhang (1990) used a single group of 32 hospitalized hypertensive patients with renal insufficiency and divided them into three groups: simple sitting, emitted chi qi by a qigong master and imitated emission by a mock qigong master. BP decreased significantly in both the qigong and mock qigong group, but the decrease was significantly greater in the real qigong master group ($P < 0.01$); no changes in BP were found in the simple sitting group ($P > 0.05$). Since this article was in abstract form it cannot be determined whether confounding variables were controlled. For example, there was no report regarding whether there was blinded outcome assessment, and we do not know whether the sham qigong master was obvious in being a sham. Because of this single and non-double blinded design, the sham practitioner may have consciously or unconsciously given off nonverbal cues (such as an obviously non-healing movement or facial expression); and the real qigong master may have given off higher levels of empathy that would indicate whether the treatment was real or mock. This confounding variable could be controlled for by asking the participants in a questionnaire afterwards whether they thought the treatment was real or mock, or by covering the eyes of the subjects.

Another study (Yasutami et al 1999) did control for this variable, even though it was not a hypertension study *per se*. Subjects lay on a reclining chair with their eyes covered by an eye-mask and ears plugged by ear-stoppers in a sound-proofed room so that they could not be aware of the beginning and end of qigong practice. Sham and external emission qigong were measured in terms of EEG and peripheral blood measurements. The major problem with this study was that there were only four subjects. Conclusions regarding efficacy are therefore difficult to make even though an increase in alpha waves was reported in three out of four subjects in the right occipital region, and there were no changes in sham qigong. There were changes in peripheral blood in two out of four experimental group subjects, whereas no changes were observed in the sham qigong group. The Yasutami study needs replication with a larger number of subjects.

DISCUSSION

Although many of the studies of qigong practice and hypertension have methodological flaws, controlling for the methodological biases listed above represents high expectations in any behavioral or clinical research. The methodological problems addressed may account for some unknown portion of improved health outcome measures, but we should be circumspect before fully discounting positive effects reported in mortality rates, incidence of strokes and retinopathy (Kuang et al 1991), and other positive outcome measurements in patients who have suffered from long-term hypertension (e.g. Jing 1988, Wu & Liu 1993), or chronic renal failure (Suzuki et al 1993). These represent significant numbers of long-term sufferers of severe hypertension. Even if methodological flaws such as expectancy biases and placebo effects contributed to positive results, the results need to be considered seriously in an area that has such significant health ramifications.

Complementary and alternative medical (CAM) methods often have associated with them a high level of belief and preference that may be part of the 'cure' (Roberts et al 1993). Further examination needs to take place regarding whether potentially effective treatments such as qigong may be unduly discarded if proportions of treatment are attributable to non-specific concomitants of the treatment such as exercise, group bonding, and empathy from the instructor.

Separating one form of treatment from others to experimentally measure it apart from others fits with a Western reductionistic need to isolate variables to measure. This notion is difficult to apply to the ideographic and holistic dimensions of Chinese medicine and qigong treatment.

Recently there has been advocacy in CAM research for a 'systems model' that attempts to identify 'the web of etiological influences' that contribute to a healing, and then with a 'holistic model' the patient's reactions are examined to multiple etiological agents and influences (Jonas & Levin 1999b). An analogy with research in plants elucidates the point that the multiple chemical agents that exist in nature, along with the active ingredient, may serve to have a positive synergistic effect, and naturally balance against side-effects. Pharmaceuticals, on the other hand, isolate the active chemical, take it out of its natural environment, perhaps increasing the strength of the treatment; this, however, may increase risk for adverse side-effects (Dey & Harbourne 1990, Dey et al 1997). Similarly, trying to isolate the active ingredient of qigong and take it away from the whole of Chinese medical treatments used, the varieties of qigong methods used, and such 'confounding variables' as the empathy of the qigong teacher may remove the natural synergistic mix that makes qigong work.

An often cited problem in CAM and behavioral research is that the practitioner's intentionality may be contributing to healing rather than the technique itself. This has led some researchers (Dossey 1997) to suggest experiments on animals or bacteria for better control of such variables. In the area of energy medicine in general, there has been research that points in the direction of intentionality effecting healing (Wirth 1990, Wirth et al 1998); and in the area of qigong there has also been much research (Cohen 1997, Subtle Energies 1990–2000) that points in this direction. Trying to control for the confounding variable of intentionality with diseases of the heart such as hypertension creates a unique problem. The human heart differs from bacteria or an animal heart. A treatment that effects the latter may not heal the former. Occam's razor may cut out the heart of the cure.

From the discussion above we can see why CAM in general is examining the research methodology issues of balancing rigor and relevance (Linde & Jonas 1999). In general, Western hypertension research (COTA 1978; Cohen 1997, p. 345), as well as Chinese qigong studies, suffer from problematic research design. In an overview of hypertension studies, Rosen states, methodological problems such as small sample sizes and lack of experimenter-blind assessment have limited the generalizability of results from most studies (Rosen et al 1998, Kaufmann et al 1988, TOHP Collaborative Research Group 1992).

Taken as a whole, many studies on hypertension do not address the criteria outlined above for reasons as varied as difficulties inherent in behavioral and CAM research itself, lack of adequate training in research methodology, general issues cited above in BP measurements, lack of funding, and the orientation of the clinician to heal rather than measure.

The treatment effects of qigong on hypertension are worthy of note and are potentially profound in their implications. Qigong fits well into the guidelines stated by a National Institutes of Health panel (NIHTAP 1996) which concluded that integrating behavioral and relaxation therapies with conventional medical treatment is imperative for successfully managing these conditions. The panel did not endorse a single technique, but stated that a variety of techniques worked in 'lowering one's breathing rate, heart rate and BP' as long as they included two features: 'a repetitive focus of a word, sound, prayer, phrase or muscular activity, and neither fighting nor focusing on intruding thoughts.'

Eastern and Integrative Methods

Many Eastern methods of stress reduction have been used successfully with hypertension. Transcendental meditation (TM) has been shown in well designed randomly assigned studies to positively affect the BP of hypertensives (Schneider et al 1995, Alexander et al 1996). Other TM studies demonstrated that significant changes in BP were even measured at times other than during the meditation period (Benson et al 1973). Positive results have been claimed in combining Vipassana meditation and stress reduction techniques at the University of Massachusetts Medical Center (Zinn 1990). When yoga was integrated into an intensive multifaceted lifestyle change program with a low fat, low cholesterol vegetarian diet, daily meditation, moderate aerobic exercise and group support, hypertension and coronary disease were reduced (Ornish 1990, Ornish et al 1990).

Since Eastern methods such as these have been shown to positively affect hypertension, it is 'plausible' (Linde & Jonas 1999) that qigong may do so also.

Like yoga (Ornish et al 1990) and other Eastern relaxation methods which have reported beneficial results in treating hypertension, qigong is a tradition that combines relaxation, breathing, and a mindful relationship to body awareness. Further research could compare yoga, qigong, exercise, and other relaxation and/or meditative traditions. Each different Eastern meditation modality may have its own advantages and disadvantages for different patients. For example, yoga may be the most appropriate exercise for patients who cannot stand, while qigong may be more beneficial for Type A, sedentary office workers who would benefit from movement. For those who would most benefit from mantra yoga, TM may prove appropriate, while those who are overly intellectual and stressed may benefit from the bodily orientation of qigong.

Qigong has the advantage for elderly hypertensives of being low impact, and therefore potentially less dangerous compared to traditional aerobic exercise (Province et al 1995). In general, a variety of factors could be considered in a given patient's choice of exercise at a given time, such as physical limitations, availability, suitability of a given instructor, life circumstances, or basic beliefs.

Finally, whether qigong alone can affect hypertension is not necessarily the most important question to be answered. If the direction that Western research points to is correct, multifaceted programs (JNC-V 1993, Kostis et al 1992, Little et al 1991, Ornish et al 1990, Rosen et al 1998) which integrate diet, aerobic exercise, relaxation techniques, social, hypnotherapeutic, and psychological dimensions may be best in treating hypertension. For example, the Heartsavers Lifestyle Program (Rosen et al 1998) treated middle aged and elderly hypertensives and found the greatest improvements in middle-aged and elderly hypertensives who followed a multifaceted program as compared with a medication and placebo control group. Quality of life also improved based upon the patients' reports of increased energy levels and improved sexual performance compared with both drug and placebo (Rosen et al 1998, p. 91).

Western psychotherapeutic and hypnotherapeutic methods have been used successfully with hypertensive patients (Benson 1983a, 1983b; Crasilneck & Hall 1985; Yanoviski 1962). The energetic dimension has long been advocated as a significant part of body–mind healing in the West (Reich 1942, Lowen 1958). It may be a useful next step to add qigong methods to this tradition. Further research has been suggested (Mayer 1994, 1996, 1997a, 1997b, 1997c, 1998) with hypertensive patients to explore and validate the integration of psychological methods such as hypnosis (Mayer 2001), self-soothing, visualization, psychodynamic interventions, and cognitive restructuring. Additional research recommendations include focusing on the felt meaning of one's hypertension (Gendlin 1978), qigong techniques such as microcosmic orbit breathing (Wilhelm 1962), and other Daoist qigong breathing methods, touching of acupressure points (Gach 1990), and belly massage from *chi nei tsang* (Chia & Wang 1990).

Qigong could have a positive role to play in multifaceted interventions in the unique way that it integrates relaxation, meditation, and exercise. Doctors (Maisel 1963) and medical hospitals, such as California Pacific Medical Center in San Francisco and Columbia Presbyterian Hospital in New York, are increasingly using qigong for their cardiology patients (Motz 1997).

CONCLUSION AND FURTHER RESEARCH RECOMMENDATIONS

The weight of evidence of 33 studies representing 5545 subjects suggests that practicing qigong has a positive effect on hypertension; however, due to inadequate addressing of methodological issues, it is difficult to determine exactly how effective qigong is, and what other factors may contribute to the positive effects reported in the studies reviewed.

We specifically recommend that future studies control for exercise as a confounding variable, report data on adherence to treatment, measure the dose–response effect to treatment, and use blinded outcome assessment. Questionnaires can be designed to further determine assessment of factors contributing to treatment effects such as lifestyle factors including diet and exercise, personality variables, belief in qigong, adjunctive treatments, and medications used by subjects.

We hope that Western researchers join hands with those in China who are investigating qigong, since all may benefit from further studies to establish whether or not qigong may provide a beneficial adjunct to other treatments.

ACKNOWLEDGMENTS

Much thanks go to Dr Kenneth Sancier, director of the Qigong Institute, for his thoughtful comments about this chapter and for his articles and Qigong Database. Great appreciation goes to Dr Larry Scherwitz, research director of the Institute for Health and Healing at the California Pacific Medical Center, for his feedback and assistance on this chapter. I am grateful for Dr Wayne Jonas's work as a leader in the field of complementary medicine, and his helping to pave the way for my contact with professionals in the field that helped to refine my work on research methodology issues. I would also like to express much gratitude to my qigong teachers who have been recognized as masters of their traditions: Fong Ha, Cai Song Fang, Han Xingyuan, Sam Tam, Ken Cohen, and Kumar Francis.

For further details please contact Dr Michael Mayer at: MM@bodymindhealing.comwww.bodymindhealing.com

REFERENCES

Alexander C A, Schneider R H, Staggers F et al 1996 Trial of stress reduction for hypertension in older African Americans. American Heart Association. Hypertension 28: 228–237

Benson H 1983a The relaxation response and norepinephrine: a new study illuminates mechanisms. Integrative Psychiaty, 1: 15–18

Benson H 1983b The relaxation response: it's subjective and objective historical precedents and physiology. Trends in Neuroscience July: 281–284

Benson H, Rosner B A, Marzetta B R 1973 Decreased systolic BP in hypertensive subjects who practice meditation. Journal of Clinical Investigation 52: 80

Bornoroni C, Genitoni V, Gori G, Gatti G, Dorigo A 1993 Treatment of 30 cases of primary hypertension by qigong techniques. 2nd World Conference for Academic Exchange of Medical Qigong, Beijing, China, p. 126 Ea

Cai S F, translated by Den M, revised by Shen T 1986 Wujishi breathing exercise. Medicine and Health Publishing, Hong Kong, China

Chai Z, Wang B 1990 Influence of qigong state on blood perfusion state of human microcirculation. 3rd National Academic Conference on Qigong Science, Guangzhou, China, p. 116 [reported in Cohen 1997, p. 61]

Chia M 1990, Chi nei tsang. Hunington, New York

Chu C 1988 Changes in blood viscosity and rheocardiogram in 44 cases with cardiovascular diseases after qigong. 1st World Conference for Academic Exchange of Medical Qigogn, Beijing, China, p. 57 E [from San Francisco Qigong Database, Sancier 1997]

Chuen L K 1991 The way of energy. Gaia Books, London, England

Cohen K 1997 The way of qigong. Ballantine Books, New York

Congressional Office of Technology Assessment 1978 Assessing the efficacy and safety of medical technologies. [quoted by Cohen 1997, p. 346]

Crasilneck H, Hall J, 1985 Clinical hypnosis: principles and applications. Grune & Straton, New York, p. 178

Dey P M, Harbourne J B 1990 Methods in plant biochemistry: enzymes of primary metabolism. Academic Press, London

Dey P M, Harbourne J B, Waterman P G 1997 Methods in plant biochemistry: alkaloids and sulphur compounds. Academic Press, London

Diepersloot J 1995 Warriors of stillness. Center for Healing and the Arts, Walnut Creek, CA

Dossey L 1997 The return of prayer. Alternative Therapies in Health and Medicine 3(6)

Eisenberg D M, Davis R B, Ettner S L et al 1998 Trends in alternative medicine use in the United States 1990–1997. Journal of the American Medical Association 289(18): 1549–1640

Francis B K 1993 Opening the energy gates of your body. North Atlantic Books, Berkeley, CA

Gach M 1990 Acupressure potent points. Bantam Books, New York

Gendlin E 1978 Focusing. Bantam Books, New York

Ha F, Olsen E 1996 Yiquan and the nature of energy. Summerhouse Publications, Berkeley, CA

Huang X 1990 Clinical observation of 204 patients with hypertension treated with qigong. Proceedings of 1st International Conference, p. 101E. [record 3590, San Francisco Qigong Database, Sancier 1997]

Huang Z 1993 Effect of qigong on heart function. Paper presented at 2nd World Conference for Academic Exchange of Medical Qigong, Beijing, China. [from San Francisco Qigong Database, Sancier 1997]

Jing G 1988 Observations on the curative effects of qigong self adjustment therapy in hypertension. Proceedings from the 1st World Conference for Academic Exchange of Medical Qigong, Beijing, China, pp. 115–117

Johnson J A 2000 Chinese medical qigong therapy. International Institute of Medical Qigong, Pacific Grove, CA

Joint National Committee on Detection, Evaluation and Treatment of High BP 1993 Fifth report. Archives of Internal Medicine 153: 154–183

Jonas W B, Levin J S (eds) 1999a Essentials of complementary and alternative medicine. Lippincott, Williams and Wilkins, Philadelphia

Jonas W B, Levin J S 1999b Introduction: models of medicine. In: Jonas W B, Levin J S (eds) Essentials of complementary and alternative, medicine. Lippincott, Williams and Wilkins, p. 8

Kaufmann P, Jacob R, Ewart C et al 1988 Hypertension intervention pooling project. Health Psychology 7(Suppl.): 209–224

Kostis J, Rosen R, Holzer B, Randolph C, Taska L, Miller M 1990 CNS side effects of centrally-active anti-hypertensive agents: a prospective placebo-controlled study of sleep, mood state and cognitive and sexual function in hypertensive males. Psychopharmacology 102: 163–170

Kostis J B, Rosen R C, Brondolo E, Taska L, Smith D E, Wilson A C 1992 Superiority of nonpharmacological therapy compared to propranolol and placebo in men with mild hypertension: a randomized prospective trial. American Heart Journal 123: 466–474

Kuang A, Chen J, Lu Y 1989 Changes of sex hormones in female type II diabetics, coronary heart disease, essential hypertension and its relations with kidney deficiency. Chih (China), 9(6): 331–334. 323 ISSN 0254 9034 [from San Francisco Qigong Database, Sancier 1997]

Kuang A, Wang C, Xu D, Qian Y 1991 Research on 'anti aging' effect of qigong. Journal of Traditional Chinese Medicine 11(2): 153–158, 11(3): 224–227

Li Z, Zhang B 1988 Group observation and experimental research on the prevention and treatment of hypertension by qigong, Proceedings of the 1st World Conference for Academic Exchange of Medical Qigong, Beijing, China, pp. 113–114

Li W, Xin Z, Pi D 1990 Effect of qigong on sympathetico-adrenomedullary function in patients with liver yang exuberance hypertension. [from San Francisco Qigong Database, Sancier 1997]

Linde K, Jonas W 1999 Evaluating complementary and alternative medicine: the balance of rigor and relevance. In: Jonas W B, Levin J S (eds) Essentials of Complementary and Alternative Medicine. Lippincott, Williams and Wilkins, Philadelphia

Little P, Girling G, Hasler A, Trafford A 1991 A controlled trial of low sodium, low fat, high fiber diet in treated hypertensive patients: effect on anti-hypertensive drug requirement in clinical practice. Journal of Human Hypertension 5: 175–181

Lowen A 1958 The language of the body. Collier Books, New York

McGee C T, Chow E P 1994 Miracle healing from China. Medipress, Coeur d'Alene, ID

Maisel E 1963 Tai chi for health. Dell, New York, p. 55

Mayer M H 1994 Trials of the heart. Celestial Arts, Berkeley, CA

Mayer M H 1996 Qigong and behavioral medicine: an integrated approach to chronic pain. Qi: The Journal of Eastern Health and Fitness 6(4): 20–31

Mayer M H 1997a Psychotherapy and qigong, partners in healing anxiety: integrative depth psychotherapy. Psychotherapy and Healing Center, Berkeley, CA

Mayer M H 1997b Combining behavioral health care and qigong with one chronic hypertensive adult. Mount Diablo Hospital-Health Medicine Forum [unpublished study; video available from Health Medicine Institute Lafayette, CA]

Mayer M H 1997c Standing meditation: doing nothing and finding contentment in being alight. Bodymind Healing Center, 2029 Durant Avenue, Suite #202, Berkeley, CA, Tel: 510-849-2878 (mm@bodymindhealing.com)

Mayer M H 1998 Bodymind qigong: a manual of methods and healing secrets. Bodymind Healing Center, Berkeley, CA [with accompanying videotape, Bodymind healing qigong. 2000. Bodymind Healing (www.bodymindhealing.com)]

Mayer M H 1999 Qigong and hypertension: a critique of research. Journal of Alternative and Complementary Medicine 5(4): 371–382

Mayer M H 2001 Find your hidden reservoir of healing energy: A guided meditation for chronic disease (Audio type). Bodymind Healing Center, Berkeley CA MM@bodymindhealing.com

Medical Research Council Working Party 1985 MRC trial of treatment of mild hypertension: principal results. British Medical Journal 291: 97–104

Motz J 1997 Work at Columbia Presbyterian Hospital reported by Van Collie S. While they sleep. Pacific Sun, April 23, 1997

National Institute of Health Technology Assessment Panel 1996 Integration of behavioral and relaxation approaches into the treatment of chronic pain and insomnia. Reported in: Journal of the American Medical Association 276(4): 313–318

Ornish D 1990, Dr Dean Ornish's program for reversing heart disease. Random House New York

Ornish D M, Brown S E, Scherwitz L W et al 1990 Can lifestyle changes reverse coronary artheriosclerosis? Lancet 336: 129–133

Pan L B, Zhang Z F 1990 Qigong treatment for hypertension caused by renal insufficiency. 3rd Nat Academic Conference on Qigong Science, Guangzhau, China, p. 90 EB. [from San Francisco Qigong Database, Sancier 1997]

Pollare T, Lithell H, Selinus I, Berne C 1989 Sensitivity to insulin during treatment with atenolol and metoprolol: a randomised double blind study of effects on carbohydrate and lipoprotein metabolism in hypertensive patients. New England Journal of Medicine 321: 868–873

Province M A, Hadley E C, Hornbrook M C et al 1995 The effects of exercise on falls in elderly patients: a preplanned meta-analysis of the FICSIT trials. Journal of the American Medical Association 273(17): 1341–1347

Qu M 1990 Taijiquan – a medical assessment. Martial Arts of China Magazine 1(5): 203–204 [reported in Cohen 1997, p. 59]

Qu Z, Wang C, Xu D, Qian Y 1998 Peripheral resistance variances and qigong therapy in hypertension of the heart-qi deficiency and blood stasis type. 7th International Symposium of Qigong, Shanghai, September 1998

Reich W 1942 Character analysis. Orgone Institute Press, New York

Roberts A H, Kewman D G, Mercier L, Hovell M 1993 The power of nonspecific effects in healing: implications for psychological and biological treatments. Clinical Psychology Review 13: 375–391

Rosen R C, Brondolo E, Kostis J B 1998 Non-pharmacological treatment of essential hypertension. In: Gatchel R J, Blanchard E B (eds) Psychophysiological disorders. American Psychological Association, Washington, pp. 85–86

Rubik B 1995 Energy medicine and the unifying concept of information. Alternative Therapies in Health and Medicine, 1(1): 34–39

Sancier K 1996a Medical applications of qigong. Alternative Therapies 2(1): 40–46

Sancier K 1996b Anti-aging benefits of qigong. Journal of the International Society of Life Information Science 14(1): 12–21

Sancier K 1997 San Francisco Qigong Database, Qigong Institute of San Francisco, Menlo Park, CA [updated May 1999] (qigonginstitute@healthy.net)

Schneider R H, Staggers F, Alexander C N et al 1995 A randomized controlled trial of stress reduction for hypertension in older African Americans. American Heart Association. Hypertension 226: 820–827

Sha Z G 2000 Zhi Neng medicine: revolutionary self-healing methods from China. Zhi Neng Press, Vancouver, BC

Shih T K, Zucker P, Ohrenstein N 1997 The effects of qigong on resting systemic BP and quality of life in hypertensive adults. Qi: the Journal of Traditional Eastern Health and Fitness 8(2): 31–33 [results reported by B Stone in Newsweek, July 28, 1997, p. 72]

Subtle Energies Journal 1990–2000 International Society for the Study of Subtle Energies and Energy Medicine, Goldco, Colorado

Suzuki M et al 1993 Clinical effectiveness of the AST Chiro method on chronic renal failure and hypertension. Japanese Mind Body Science 2(1): 15–22 [0918–2489, from San Francisco Qigong Database, Sancier 1997]

Tianjin Research Institute of Traditional Chinese Medicine 1988 Group observation and experimental research on the prevention and treatment of hypertension by qigong. Paper presented at 1st World Conference for Academic Exchange of Medical Qigong, Beijing, China, p. 113 [cited in Cohen 1997]

Trials of Hypertension Prevention, Collaborative Research Group 1992 The effects of non-pharmacologic interventions on BP of persons with high normal levels. Journal of the American Medical Association 267: 1213–1220

Wang B, Chia Z Shen X, Chai X 1990 The influence of qigong state on the volume of human peripheral vascular blood flow. 3rd National Academic Conference on Qigong Science, Guangzhou, China, November 1990, pp. 11–12 [reported in Cohen 1997, pp. 60–61]

Wang C, Xu D, Qian Y, Kuang A 1990 The beneficial effects of qigong on hypertension and heart disease. Proceedings from the 3rd International Symposium on Qigong, Shanghai Institute of Hypertension, Shanghai, China, p. 40

Wang C, Xu D, Qian Y, Shi W 1993 Effects of qigong on preventing stroke and alleviating the multiple cerebro-cardiovascular risk factors: a follow-up report on 242 hypertensive cases over 30 years. Proceedings from the 2nd World Conference for Academic Exchange of Medical Qigong, Beijing, China, pp. 123–124

Wang C, Xu D, Quian Y, Shi W 1994 Beneficial effects of qigong on the ventricular function and microcirculation of deficiency in heart-energy hypertensive patients. [private communication reported in Sancier 1996b, p. 15]

Wang C, Xu D, Qian Y, Shi W, Bao Y, Kuang A 1995 The beneficial effects of qigong on the ventricular function and micorcirculation of deficiency in heart energy hypertensive patients. Chinese Journal of Internal Medicine 1(1): 21–23

Wen D E 1998 Static qigong, cross-legged sitting posture and blood redistribution. 4th Conference for Academic Exchange of Medical Qigong, pp. 201–202 [from San Francisco Qigong Database, Sancier 1997]

Wickramesekera I 1998 Secrets kept from the mind but not the body or behavior. Advances in Mind-Body Medicine 14: 81–132

Wilhelm R 1962. The secret of the golden flower. Harcourt Brace Janovich, New York

Wirth D 1990 The effect of non-contact therapeutic touch on the healing rate of full thickness dermal wounds. Subtle Energies 1(1): 1–20

Wirth D P, Richardson J T, Martinez R D, Eidelman W S, Lopez M E 1998 Non-contact therapeutic touch intervention and full-thickness cutaneous wounds: a replication. Complementary Therapies in Medicine 4: 237–240

Wollam G, Hall W (eds) 1988 Hypertension management: clinical practice and therapeutic dilemmas. Yearbook Publishers, Chicago

Wu R, Liu Z 1993 Study of qigong on hypertension and reduction of hypotension: Proceedings of 2nd World Conference for Academic Exchange of Medical Qigong, Beijing, China, p. 125 [from San Francisco Qigong Database, record 7970, Sancier 1997; full article provided by author translated into English]

Xian B H 1990 Clinical observation of 204 patients with hypertension treated with Chinese Qigong. Paper presented at 5th International Congress of Qigong, Berkeley, California, p. 101 [reported in Cohen 1997]

Xing Z H, Li W 1997 Effect of qigong on blood pressure and life quality of essential hypertensive patients. [from San Francisco Qigong Database, Sancier 1997]

Xu D, Wang C A 1993 Study of the recuperation function of qigong on hypertension target organ impairment. Shanghai Insitute of Hypertension. 2nd World Conference on Medical Qigong, Beijing, China

Xu D, Wang C 1994 Clinical study of delaying effect on senility of hypertensive patients by practicing Yang Jing Yi Shen Gong. Proceedings from the 5th International Symposium on Qigong, Shangai China, p. 1994:109 [cited in Sancier 1996a pp. 15–16]

Yanovski A 1962 The feasibility of alteration of cardiovascular manifestations in hypnosis. American Journal of Clinical Hypnosis 4: 8–16

Yasutami T, Hisanobu S, Shigenori S 1999 Does suggestion change the effects of qigong? Journal of International Society of Life Information Science 17(2): 284–285

Young D R, Appel L J, Jee S H 1998 The effects of aerobic exercise and tai chi on BP in the elderly. Unpublished study, reported in Natural Health, September 1998, p. 21

Yuan S, Xia B, Wang Z, Shu Y, He W, Tang J 1996 The effect of qigong on BP and vascative substances in patients with chronic nephritic hypertension. 6th International Symposium on Qigong, Shangai, China, pp. 41–42 [from San Francisco Qigong Database, Sancier 1997]

Zdravkovic G, Marciniak Z, Trocyneka, Zdrekivic U, Vukaan V 1998 Sport Medicine and Rehabilitation Clinic Risk Modification Center, St. Michael's Hospital, Toronto, Canada. Reported at 2nd World Congress on Qigong, 1998, San Francisco

Zhang T, Hou S 1993 Patients of hypertension should exercise qigong carefully. Institute of Space Medical Engineering, Rehabilitation Hospital of Qigong. Presented at 2nd World Conference for Academic Exchange of Medical Qigong, Beijing, China, p. 126e

Zinn J K 1990 Full catastrophe living: using the wisdom of your body and mind to face stress, pain and illness. Bantam Doubleday, New York

11

Laboratory research on bioenergy healing[1]

Andrew G Sparber
Cindy C Crawford
Wayne B Jonas

This chapter critically reviews laboratory research done on spiritual healing and bioenergy healing methods and gives recommendations for improvement of this research.

Most clinicians and investigators do not realize that there is a small but significant body of laboratory research on bioenergy healing in the West. This research has focused on a variety of laboratory models such as wound healing, goiter in mice, recovery times from anesthesia, and the effect of bioenergy healing on cell and plant growth. A number of authors have described this literature, but no attempt to evaluate its quality has been attempted. Most authors take the investigators' results on face value. This is risky as most of this research is done by advocates, on low budgets, and with limited review or expert input on study design and analysis. In addition, baseline variability in laboratory studies can be substantial, making multiple and independent replication attempts essential.

In this chapter, Andrew Sparber, Cindy Crawford and Wayne Jonas use pre-established criteria for evaluating the quality of laboratory research on bioenergy effects in laboratory models. These criteria include adequacy of controls,

[1]The views, opinions and assertions expressed in this chapter are those of the authors and do not reflect official policy of the Department of Defense, the Department of Health and Human Services, the National Institutes of Health, or the US government.

blinding, outcome measures, statistical analysis, lost data and independent replication. Unlike qigong literature evaluation, in which all studies were evaluated, only randomized studies with parallel control groups were selected for this data set. Thus, lower quality studies were already eliminated from the evaluation. While there are a surprising number of positive studies, even among those that met most quality criteria, the great diversity of healers used, models used, and outcomes selected prevent definitive conclusions. An independent replication was done in only a single high-quality study.   **WBJ**

BACKGROUND

The capacity of healers to use focused intention to influence biological systems has been known by ancient religious and spiritual orders throughout the world for centuries (Rein 1985, Rauscher 1980). The belief that certain individuals mediate 'supernatural' healing powers is prevalent in human cultures, whether ancient or modern, primitive or advanced (Grad et al 1961). A universal goal for these healers is to alleviate symptoms, arrest progressive disease and accelerate recuperation from all illnesses known to man (Benor 1990).

This focused intention is referred to by a number of terms, including: paranormal healing, psychic healing, psychokinesis (PK), laying-on of hands, bio-PK, external hands-on healing, non-contact therapeutic touch, healing and therapeutic touch, healing with intent, spiritual healing, bioenergy, biofield therapy, telekinesis, natural healing, distant or remote mental influence on living systems (DMILS) or Reiki (Bunnel 1999). For the purpose of simplicity the authors of this chapter will refer to these practices by the term 'bioenergy'.

Interest in the pre-scientific healing practices of non-Western communities was limited to the missionary, the venturing traveler and the anthropologist (Grad 1976). Though scientists have explored healing for over 200 years, quality methodology and technology have not been available until more recently. For at least the past 40 years investigators have systematically searched for answers concerning the claims made by psychic healers of their bioenergy abilities, in order to either corroborate or dismiss other conceivable causes of these effects.

Investigators have asked a wide range of questions about the healing effects of bioenergy in biological models. While there is ample evidence to support the hypothesis of suggestion or placebo, this does not rule out the likelihood that other mechanisms might also be operative (Grad 1961). The majority of investigators are trained in Western science, and therefore the choice of models to study and the use of measurement tools have largely come from the mainstream of biological research. Studies of growth have focused on seeds, fungi, and rodents, as well as the growth and mobility of bacteria. The secondary healing properties of bioenergy-treated water and plant growth, and the hemolysis of healthy human blood cells have also been investigated.

The healing of cancer is an age-old question that rightfully stirs much controversy. Investigators have measured the survival time of cancerous rats, alteration of the properties of cancer cells, and tumor cell proliferation, as well as goiter and amyloidosis. *In vivo* studies focused on human wound healing and regeneration of salamander limbs have also been conducted.

Another area of interest has been whether bioenergy could affect the arousal rate of anesthetized mice. Advances in immunology and molecular biology have opened up new horizons for bioenergy investigation. Some of these include the effect of bioenergy on neurotransmitters, enzymes, dihydroepiandrosterone (DHEA), cortisol, nitric oxide, calcium dynamics, and the conformation of DNA.

The purpose of this chapter is to summarize how bioenergy effects have been scientifically investigated in the laboratory and to evaluate the quality of that research. While summaries of these studies have been reported, no evaluation of study quality has been conducted. The quality of current laboratory and clinical research must be critically evaluated for factors that can reduce potential bias thus increasing the usefulness of the research information that is generated.

LITERATURE SEARCH

For the production of the bibliography on basic and laboratory research involving healing and bioenergy research we used expert summaries produced by investigators who participated in the Science and Spirituality of Healing conference held at Wake Forest University and Home Moravia Church in Winston-Salem, North Carolina, in 2000. We also conducted a comprehensive literature search on spiritual healing in MEDLINE, PSYCH LIT, EMBASE, CISCOM, and the Cochrane Library from their inception to the present. Terms used were: spiritual healing, intentionality, mental intention, energy medicine, subtle energies, faith healing, folk healing, prayer, therapeutic and healing touch, Reiki, distant healing, psychic healing, and laying-on of hands. In addition, leading researchers in the field were contacted to identify studies not found via our own searches.

Study Selection

From these, we selected studies that involved *in vitro* or *in vivo* laboratory experiments with randomization and controlled groups. Excluded from the analysis were: research briefs with minimal information; reports not available in English; studies which did not incorporate a healer; studies which did not have a parallel control group; studies which did not randomize samples between comparison groups; and studies where, after numerous attempts, the complete reference could not be obtained. We also excluded studies of the Chinese energy practice qigong and clinical trials of healing treatment of human illness as these are reviewed elsewhere in this book.

Internal Validity

We felt that a detailed evaluation of study parameters to assess the likelihood that bias might explain reported results was needed. The evaluation of study quality in systematic reviews has been extensively developed in clinical medicine though it is rarely used in laboratory research. Although evaluation criteria vary

somewhat in clinical methods, a basic set of criteria to assess what is often termed 'internal validity' has been developed (Balk et al 2002). These criteria have been assembled and applied to complementary medicine with a comprehensive scoring sheet called the 'likelihood of validity evaluations' (LOVE) scale, developed by Jonas & Linde (2002). We adapted this tool to evaluate laboratory research using the selected criteria (described below). This process was carried out by examining the presence of a variety of quality criteria in each study. We considered the percentage of positive responses to all criteria to obtain an internal validity score for each laboratory study. General categories for the LOVE scale (Table 11.1) are:

1. controls
2. randomization
3. group baseline comparability
4. blinding
5. loss of data
6. intervention
7. outcomes
8. statistical analysis
9. reproducibility.

One point is given for each of the 22 criteria of these nine categories except for a possible two points for controls depending on the composition of interveners. Subcategories are discussed in the analysis section of this chapter. Inter-rater reliability was tested with the kappa statistic on a subset of studies scored independently by two reviewers.

Though typically used for review of clinical studies, we explored the use of the Jadad scale (0–5) for quality of reporting (Jadad 1996). In this scale, one point is given for each positive response to the following questions:

1. Was the study described as randomized?
2. Was the method to generate the sequence of randomization described and was it appropriate?
3. Was the study described as double blind?
4. Was the method of double blinding described and was it appropriate?
5. Was there a description of withdrawals and drop-outs?

Table 11.1 Laboratory LOVE scale: Internal validity. How likely it is that the effects reported are due to the treatment?

		Yes	No	Unk
Controls	Comparison/control group present?			
	Parallel groups (data collected at the same time)?			
	Reasonable and convincing control procedure (2 pts mock, 1pt no mock, 0 nothing)?			
Randomization	Randomization done and method described?			
Group baseline comparability	Group comparability checked/balanced (dose animal size, age, growth or expression rates in controls, etc.)?			
Blinding	Sample allocation (cells/animals) done blind?			
	Adequacy checked?			
	Analysis done blind?			
Loss of data	Sample loss < 20%?			
	Clear distinction between pilot and confirmatory data sets?			
Intervention	Clearly detailed description (dose, time, procedure)?			
Outcomes	Clearly defined and explicit?			
	Reliability established (by reference or measured in study)?			
	Sensitivity of measurements assessed?			
	Objective measurement?			
Statistical analysis	Power calculation done and sample size achieved?			
	Descriptive stats used and effect size reported?			
	P value statistics used?			
	Confidence intervals provided?			
	Multiple outcomes corrected or NA?			
Reproducibility	More than one therapist within study?			
	Is this study an independent replication of a previous study by a different investigator?			

Total scores: yes = 1; no = 0; unk = 0. Report on % Yes

RESULTS

A search for *in vivo* and *in vitro* biological and bioenergy experiments resulted in a total of 111 studies published between the years 1956 and 2002 (Table 11.2). One hundred and eleven studies were obtained from six parapsychology journals, six 'mainstream' peer reviewed publications and a non-published graduate thesis. Of these articles 45 met the criteria for this review. No difference was found in the quality of investigations by publication date, as opposed to Astin (2002), who observed that more recent studies on 'Intercessory and healing prayer in humans' were significantly more likely to be of higher quality.

It is not possible to combine results of both the *in vivo* and *in vitro* studies because the sampling designs and models are so varied. The number of subjects of trials based on individual targets or

subjects is: animal studies (range 2–300, mean = 72.8); and seeds (range 24–1200, mean = 178.4).

A total of 38 *in vivo* and seven *in vitro* studies were identified (Table 11.3). *In vivo* studies included 15 on seeds (barley, corn, radishes, wheat, rye); eight on animals (hamster, mice, rat); five on cells (tumor, T cells, lymphocytes, red blood cells); three on bacteria (*Salmonella*, *Escherichia coli*); three on molecular (cortisol, dopamine, nitrite, DHEA, cytokines, immunoglobin A); and one on fungus (*Stereum purpureum* and *Rhizictonia solani*). *In vitro* trials included five on cells (tumor, HeLa); and two on molecular (DNA, enzymes: MAO, trypsin, pepsin).

Study Quality

Quality scores for all reviewed studies measured by the modified LOVE scale resulted in a range

Table 11.2 Results of literature search

Author	Year of publication	Model	Intervention	Quality	Author's results	Comments
Grad B	1961	animal	HT	19	++	Gentling alone does not explain healing effect
Grad B	1963	seeds	TK	18	++	Significance on day 7
Grad B	1964	seeds	TK	20	?	4 exp mean ht. and yield with saline/hands incr. 3/4 sign.
Grad B	1976	seeds	LOH	20	++	Significant effect – just holding water used in plants
Watkins G	1971	animal	PK	19	++	Experimental animal requires 87% as much time to arouse
Smith M	1972	molecular	HE	17	?	Significance – no P
Wells R	1972	animal	PK	19	+	Ave. diff. of 5.52 seconds. Exp vs. control mouse aroused
Wells R	1974	animal	PK	19	+	Significant lingering effects
McDonald R	1976	seeds	PK	18	+	27% growth and 18% growth
Lenington S	1979	seeds	Touch	16	–	Poor design
Rauscher E	1980	bacteria	HT	17	++	23% ave. diff of healer vs. control
Tedder W	1980	fungus	PK	18	++	Significant growth
Kmetz J	1981	cells	PK	17	++	Increase effect, increase in cells
Nash C	1982	bacteria	Att	18	+	Promoted and inhibited control
Solfvin, G	1982	animal	Exp	16	++	Increase effect, illness expectancy
Solfvin, G	1982	animal	Exp	17	+	Actual illness influenced expectance
Solfvin, G	1982	seeds	PK	19	–	Study design flawed
Solfvin, G	1982	seeds	PK	18	–	Study design flawed
Solfvin, G	1982	seeds	PK	19	–	Study design flawed
Solfvin G	1982	seeds	PK	17	–	Study design flawed
Solfvin, G	1982	seeds	PK	16	–	Study design flawed
Solfvin, G	1982	seeds	PK	17	–	Study design flawed
Snel, F	1983	animal	PK	18	++	Significant change in lactate dehydrase and bands
Snel, F	1983	animal	PK	19	–	Healers complained of little time given to heal
Wallack, J	1984	seeds	LOH	18	–	Unsure if negative results due to design or healer's skills
Nash, C	1984	bacteria	PK	17	++	Mutant ratio of bacteria > in promoted tubes than inhibited
Rein, G	1985	molecular	HT	20	++	Activity of enzyme decreased between 34% and 49%
Saklani, A	1989	seeds	PK	16	+	Marginal growth
Saklani, A	1989	seeds	PK	16	++	Significant height
Braud, W	1990	cells	DMILS	20	?	Significant diff $P = 1.91 \times 10^{-5}$ whose cells did not matter
Wirth, D	1990	dermal healing	TT	18	++	Significant healing
Bush, A	1992	seeds	TT	17	–	Closed seed container may have affected outcome

Continued

Table 11.2 *Continued*

Author	Year of publication	Model	Intervention	Quality	Author's results	Comments
Wirth, D	1993	dermal healing	TT	19	++	Scar formation, pigmentation and cosmetic appearance
Frans W	1995	cell	HE	18	–	Tumor weight for kind of tumor not a good measure
Frans W	1995	cell	HE	18	–	Tumor weight for kind of tumor not a good measure
Frans W	1995	cell	HE/gentling	19	–	Tumor weight for kind of tumor not a good measure
Frans w	1995	cell	DMILS	19	–	Tumor weight for kind of tumor not a good measure
Wirth D	1996	dermal healing	TT	19	+	Day 10 significant healing
Shah S	1999	cells	HE	21	++	Significant inhibition
Shah, S	1999	cells	HE	21	++	Significant inhibition
Shah, S	1999	cells	HE	21	–	Large random error
Lafmiere, K	1999	molecular	TT	17	+	Significant increase in NO by 3rd session – not other indications
Robins, J	1999	molecular	HT	18	–	No impact on care of HIV patients
Cha, K	2001	cell	Prayer	18	++	Significant increase in pregnancy
Wilkinson, D	2002	molecular	HT	19	++	Significant change – more HT training better effect

$(++) = < 0.01$
$(+) = < 0.05$
$(–) = > 0.05$
$(?)$ = uncertain

LOH = laying-on of hands
HT = Healing touch
TT = Therapeutic touch
DMILS = distance mental influence on living systems
PK = psychokinetics
HE = healing energy
Exp = expectance
TK = Teleninetic
Att = Attention

from 16 to 21 out of a maximum of 23, with a mean score of 18/23 (79%). The mean quality score by type of experiment was 18 for both *in vivo* and *in vitro* studies. There was no difference in quality score by positive/negative results, or hands-on/distant healing. Inter-rater reliability of LOVE scoring was moderate (kappa = 0.472) prior to one reviewer's training, and was excellent with a kappa score for rater agreement beyond chance of 0.942 between two independent investigators on a subset of studies once training was accomplished.

The overall mean for the Jadad scores was 2.84/5 (57%). There was no difference for the Jadad score by positive/negative results, *in vivo/in vitro*, or for hands-on or distant healing. The one Jadad item not included in the LOVE scale was a description of subjects who had withdrawn from the study (*N* = 12).

LOVE scale analysis

A surprisingly high level of internal validity was demonstrated by these studies. The following analysis presents results according to individual quality criteria evaluated to enable the reader to get a sense of how often these items were applied. A majority of the studies attempted to aim for the gold standard of research, namely randomized, controlled and blind; however, there were a few investigators who had consciously chosen alternative, yet acceptable study designs which they believed were better suited for this kind of research.

Controls. All reviewed studies used control and parallel groups to compare interventions as this was an inclusion criterion for this review. The control procedure was scored by whether there was no sham condition and the healer(s) were the only interveners (Mach I), or a true sham where an untrained 'pseudo' healer was also included to treat the control group (Mach II) to increase the quality of the study. From a total of 45 studies, there were 30 (67%) Mach I, 12 (27%) Mach II and three (6%) studies that did not have either design; thus most did not have a true sham. Mach I accounted for 18/28 (64%) positive and 12/17 (71%) negative results. Positive

studies for Mach II designs was 7/28 (25%) and 5/17 (29%) for negative trials. Investigations with neither Mach design had 3/28 (11%) positives and no negatives.

Randomization. All investigations used some kind of randomization in their overall methodology as this was an inclusion criterion.

Group baseline comparability. It is vital to have study groups checked and balanced for comparability. To help assure the validity of a study it is critical to establish a qualitative and quantitative balance of subjects and healing interventions. All of the studies met these criteria.

Blinding. Thirty-three (73%) studies stated that neither the analyst nor the practitioners and evaluators were aware of who received treatment. Twenty-eight (62%) studies checked for adequacy of the blind. Twenty-eight (62%) conducted a blind analysis. Of the 33 studies that reported sample allocation blinding, 21 were positive (63.6%), while 12 were negative (36.4%). Of the 12 studies that were not blinded, seven were positive (58%), and five were negative (41.6%). However, there was insufficient information available to adequately assess the effects of blinding.

Loss of data. Twenty-seven (60%) of the studies reported a loss of less than 20% of their data with 39 (87%) having a clear distinction between pilot and confirmatory data.

Outcomes. All 45 studies had clearly defined and explicit outcomes and used objective measures. Reliability was established for 37 (82%) and sensitivity of measurement for 37 (82%).

Statistical analysis. One of the key reasons for the high quality of these trials can be attributed to the fact that we excluded studies that were not randomized. As a result all studies used some type of statistical evaluation. All of the studies utilized descriptive statistics. The majority, 42 (93%), calculated *P* values, 27 (69%) used confidence intervals, and 44 (98%) either made corrections for multiple outcomes or were not required to make corrections due to the use of a single variable outcome. Seven studies (16%) reported the use of power calculations. This would probably be seen as a major limitation unless most of

Table 11.3 Models and designs

Models	In vivo N = 38	In vitro N = 7
Seeds	15	0
Animal	8	0
Cells	5	5
Bacteria	3	0
Molecular	3	2
Fungi	1	0

the studies were pilot or the sample or effect size were large.

Reproducibility. Thirty eight (84%) conducted a combination of experiments and 16 (36%) conducted independent replications of the investigations of others. There was little difference in results for the independently replicated studies with the quality scores averaging 18/23 (78%). However, there was only one independent replication of a single model by separate investigators that was high quality (top quartile of the LOVE score). Thus, there is a paucity of quality replication attempts in this literature by independent investigators.

Table 11.4 lists and compares all the reviewed studies as well as the top and bottom quality quartiles. In addition, it compares by type of experiment, results, and distance of healing from the target. The overall quality score of 18 is contrasted with the top quartile score of 20, and 17 for the bottom quartile. Individual differences between all of the studies and the top quartile show that for the top quartile there was higher rate of: checking adequacy of the blind, blinding of sample, inclusion of more than one experiment, use of confidence intervals, analysis blinded, and power calculations.

A comparison between the top and bottom quality quartiles shows the differences as: group baseline comparability, corrections for multiple outcomes, use of more than one therapist, and provision of confidence intervals. The three subcategories for blinding (marked in the table by an asterisk) represented the major difference between the two quartiles.

Overall, investigators reported significance ($P < 0.05$) for 28 (62%) studies which were positive (Table 11.5) and 17 (38%) investigations

generated negative or inconclusive results. All modalities of healing were categorized as either 'hands-on (physical touch or off the skin contact) or at a distance (another room and beyond) from the subjects. Results for both of these observations can be seen in Table 11.5.

SUMMARY AND DISCUSSION

A major distinction between Eastern and Western thought is the underlying philosophical differences concerning the body and healing that have arisen in their respective cultures. Eastern thought is holistic and based on an internal naturalistic appreciation of the body and nature. The Western view is rooted in a dyadic cause and effect relationship based on external observations and being separate from nature. These oppositional philosophical beliefs have paved the way for the respective medical and scientific practices of the two cultures.

There are some obvious limitations to this review. The majority of the investigations studied are small-scale studies, conducted by people interested in bioenergy healing. Though laboratory experiments are more cost-effective, there is the potential for investigators to be biased in their data selection. However, we found a fair degree of investigator integrity in the reporting of lost data.

The delivery of bioenergy appears to be far more effective if the healer is in close proximity (on-hands) to the subject or target (mean difference 54%, 95% CI from 31–76%, 1 d.f., chi-square 15.997, $P < 0.005$). Positive results for in vivo studies are more likely than for in vitro experiments, although this was not of statistical significance (mean difference of 25%, 95% CI from − 14% to 65%, 1 d.f., chi-square 1.696, $P = 0.189$). One of the gold standards in the design of this kind of research is the use of a 'mimic healer' or sham, therefore we expected that the Mach II would produce more significant results. However, our data did not bear this out. Having a body present may influence the outcome of a laboratory result even if that person does not purport to be a healer or emit 'energy', and some of the effects reported in healing studies appear to be due to simply the

Table 11.4 Comparison of all studies by quality scores (*N* (%)) and methods with top and bottom quartile studies

	Quartile		
	Total *N* = 45	Top *N* = 8	Bottom *N* = 8
Control group	45 (100)	8 (100)	8 (100)
Parallel groups	45 (100)	8 (100)	8 (100)
Group baseline comparability	45 (100)	8 (100)7	7 (88)
Adequacy checked*	28 (62)	(88)	3 (7)
Description of intervention	43 (96)	8 (100)7	7 (88)
Sample blinded*	33 (73)	(88)	2 (25)
Objective measurement	45 (100)	8 (100)	8 (100)
Descriptive statistics	45 (100)	8 (100)	8 (100)
P value statistics	42 (93)	8 (100)	7 (88)
Multiple outcomes corrected/NA	44 (98)	8 (100)	7 (88)
Outcomes clearly def/explicit	45 (100)	8 (100)	8 (100)
Randomized	45 (100)	8 (100)	8 (100)
Sensitivity of measure assessed	39 (87)	7 (88)	7 (88)
More than one experiment	38 (84)	8 (100) 3	6 (75)
Independent replication	16 (36)	(38)	2 (25)
Confidence interval provided*	27 (60)	7 (88)	4 (50)
Analysis blinded*	25 (56)	6 (75)	1 (13)
Reliability established	37 (82)	5 (63)	6 (75)
Distinction: pilot/study data sets.	39 (87)	6 (75)	7 (88)
Sample loss < 20%	27 (60)	5 (63)	5 (63)
Control procedure*			
MACH I	30 (67)	3 (38)	6 (75)
MACH II	12 (27)	5 (11)	1 (13)
Other	3 (7)	0	1
Power calculation/size met	7 (16)	2 (25)	0
Mean LOVE score	18 (80)	20 (85)	17 (73)
In vivo	38 (84)	7 (88)	6 (75)
In vitro	7 (16)	1 (13)	2 (25)
Positive	28 (62)	8 (100)	6 (75)
Hands-on	25 (56)	6 (75)	5 (63)
Distant healing	20 (44)	2 (25)	3 (38)

*Subcategories for blinding and controls (see text).

presence of a person. There is certainly a need to continue to evaluate this methodological issue. Finally, blinding did not influence the frequency of positive outcomes reported. While not often used in laboratory research, it is generally agreed to be important when investigating controversial areas such as bioenergy healing. The inclusion criteria for this study resulted in a somewhat skewed picture. However, it is expected that this review will assist in the further development of evaluation criteria and scales to measure the quality of CAM laboratory research.

Because of the more stringent selection criteria for this review, the quality of these investigations were higher than those reported in the evaluation of the qigong laboratory research reviewed

Table 11.5 Study designs, bioenergy interventions and results

N = 45	Positive *N* (%)	Negative *N* (%)
P = < 0.05	28 (62)	17 (38)
In vivo (38)	25 (66)	13 (34)
In vitro (7)	3 (43)	4 (57)
Hands-on (25)	23 (92)	2 (8)
Distant (20)	5 (25)	15 (75)

elsewhere in this book. Overall, there were a significant number of positive results from these randomized and controlled studies. Though other chapters in this book also reviewed randomized controlled studies, it is not possible to compare this analysis to those sections. However it does provide a baseline that can be used for establishing criteria for future research. Publication bias is certainly an important issue here as evidence suggests that such biases are quite common and can significantly alter the results of meta-analyses and systematic reviews. It should also be noted that reverse publication bias, particularly in a controversial area such as bioenergy, does occur (Resch 2000). Furthermore, there are also a limited number of investigators in the field which has resulted in few high-quality independent replications.

An unanswered yet significant concern pertinent to all biomedical research is determining when there is adequate verification regarding efficacy of a specific intervention. The case against the claims made by those in the bioenergy field is for the need of 'extraordinary evidence.' There must be a level field in which objectively to evaluate the 'extraordinary' assertions made by healers and investigators. There is no room for a double standard as all therapies should be evaluated by their outcomes. Certainly independent replications should be a criterion for acceptance, but the amount of research done in this field so far has not provided for that. Because bioenergy laboratory experiments can be conducted under tightly controlled laboratory conditions at a relatively low cost, they may serve as convenient models for such replication and to help us better understand the relevant conditions and mechanism of bioenergy healing (Astin, 2002).

If there were a negative correlation between measures of methodological quality and study outcomes, it would imply that apparently significant results were potentially due to flaws in experimental design. Alternatively, significant investigations tend to be published in more detail than non-significant studies, in which case one might anticipate seeing a positive correlation between study quality and outcomes. If instead no correlation were observed between quality and study effects, then it would seem that methodological quality was not a significant factor in producing non-random results (Astin 2002). Our results support the notion that there are many well-designed and implemented bioenergy healing laboratory experiments. Positive results were documented even in the most rigorous and elegantly designed studies.

For clinicians, there is always the question of the relevance and transferability of basic laboratory research to clinical care. The future and acceptance of bioenergy research may be based on studies that can simultaneous measure biological indicators with clinical outcomes. The field of molecular biology is already providing new tools which will begin to bridge the 'believability gap.' An example of this new direction is the study by Kiang et al (2002) on the effects of bioenergy on intracellular free calcium concentration as it relates to cellular response to heat stress. These investigators found that that bioenergy can upregulate $[Ca^{2+}]$ and downregulate the cellular response to stress which may be a helpful indicator for the presence of this phenomenon. Though understanding the underlying mechanism of action may take time, other important questions will begin to be answered. Better research designs are needed that can decrease baseline variability. Qian (2000) designed a study where alternating trials compared control treatment to simultaneous controls (sham/sham trials) with trials comparing qigong treatment to simultaneous controls (qigong/sham trials). This design helped to further rule out 'other causes' for bioenergy and supported the assertion that changes in the growth of cultured human brain cells can be measured following qigong.

FUTURE DIRECTIONS

Whether investigators were able successfully to answer key research issues or not, we are left with a list of challenging questions that are in the process of being addressed. Because of the nature of bioenergy there is a need to further explore the bidirectional relationship that can exist between healer and client. We hear much about practitioner consciousness and the impact of different states of consciousness. There is a suggestion that there is a lingering effect that remains in the area or on the subject after healing. How can we design studies to measure this phenomenon and what are the implications for bioenergy research? Are there cumulative effects of bioenergy and how can we understand the qualitative and quantitative differences between distant and 'hands-on' healing? There is also a question about the use of blinding. Will this gold standard stand up to the test of bioenergy investigation? Measurement is one of the keys to success. The field needs reliable and sensitive measurement tools that can help bridge the believability gap. One of the common themes in CAM research is Western science's goal to reduce therapy to a simple and repeatable intervention. There is a need to design studies that can more closely resemble how modalities in healing are actually used by practitioners in the field rather than by an agreed upon formula. Scientists investigating the healing effects of bioenergy can now join the good company of adventure seeking missionaries, venturing travelers and anthropologists. A growing body of knowledge, supported by well-designed studies, highlights the complexities of studying the healing effects of bioenergy in the laboratory. Perhaps this evidence will ultimately provide the support necessary to bring these studies from the bench to the bedside, alleviating the symptoms and progression of disease, improving quality of life, and accelerating the recuperation time from illness.

REFERENCES

Astin J 2002 Intercessory prayer and healing prayer in humans: a systematic review of randomized placebo-controlled studies. In: Chez R (ed) Proceedings October 2000: the science and spirituality of healing. pp. 20–31, 277–285

Balk E M, Bonis P A L, Moskowitz H et al 2002 Correlation of quality measures with estimates of treatment effect in meta-analyses of randomized controlled trials. Journal of the American Medical Association 287: 2973–2982

Benor D J 1990 Survey of spiritual healing research. Complementary Medicine Research 4(3): 9–33

Braud W 1990 Distant mental influence of rate of hemolysis of human red blood cells. Journal of the American Society for Psychical Research 84(1): 1–24

Braud W, Davis G, Wood R 1979 Experiments with Mathew Manning. Journal of the American Society for Psychical Research 50(782): 199–223

Braud W, Shafer D, Andrews S 1992 Further studies of autonomic detection of remote staring: replication of new control procedure and personality correlations. In: Roll W, Morris R, Morris J (eds) Research in Parapsychology. Scarecrow Press, Metuchen, NJ, pp. 1–6

Bunnell T 1999 The effect of 'healing with intent' on pepsin activity. Journal of Scientific Exploration 13: 139–148

Bush A, Geist C 1992 Geophysical variables and behavior: LXX, PK effect of TT on germinating corn seed. Psychological Reports 70: 891–896

Cha K, Wirth D, Lobo R 2001 Does prayer influence the success of in vitro fertilization-embryo. Journal of Reproductive Medicine 46(9): 781–787

Grad B 1963 A telekinetic effect on plant growth. Internal Journal of Parapsychology 5 (Spring): 117–133

Grad B 1964 A telekinetic effect on plant growth: 11. Experiments involving treatment of saline in stoppered bottles. International Journal of Parapsychology 6(Autumn): 473–498

Grad B 1976 The laying on of hands: implication for psychotherapy, gentling and the placebo effect. Journal of the American Society for Psychical Research 61(4): 287–305

Grad B, Cadoret R, Paul G I 1961 An unorthodox method of treatment on wound healing in mice. Internal Journal of Parapsychology 4, 5–19

Jadad A R, Moore R A, Jenkinson C et al 1996 Assessing the quality of reports of randomized clinical trials: is blinding necessary? Control Clinical Trials 17: 1–12

Jonas W B, Linde K 2002 Conducting and evaluating clinical research in complementary and alternative medicine. In: Gallin J (ed) Principles and practice of clinical research. Academic Press, New York, pp 401–426

Kiang J, Marotta D, Wirkus M, Wirkus M, Jonas W 2002 External bioenergy increases intracellular free calcium concentration and reduces cellular response to heat stress. Journal of Investigative Medicine 50(1): 38–45

Kmetz J 1981 Effects of healing on cancer cells (Appendix). In: Kraft D (ed) Portrait of a psychic healer. Putnam, New York, pp. 181–185

Lafrniere K, Mutus B, Cameron S et al 1999 Effects of TT on biochemical and mood indications in women mood indicators. Journal of Alternative and Complementary Medicine 5(4): 367–370

Lenington S 1979 Effect of holy water on the growth of radish plants. Psychological Reports 45: 381–382

McDonald R G, Hickman J L, Dakin H S 1976 Preliminary studies with three alleged psychic healers. In: Roll W, Morris R, Morris J (eds) Research in parapsychology. Scarecrow Press, Metuchen, NJ, pp. 74–76

Nash C B 1982 Psychokinetic control of bacterial growth. Journal of the American Society for Psychical Research 51: 217–221

Nash C B 1984 Test of psychokinetic control of bacterial growth. Journal of the American Society for Psychical Research 78(2): 145–152

Qian Y, Solfvin J, Yount G 2000 Methods and issues of laboratory research. In: Chez R (ed) Proceedings October 2000: the science and spirituality of healing. pp. 277–285

Rauscher E 1980 Human volitional effects on a model bacterial system. Subtle Energies 1(1): 21–41

Rein G 1985 A PK effect on neurotransmitter metabolic alterations in the degradation of enzymes, MAO. In: Roll W, Morris R, Morris J (eds) Research in parapsychology. Scarecrow Press, Metuchen, NJ, pp. 77–79

Resch K I, Ernst E, Garrow J 2000 A randomized controlled study of reviewer bias against an unconventional therapy. Journal of the Royal Society of Medicine 93(4): 164–167

Robins J 1999 Psychoneuroimmunology and healing touch in HIV disease. Unpublished Doctoral dissertation, Virginia Commonwealth University Ricunoud, Virginia, USA

Saklani A 1989 PK effects on plant growth: further studies. In: Roll W, Morris R, Morris J (eds) Research in parapsychology. Scarecrow Press, Metuchen, NJ, pp. 37–41

Schmidt S, Schneider R, Binder M et al (in press) Investigating methodology issues in EDA-DMILS: results from a pilot study. Journal of Parapsychology

Shah S, Ogden A, Pettker C, Raffo A, Itescu S, Oz M 1999 A study of the effect of energy healing on *in vitro* tumor cell proliferation. Journal of Alternative and Complementary Medicine 5(4): 359–365

Smith M J 1972 Paranormal effects on enzyme activity. Human Dimensions 1: 15–19

Snell F 1983 PK experiments in case induced amyloidosis on the hamster. European Journal of Parapsychology 5: 51–76

Snel F, Van Der Sude P 1995 The effect of paranormal healing on tumor growth. Journal of Scientific Exploration 9(2): 209–221

Solfvin G F 1982 PSI expectancy effects in psychic healing studies with malarial mice. European Journal of Parapsychology 4(3): 159–197

Solfvin G 1982 Studies of the effects of mental healing and expectations on the growth of corn seedlings. European Journal of Parapsychology 4(3): 287–323

Tedder W, Monty M 1980 Exploration of long-distance PK: a conceptual replication of the influence on a biological system. In: Roll W, Morris R, Morris J (eds) Research in parapsychology. Scarecrow Press, Metuchen, NJ, pp. 90–93

Wallack J M 1984 Testing for a PK effect on plants: effect of laying on of hands on germinating seeds. Psychological Reports 55: 15–18

Watkins G K, Watkins A M 1971 Possible PK influence on the resuscitation of anesthetized mice. Journal of Parapsychology 35(4): 257–272

Wells R, Klein J 1972 A replication of a psychic healing paradigm. Journal of Parapsychology 36: 144–149

Wells R, Watkins G 1974–5 Lingering effects in several PK experiments. In: Roll W, Morris R, Morris J (eds) Research in parapsychology. Scarecrow Press, Metuchen, NJ, pp. 143–147

Wilkinson D, Knox P, Chatman J et al 2002 The clinical effectiveness of healing touch. Journal of Alternative and Complementary Medicine 8(1): 33–47

Wirth D 1990 The effect of non-contact TT on the healing rate of full thickness dermal wounds. Subtle Energies 1(1): 1–20

Wirth D 1996 The effect of non-contact TT on the healing rate of full thickness dermal wounds: a replication. Complementary Therapies in Medicine 4: 237–240

Wirth D, Richardson J T, Eidelman W S et al 1993 The effect of non-contact TT on the healing rate of full thickness dermal wounds: a replication and extension. Complementary Therapies in Medicine 1: 127–132

12

The therapeutic effects of music

David Aldridge

This chapter summarizes the current research on the therapeutic effect of music.

Many healing rituals and spiritual practices use music to convey mood and communicate non-verbal messages. Music is truly informational in the sense that the same amount of energy is similar from tune to tune, but the difference in effect can be profound. In this chapter, David Aldridge provides a narrative review of what are mostly observational (non-controlled) studies on the theraputic effect of music.　**WBJ**

INTRODUCTION

Music therapy has risen to the challenge of research in recent years. Not only is there a tradition of quantitative research but qualitative research approaches have also been incoprorated within the discipline, as is necessary for a clinical approach that involves both science and art (Aldridge D 1996, Dileo 1999, Pratt & Erdonmez-Grocke 1999, Pratt & Spintge 1996, Wigram et al 1995b).

HOSPITAL BASED OVERVIEWS

After the Second World War, music therapy was intensively developed in American hospitals. Since then, some hospitals, particularly in mainland Europe, have incorporated music therapy within their practice carrying on a tradition of European hospital based research and practice.

The nursing profession particularly in the United States, has seen the value of music therapy, and championed its use as an important nursing intervention even when music therapists are not available. Indeed, a clinical nurse specialist has produced an overview of 14 articles on audioanalgesia (Bechler-Karsch 1993). She reports a confusing picture of changes related to heart rate, but a clearer picture emerges on physiological parameters related to pain and anxiety, and she concludes that music has no adverse effects on ill patients when used as an adjunctive non-invasive therapy.

Standley (1986, 1995), who has consistently reviewed the literature relating to music therapy applications in medical settings, carried out a meta-analysis of the current findings from 55 studies utilizing 129 dependent variables (Standley 1995). Standley concludes (p. 4) that the average therapeutic effect of music in medical treatment is almost one standard deviation greater than treatment without music (0.88). From these results she generalizes that women react more favorably to music than men, as do children compared with adults. While music is less effective for severe pain, it is indicated for chronic pain. Live music administered by a music therapist has a greater effect than recorded music and the effect sizes vary according to the dependent measure being used, physiological measures being stronger than subjective assessment.

During the 1990s there were numerous writings relating to the clinical application of music therapy, often from symposia (Pratt & Erdonmez-Grocke 1999, Pratt & Spintge 1996), and the development of research strategies suitable to clinical application (Aldridge D 1996, Wheeler 1995).

PSYCHIATRY AND PSYCHOTHERAPY

The published work covering psychiatry has its basis in hospital treatment (Wigram et al 1995a).

In a study of chronic psychiatric patients who exhibited disruptive and violent behavior at meal times, the playing of taped music as a background stimulus with the intention of providing a relaxed atmosphere reduced the disruptive behavior (Courtright et al 1990). Meschede and colleagues (1983) observed the behavior of a group of chronic psychiatric patients over 8 weeks of active music-making sessions and discovered that the subjective feelings of the patients had no correlation with the observations of the group leaders about the outward expression of those feelings.

Continental Europe has encouraged the use of music, particularly in terms of individual and group psychotherapy, to encourage the awakening of the emotions of patients and to help them cope with unconscious intrapsychic conflicts. This is unsurprising given that the roots of psychoanalysis are middle European. Group psychotherapy has been used on both an inpatient and an outpatient basis

Schizophrenia

Schizophrenia has been the subject of varying studies in applied music therapy (Aigen 1990, Glicksohn & Cohen 2000, Hadsell 1974, Pavlicevic & Trevarthen 1989, Pavlicevic et al 1994, Tang et al 1994).

Within recent years, researchers have attempted to understand the musical production of schizophrenic patients (Steinberg & Raith 1985a, 1985b; Steinberg et al 1985) in terms of emotional response. The underlying reasoning in this work is: first, to produce music depends upon the mastery of underlying feelings; and second, in psychiatric patients musical expression is negatively influenced by the disease. Steinberg and colleagues found that in the musical playing of endogenous-depressive patients there were weakened motoric qualities influencing stability and rhythmicity, while manic patients also exhibited difficulties in ending a phrase with falling intensity. Tempo appeared uninfluenced by depression, but was susceptible to the influence of medication. Schizophrenic patients exhibited changes in the dimensions of musical logic and order.

More recently, Pavlicevic & Trevarthen (1989) compared the musical playing of 15 schizophrenic patients, 15 depressed patients, and 15 clinically normal controls. Significant differences in musical interaction between therapist and patient were found between the groups on a self-developed scale to test musical interaction. This musical interaction scale was developed to assess the emotional contact between therapist and partner according to musical criteria based upon six levels of interaction ranging from no contact (level 1) to established mutual contact (level 6). A critical element of the musical contact is the establishment of a common musical pulse which is defined as a series of regular beats.

In the above study, schizophrenic patients appeared musically unresponsive and idiosyncratic in their playing, which correlates with other studies of schizophrenia (Fraser et al 1986, Lindsay 1993). The depressed patients appeared to make fewer initiatives in the music although it was possible for the therapist to make contact with them. Controls were able to enter into a musical partnership with the therapist and take musical initiatives. The lack of reciprocity from the schizophrenic patients seemed to be the factor which prevented contact and thereby disturbed communication. However, this finding with individual patients is in contrast to the previously mentioned group studies which refer to 'open' communication within the group. The strength of the Pavlicevic & Trevarthen paper is that it is firmly grounded in empirical data and, unlike many of the group therapy papers, gives clear evidence of how conclusions have been reached.

The peculiarities of language which accompany some forms of schizophrenia have led to the inevitable link between speech disorders and musical components of language and the processing of language and musical information. Fraser's study (Fraser et al 1986) suggested that the speech of schizophrenics had fewer well formed sentences, often contained errors with many false starts, and was simpler than the speech of controls which was fluent, error free, and complex. Lindsay (1980) argues that social behavior is dependent upon social language skills of communication. Withdrawn patients speak with less spontaneous speech utterances, and their speech is improved by matching their utterances and building up dialogues from simple interactions to complex sequences, which is a feature of dialogic playing in improvised music therapy.

Adolescent psychiatry

Group music therapy is the principal music therapy approach to the treatment of adolescents. Friedman & Glickman (1986) recommend the use of creative therapies in general for the treatment of drug abuse in adolescents as it encourages spontaneous activity, motivates the client's response, and fosters a culture of free expression.

Phillips (1988), as psychotherapist and jazz fan, provides an overview of improvization in psychotherapy and the way in which it relates to adolescent patients. He identifies four important qualities as bases which enable the therapist to improvize in clinical practice:

1. to have access to his or her past
2. to be able to focus attention solely on the present
3. to be comfortable enough to give up control over the outcome of the task to experiment during the session
4. to recognize the significance of accidental expression (p. 184).

He relates this ability to improvize to the therapeutic task of treating adolescents who call upon a wide range of responses which relate to the past experience of the therapist and which may require quite novel solutions.

Culture

References to the use of music therapy in medicine are predominantly Western, although the use of music as a therapeutic medium is found in most cultures. Two papers (Benjamin 1983, Devisch & Vervaeck 1986) describe the use of music in African hospitals, both locating the use of music within a cultural context, and combining this music with drama and dance. As in other group therapy methods, music is used as a vehicle to reach those who are isolated and withdrawn and reintegrate them into social relationships.

In South Africa (Benjamin 1983) the group consisted of about 100 female patients sitting in a circle directed by a doctor. Music, through increasing tempo in singing and dancing, was used as an activator for the psychodrama techniques of Moreno (1946).

A Tunisian approach was far more radical in terms of psychiatry. Through 'art group therapy' (Devisch & Vervaeck 1986) utilizing dance, painting, clay, role play and singing, patients were encouraged to integrate personal experiences and emotions within a social context of relationships. The explanatory principle behind this work is that of 'the door' whereby fixed barriers between experiences are broken down, but the concept of threshold between experiences remains. In support of this integration family members of patients can be included in the singing and dancing to facilitate the patient returning to a family or wider social environment. For the individual patient it is argued that individual expression, when given the form of a work of art (to include singing and dancing), allows people to experience themselves as orderly and subjective, and, like a door, able to be opened or closed to others and participate in interaction. This ability to discriminate between activities was called by the authors (social anthropologists) 'the liminal or threshold function of the body and the door' (p. 543). Such an approach attempts to establish a meaningful relationship between the inner rhythms of the body, outer rhythms of personal interaction, and broader patterns of cultural activity.

The Arab tradition, which regards the body as the meeting place of psyche and soma, and locates psychiatric illness within social relationships, gives cultural support to the ideas practiced in such an institution. Culture is a source of meaning which acts not only through cognition, but also through personal interaction. The way in which people greet each other, listen to each other, and play with each other structures the meaning of that interaction and has a direct experience on the body. Similarly, bodily experiences shape social contact. The act of kissing as a greeting, for example, has an external effect on a relationship, and an internal effect on the emotional experiences of the body. This symbolic reality is not restricted solely to cognitive activity. We can further infer that the playing of music, and encouraging someone to express themselves in an articulate form within a relationship, promotes experiences which integrate the person inwardly within themselves, and outwardly with others independent from cognition.

Rehabilitation

Strategies for rehabilitating psychiatric patients using group and family approaches are not solely confined to African traditions (Barker & Brunk 1991, Glassman 1991, Longhofer & Floersch 1993) and music therapy has a broad base within the tradition of psychiatric and general rehabilitation (Aldridge 1993b, Pavlicevic et al 1994, Pratt & Spintge 1996, Purdie & Baldwin 1995, Purdie et al 1997).

Haag & Lucius (1984) discuss theories including psychosocial factors involved in the development of, and coping with, disability. Psychological intervention approaches are set out, focusing on their particular relevance to rehabilitation. Music therapy is also recommended for the rehabilitation of patients who have difficulty in expressing their feelings and communicating with others.

Psychosomatics

Where both physical and mental processes overlap within medicine (i.e. the field of psychosomatics), then individual and group music therapy appears to play an important role.

Multiple sclerosis is a chronic neurological disease of unknown origin which can result in severe neuropsychological symptoms. Difficulties of anxiety, resignation, isolation, and failing self-esteem seen in this disease are not easily relieved by symptom-oriented medication or physiotherapy. Lengdobler & Kiessling (1989) set out to treat in a clinic, over a 2 year period, 225 patients with multiple sclerosis with group music therapy. Each treatment period lasted 4–6 weeks. A further part of their work was to discover the musical parameters of the playing of such patients using methods which were based on active improvization: group instrumental playing, singing, listening, and free-painting to music. Unfortunately the size of the groups is not recorded, patient attendance at the groups was uncontrolled, and the reports made by the patients were unstructured. The vagueness of the reports has prompted other clinicians to pursue more rigorous research (Magee 1998, O'Callaghan 1996, O'Callaghan & Turnbull 1987).

THE ELDERLY

The psychosocial rehabilitation of older people is one of the main problems in health policy. About one-quarter of those aged over 65 face psychosocial problems without receiving adequate treatment and rehabilitative care. Substantial deficits exist above all in the outpatient and non-residential service sector, and the development of ambulatory, community-based services as well as intensive support for existing self-help efforts are necessary. Music therapy has been suggested as a valuable part of a combined treatment policy for the elderly (Aldridge 2000).

Music and Dementia in the Elderly

The responsiveness to music of patients with Alzheimer's disease is a remarkable phenomenon (Aldridge 1993a, 1994, 1995; Aldridge & Brandt 1991). While language deterioration is a feature of cognitive deficit, musical abilities appear to be preserved. Beatty et al (1988) describe a woman who had severe impairments in terms of aphasia, memory dysfunction, and apraxia, yet was able to sight read an unfamiliar song and perform on the xylophone which to her was an unconventional instrument. In a doctoral thesis Foster (1998) demonstrated an improvement in autobiographical memory in dementia sufferers compared to normal controls with an auditory background condition of music. He suggests that it is the arousal due to experiencing music that facilitates improved cognition and that the patient is dependent upon environmental cues.

Certainly the anecdotal evidence suggests that the quality of life of Alzheimer's patients is significantly improved with music therapy, accompanied by the overall social benefits of acceptance and sense of belonging gained by communicating with others. Prinsley (1986) recommends music therapy for geriatric care in that it reduces the individual prescription of tranquilizing medica-

tion, reduces the use of hypnotics on the hospital ward, and helps overall rehabilitation. Music therapy is based on treatment objectives: social goals of interaction and cooperation; psychological goals of mood improvement and self-expression; intellectual goals of the stimulation of speech and organization of mental processes; and physical goals of sensory stimulation and motor integration. Such approaches also emphasize the benefit of music programs for the professional carers and families of elderly patients.

There has been recent research related to music and its influence upon patients suffering with various forms of dementia, and particularly the influence of music therapy in the treatment of Alzheimer's disease (Aldridge 2000).

Research Approaches to New Treatments

Until recently, psychotherapy and counseling techniques had rarely been used with people with dementia. However, the change in emphasis within dementia care towards a person-centered approach, and often a non-pharmacological approach, has meant that there is a growing clinical interest in the use of these techniques (Beck 1998, Bender & Cheston 1997, Bonder 1994, Cheston 1998, Johnson et al 1992, Richarz 1997). This has also meant an increase in studies using creative arts therapies (Kamar 1997, Mango 1992) and overviews of music therapy as a treatment approach to Alzheimer's disease have already been written (Aldridge 2000, Brotons et al 1997, Brotons & Pickettcooper 1996, Smeijsters 1997). What music therapy offers is an improvement in communication skills for both sufferer and family caregiver, and possibilities for managing the disruption and agitation often found in the later stages of disease.

People with Alzheimer's disease often experience depression, anger, and other psychological symptoms. Various forms of psychotherapy have been attempted with these individuals, including insight-oriented therapy and less verbal therapies such as music therapy and art therapy. Although there are few databased outcome studies that support the effectiveness of these interventions, case studies and descriptive information suggest that they can be helpful in alleviating negative emotions and minimizing problematic behaviors (Bonder 1994).

Although there is a developing clinical literature on intervention techniques drawn from all the main psychotherapeutic approaches, there has been little research into the effectiveness of this work and such research as does exist often uses methodologies that are inappropriate for such an early stage of clinical development. While some authors (Cheston 1998) argue that clinical research should adopt case study or single-case designs, some researchers are also planning group designs for evaluating new clinical developments. My argument is for a broad spectrum of research designs that will satisfy differing needs. We know from experience that music therapy brings benefits to sufferers and the challenge is to convert this knowledge into evidential studies.

Annenmiek Vink (Aldridge 2000) focuses on the treatment of agitation in Alzheimer's disease using music therapy and her current work is in the administration of a controlled study in The Netherlands. The success of such a venture may have a profound effect upon the political acceptance of music therapy as a non-pharmacological treatment modality, should the results be of significance. I am tentative about suggesting how strong the impact of such research trials will be as there is never any guarantee that such studies will be heeded. More importantly, if such a study discovers that a control musical condition is almost as effective as music therapy then there may be support for using music in treatment settings but not necessarily music therapists. Given that music therapists are a professional group with their own pay scales then while the argument for using musical initiative may be strong, the argument for employing music specialists may be weak. Research, and its results, are rarely neutral in their effect.

However, qualitative understanding of how musical playing changes also offers profound insights into the relief of suffering. We simply cannot restrict our endeavors to one particular form of understanding. Differing research approaches will inform one another and the challenge is for us to coordinate our approaches so that the knowledge gained is pooled and shared. It is to such an end that this book is aimed.

Patients and Caregivers in Dementia Care

In the absence of definitive treatments for Alzheimer's disease and related dementias, researchers in a variety of disciplines are developing psychosocial and behavioral intervention strategies to help patients and caregivers better manage and cope with the troublesome symptoms common in these conditions. These strategies include cognitive interventions, functional performance interventions, environmental interventions, integration of self-interventions, and pleasure-inducing interventions. Although we have seen that more research is needed to further develop these strategies and establish their best use, psychosocial and behavioral interventions hold great promise for improving the quality of life and well-being of dementia patients and their family caregivers (Beck 1998).

We know that people who are suffering do not suffer alone (Aldridge 1998, 1999). It is in a primary care setting that dementia is generally recognized, and early recognition is important for initiating treatment interventions before a person becomes permanently or semi-permanently institutionalized and to minimize disability (Larson 1998). There is an increasing expectation that the community will care for its elderly infirm, although this expectation is rarely met by financial resources to support such caregiving, placing the caregivers under stress, while relieving the community budget in the short term.

Recent research on caregiver stress focuses extensively on its predictors and health consequences, especially for family members of those with dementia. Gwyther & Strulowitz (1998) suggest four areas of caregiver stress research: caregiver health outcomes, differential impacts of social support, caregiving for family members with dementia, and balancing work and caregiving responsibilities.

In a study by Harris (Harris 1998), in-depth interviews with 30 sons actively involved in caring for a parent with dementia elicit the understanding of a son's caregiving experiences. Common themes that emerge from such narratives are a sense of duty, acceptance of the situation, and having to take charge, as well as issues regarding loss, a change in relationships with other brothers and sisters, the reversal of role based on having to take charge, and the necessity to develop coping strategies.

In another study of the psychological well-being of caregivers of demented elderly people (Pot et al 1997), three groups of caregivers were identified: those providing care for 2 years after baseline; those whose care-recipient died within the first year after baseline; and those whose care-recipient was institutionalized within the first year. All three groups showed a great deal of psychological distress compared to a general population sample, with an overall deterioration of psychological well-being. As the elderly patient declined and the caregiving at home continued, then psychological distress increased. For caregivers whose demented care-recipient had died or was institutionalized in the first year after baseline then there was no deterioration. There is, then, a high level of psychological distress and deterioration in psychological well-being among informal caregivers of dementia patients and we may have to reconsider the personal and social costs of demented older people living on their own as long as possible if we are not able to release adequate resources to support the caregivers.

Part of this support will include sharing information and developing methods of counseling appropriate to caregivers. Increasing public awareness, coupled with the wider availability of drug therapies for some dementing conditions, means that carers are often informed of the diagnosis of dementia. However, it is unclear how many of the sufferers of dementia are told about the diagnosis. In a study of how sufferers of dementia were given diagnostic information among 71 carers recruited through old age psychiatry services in East Anglia, England, only half of the sufferers had learned their diagnosis, more from their carers than their doctors (Heal & Husband 1998). The age of the sufferer was found to be related to whether or not doctors told them their diagnosis, which supports a suspicion that there is a prejudice among doctors

regarding the elderly and what they can understand. Only 21% of carers were given an opportunity to discuss the issues involved and younger carers were significantly more likely to feel that such an opportunity would have been useful. Most of the carers who had informed the sufferer said that the sufferer had wanted to know, or needed a meaningful explanation for their difficulties, rather than giving more practical legal or financial reasons. Carers who had not disclosed feared that diagnostic information would cause too much distress, or that the sufferer's cognitive impairments were too great an obstacle.

Emotional context and ability

As the course of degenerative disease progresses there is a decline in the ability to comprehend and express emotion that is linked with mental impairment (Benke et al 1998). The creative arts therapies have based some of their interventions on the potential for promoting emotional expression and retaining expressive abilities.

Depression

Depression is a common disorder in the elderly (Forsell 1998). The rate of treatment of depression in the very elderly is low, exaggerated among dementia sufferers, and the course is chronic or relapsing in almost half of the cases. The interface between depression and dementia is complex and has been studied primarily in Alzheimer's disease (Aldridge 1993b) where depression may be a risk factor for the expression of Alzheimer's disease in later life (Raskind 1998). A contributory factor to this depression is the patients' perceptions of their own deficits, although these may be ill-founded (Tierney et al 1996). Emotional context is an important factor and this will be linked to the way in which the patient sees his or her current life situation and understanding of what life holds in the near future.

Hearing impairment

If depression is a confounding factor in recognizing cognitive degeneration, then hearing impairment is another contributory factor. Central auditory test abnormalities may predict the onset of clinical dementia or cognitive decline. Hearing loss significantly lowered performance on the verbal parts of the Mini-Mental State Examination, a standard test for the presence of dementia (Gates et al 1996). Central auditory dysfunction precedes senile dementia in a significant number of cases and may be an early marker for senile dementia. Gates et al recommend that hearing tests should be included in the evaluation of people older than 60 years and in those suspected of having cognitive dysfunction. If this is so then we may have to include this consideration in designs of research studies of music therapy as perhaps the patients are not actually hearing what is being played but responding to social contact and gesture. However, encouraging musical participation may foster residual hearing abilities and those abilities that the tests cannot measure. Returning to developmentally-challenged children, where hearing disability was ever present, it was the joint attention involved in making music that brought about an improvement in listening that appeared as an improvement in hearing. This is perhaps a feature of active music therapy that needs to be further investigated.

What Happens in Treating Dementia Patients with Music Therapy

Most music therapists have concentrated on the pragmatic effects of music therapy. As we will see, practitioners and researchers alike are concerned with demonstrating the benefits of music therapy for dementia sufferers. However, how music therapy actually achieves its effects is relatively unresearched.

My hypothesis is that music offers an alternative form for structuring time that fails in working memory. Just as developmentally delayed children achieve a working memory that enhances their cognitive ability, then the reverse process occurs in dementia sufferers.

While several components of working memory may be affected, not all aspects of the central executive mechanism are necessarily influenced (Collette et al 1998). White & Murphy (1998) suggest that tone perception remains intact, but

there is a progressive decline in working memory for auditory non-verbal information with advancing Alzheimer's disease. A similar decline was also noted on a task assessing working memory for auditory presented verbal information. This ties in with what we know about hearing impairment and again encourages a test of hearing capabilities before music therapy is used as a treatment modality but also suggests that music therapy may promote improved hearing.

Temporal coherence

I argued earlier that music therapy offers an external sense of temporal coherence that is failing in the patient. Ellis (1996) reports on the linguistic features and patterns of coherence in the discourse of mild and advanced Alzheimer's patients. As the disease progresses, the discourse of Alzheimer's patients becomes pre-grammatical in that it is vocabulary driven and reliant on meaning-based features of discourse rather than grammatically based features. Temporal coherence fails. Knott et al (1997), considering the short-term memory performance of patients with semantic dementia, suggest that impaired semantic processing reduces the 'glue' or 'binding' that helps to maintain a structured sequence of phonemes in short-term memory. We may speculate that this temporal coherence, the metaphoric glue or binding, is replaced by musical form. As we know, some songs stick to our memories.

No loss of semantic memory

Repetition ability depends in part on semantic memory remaining intact. If the conceptual contents of semantic memory are lost as a function of Alzheimer's disease, meaningfulness of stimuli should have progressively less effect on the ability to repeat as the disease worsens. A study by Bayles et al (1996) was designed to evaluate the effects of meaningfulness and length of phrasal stimuli on repetition ability in mild and moderate Alzheimer's disease patients and normal elderly subjects. Fifty-seven Alzheimer's disease patients and 52 normal subjects were given six- and nine-syllable phrases that were meaningful, improbable in meaning, or meaningless. Cross-sectional and longitudinal data analyses were conducted and results failed to confirm a performance pattern consistent with a semantic memory loss theory.

Several lines of evidence suggest that in Alzheimer's disease there is a progressive degradation of the hierarchical organization of semantic memory. When clustering and switching on phonemic and semantic fluency tasks were correlated with the numbers of correct words generated on both fluency tests, the contribution of clustering was greater on the semantic task. Patients with Alzheimer's disease generated fewer correct words and made fewer switches than controls on both fluency tests. The average size of their semantic clusters was smaller and the contribution of clustering to word generation was less than for controls. Severity of dementia was correlated with the numbers of correct words and switches, but not with cluster size. The structure of semantic memory in Alzheimer's disease is probably degraded but there is no evidence that this process is progressive. Instead, progressive worsening of verbal fluency in Alzheimer's disease seems to be associated with the deterioration of mechanisms that govern initiation of search for appropriate subcategories (Beatty et al 1997). This pattern can be interpreted as reflecting significantly impaired procedural routines in Alzheimer's disease, with relative sparing of the structure of semantic memory (Chenery 1996).

No loss of source memory

A source memory task, using everyday objects in actions performed by either the participant or the experimenter, was given to probable Alzheimer's disease and elderly normal individuals. When the overall recognition performance of the two groups was made equivalent by increasing the test delay intervals for the control group, both groups of participants showed similar patterns of correct and incorrect responses. Moreover, both groups showed evidence of a generation effect and of an advantage for items repeated at study. The findings of this study suggest that, for a given level of event memory, memory for the source of the events is comparable between the elderly normal and individuals with Alzheimer's disease (Brustrom & Ober 1996).

Contextual cues

Two experiments examined whether impairments in recognition memory in early stage Alzheimer's disease were due to deficits in encoding contextual information (Rickert et al 1998). Normal elderly people and patients diagnosed with mild Alzheimer's disease learned one of two tasks. In an initial experiment, correct recognition memory required participants to remember not only what items they had experienced on a given trial but also when they had experienced them. A second experiment required that participants remembered only what they had seen, not when they had seen it. Large recognition memory differences were found between the Alzheimer's disease and the normal elderly groups in the experiment where time tagging was crucial for successful performance. In the second experiment, where the only requisite for successful recognition was remembering what one had experienced, memory of the temporal record was not necessary for successful performance. In this instance, recognition memory for the both groups was identical. Memory deficits found in early stage Alzheimer's disease may be partly due to impaired processing of contextual cues that provide crucial information about when events occur.

Foster (1998) carried out a series of studies of background auditory conditions that provided such a context, and their influence upon autobiographical memory. While the use of background music has no effect on word-list recall in the normal elderly, there is a constant beneficial effect of music for autobiographical memory for patients with Alzheimer's disease. This music did not have to be familiar to the sufferer, nor did it reduce anxiety. The effect of music is stronger in cognitively impaired participants, thus promoting another reason for using music-based interventions in treatment initiatives. Foster, like Aldridge (Aldridge 1993c), argues for the use of music in assessment procedures.

As part of a program of studies investigating memory for everyday tasks, Rusted et al (1997) examined the potential of auditory and olfactory sensory cues to improve free recall of an action event (cooking an omelet) by individuals with dementia of the Alzheimer's type. Both healthy elderly people and volunteers with Alzheimer's disease recalled more of the individual actions which comprised the event when they listened, prior to recall, to a tape of sounds associated with the event. Olfactory cues which accompanied auditory cues did not produce additional benefits over auditory cues alone. The pattern of recall suggests that the auditory cues improved recall of the whole event, and were not merely increasing recall of the specific actions associated with the sound cues. Individuals with Alzheimer's disease continue to encode experiences using a combination of senses, and can subsequently use this sensory information to aid memory. These findings have practical implications for accessing residual memory for a wide range of therapeutic activities using the creative arts that emphasize sensory abilities.

Functional plasticity

Conscious recall of past events that have specific temporal and spatial contexts, termed episodic memory, is mediated by a system of interrelated brain regions. In Alzheimer's disease this system breaks down, resulting in an inability to recall events from the immediate past. Using brain scanning techniques of cerebral blood flow, Becker et al (1996) demonstrated that Alzheimer's disease patients show a greater activation of regions of the cerebral cortex normally involved in auditory-verbal memory, as well as activation of cortical areas not activated by normal elderly subjects. These results provide clear evidence of functional plasticity in the brain of sufferers, even if those changes do not result in normal memory function, and provide insights into the mechanisms by which the brain attempts to compensate for neurodegeneration. Similarly, it has been demonstrated that people with Alzheimer's disease can effectively learn and retain a motor skill for at least 1 month (Dick et al 1995).

Both anterograde and retrograde procedural memory appear to be spared in Alzheimer's disease (Crystal et al 1989). An 82-year-old musician with Alzheimer's disease showed a preserved ability to play previously learned piano compositions from memory while being unable to identify the composer or titles of each work. He also showed a preserved ability to learn the new skill of mirror reading while being unable to recall or recognize new information.

Communication

Characteristic features of communication breakdown and repair among individuals with dementia of the Alzheimer's type and their caregivers have been described (Orange et al 1998). The nature of communication breakdown, how it is signaled, how it is repaired, and the outcome of the repair process appear to be disease stage-dependent. Couples in the early and middle stages of the disease achieve success in resolving communication breakdowns despite declining cognitive, linguistic, and conversational abilities of the individual with the disease. This has important implications for understanding the influence of the progression of Alzheimer's disease on conversational performance and for advancing the development of communication enhancement education and training programs for spousal caregivers of individuals with Alzheimer's disease.

Music therapy will have an important role to play here as the ground of communication, as we have seen, is inherently musical. Dementia sufferers appear to be open to musical stimuli and responsive to music making, thus implementation of musical elements in facilitating communication and expression can be enhanced as the disease progresses. If music enhances communicative abilities – indeed, is the fundamental of communication – and spousal caregivers are important in managing the progress of the disease, then have to return to the idea that it is the caregivers who will benefit from music therapy.

MUSICAL HALLUCINATIONS

Hallucinations may occur in any of our senses, and auditory hallucinations take various forms: as voices, cries, noises, or rarely, music. However, the appearance of musical hallucinations, often in elderly patients, has generated interest in the medical literature (Berrios 1990, Brasic 1998, Mahowald et al 1998, Wengel et al 1989). When such hallucinations do occur they are described as highly organized vocal or instrumental music. In contrast, tinnitus is characterized by unformed sounds or noises that may possess musical qualities (Wengel et al 1989).

The case histories of patients with musical hallucinations suggest an underlying psychiatric disorder (Aizenberg et al 1986, Wengel et al 1989); this may be exacerbated by dementing illness occurring with brain deterioration (Gilchrist & Kalucy 1983), or it may be that patients with musical hallucinations and hearing loss become anxious and depressed (Fenton & McRae 1989). Fenton challenges the association of psychosis and previous mental illness, preferring an explanation that relies upon the degeneration of the aural end-organ whereby sensory input, which suppresses much non-essential information, fails to inhibit information from other perception-bearing circuits. Other investigators (Gilchrist & Kalucy 1983) argue for a central brain dysfunction as evidenced by measures of brain function. In a sample of 46 subjects experiencing musical hallucinations, the hallucinations were far more common in women; age, deafness, and brain disease affecting the non-dominant hemisphere played an important role in the development of hallucinations; and psychiatric illness and personality factors were found to be unimportant (Wengel et al 1989).

For these patients the application of music therapy to raise the ambient noise level, to organize aural sensory input by giving it a musical sense and counter sensory deprivation, and to stimulate and motivate the patient seems a reasonable approach.

MUSIC THERAPY, HEART RATE, AND RESPIRATION

The effect of music on the heart and blood pressure has been a favorite theme throughout history.

In an early issue of the medical journal *The Lancet* (Vincent & Thompson 1929) an attempt was made to discover the influence of listening to gramophone and radio music on blood pressure. The effects of music were influenced by how much the subjects appreciated music. Differing groups of musical competence responded in relation to volume, melody, rhythm, pitch, and type of music. Interest in the music was an important factor influencing response. Melody produced the most marked effect in the musical group. Volume produced the most apparent effect in the moderately musical group. In general, listening to music was accompanied by a slight rise in blood pressure in the listener.

If music produces physiological and psychological effects in healthy listeners then it may be assumed that individuals with various diseases respond to music in specific ways. A particular hypothesis, which has yet to be substantiated empirically, is that people with known diseases respond to music in a way which is mediated by that disease. Hence, we might find that the musical parameters of improvised playing are restricted by disease. Also, in terms of music therapy, if music is known to influence a physiological parameter such as heart rate or blood pressure, then perhaps music can be used therapeutically for patients who have problems with heart disease or hypertension.

Bason & Celler (1972) found that the human heart rate could be varied over a certain range by entrainment of the sinus rhythm with external auditory stimulus which presumably acted through the nervous control mechanisms, and resulted from a neural coupling into the cardiac centers of the brain. An audible click was played to the subject at a precise time in the cardiac cycle. When it came within a critical range then the heart rate could be increased or decreased up to 12% over a period of time up to 3 minutes. Fluctuations caused by breathing remained, but these tended to be less when the heart was entrained with the audible stimulus. When the click was not within the time range of the cardiac cycle then no influence could be discerned. This paper is important for supporting the proposition often made by music therapists that meeting the tempo of the patient influences their musical playing and is the initial key to therapeutic change.

An extension of this premise, that musical rhythm is a pacemaker, was investigated by Haas and colleagues (Haas et al 1986) in terms of the effects of perceived rhythm on respiratory pattern, a pattern which serves both metabolic and behavioral functions. Metabolic respiratory pathways are located in the reticular formation of the lower pons and medulla, whereas the behavioral respiratory pathways are located mainly in the limbic forebrain structures which lead to vocalization and complex behavior. There appear to be both hypothalamic and spinal pattern generators capable of synchronizing this respiratory and locomotor activity. Therefore, Haas et al hypothesized that an external rhythmical musical activity, in this case listening to taped music, would have an influence on respiratory pattern while keeping metabolic changes and afferent stimuli (i.e. no gross motor movements) to a minimum.

Twenty subjects were involved in this experiment, four of whom were experienced musicians and practicing musicians, six had formal musical training but no longer played a musical instrument, and the remaining 10 had no musical training. Respiratory data, including respiration frequency and airflow volume, were collected alongside heart rate and end-tidal CO_2. Subjects listened to a metronome set at 60 b.p.m. and tapped to that beat on a microphone after a baseline period. The subjects were then randomly presented with four musical excerpts and a period of silence with which they tapped along to. There were no appreciable changes in heart rate during the experiment, but there was an appreciable change in respiratory frequency and a significant decrease in the coefficient of variation for all respiratory parameters during the finger tapping. For non-musically trained subjects there was little coordination between breathing and musical rhythm, while for trained musicians there was a coupling of breathing and rhythm. That singers have more efficient pulmonary strategies than non-trained musicians, even when talking, is supported elsewhere in the literature (Formby et al 1989).

Auditory cues, then, appear to be important in the synchronization of respiration and other motor activity. It is this aspect of organization of behavioral events that appears to be the important aspect of music and central to music therapy (Aldridge 2000).

Coronary Care

Several authors have investigated this relationship in the setting of hospital care (Aldridge 1993b, Bonny 1983, Davis-Rollans & Cunningham 1987, Elliott 1994, Fitzsimmons et al 1991, Guzzetta 1989, Philip 1989, Zimmerman et al 1988), often with the intent of reducing anxiety in chronically ill patients (Gross & Swartz 1982, Standley 1986), for treating anxiety in general (Robb 2000), or specifically in musicians (Brodsky & Sloboda 1997).

A hospital situation which is fraught with anxiety for the patient is the intensive care unit. For patients after a heart attack, where heart rhythms are potentially unstable, the setting of coronary care is itself anxiety-provoking which recursively influences the physiological and psychological reactions of the patient. In these situations several authors, in varying hospital intensive care or coronary care clinics, have assessed the use of tape-recorded music delivered through headphones as an anxiolytic with the intention of reducing stress (Updike 1990). Bonny (1983) has suggested a series of musical selections for tape recordings which can be chosen for their sedative effects and according to other mood criteria, associative imagery, and relaxation potential (Bonny 1978); none of this has been empirically confirmed, although Updike (1990), in an observational study, confirms Bonny's impression that there is a decreased systolic blood pressure and a beneficial mood change from anxiety to relaxed calm when sedative music is played.

Rider (1985a, 1985b) proposed that disease-related stress was caused by the desynchronization of circadian oscillators and that listening to sedative music, with a guided imagery induction, would promote the entrainment of circadian rhythms as expressed in temperature and corticosteroid levels of nursing staff. This study found no conclusive results, mainly because there was no control group and the study design was confused, highlighting the essential difference between music when applied as a music therapy discipline, and music as an adjunct to psychotherapy or biofeedback.

Davis-Rollans & Cunningham (1987) describe the use of a 37-minute tape recording of selected classical music[1] on the heart rate and rhythm of coronary care unit patients. Twelve of the patients had had heart attacks and another 12 had a chronic heart condition. Patients were exposed to two randomly varied 42-minute periods of continuous monitoring: one period with music delivered through headphones, the other, control, period without music and containing background noise of the unit as heard through silent headphones. Eight patients reported a significant change to a happier emotional state after listening to the music (a result replicated by Updike (1990)), although there were no significant changes in specific physiological variables during the music periods. A change in mood, however, which relieves depression is believed to be beneficial to the overall status of coronary care patients (Cassem & Hackett 1971).

Bolwerk (Bolwerk 1990) set out relieve the state anxiety of patients in a myocardial infarction ward using recorded classical music.[2] Forty adults were randomly assigned to two equal groups, one of which listened to relaxing music during the first 4 days of hospitalization, while the other received no music. There was no controlled 'silent condition.' While there was a significant reduction in state anxiety in the treatment group, state anxiety was also reduced in the control group. The reasons for this overall reduction in anxiety may have been that after 4 days the situation had become less acute, the situation was not so strange for the patient, and by then a diagnosis had been confirmed.

State anxiety is an individual's anxiety at a particular state in time, as opposed to trait anxiety which is an overall prevailing condition of anxiety unbounded by time and determined by personality. The relationship between stress and anxiety is that stimulus conditions, or stressors, produce anxiety reactions – i.e. the state of anxiety. Anxiety as a state is characterized by subjective feelings of tension, worry, and nervousness which are accompanied by physiological changes of heart rate, blood pressure, myocardial oxygen consumption, lethal cardiac dysrhythmias, and reductions in peripheral and renal perfusion. Admission to a coronary care unit is in itself a stressor, and the environment produces further stress; hence the importance of managing state anxiety.

The purpose of a study by Guzzetta (1989) was to determine whether relaxation and music therapy were effective in reducing stress in patients admitted to a coronary care unit with the presumptive diagnosis of acute myocardial infarction. In this experimental study, 80 patients were randomly assigned to a relaxation, music therapy, or control group. The relaxation and music therapy groups participated in three sessions over a 2-day period. Music therapy comprised a relaxation induction and listening to a 20-minute musical cassette tape selected from three alternative musical styles: soothing classical music, soothing popular music, and non-traditional music (defined as 'compositions having no vocalization or meter, periods of silence and an asymmetric rhythm' (p. 611). Stress was evaluated by apical heart rates, peripheral temperatures, cardiac complications, and qualitative patient evaluative data. Data analysis revealed that lowering apical heart rates and raising peripheral temperatures were more successful in the relaxation and music therapy groups than in the control group. The incidence of cardiac complications was found to be lower in the intervention groups, and most intervention subjects believed that such therapy was helpful. Both relaxation and music therapy were found to be effective modalities of reducing stress in these patients, and music listening was more effective than relaxation alone. Furthermore, apical heart rates were lowered in response to music over a series of sessions, thus supporting the argument

---

[1]Beethoven *Symphony No. 6* (first movement); Mozart, *Eine kleine Nachtmusik* (first and fourth movements), and Smetana, *The Moldau.*
[2]Bach, Largo; Beethoven, Largo; Debussy, Prelude to the Afternoon of a Faun.

that the assessment of music therapy on physiological parameters is dependent upon adaptation over time. Further research strategies may wish to make longitudinal studies of the influence of music on physiological parameters.

The positive finding above was in contrast to Zimmerman et al (1988), who failed to find an influence of music on heart rate, peripheral temperature, blood pressure, or anxiety score. However, Zimmerman's study only allowed for one intervention of music. In this experimental study the authors examined the effects of listening to relaxation-type music on self-reported anxiety and on selected physiologic indices of relaxation in patients with suspected myocardial infarction. Seventy-five patients were randomly assigned to one of two experimental groups, one listening to taped music and the other to 'white noise'[3] through headphones, or to a control group. The Spielberger state anxiety inventory (Spielberger 1983) was administered before and after each testing session, and blood pressure, heart rate, and digital skin temperature were measured at baseline and at 10-minute intervals for the 30-minute session. There was no significant difference among the three groups for state anxiety scores or physiologic parameters. Because no differences were found, analyses were conducted of the groups combined. Significant improvement in all of the physiologic parameters was found to have occurred. This finding reinforces the benefit of rest and careful monitoring of patients in the coronary care unit, but adds little to the understanding of music interventions. Time to listen, separated from the surrounding influence of the hospital unit by the use of headphones, may itself be an important intervention. Although Rider (1985a) did not reach this conclusion, he found that perceived pain was reduced in a hospital situation in response to classical music delivered through headphones. It could be concluded from his work that isolation from environmental sounds, canceling out external noise, has a positive benefit for the patient regardless of inner content – i.e. music, relaxation induction, or silence.

Given that the study by Bason & Celler (1972) could influence heart rate by matching the heart rate of the patient, then we must conclude that studies of the influence of music on heart rate must match the music to the individual patient. This also makes psychological sense as different people have varied reactions to the same music. Furthermore, improvised music playing, which takes meeting the tempo of the patient as one of its main principles, may have an impact other than the passive listening to music. In addition, the work of Haas et al (1986) mentioned above showed that listening, coupled with tapping, synchronizes respiration pattern with musical rhythm, further emphasizing that active music playing can be used to influence physiological parameters and that this synchronization can be learned. Thaut (1985) also found that children with gross motor dysfunction achieved significantly better motor rhythm accuracy when aided by auditory rhythm and rhythmic speech.

Gustorff has successfully used music therapy in the treatment of coma patients in the context of intensive care (Aldridge et al 1990). This work has also been extended to persistent vegetative state where patients who are seemingly unaware of their environment begin to respond to the human singing voice (Aldridge 1991, Ansdell 1995, Gustorff 1990).

Anaesthesia

The ability of music to induce calm and well-being has been used in general anaesthesia. Patients express their pleasure at awakening to music in the operating suite (Bonny & McCarron 1984) where music was played openly at first, and then through earphones during the operation. In a study by Lehmann et al (1985) patients undergoing elective orthopedic or lower abdominal surgery were given placebo infusion (0.9% NaCl) instead of tramadol in a randomized and double blind manner in order to evaluate tramadol efficacy as one component of balanced anaesthesia. Postoperative analgesic requirement and awareness of intra-operative events

[3]'White noise' or 'synthetic silence' is an attempt to block out environmental noise. In this case it was a tape recording of sea sounds, which themselves were rhythmic.

(tape recorded music offered via earphones) were further used to assess tramadol effects. Although anaesthesia proved to be quite comparable in both groups, striking differences between the two groups were shown with respect to intra-operative awareness: while patients receiving placebo proved to be amnesic, 65% of tramadol patients were aware of intra-operative music. The ability to hear music during an operation is also reported by Bonny & McCarron (1984).

CANCER THERAPY, PAIN MANAGEMENT, AND HOSPICE CARE

Cancer and chronic pain care require complex coordinated resources which are not only medical but psychological, social, and communal. Hospice care in the United States and Britain has attempted to meet this need for palliative and supportive services which provide physical, psychological and spiritual care for dying people and their families. Such a service is based upon an interdisciplinary team of health care professionals and volunteers and often involves outpatient and inpatient care.

In the supportive care program of the pain service to the neurology department of Sloan-Kettering Cancer Center, New York, a music therapist is part of that supportive team, along with a psychiatrist, nurse-clinician, neuro-oncologist, chaplain, and social worker (Bailey 1984, Coyle 1987). Music therapy is used to promote relaxation, reduce anxiety, supplement other pain control methods, and enhance communication between patient and family (Bailey 1983, 1984). As depression is a common feature of the patients within this program, then music therapy is hypothetically an influence on this parameter and in enhancing quality of life. Although quality of life has assumed a position of importance in cancer care in recent years, and music therapy, along with other art therapies, is thought to be important, the evidence for this belief is largely anecdotal and unstructured. Bailey (1983) discovered a significant improvement in mood when playing live music to cancer patients as opposed to playing taped music,

a factor she attributes to the human element being involved. Gudrun Aldridge (Aldridge G 1996), in a single case study, emphasizes the benefits of expression facilitated by playing music for the postoperative care of a woman after mastectomy.

A better researched phenomenon is the use of music in the control of chronic cancer pain, although such studies abdicate the human element of live performance in favor of tape recorded interventions.

In addition to reducing pain, particularly in pain clinics, music as relaxation and distraction has been tried during chemotherapy to bring overall relief (Kerkvliet 1990), and to reduce nausea and vomiting (Frank 1985). Using taped music and guided imagery in combination with pharmacological antiemetics, Frank (1985) found that state anxiety was significantly reduced resulting in a perceived degree of reduced vomiting, although the nausea remained the same. As this study was not controlled the reduced anxiety may have been a result of the natural fall in anxiety levels when chemotherapy treatment ended. However, the study consisted of patients who had previously experienced chemotherapy and were conditioned to experience nausea or vomiting in conjunction with it. That the subjects of the study felt relief was seen as an encouraging sign in the use of music therapy as a treatment modality.

There is a rapidly developing literature related to working with children with cancer (Aldridge 1999, Fagen 1982, Standley & Hanser 1995) that also focuses on specific issues such as the management of pediatric pain (Frager 1997, Loewy 1997), hospitalization (Froehlich 1996) special needs groups (McCauley 1996) and the use of songs (Aasgaard 1994, O'Callaghan 1996).

Some music therapists work in situations with adult patients (Bunt 1995), or clients who are living with challenge of the HIV (Aldridge 1993a, 1995, 1999; Aldridge & Aldridge 1999; Hartley 1994; Schnürer et al 1995). There is a pioneering literature in this field of the work that has been carried out by Lee (1995, 1996) and Bruscia (1991, 1995), and their texts demonstrate how other therapists have also been advancing the use of music therapy to meet this challenge.

NEUROLOGICAL PROBLEMS

In many cases neurological diseases become traumatic because of their abrupt appearance resulting in physical and/or mental impairment (Jochims 1990). Music appears to be a key in the recovery of former capabilities in the light of what at first can seem like hopeless neurological devastation (Aldridge 1991; Jones 1990; Magee 1995a, 1995b; Sacks 1986).

For some patients with brain damage following head trauma the problem may be a temporary loss of speech (aphasia). Music therapy can play a valuable role in aphasia rehabilitation (Lucia 1987). Melodic intonation therapy (Naeser & Helm-Estabrooks 1985, O'Boyle & Sanford 1988) has been developed to fulfil such a rehabilitative role and involves embedding short propositional phrases into simple, often repeated, melody patterns accompanied by finger tapping. The inflection patterns of pitch changes and rhythms of speech are selected to parallel the natural speech prosody of the sentence. The singing of previously familiar songs is also encouraged as it encourages articulation, fluency, and the shaping procedures of language which are akin to musical phrasing. In addition the stimulation of singing within a context of communication motivates the patient to communicate and, it is hypothesized, promotes the activation of intentional verbal behavior. In infants the ability to reciprocate or compensate a partner's communicative response is an important element of communicative competence (Murray & Trevarthen 1986, Street & Cappella 1989) and vital in speech acquisition (Glenn & Cunningham 1984). Music therapy strategies in adults may be used in a similar way with the expectation that they will stimulate those brain functions which support, precede, and extend functional speech recovery, functions which are essentially musical and rely upon brain plasticity. Combined with the ability to enhance word retrieval, music can also be used to improve breath capacity, encourage respiration-phonation patterns, correct articulation errors caused by

inappropriate rhythm or speed, and prepare the patient for articulatory movements. In this sense music offers a sense of time which is not chronological, which is fugitive to measurement and vital for the coordination of human communication (Aldridge D 1996).

Evidence of the global strategy of music processing in the brain is found in the clinical literature. In two cases of aphasia (Morgan & Tilluckdharry 1982) singing was seen as a welcome release from the helplessness of being a patient. The authors hypothesized that singing was a means to communicate thoughts externally. Although the 'newer aspect' of speech was lost, the older function of music was retained, possibly because music is a function distributed over both hemispheres. Berman (1981) suggests that recovery from aphasia is not a matter of new learning by the non-dominant hemisphere but a taking over of responsibility for language by that hemisphere. The non-dominant hemisphere may be a reserve of functions in case of regional failure indicating an overall brain plasticity, and language functions may shift with multilinguals as compared with monolinguals, or as a result of learning and cultural exposure where music and language share common properties (Tsunoda 1983).

That singing is an activity correlated with certain creative productive aspects of language is shown in the case of a 2-year-old boy of above-average intelligence who experienced seizures, manifested by tic-like turning movements of the head, which were induced consistently by his own singing, but not by listening to or imagining music. His seizures were also induced by his recitation and by his use of silly or witty language such as punning. Seizure activity on an EEG was present in both temporocentral regions, especially on the right side, and was correlated with clinical attacks (Herskowitz et al 1984).

Aphasia is also found in elderly stroke patients, and music therapy, as reported in case studies, has been used effectively in combination with speech therapy.

Gustorff (Aldridge et al 1990, Gustorff & Hannich 2000) has successfully applied creative music therapy to coma patients who were otherwise unresponsive. Matching her singing with the breathing patterns of the patient, she has stimulated changes in consciousness which are both measurable on a coma rating scale and apparent to the eye of the clinician.

Mentally Handicapped Adults

Music appears to be an effective way of engaging profoundly mentally handicapped adults in activity (Wigram 1988). The functional properties of music have implications for the treatment of adults with learning disability in that:

1. exposure to sound arouses sensory processes
2. a musical event is an organized temporal auditory structure with a beginning and an end
3. music facilitates memory recall and expectation ('the signature tune effect')
4. a sequence of musical themes can enhance memory recall and the organization of a sequence of cognitive activities (Knill 1983).

Music therapy was used to encourage profoundly mentally handicapped adults to attempt movements and actions and achieve non-musical aims within music therapy sessions (Oldfield & Adams 1990). Music therapy was compared with play activity using two groups of subjects. Each group received either music therapy or play activity for 6 months, at which time the groups were reversed to receive the comparison treatment. As the handicaps were so profound and varied between individuals, a separate behavioral index was formulated for each subject. It was hypothesized that each objective would be achieved to a greater extent in the music therapy group than in play activity. While the study was restricted in terms of numbers, and the behavioral indices were varied, there was a significant difference in the performance in music therapy than in play therapy. This improved performance was not attributable to greater attention in the music therapy group. The type of input was noticeably different in the two groups; in the music therapy group improvisations were based on the subjects' own musical productions. However, for one subject there was greater improvement in the play activity which came before the music therapy treatment.

CHILDREN

Much of modern music therapy was developed in working with children and the diversity and richness of this work is reflected in the literature.

Stern (1989) emphasizes the importance of the creative arts in general to child development as they involve the child's natural curiosity. However, she also proposes that in terms of child development then therapies must involve the family of the child, particularly in the case of child disability. For children with multiple disabilities there is need for stimulation and this can be achieved using music which also provides a sense of fun and enjoyment. Stern's approach suggests that songs stimulate a bond between therapist and patient, and that for one particular disabled patient, 'The music entered Susan's frame of reference' (p. 649). An alternative explanation could be that music *was* Susan's frame of reference by which she coordinated her own activities, and those activities with another person. It may well be that families of handicapped children need to learn the rudiments of music therapy, as organized rhythmic communication, such that they can provide a structure for their mutual communications (Aldridge 1989). It makes sense for therapists to work with both parents and children.

Songs, both composed and improvised, provide the vehicle for working with hospitalized children (Aasgaard 1999, Dunn 1999).

Songs were also used in the preoperative preparation of children in an attempt to relieve fear and anxiety by transmitting surgery-related information. To ascertain the efficacy of using information alone, or information with songs, three groups of children were prepared on the day before surgery, one group with information alone, one group with information followed by specially prepared songs based on that information, and a third group which also had information followed by songs with an additional session of songs in the immediate preoperative phase on the day of the operation. The group receiving music therapy on the morning before the induction of pre-operative medication showed significantly less anxiety based on a number of observed variables. Lessons to be learned from this research may be that although information is made available, this does not mean that the child will be able to use this information when it is needed; no amount of information will make a procedure less painful, and a cognitive understanding of pain made during a therapy session is not necessarily translated into physical or emotional relief during the context of surgical preparation. Music therapy in its immediacy may have been a critical factor in reducing anxiety, as anecdotal reports suggest, but in this study no group received music therapy alone.

In a general study of music therapy as applied to newborns and infants in hospital (Marley 1984), music appeared beneficial as a calming effect inducing sleep and relaxation. The methods ranged from simple tapping on the back to simulate a heartbeat, through rocking of children in time to played music, to receptive music therapy. It is difficult to understand the nature of this work as music therapy. The researcher reports that in 13 of the rooms the television was off, and in 14 rooms the television was on. When the television was on, in most cases the sound was either too low or too loud. It must be added that the children were between the ages of 5 weeks and 36 months. With continuous sound stimulation, it is little wonder the children responded to the television being switched off and guitar music being played to them.

Fagen (1982), working with terminally ill pediatric patients, also emphasizes the psychosocial setting of the family and the hospital as important. Music therapy in this setting was used to improve the quality of life of the patients in an attempt to broaden and deepen their range of living. However no quality-of-life scale was used, nor are the criteria for assessing the quality of life in dying children made clear. This is not surprising, as no quality-of-life scales for children with terminal illness exist at present. In her music therapy practice Fagen was eclectically borrowing from various music therapy schools but concentrating on songs to confront the issues of hospitalization and dying. These songs often had improvised lyrics according to the needs of the situation, or songs which had given meanings

and were appropriate to the patient. No attempt was made to force patients to confront their own dying.

Aasgard has pursued the theme of music therapy in pediatric oncology further. He uses songs to facilitate a return to health, where health is seen as a performed activity within an ecology of care (Aasgaard 1999). These songs are not, however, privatized productions, but shared pieces of music that are sung by siblings, family members, and hospital staff.

Creative expression, as reported in the work with children, is generally accepted as a means of coping whereby pain and anxiety are channeled into activities (Lavigne et al 1986). In an attempt to encourage children to cope with the trauma of hospitalization by verbalizing their experiences, Froehlich (1984) compared the use of play therapy and music therapy as facilitators of verbalization. When specifically structured questions about hospitalization were asked of the children after sessions of music therapy or play therapy, music therapy elicited more 'answers' than 'no answers' and a more involved type of verbalization involving elaborated answers than play therapy.

Autism

Music therapy allows children without language to communicate and possibly to orient themselves within time and space. It has developed a significant place in the treatment of mental handicap in children.

Children exhibiting autistic behavior appeared to prefer a musical stimulus rather than a visual stimulus when compared with normal children (Thaut 1987). Although the significance of this finding was not statistically valid, the study does report that autistic children showed more motor reactions during periods of music than normal children, and that autistic children appeared to listen to music longer than their normal peers who preferred visual displays.

In a later study comparing autistic children and their normal peers (Thaut 1988), autistic children produced spontaneous tone sequences almost as well as normal children and significantly better than a control group of mentally handicapped children. Each child sat at a xylophone with two beaters, after having had a short demonstration from the researcher, who then asked them to play spontaneously for as long as they liked until they came to a natural ending. The musical parameters of the first sixteen tones of these improvisations, which were assessed and used as the basis for group comparisons were: rhythm (representing the imposition and adherence to temporal order); restriction (representing the use of all available tonal elements); complexity (representing the generation of recurring melodic patterns; rule adherence (representing the application of melodic patterns to the total sound sequence); and, originality (representing the production of melodic patterns that occurred only once but fulfilled criteria of melodic and rhythmic shape). Autistic children perceived and explored the xylophone as normal children did in terms of originality and restriction, but tended to play with short recurring motives rather like the mentally handicapped children. Thaut (1988) concludes that 'The low performances on complexity and rule adherence of such children suggest an inability to organize and retain complex temporal sequences' (p. 567). This relationship between cognition and motor behavior as it is coordinated in rhythmical performance, as we have read above in terms of heart rate, breathing, muscle performance and speech rehabilitation, would appear to be worthy of investigation in a wide variety of patients with communication difficulties, regardless of the source of those difficulties.

Music therapy has been used extensively in the treatment of developmental delay. In a crossover study (Aldridge et al 1995), the children in the initially treated group changed more than the children on the waiting list. When those waiting-list control group children were then treated with music therapy, and the formerly treated children rested, then the newly treated children caught up in their development. Such changes were demonstrated at a level of clinical significance. There was a continuing improvement in hearing and speech, hand–eye coordination, and personal-social interaction. While active listening and performing were seen to be central to the developmental process, it was the importance of hand–eye coordination skills emphasized in the active musical playing which were instrumental in encouraging cognitive change.

CONCLUSION

There is a broad literature covering the application of music therapy as reported in the medical press and a growing resource of valid clinical research material from which substantive conclusions can be drawn. The obscure observations in the realm of psychotherapy highlight a critical feature of music therapy research: well intentioned, and often rigorous work is spoiled by failures in research methodology. This is not to say that all music therapy clinical research should conform to a common methodology (Aldridge D 1996, 1999, 2000), or that it should be medical research; rather, that standard research tools and methods of clinical assessment should be developed which can be replicated and which are appropriate to music therapy, and a link developed with other forms of clinical practice. In this way we can devise working tools which allow us to inform both ourselves and others. There is a lively debate in music therapy circles about which methods are appropriate and a variety of books have addressed themselves to presenting research material and methods (Wheeler 1995).

The research which has been produced is notably lacking in follow-up data, without which it is impossible to make any valid statements about clinical value. The assessment instruments are generally lacking by which internal or external validity can be conferred. For example, as 'depression' appears to feature in many chronic diseases, then it would be appropriate to include a clinical rating of depression, using a validated scale, in future research design. If this assessment of depression could be combined with an overall assessment of life-quality, then a significant step forward would have been made in establishing a minimal data set for assessing clinical change.

Much of the research work so far has been developed within the field of nursing where music is accepted as a useful therapeutic adjunct. Not surprisingly, the work from this field has concentrated on medical scientific perspectives. There is an almost complete absence of cross-cultural studies and the use of anthropological methods which would bring other insights into music therapy. That music has been used therapeutically in other cultures cannot be denied, and other perspectives regarding the application of music therapeutically would highlight the limitations of modern Western scientific approaches when used as the sole means of research.

REFERENCES

Aasgaard T 1994 Music therapy at the end of life – and at the funeral. Nordisk Tidsskrift for Musikkterapi 3(2): 86–88

Aasgaard T 1999 Music therapy as milieu in the hospice and paediatric oncology ward. In: Aldridge D (ed) Music therapy and palliative care. Jessica Kingsley, London

Aigen K 1990 Echoes of silence. Music Therapy 9(1): 44–61

Aizenberg D, Schwartz B, Modai I 1986 Musical hallucinations, acquired deafness, and depression. Journal of Mental and Nervous Disorders 174(5): 309–311

Aldridge D 1989 Music, communication and medicine: discussion paper. Journal of the Royal Society of Medicine 82(12): 743–746

Aldridge D 1991 Creativity and consciousness: music therapy in intensive care. Arts in Psychotherapy 18(4): 359–362

Aldridge D 1993a Music and Alzheimers' disease – assessment and therapy: a discussion paper. Journal of the Arts in Psychotherapy 86: 93–95

Aldridge D 1993b Music therapy research: I. A review of the medical research literature within a general context of music therapy research. Special Issue: Research in the Creative Arts Therapies 20(1): 11–35

Aldridge D 1993c The music of the body: music therapy in medical settings. Advances 9(1): 17–35

Aldridge D 1994 Alzheimer's disease: rhythm, timimg and music as therapy. Biomedicine and Pharmacotherapy 48(7): 275–281

Aldridge D 1995 Music therapy and the treatment of Alzheimer's disease. Clinical Gerontologist 16(1): 41–57

Aldridge D 1996 Music therapy research and practice in medicine: from out of the silence. Jessica Kingsley, London

Aldridge D 1998 Suicide: the tragedy of hopelessness. Jessica Kingsley, London

Aldridge D 1999 Music therapy in palliative care: new voices. Jessica Kingsley, London

Aldridge D 2000 Music therapy in dementia care. Jessica Kinglsey, London

Aldridge D, Aldridge G 1999 Life as jazz: hope, meaning and music therapy in the treatment of life-threatening illness. In: Dileo C (ed) Music therapy and medicine. American Music Therapy Association, Silver Spring, MD, pp. 79–94

Aldridge D, Brandt G 1991 Music therapy and Alzheimer's disease. Journal of the Arts in Psychotherapy 5(2): 28–63

Aldridge D, Gustorff D, Hannich H-J 1990 Where am I? Music therapy applied to coma patients. Journal of the Royal Society of Medicine 83(6): 345–346

Aldridge D, Gustorff D, Neugebauer L 1995 A pilot study of music therapy in the treatment of children with developmental delay. Complementary Therapies in Medicine 3: 197–205

Aldridge G 1996 'A walk through Paris': the development of melodic expression in music therapy with a breast-cancer patient. Arts in Psychotherapy 23: 207–223

Ansdell G 1995 Music for life: aspects of creative music therapy with adult clients. Jessica Kingsley, London

Bailey L M 1983 The effects of live music versus tape-recorded music on hospitalised cancer patients. Music Therapy 3(1): 17–28

Bailey L M 1984 The use of songs with cancer patients and their families. Music Therapy 4(1): 5–17

Barker V L, Brunk B 1991 The role of a creative arts group in the treatment of clients with traumatic brain injury. Music Therapy Perspectives 9: 26–31

Bason B, Celler B 1972 Control of the heart rate by external stimuli. Nature 4: 279–280

Bayles K, Tomoeda C, Rein J 1996 Phrase repetition in Alzheimer's disease: effect of meaning and length. Brain and Language 54(2): 246–261

Beatty W W, Zavadil K D, Bailly R et al 1988 Preserved musical skills in a severely demented patient. International Journal of Clinical Neuropsychology 10: 158–164

Beatty W W, Testa J A, English S, Winn P 1997 Influences of clustering and switching on the verbal fluency performance of patients with Alzheimer's disease. Aging Neuropsychology and Cognition 4(4): 273–279

Bechler-Karsch A 1993 The therapeutic use of music. Online Journal of Knowledge Synthesis for Nursing 1(4): U1–U21

Beck A T, Steer R A, Beck J S, Newman C F 1993 Hopelessness, depression, suicidal ideation, and clinical diagnosis of depression. Suicide and Life-Threatening Behavior 23(2): 139–145

Beck C 1998 Psychosocial and behavioural interventions for Alzheimer's disease patients and their families. American Journal of Geriatric Psychiatry 6(2): S41–S48

Becker J T, Mintun M A, Aleva K, Wiseman M B, Nichols T, Dekosky S T 1996 Compensatory reallocation of brain resources supporting verbal episodic memory in Alzheimer's disease. Neurology 46(3): 692–700

Bender M, Cheston R 1997 Inhabitants of a lost kingdom: a model of the subjective experiences of dementia. Ageing and Society 17: 513–532

Benjamin B 1983 'The singing hospital': integrated group therapy in the black mentally ill. South African Medical Journal 63(23): 897–899

Benke T, Bosch S et al 1998 A study of emotional processing in Parkinson's disease. Brain and Cognition 38(1): 36–52

Berman I 1981 Musical functioning, speech lateralization and the amusias. South African Medical Journal 59: 78–81

Berrios G 1990 Musical hallucinations: a historical and clinical study. British Journal of Psychiatry 156: 188–194

Bolwerk C A 1990 Effects of relaxing music on state anxiety in myocardial infarction patients. Critical Care Nursing Quarterly 13(2): 63–72

Bonder B 1994 Psychotherapy for individuals with Alzheimer disease. Alzheimer Disease and Associated Disorders 8(Suppl. 3): 75–81

Bonny H 1978 GIM Monograph No. 2. The role of taped music programs in the GIM process. ICM Press, Baltimore

Bonny H 1983 Music listening for intensive coronary care units: a pilot project. Music Therapy 3(1): 4–16

Bonny H, McCarron N 1984 Music as an adjunct to anesthesia in operative procedures. Journal of the American Association of Nurse Anesthetists February: 55–57

Brasic J 1998 Hallucinations. Perceptual and Motor Skills 86(3): 851–877

Brodsky W, Sloboda J A 1997 Clinical trial of a music generated vibrotactile therapeutic environment for musicians: main effects and outcome differences between therapy subgroups. Journal of Music Therapy 34(1): 2–32

Brotons M, Pickettcooper P K 1996 The effects of music therapy intervention on agitation behaviors of Alzheimer's disease patients. Journal of Music Therapy 33(1): 2–18

Brotons M, Koger S M, Pickettcooper P 1997 Music and dementias: a review of literature. Journal of Music Therapy 34(4): 204–245

Bruscia K 1991 Embracing life with AIDS: psychotherapy through guided imagery and music. In: Bruscia K Case studies in music therapy. Barcelona Publishers, Phoenixville, PA

Bruscia K 1995 Images in AIDS. In: Lee C Lonely waters. Sobell Publications, Oxford, pp. 119–123

Brustrom J E, Ober B A 1996 Source memory for actions in Alzheimer's disease. Aging Neuropsychology and Cognition 3(1): 56–66

Bunt L 1995 Where words fail music takes over: a collaborative study by a music therapist and a counselor in the context of cancer care. Music Therapy Perspectives 13: 46–50

Cassem N H, Hackett T P 1971 Psychiatric consultation in a coronary care unit. Annals of Internal Medicine 75: 9

Chenery H J 1996 Semantic priming in Alzheimer's dementia. Aphasiology 10(1): 1–20

Cheston R 1998 Psychotherapeutic work with people with dementia: a review of the literature. British Journal of Medical Psychology 71: 211–231

Collette F, VanderLinden M, Bechet S, Belleville S, Salmon E 1998 Working memory deficits in Alzheimer's disease. Brain Cognition 37(1): 147–149

Courtright P, Johnson S, Baumgartner M A, Jordan M, Webster J C 1990 Dinner music: does it affect the behavior of psychiatric inpatients? Journal of Psychosocial Nursing and Mental Health Sevices 28(3): 37–40

Coyle N 1987 A model of continuity of care for cancer patients with chronic pain. Medical Clinics of North America 71(2): 259–270

Crystal H A, Grober E, Masur D 1989 Preservation of musical memory in Alzheimer's disease. Journal of

Neurology, Neurosurgery and Psychiatry 52(12): 1415–1416

Davis-Rollans C, Cunningham S 1987 Physiologic responses of coronary care patients to selected music. Heart and Lung 16(4): 370–378

Devisch R, Vervaeck B 1986 Doors and thresholds: Jeddi's approach to psychiatric disorders. Social Science and Medicine 22(5): 541–551

Dick M B, Neilson K A, Beth R E, Shankle W R, Cotman C W 1995 Acquisition and long-term retention of fine motor skill in Alzheimer's disease. Brain and Cognition 29(3): 294–306

Dileo C 1999 Music therapy and medicine. American Music Therapy Association, Silver Spring

Dunn B 1999 Creativity and communication aspects of music therapy in a children's hospital. In: Aldridge D (ed) Music therapy and palliative care. Jessica Kingsley, London.

Elliott D 1994 The effects of music and muscle relaxation on patient anxiety in a coronary care unit. Heart and Lung 23(1): 27–35

Ellis D G 1996 Coherence patterns in Alzheimer's discourse. Communication Research 23(4): 472–495

Fagen T S 1982 Music therapy in the treatment of anxiety and fear in terminal pediatric patients. Music Therapy 2(1): 13–23

Fenton G W, McRae D A 1989 Musical hallucinations in a deaf elderly woman. British Journal of Psychiatry 155: 401–403

Fitzsimmons L, Shively M, Verderber A 1991 Variables influencing cardiovascular function. Journal of Cardiovascular Nursing 5(4): 87–89

Formby C, Thomas R G, Halsey J H J 1989 Regional cerebral blood flow for singers and nonsingers while speaking, singing, and humming a rote passage. Brain and Language 36(4): 690–698

Forsell Y, Jorm A F, Winblad B 1998 The outcome of depression and dysthymia in a very elderly population: results from a three-year follow-up study. Aging and Mental Health 2(2): 100–104

Foster N 1998 An examination of the facilitatory effect of music on recall, with special reference to dementia sufferers. Psychology at Royal Holloway, University of London

Frager G 1997 Palliative care and terminal care of children. Child and Adolescent Psychiatric Clinics of North America 6(4): 889

Frank J M 1985 The effects of music therapy and guided visual imagery on chemotherapy induced nausea and vomiting. Oncology Nursing Forum 12(5): 47–52

Fraser W, King K, Thomas P, Kendell R 1986 The diagnosis of schizophrenia by language analysis. British Journal of Pyschiatry 148: 275–278

Friedman A S, Glickman N W 1986 Program characteristics for successful treatment of adolescent drug abuse. Journal of Mental and Nervous Disorders 174(11): 669–679

Froehlich M 1984 A comparison of the effect of music therapy and medical play therapy on the verbalization behavior of pediatric patients. Journal of Music Therapy 21(1): 2–15

Froehlich M-A 1996 Music therapy with the terminally ill child. In: Froelich M-A Music therapy with hospitalized children. Jeffrey Books, Cherry Hill, NJ

Gates G A, Cobb J L, Linn R T, Rees T, Wolf P A, Dagostino R B 1996 Central auditory dysfunction, cognitive dysfunction, and dementia in older people. Archives of Otolaryngology – Head and Neck Surgery 122(2): 161–167

Gilchrist P N, Kalucy R S 1983 Musical hallucinations in the elderly: a variation on the theme. Australian and New Zealand Journal of Psychiatry 17(3): 286–287

Glassman L 1991 Music therapy and bibliotherapy in the rehabilitation of traumatic brain injury: a case study. Arts in Psychotherapy 18(2): 149–156

Glenn S, Cunningham C 1984 Nursery rhymes and early language acquisition by mentally handicapped children. Exceptional Children 51(1): 72–74

Glicksohn J, Cohen Y 2000 Can music alleviate cognitive dysfunction in schizophrenia? Psychopathology 33(1): 43–47

Gross J-L, Swartz R 1982 The effects of music therapy on anxiety in chronically ill patients. Music Therapy 2(1): 43–52

Gustorff D 1990 Lieder ohne Worte. Musiktherapeutische Umschau 11: 120–126

Gustorff D, Hannich H-J 2000 Jenseit des Wortes. Verlag Hans Huber, Bern

Guzzetta C E 1989 Effects of relaxation and music therapy on patients in a coronary care unit with presumptive acute myocardial infarction. Heart and Lung 18(6): 609–616

Gwyther L P, Strulowitz S Y 1998 Caregiver stress. Current Opinion in Psychiatry 11(4): 431–434

Haag G, Lucius G 1984 Psychology in rehabilitation. Psychologie in der Rehabilitation. Rehabilitation-Stuttgart 23(1): 1–9

Haas F, Distenfeld S, Axen K 1986 Effects of perceived musical rhythm on respiratory pattern. Journal of Appied Physiology 61(3): 1185–1191

Hadsell N 1974 A sociological theory and approach to music therapy with adult psychiatric patients. Journal of Music Therapy 11(3): 113–124

Hartley N 1994 In retrospect, in prospect. Music therapy with those who are living with or who are affected by HIV/AIDS. International Conference, Music Therapy in Palliative Care, Sobell House, Oxford

Heal H C, Husband H J 1998. Disclosing a diagnosis of dementia: is age a factor? Aging and Mental Health 2(2): 144–150

Herskowitz J, Rosman N, Geschwind N 1984 Seizures induced by singing and recitation: a unique form of reflex epilepsy in childhood. Archives of Neurology 41(10): 1102–1103

Jochims S 1990 Coping with illness in the early phase of severe neurologic diseases: a contribution of music therapy to psychological management in selected neurologic disease pictures. Krankheitsverarbeitung in der Fruhphase schwerer neurologischer Erkrankungen. Ein Beitrag der Musiktherapie zur psychischen Betreuung bei ausgewahlten neurologischen Krankheitsbildern. Psychotherapie, Psychosomatik Medizinische Psychologie 40(3–4): 115–122

Johnson C, Lahey P, Shore A 1992 An exploration of creative arts therapeutic group work on an Alzheimer's unit. Arts in Psychotherapy 19(4): 269–277

Jones C 1990 Spark of life. Geriatric Nursing New York 11(4): 194–196

Kamar O 1997 Light and death: art therapy with a patient with Alzheimer's disease. American Journal of Art Therapy 35(4): 118–124

Kerkvliet G J 1990 Music therapy may help control cancer pain news. Journal of the National Cancer Institute 82(5): 350–352

Knill C 1983 Body awareness, communication and development: a programme employing music with the profoundly handicapped. International Journal of Rehabilitation Research 6(4): 489–492

Knott R, Patterson K, Hodges J R 1997 Lexical and semantic binding effects in short-term memory: evidence from semantic dementia. Cognitive Neuropsychology 14(8): 1165–1218

Larson E B 1998 Management of Alzheimer's disease in a primary care setting. American Journal of Geriatric Psychiatry 6(2): S34–S40

Lavigne J, Schulein M, Hahn Y 1986 Psychological aspects of painful medical conditions in children. II. Personality factors, family characteristics and treatment. Pain 27(2): 147–169

Lee C 1995 Lonely waters. Sobell House, Oxford

Lee C 1996 Music at the edge: the music therapy experiences of a musician with AIDS. Routledge, London

Lehmann K A, Horrichs G, Hoeckle W 1985 The significance of tramadol as an intraoperative analgesic: a randomized double-blind study in comparison with placebo. Zur Bedeutung von Tramadol als intraoperativem Analgetikum. Eine randomisierte Doppelblindstudie im Vergleich zu Placebo. Anaesthesist 34(1): 11–19

Lengdobler H, Kiessling W R 1989 Group music therapy in multiple sclerosis: initial report of experience. Gruppenmusiktherapie bei multipler Sklerose: Ein erster Erfahrungsbericht. Psychotherapeutic, Psychosomatic and Medical Psychology 39(9–10): 369–373

Lindsay W 1980 The training and generalization of conversation behaviours in psychiatric inpatients: a controlled study employing multiple measures across settings. British Journal of Social and Clinical Psychology 19: 85–98

Lindsay S 1993 Music in hospitals. British Journal of Hospital Medicine 50(11): 660–662

Loewy J 1997 Music therapy and paediatric pain. Jeffrey Books, Cherry Hill, NJ

Longhofer J, Floersch J 1993 African drumming and psychiatric rehabilitation. Psychosocial Rehabilitation Journal 16(4): 3–10

Lucia C M 1987 Toward developing a model of music therapy intervention in the rehabilitation of head trauma patients. Music Therapy Perspectives 4: 34–39

McCauley K 1996 Music therapy with pediatric AIDS patients. In: Froehlich M-A Music therapy with hospitalized children. Jeffrey Books, Cherry Hill, NJ

Magee W 1995a Case studies in Huntington's disease: music therapy assessment and treatment in the early to advanced stages. British Journal of Music Therapy 9(2): 13–19

Magee W 1995b Music therapy as part of assessment and treatment for people living with Huntingtons's disease. In: Lee C Lonely waters. Sobell House, Oxford, pp. 173–183

Magee W 1998 A comparative study of familiar pre-composed music and unfamiliar improvised music in clinical music therapy with adults with multiple sclerosis. Unpublished doctoral thesis, University of London

Mahowald M, Woods S R, Schenck C H 1998 Sleeping dreams, waking hallucinations, and the central nervous system. Dreaming 8(2): 89–102

Mango C 1992 Emma: art therapy illustrating personal and universal images of loss. Omega Journal of Death and Dying 25(4): 259–269

Marley L 1984 The use of music with hospitalized infants and toddlers: a descriptive study. Journal of Music Therapy 21: 126–132

Meschede H G, Bender W, Pfeiffer H 1983 Music therapy with psychiatric problem patients. Musiktherapie mit psychiatrischen Problempatienten. Psychotherapeutic, Psychosomatic and Medical Psychology 33(3): 101–106

Moreno J L 1946 Psychodrama. Beacon House, New York

Morgano, Tilluckdharry R 1982 Presentation of singing function in severe aphasia. West Indian Medical Journal 31: 159–161

Murray L, Trevarthen C 1986 The infant's role in mother-infant communications. Journal of Child Language 13: 15–29

Naeser M, Helm-Estabrooks N 1985 CT scan lesion localization and response to melodic intonation therapy with nonfluent aphasia cases. Cortex 21(2): 203–223

O'Boyle M W, Sanford M 1988 Hemispheric asymmetry in the matching of melodies to rhythm sequences tapped in the right and left palms. Cortex 24(2): 211–221

O'Callaghan C 1996 Lyrical themes in songs written by palliative care patients. Journal of Music Therapy 33(2): 74–92

O'Callaghan C, Turnbull G 1987 The application of a neuropsychological knowledge base in the use of music therapy with severely brain damaged adynamic multiple sclerosis patients. Conference proceedings of the Australian Music Therapy Association, Melbourne, Australia, pp. 6–9

Oldfield A, Adams M 1990 The effects of music therapy on a group of profoundly mentally handicapped adults. Journal of Mental Deficiency Research 34(2): 107–125

Orange J B, VanGennep K M, Miller L, Johnson A M 1998 Resolution of communication breakdown in dementia of the Alzheimer's type: a longitudinal study. Journal of Applied Communication Research 26(1): 120–138

Pavlicevic M, Trevarthen C 1989 A musical assessment of psychiatric states in adults. Psychopathology 22(6): 325–334

Pavlicevic M, Trevarthen C, Duncan J 1994 Improvisational music therapy and the rehabilitation of persons suffering from chronic schizophrenia. Journal of Music Therapy 31(2): 86–104

Philip Y T 1989 Effects of music on patient anxiety in coronary care units letter. Heart and Lung 18(3): 322

Phillips R 1988 The creative moment: improvising in jazz and psychotherapy. Adolescent Psychiatry 15: 182–193

Pot A, Deeg D, VanDyck R 1997 Psychological well-being of informal caregivers of elderly people with dementia: changes over time. Aging and Mental Health 1(3): 261–268

Pratt R R, Erdonmez-Grocke D 1999 MusicMedicine 3. University of Melbourne, Melbourne

Pratt R R, Spintge R (ed) 1996 MusicMedicine II. MMB Music, St Louis

Prinsley D 1986 Music therapy in geriatric care. Australian Nurses Journal 15(9): 48–49

Purdie H, Baldwin S 1995 Models of music therapy intervention in stroke rehabilitation. International Journal of Rehabilitation Research 18(4): 341–350

Purdie H, Hamilton S, Baldwin S 1997 Music therapy: facilitating behavioural and psychological change in people with stroke: a pilot study. International Journal of Rehabilitation Research 20(3): 325–327

Raskind M A 1998 The clinical interface of depression and dementia. Journal of Clinical Psychiatry 59: 9–12

Richarz B 1997 Considerations to the psychosomatics of Alzheimer's disease. Dynamische Psychiatrie 30(5–6): 340–355

Rickert E, Duke L, Putzke J, Marson D, Graham K 1998 Early stage Alzheimer's disease disrupts encoding of contextual information. Aging Neuropsychology and Cognition 5(1): 73–81

Rider M S 1985a The effects of music imagery and relaxation on adrenal corticosteroids and the re-entrainment of circadian rhythms. Journal of Music Therapy 22(1): 46–56

Rider M S 1985b Entrainment mechanisms are involved in pain reduction, muscle relaxation, and music-mediated imagery. Journal of Music Therapy 22(4): 183–192

Robb S L 2000 Music assisted progressive muscle relaxation, progressive muscle relaxation, music listening, and silence: a comparison of relaxation techniques. Journal of Music Therapy 37(1): 2–21

Rusted J, Marsh R, Bledski L, Sheppard L 1997 Alzheimer patients' use of auditory and olfactory cues to aid verbal memory. Aging and Mental Health 1(4): 364–371

Sacks O 1986 The man who mistook his wife for a hat. Pan, London

Sachs L 1995 Is there a pathology of prevention? The implications of visualizing the invisible in screening programs. Culture, Medicine and Psychiatry 19: 503–525

Schnürer C, Aldridge D, Altmaier M, Neugebauer L, Kleinrath U, Steinke U 1995 Kreativität, Individualität-Wege in der AIDS-Therapie? AIDS-Forschung (AIFO) 10(1): 15–35

Smeijsters H 1997 Musiktherapie bei Alzheimerpatienten. Eine Meta-Analyse von Forschungsergebnissen. [Music therapy in the treatment of Alzheimer patient. A meta-analysis of research results.] Musiktherapeutische Umschau 1997(4): 268–283

Spielberger C 1983 Manual for state trait anxiety inventory. Consulting Psychologists' Press, Palo Alto, CA

Standley J M 1986 Music research in medical/dental treatment: meta-analysis and clinical applications. Journal of Music Therapy 23(2): 56–122

Standley J 1995 Music as a therapeutic intervention in medical and dental settings. In: Wigram T, Saperston B, West R (ed) Art and science of music therapy. Harwood Academic Publishers, Chur, Switzerland

Standley J, Hanser S 1995 Music therapy research and applications in pediatric oncology treatment. Journal of Paediatric Oncology Nursing 12(1): 3–8, 9–10

Steinberg R, Raith L 1985a Music psychopathology. I. Musical tempo and psychiatric disease. Psychopathology 18(5–6): 254–264

Steinberg R, Raith L 1985b Music psychopathology. II. Assessment of musical expression. Psydropathology 18(5–6): 265–273

Steinberg R, Raith L, Rossnagl G, Eben E 1985 Music psychopathology. III. Musical expression and psychiatric disease. Psychopathology 18(5–6): 274–285

Stern R S 1989 Many ways to grow: creative art therapies. Pediatric Annals 18(10): 645, 649–652

Street R, Cappella J 1989 Social and linguistic factors influencing adaptation in children's speech. Journal of Psycholinguistic Research 18(5): 497–519

Tang W H, Yao X W, Zheng Z P 1994 Rehabilitative effect of music therapy for residual schizophrenia: a one-month randomised controlled trial in Shanghai. British Journal of Psychiatry 165 (Suppl. 24): 38–44

Thaut M H 1985 The use of auditory rhythm and rhythmic speech to aid temporal muscular control in children with gross motor dysfunction. Journal of Music Therapy 22: 129–145

Thaut M H 1987 Visual versus auditory (musical) stimulus preferences in autistic children: a pilot study. Journal of Austism and Developmental Disorder 17(3): 425–432

Thaut M H 1988 Measuring musical responsiveness in autistic children: a comparative analysis of improvised musical tone sequences of autistic, normal, and mentally retarded individuals. Journal of Austism and Developmental Disorder 18(4): 561–571

Tierney M C, Szalai J P, Snow W, Fisher R 1996 The prediction of Alzheimer disease: the role of patient and informant perceptions of cognitive deficits. Archives of Neurology 53(5): 423–427

Tsunoda T 1983 The difference in the cerebral processing mechanism for musical sounds between Japanese and non-Japanese and its relation to mother tongue. In: Spintge R, Droh R (eds) Musik in der Medizin Springer Verlag, Berlin

Updike P 1990 Music therapy results for ICU patients. Dimensions of Critical Care Nursing 9(1): 39–45

Vincent S, Thompson J 1929 The effects of music on the human blood pressure. Lancet 1 (March 9): 534–537

Wengel S, Burke W, Holemon D 1989 Musical hallucinations. The sounds of silence? Journal of the American Geriatric Association 37(2): 163–166

Wheeler B 1995 Music therapy research: quantitative and qualitative perspectives. Barcelona Publishers, Phoenixville

White, D, Murphy C 1998 Working memory for nonverbal auditory information in dementia of the Alzheimer type. Archives of Clinical Neuropsychology 13(4): 339–347

Wigram A L 1988 Music therapy: developments in mental handicap. Special Issue: Music Therapy. Psychology of Music 16(1): 42–51

Wigram T, Saperston B, West R 1995a Art and science of music therapy. Harwood Academic Publishers, Chur, Switzerland

Wigram T, Saperston B, West R 1995b The art and science of music therapy: a handbook. Harwood Academic Publishes Chur, Switzerland

Zimmerman L M, Pierson M A, Marker J 1988 Effects of music on patient anxiety in coronary care units. Heart-Lung 17(5): 560–566

The impact of healing in a clinical setting

Tim Harlow

Does healing make a difference in a conventional medical practice? Attempts to 'prove' that energy exists or healing prayer works are fraught with conceptual and methological problems. Clinical research is often too insensitive to answer such questions. One option is pragmatic controlled trials or carefully done observational studies to assess the impact of healing as it is usually delivered.

This paper summarizes the impact of bringing a healer into a conventional practice in the context of doing a quasi-randomized, wait-list trial of healing on chronically ill patients. While over half the patients improved and costs were reduced, the most important observation may be the effect of the healer on doctor–patient communication. Patients began to more openly discuss with their doctors their use of complementary medicine interventions and doctors began to see the importance of listening to and touching patients after the healer entered the practice.   **WBJ**

INTRODUCTION

From May 1992 up to the time of writing (September 2000), and continuing, there has been initially one healer and then two working alongside the doctors in our conventional general medical practice, at College Surgery, Devon, England. This has provided the opportunity to carry out research into the efficacy of healing in this context. Two published research trials have been performed. Equally important, we have begun to learn something of the place of healing in conventional practice and which conditions seem to respond best to such an approach.

We also have been helped to look critically at the much neglected role of the doctor as a healer. Much work remains to be done, especially to see how much of any beneficial effect is placebo and what aspects can be learned and applied by conventional therapists such as doctors.

Coming as we do from a conventional scientific background, it has been important to ensure that scientific tests of efficacy are used. This seems important not only so that we can advise our patients adequately but also for the purposes of fundamental research. If there really is an effect inexplicable by our conventional scientific model, then either the observation is wrong or, fascinatingly, our scientific model is incomplete. To be able to combine these two aspects, both helping patients and conducting research, in general clinical practice is a rare treat.

DEFINITION OF HEALING

There are various definitions of the term 'healing' and a pragmatic one, used in this discussion, is: the focused interaction between one person, the healer, and another who is unwell with the intention of improving the health of the ill person. This may result from an as yet poorly characterized energy transfer or channeling.

HISTORY OF HEALING AT COLLEGE SURGERY

Gill White started working at the surgery in 1992, seeing five patients one morning a week. This was initially a trial period, at the invitation of Michael Dixon, a partner at the surgery, and as part of a trial funded by local research grant (Dixon 1991) (details of the trial are discussed below). The trial ran from May 1992 to June 1993. It was clear that there was enough benefit to our patients to justify Gill's continuing work in the surgery. The number of patients who could benefit soon made it sensible to include a second healer and Teresa Seward joined the healing clinic in September 1994.

The initial research findings were sufficiently interesting to prompt a second trial, including this time a control group (Dixon 1998). This second trial ran from September 1994 to September 1996 and also attempted to look at possible underlying cellular changes during healing.

Since then both healers have continued to work in the surgery as an integral part of the team. There are plans for further research to look at mechanisms of healing and differentiation from placebo effect. The practice has close links with Professor Edzard Ernst and his Department of Complementary Medicine at Exeter University in Devon.

THE FIRST STUDY

Method

When patient and doctor felt it was appropriate, baseline information was recorded. This included the main symptom, treatment to date and current treatment, and number of consultations with a doctor in the last 12 months. It was also recorded whether the patient was in work. A symptom score was made by both doctor and patient. The symptom score ranged from zero (no symptoms) to 4 (very bad indeed) with 5 being variable.

The main symptom had to be chronic (of 6 months or more duration) and had also to be fully evaluated conventionally so that even if a clear diagnosis was impossible, there was confidence that no serious underlying disease had been missed.

Healing was given by Gill White for an average of eight weekly sessions of 45 minutes each. The range was from 3 to 18 sessions. A total of 25 patients were seen and the symptom scores were repeated, together with an assessment by the patient as to how their symptom had changed. This scale was from -4 (could not be worse) to $+4$ (no symptoms at all any more) with 0 being unchanged.

As the study progressed it became possible to follow up some patients for longer and so at 6 months after treatment a further set of scores were obtained for nine patients.

Results

The average symptom score was 3 (very bad) at the start of the trial. Seven patients (28%) showed no improvement, the other 18 (72%) showed some improvement. Of these, eight (32%) showed substantial improvement. It seemed that those with lower initial symptom scores did better than those with higher initial scores.

The patient's change score showed eight (32%) no change, four (16%) slight improvement, five (20%) much better and eight (32%) felt very much better.

The doctor's change scores showed similar patterns to the patients change scores. One notable discrepancy was a patient who initially felt only slightly better even though her doctor felt she was much better. At the 6 month follow-up she remarked that she had felt better without being able to recognize this. Thus without her being aware of the doctor's score her later score was much closer to his original one.

Discussion

Joint pain, stress, skin disease, and abdominal pain appeared to respond especially well. Back pain, depression, and ME /chronic fatigue syndrome were more variable in response, while headaches and agoraphobia seemed unresponsive.

One of the limitations of the study design was in using just one cardinal symptom as a measure of success. This did, however, demonstrate that there was a noticeable effect and that this was an effective treatment. Looking only at this aspect of the study would underestimate the other benefits shown. All but one of the patients (96%) reported that the experience of healing had been useful and pleasurable even if their main symptom was unaffected.

Many favourable comments were made, such as 'I have altered my whole outlook on life' and 'She encouraged me to help myself.' Some clue to the other aspects can be found in the longer-term follow-up including consultation rate and medication use.

The nine patients followed up for 6 months after healing were high users of surgery consultations with an average of 12.5 per annum (the practice average is 3 per annum). Even though many of those followed up did not show improvement in symptom score with healing, their consultation rate dropped by 4 consultations per annum to 7.16. This is both significant ($P < 0.01$) and represents a saving of 100 or so consultations a year. Even a year later the consultation rate was still reduced at 8.04 ($P < 0.05$). Eight patients reduced or stopped their medication while attending the healing clinic. This represented a saving of around £ 1164 per annum. This is clearly desirable both from the point of view of patients' well-being and in cost terms.

Longer-term follow-up of this study was extended to 50 patients and the results were confirmed. Skin conditions (eczema and psoriasis) showed most improvement with all five patients much better or very much better and with four stopping treatment completely.

This study demonstrated that the concept of a healer working in a general clinical practice was a good one with real benefits for patients. The doctors commented that medical consultations after healing had become more positive and less wearying. There were benefits too for the doctors which will be discussed later in the chapter.

THE SECOND STUDY

Complementary treatments can be difficult to subject to controlled trials and after the previous observational study it was felt important to try to introduce a control group. Using a group of patients on a waiting list for healing was a useful way of introducing a control group. However, there were some drawbacks (Kirk-Smith 1998); these included expectational effect (the knowledge that nothing was being done but soon would be) and feeling an obligation to provide positive reports to the therapist. Nonetheless, it did allow some comparison between groups with interesting results.

It was also interesting to see if the cellular mechanisms behind healing could be examined. Research into psychoneuroimmunology has suggested that natural killer cells (CD16, CD56) might be involved in beneficial effects of healing (Fawzey et al 1990). One of the objectives of this study was to see whether there were immunological changes that might correlate with response to healing.

Chronic illness is difficult for both patient and primary care physician. There is a paucity of data on the effectiveness of healing in primary care, though some evidence to suggest that chronic idiopathic pain is not helped much by healing. Psychological state is known to influence physical health as well as being important in its own right; thus it seemed sensible to look specifically at changes in anxiety and depression during healing. Good instruments already exist to measure these variables such as the hospital anxiety and depression (HAD) scale (Zigmond & Snaith 1983). An attempt was made to measure the much more general changes which patients had reported in previous studies. The Nottingham health profile (NHP), a measure of general functional ability, both physical and mental, was used in our study (Hunt 1985).

Method

This second study ran from September 1994 to September 1996 and took place at College Surgery. As before, the patients were referred by the seven doctors in the practice when both patient and doctor felt it appropriate. A total of 57 patients entered the trial and were consecutively allocated alternately to study and control groups. The study group received 10 weekly healing sessions on a Thursday morning while the control group had their healing deferred by 6 months. As is usual in general practice consultations, there were more women than men in both groups. The groups were similar in symptomatology with half having had symptoms for at least 5 years. There was a good match in all the main indices between the two groups at the beginning of the trial. All the patients were people who had been conventionally well worked up as in the first study.

Results

After 3 months of healing patients showed an improvement in median symptom score of 1.0 compared with 0 for controls ($P < 0.05$). There was no significant difference at 6 months. Of 27 patients who had healing, five thought their symptoms the same, eight felt slightly better, seven felt much better, six felt very much better and one had no symptoms at all. Thus 21 (81%) felt their symptoms improved, 15 (55%) felt them improved substantially. The study group did better in their perception of symptom improvement than controls and this was still significantly different at 6 months ($P < 0.05$). Thus there was a marked improvement in patients with a chronic condition who had already had a lot of unsuccessful conventional treatment.

There were improvements too in anxiety and depression at 3 months in the study group with minimal change in the control group. The HAD anxiety scale showed a significant ($P < 0.01$) improvement compared with controls. The HAD depression scale showed a similar effect with significant improvement ($P < 0.05$). At 6 months of the trial (3 months after finishing healing) the improvement in the treated group was better than that of the controls for both anxiety ($P < 0.01$) and depression ($P < 0.05$). Thus there were significant differences which persisted well after the healing had finished.

When general function was considered with the NHP, the same trend appeared. There was a significant ($P < 0.01$) improvement with the treated group compared to the controls. Interestingly, the treated patients had maintained an improvement at 6 months but the difference between them and the controls was not statistically significant.

There was a problem with the study of natural killer cells as during the trial it became clear that the reagent for the CD16 cells was faulty and that there was no short-term change in the other line (CD56). The replacement reagent meant that the patients in the second half of the study had their healing delayed for 6 rather than 3 months so that they could have their results compared with the treatment group at the completion of their healing and after 3 months. There was no significant change or difference with healing in the level of CD16 or CD56 killer cells.

Consultation rates had been shown to change after the first study and this was an area to explore again. The patients in both healing and control groups had higher than average annual consultation rates of 12 p.a. compared with practice average of 3.4, reflecting the chronic symptomatology. This study did not show any significant difference either between the groups or after healing. There were patient self reports of a greater likelihood of reducing medication if patients were in the treatment group. The study did not specifically look at this point and there is therefore no independent measure of this intriguing possibility.

Discussion

This trial, the first research from primary care to look at healing in a controlled way, suggests that there may be an improvement in a variety of measures of ill health in chronically ill people. Symptoms, anxiety, depression, and general functioning all improved. A majority (52%) of patients felt substantially better after healing and this improvement was maintained after 3 months. It seems that these general effects on well-being are maintained better long term than specific changes in symptoms. This fits in with previous work from Lourdes (Morris 1982).

The lack of immunological response may mean either that the responses seen were not reflected in immunological change or that the wrong parameters were measured. There was no attempt to distinguish between general effects from patients being given time in a caring way and between any specific effect of healing.

A major factor which should be emphasized at this point was the complete lack of adverse effects due to healing. For an effective and relatively inexpensive treatment to seem to be entirely free of adverse side-effects is remarkable.

A variety of questions remain unanswered by this research and some others are generated by it. The most pressing one seems to be whether there is a specific benefit due to healing not found in other interactions. Related to that question is the more pragmatic one of how these benefits (however caused) can best be used in general medical practice. Can physicians learn to be healers in the sense meant here or at least learn to exploit their

placebo and therapeutic effect to maximize the help they give to their patients? With the background of these studies as a scientific underpinning, further discussion on the actual experience of healing in this context is possible.

THE EXPERIENCE OF HEALING FOR OUR PRACTICE

The College Surgery has always had a tradition of complementary medicine. Individuals among the doctors have combined acupuncture, homeopathy, and hypnotherapy with their conventional medical practice. Some of the doctors are skeptical about complementary treatments but are tolerant of them and so fortunately there is no outright opposition. In general we are in favour of anything that helps our patients. Conventional medicine has many triumphs but we are daily confronted with its limitations. Daily too we see patients who tell us of the help they have had from complementary practitioners.

Thus when Michael Dixon came to the practice with the idea of introducing Gill White as a healer we were at least prepared to be open minded. He had met Gill on a course about healing and was captivated by the possibilities not only of help for our patients but also of research into an area even more poorly understood then than now. He has been the driving force and vision behind the healing research in our practice; much of the work is his, and I have been lucky enough to be involved with him on this and other, current, research.

There are five ways in which this experience of healing has affected our medical practice. The first and most obvious is the extra point of referral now available. We have a further option for those patients we are often least able to help conventionally. This can be most valuable in enabling us to continue to deal with patients whom we, as conventional doctors, have failed to 'cure'.

This can be an especially difficult group of patients, sometimes termed the 'heartsink' patients. We dread seeing them not of themselves but because our conventional medical model is so poor at understanding their problems and seems unable satisfactorily to resolve them. The patients, expectations raised by the mirage of omnipotent doctors, are bitterly disappointed by our inability to deal with their symptoms. As doctors we are frustrated by the way the conditions of these patients defy the neat categorization of our reductionist methods and by how poor our therapies can be.

The benefit of being allowed to escape from this impasse is enormous. It is vital to be clear about why we are referring patients for healing. Just 'offloading' problem patients is unfair on everyone. It is important to see when the moment is truly right to suggest healing and to ensure the patient is part of the decision process. That the healing is taking place in the surgery is a help; we are able to ensure the patient feels still cared for by the surgery and does not feel rejected by the decision.

The second way in which our practice has been affected by healing is in the positive way our attitude to complementary medicine is viewed by our patients. Some patients are reluctant to tell us of complementary treatments they are having for fear of disapproval. This is a hindrance when discussing treatment options: the mere fact of our using healers in a high profile way allows open discussion of such subjects. Paradoxically, our being ready to accept complementary treatments seems to make patients readier to accept our offer of conventional therapy. If we seem genuinely ready to consider all helpful avenues then it gives a credibility to our suggestions of treatment. Conversely if a patient has had a positive experience of a complementary therapy and yet we appear to dismiss it out of hand the patient would be justified in doubting our objectivity and advice.

Third in the effects of healing on our practice is the impact of research. It is easy to be so caught up with day-to-day practice that one loses sight of the larger picture; we continue to do the same things we have always done and can be blind to other approaches. Research is easily left to those in ivory towers who have the time and resources. They, of course, end up not addressing the real world of clinical medicine and important issues in everyday practice.

One way to ensure that research is relevant to our daily practice is to do the research ourselves.

The mere act of looking critically at a part of that practice is helpful, as is being able to ask real and pertinent questions with robust enough conclusions to ensure usefulness. The change of culture within the practice has been gradual but has gathered pace. Now that we have an established track record of research, funding is easier, and we expect to be involved in further research. As well as conventional research with the Medical Research Council we are involved with the department of complementary medicine of the University of Exeter in other work, for example the use of magnetic bracelets for joint pain and vitamin B for tiredness.

There is the 'Hawthorn effect' where the act of looking critically at an area is in itself a way of producing improvement. Once, as conventional physicians, we begin to look at complementary treatments we are able to start advising our patients how particular therapies may fit their health needs.

This leads us to the fourth way in which the experience of healing has impacted on our practice. Conventional medical training provides no information about which complementary treatments might be particularly helpful in certain conditions or for certain patients. In general there is very little discussion about how different patient types will respond to different therapies. We have begun to learn that this is a key factor in the success of, for example, healing.

It has become clear to us, both from the research already discussed and through our experience with healing, that some problems are especially suitable for this approach. We see that skin conditions such as eczema and psoriasis respond well to healing. Our conventional experience tells us that these conditions flare up in response to stress; that hypnotherapy can be a useful therapeutic adjunct seems to fit with a whole-person approach such as healing.

Problems of impaired immunity such as recurrent cold sores and viral infections are also helped, which might also be predicted by experience of such conditions being commoner in exhausted or emotionally drained patients. Babies with colic have been helped and our practice health visitors often refer them. The healers feel that much of the healing is going to the mother who, by the time she has sought professional help, is often very run down herself.

Some things seem to respond less well, at least in the setting of our community in Devon. Chronic fatigue syndrome is an area for which we initially had high hopes of healing. People do feel better in general terms, and overall are positive about the experience, but the symptoms themselves seem to respond poorly.

Anxiety and depression can be helped but one healer feels that the presence of antidepressant medication can be a barrier to healing. As conventional doctors we are then in a difficult position. Depression is an illness with a worrying mortality and morbidity, and antidepressants are an effective and recognized treatment. If we were to diagnose a serious depressive illness and either fail to use, or stop a proven treatment we would be in a weak position both personally and medico-legally if, for instance, the person were to commit suicide. We also feel the need to protect our healers from such a situation. In reality milder cases or those recovering can receive much benefit from healing.

A fifth (and to me surprising) way that healing has altered our practice is the way it has changed some of us as doctors. In the distant past there were limited treatments for many conditions and much of a doctor's ability to help came from either placebo or possibly a form of healing – placebo here, it must be emphasized, is by no means intended to be a disparaging term. Placebo is one of the most powerful and ill understood ways of one person helping another. This fact is often neglected now so that most conventional physicians would see themselves as simply applying the correct one of a range of specific and potent treatments. Well and good when the condition or patient responds and can be neatly categorized.

Real problems arise, however, when, as so often in real life, things are not that simple. Our training ill equips us either to be a compassionate observer of disease and the human condition or to use to the full such placebo and natural healing powers as we possess. This an area we must learn to maximize if we are to be of most help to our patients. Healing has, for me, brought to the fore this side of my profession and is a constant reminder of my need to remain aware of it. Having healers in the building, meeting them, seeing patients who have been treated, and being aware of healing as a referral possibility are all hugely helpful to me.

Some benefits were also experienced by the healers in this joint venture. Knowing that there had been a conventional medical work up was a help, for example reducing the chances of a serious undiagnosed illness. The healers found conventional back-up useful and the joint discussions about cases were mutually illuminating. We each discovered aspects of cases that we would have failed to perceive without that partnership.

PRACTICALITIES

As a practice we were initially unsure of some of the practicalities of using healing. I have discussed the way we learned something of the kinds of conditions that might respond best, but not the kind of people who respond best. There is no formal work on this yet but some tentative thoughts are possible.

There first needs to be a willingness in the patient to try the therapy with an open mind; a healthy skepticism is compatible with healing but a defiant patient who has gone along merely out of duty is difficult. Someone who is totally passive and wishes to transfer all responsibility onto the therapist is also a problem. There are some patients who are not ready to be well. These people seem almost to need their illness, or at least the sick role, and must be helped to deal with this by other means before healing can be useful. Other than these, there seem to be no real groups in whom healing is unwise except the very ill with whom we have too little experience to be confident.

At first we worried about how to raise the subject of healing with a patient in the course of a conventional consultation. In reality there was no difficulty provided we had already spent enough effort to ensure that we had properly worked out the situation and the patient felt that too. Then patients seemed ready to embrace the idea and did not feel 'fobbed off.'

Both healers in our surgery are practicing Christians and see their healing in that context, as coming from the Divine. The doctors and patients in the practice have a variety of religous beliefs and unbeliefs. This seems not to matter. When I discuss the referral with a patient I tell them the religous position of the healers but emphasize that they wish only to help and that there will be no pressure to conform with their beliefs at all.

HEALING AND SCIENCE

Rigorous science is vital if we are to help our patients best and to use finite resources to maximum advantage. As yet conventional science has no coherent explanation to account for healing. Some scientists therefore assume that because current scientific understanding is not able to explain healing, it cannot be happening. This is a profoundly unscientific view. If an observation is made, such as the effect of healing, and the current scientific model does not allow or explain the observation, then there are only two possibilities: either the observation is wrong or the scientific model is incomplete. There is a great deal of anecdotal evidence, much of which we see regularly in clinical practice, that there is something happening in healing. Now there is also hard scientific evidence that healing has a definite effect. Thus it is illogical not to accept the possibility that our scientific model may need to be modified. 'Every Newton awaits his Einstein.'

We tend to think of scientific truth as absolute. For everyday purposes that may be adequate, so that Newtonian physics is still useful for designing, say, kitchen scales or a car bumper. But quantum mechanics and Einsteinian physics show that Newtonian methods are only an approximation and for other purposes such as nuclear power they are inadequate. Thus it is in this field.

THE FUTURE

Nationally there is much interest in healing in the UK with 20 000 spiritual healers registered with the main healing organizations; this makes it now the most prevalent therapy in the UK (Daniel 2000). There is evidence that healing stands up to scientific scrutiny; and there are moves afoot to try and incorporate proven complementary therapies into the National Health Service which is most exciting (Royal Society of Medicine 2000).

Locally we are planning research into the mechanism of healing to try and tease out the effect from healing alone, as opposed to that from placebo. This is not to suggest that placebo is not extremely powerful. There is a placebo effect even in very effective and well-established conventional treatments such as morphine for the relief of pain. There is a tendency to dimiss the placebo effect as somehow improper, as a form of theraputic cheating. We should seek rather to explore how the placebo effect actually works and how it differs from the effect of healing. Rather as recent work has shown that homeopathy can have an effect (Taylor et al 2000), this might cause scientists to see the limits of our present understanding of the world. It will be important also to continue with as rigorous a scientific method as possible, there is no place for pseudo-science when planning health care.

SUMMARY

Healing does not make antibiotics, heart transplants, or genetically engineered vaccines irrelevant, it simply shows us another way which can be complementary to our conventional methods. I believe there are great advances to be made in the interface between conventional and complementary medicine. We also, as conventional physicians, need to relearn the power of healing we have in ourselves and learn to maximize this for our patients' benefit.

There is much still to be discovered about the mechanism of healing and research is planned. We would be unwise to stop using healing just because we do not completely understand it. There is a great deal to be said for a pragmatic approach which accepts the benefits and seeks to apply them without being inhibited by a lack of understanding of the fundamental mechanisms.

REFERENCES

Daniel R 2000 The place of healing in medicine today. Healing Today Jan: 8–13

Dixon M 1991 A healer in the practice. British Journal of General Practice 45: 396

Dixon M 1998 Does 'healing' benefit patients with chronic symptoms? A quasi-randomized trial in general practice. Journal of the Royal Society of Medicine 91: 183–188

Fawzy F L, Kemen M E, Fawzy N W, et al 1990 A structured psychiatric intervention for cancer patients. 11. Changes over time in immunological measures. Archives of General Psychiatry 47: 729–735

Hunt S M 1985 Measuring health status: a new tool for clinicians and epidemiologists. Journal of General Practice 35: 185–188

Kirk-Smith M 1998 Healing and expection. *Journal of the Royal Society of Medicine 91: 400*

Morris P A 1982 The effect of pilgrimage on anxiety, depression and religous attitude. Psychological Medicine 12: 291–294

Taylor M A, Reilly D, Llewellyn-Jones R H, McSharry C, Aitchison, T 2000 Randomised controlled trial of homeopathy versus placebo in perennial allergic rhinitis with overview of four trial series. British Medical Journal 321: 471–476

Royal Society of Medicine 2000 Complementary medicine, primary care and the new NHS: applying the evidence. Conference at the Royal Society of Medicine, London, September 26, 2000

Zigmond A S, Snaith R D 1983 The hospital anxiety and depression scale. Acta Psychiatica Scandinavica 67: 361–370

Methods and challenges for research on healing

14

The phenomenology of paranormal healing practices

M. Allan Cooperstein

This chapter describes published efforts to describe and classify types of metal energy and spiritual healing practice.

All research starts with observation and description. Accurate description is required before categories can be established for classification and measurement tools developed to quantify those classifications. This is the role of phenomenology. Replication by others, a hallmark of science, also builds on accurate description. Unfortunately, accurate and detailed observation and description is an often neglected area of research. Too frequently we jump to the more fascinating questions such as 'does mental energy and spiritual healing work' or 'is consciousness non-local' without knowing what we and others mean by 'consciousness,' 'spiritual' energy or 'healing.' When the basics of description and classification are neglected in clinical trial research, inconsistent and confusing results are likely. In this chapter, M. Allan Cooperstein outlines the process of phenomenology and describes the few systematic efforts conducted to describe and classify healing behavior and practices.   **WBJ**

INTRODUCTION

The term 'healing' is used in this chapter to refer to purported paranormal healing, or the effects of intentional paranormal influencing. Such alternative healing methods are considered anomalous, do not necessarily use material objects, rely chiefly upon the healers' beliefs in scientifically non-validated energies, intervention by spiritual or spiritistic entities, or existence of non-ordinary human potentials.

Many labels have been applied to anomalous healing by scholars and healers, for example faith healing, laying-on of hands, prayer healing, psychic healing or, as in my research, transpersonal healing. The genesis of these methods appears rooted in folk healing and shamanic, magico-religious tradition, extending back 15–40 000 years (Eliade 1974, Halifax 1982).

There is a dearth of investigations into healers' phenomenology and intrapsychic processes. I undertook a comprehensive literature search with the assistance of the internet and other researchers in the field.[1] The results led to the conclusion that, in contrast to studies attempting to measure healing/influencing effects, too little research attention has been focused on the psychological means used by healers to produce effects under controlled or clinical conditions.

Below, I examine mainly three phenomenological studies: those by LeShan (1969, 1975), Van Dragt (1980) and myself (Cooperstein 1990). Although LeShan's findings were incorporated in my study, I was unaware of Van Dragt's unpublished dissertation.

PHENOMENOLOGICAL STUDIES

Lawrence LeShan

Psychologist LeShan's contribution stemmed from his primary goal of developing a general theory of the paranormal. Starting with a single-case study of Eileen Garrett, a 'sensitive,' he learned that sensitives experience altered consciousness in which their concept of reality differs markedly

from the ordinary. He proposed that two realities were used by sensitives, their relationship viewed as overlapping, each representing a different aspect of a greater whole.

The first, sensory reality, is formed from sense perceptions of the uniqueness and separateness (via time and space) of objects. In this reality, communications are limited to transmission and reception of sensory data; time is experienced as a flow of events; personal values are attributed to events and actions; there is a sense of free will and self-determination; and personal will directs actions. Space and time separations preclude information or energy exchange.

In clairvoyant reality, on the other hand, the separateness of the other reality is illusory, as all objects are part of a greater whole. Information about another, apparently discrete individual is directly accessible when individuals merge within the greater unity. Here a timeless present is experienced; personal values are not attributed to events; personal will does not exist as events are already determined; and perception is not directed by personal will. Information is received non-ordinarily via one's immersion in events. Space and time are irrelevant in transmitting information or energy, as both are illusory.

LeShan selected psychic healing to test whether a parapsychological skill could be acquired through immersion in the two realities. Seeking serious psychic healers – those believed to be effective, who practiced consistently, and about whom biographical or autobiographical materials existed – he isolated common methods and developed a typology (presented later in the chapter).

Bryan Van Dragt

Van Dragt (1980), a psychologist, limited his doctoral research to 10 individuals who identified themselves as 'psychic,' 'spiritual,' parapsychological, and 'prayer healing' healers and were recognized by their peers as having genuine skills. He applied a phenomenological methodology in a three-phase approach (Fig. 14.1).

Healers were asked a general question, followed by more categorical questions to prompt responses. A summary and comparison of Van

---

[1]Patrice Keene of the American Association of Psychical Research (ASPR), the librarian at the Parapsychology Foundation, Penny Hiernu of the International Society for the Study of Subtle Energies and Energy Medicine (ISSSEEM), Savely Savva of the Monterey Institute for the Study of Alternative Healing Arts (MISAHA), and personal contacts with Drs Bernard Grad, Steven Fahrion (ISSSEEM), Michaleen Maher, Joanne McMahon, Norman Shealy, Joyce Goodrich, Daniel Benor, and Elmer Green.

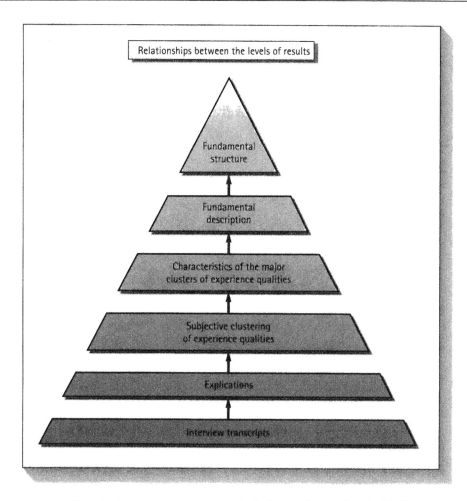

Figure 14.1 Van Dragt's phenomenological methodology (Van Dragt 1980).

Dragt's findings are presented in the appendix to this chapter (Appendix 1).

In other research, Tilley (1989), a pastor, used a sample of 10 healers chosen for healing exclusively within the Christian tradition and based on their established reputation. His findings are also found in Appendix 1. Despite Tilley's claim to replicate Van Dragt's work, his research is replete with inherent biases and lacks the detailed description and articulation offered by Van Dragt and will not be addressed in detail.

M. Allan Cooperstein

Without knowledge of Van Dragt or Tilley, the principal goals of Cooperstein's (1990) research were,

first, to discover and describe the nature of the psychological processes used by healers during healing, and second, to develop a typological system that could differentiate between healers based upon their psychologies, rather than misleading labels.

Cooperstein used a multiphasic phenomenological approach, attempting to bridge healers' unsupported statements and ground findings in research participants who had demonstrated experimental or clinical results. Research steps 1–3 (Figure 14.2) led to the following dimensions. This enabled the development and refinement of an extensive, structured protocol used to analyze the content of:

- 10 texts by healers
- 10 interviews of healers who demonstrated experimental or clinical effects.

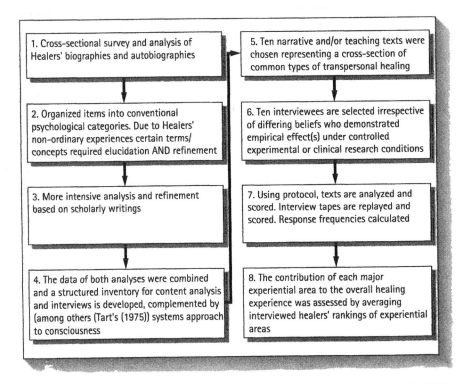

Figure 14.2 Cooperstein's multiphasic phenomenological methodology (Cooperstein 1990).

Upon completing the content analyses and interviews, interviewees ranked the importance of experiential areas to their healing experience. A correlation between texts and interviews was performed, but has inherent limitations due to the use of texts (Box 14.1).

Research Results

Results indicate that, during consciously intended transpersonal healing, attention is first personally controlled, or self-regulated, effortfully through selective attention, or concentration at treatment onset. Non-relevant sensory input is rejected. Withdrawn from the environment, attention is focused upon inner experience. There is a shift in consciousness sufficiently atypical, stable, and long-lasting to be considered an altered state. This alternate awareness is distinguished by decreased effort, enhanced awareness of, and sensitivity towards inner processes, without complete exclusion of the external world, and intense absorption within, or surrender to the object of attention. Once the process is activated, personal control may be decreased or surrendered.

The alterations described lead to emergence of appositional processes of ordinary, rational and non-ordinary, non-rational cognition. Thinking is more non-analytical, non-critical, and expectational relative to the healer's goal setting. The rate of thinking may seem ordinary or increased. Discursive thought decreases and may reach 'inner silence.' There is increased tolerance of ambiguity. General or specific goals are established for the healer and healee. The chief methods of realization, or 'making real' the healer's intent is through the use of verbal affirmations, non-imaginal beliefs, and mental imagery. Mental imagery is important, but not essential. Images aid in inducing the healing state, treatment, and goal visualization. Among non-visual imagery, somesthetic types manifest frequently, often expressed as non-ordinary heat or cold.

Visual images increase in quantity, become more vivid and dynamic. Visual images are

Box 14.1   Interviewed healers averaged rank order of transpersonal healing experiential areas and correlations between author and interviewee responses

Rank	Areas of consciousness	Averages	r
1	Attention	2.6	0.87
2	Cognitive processes	4.1	0.86*
3	Sense of self	5.9	0.66
4	Beliefs and assumptions	6.2	0.89
5	Somatic and physiological features	6.9	0.63
6	Preparation and induction of 'healing state'	6.9	0.81
7	Emotions	7.5	0.57
8	Attitudes	7.6	0.65
9	Subconscious processes	8.1	0.04*
10	Awareness of and contact with external environment	8.8	0.63*
11	Time sense	9.4	0.87
12	Purported paranormal experiences	9.9	0.81
13	Meaning	10.4	− 0.81
14	Motor activity	10.7	0.84*

*Depending upon the number of items available for scoring, authors not addressing aspects or areas of the healing experience affected some correlations. This occurred in environmental awareness, motor activity, subconscious activity and cognitive processing. Interviewees responded to all areas. In some instances, the number of items within an area was sufficient to compensate for authors' deficits and still produce substantial correlations. For example, cognitive processes, a broad area of enquiry with many items, was unaffected, while the correlation for subconscious processes was affected due to authors' lack of response.

predominantly realistic or quasi-realistic and consciously selected by the healer or emerge spontaneously as a function of the depth of the healing state. Intuitions are experienced as hunches or feelings, proving to be accurate but not deduced through analytical thinking. Imagination is expressed in the combined use of imagery and belief constructs. The categories of beliefs used to extend conceptual boundaries and the limits of sensory reality include energies, powers, and forces, discarnate (spiritual and spiritistic) beings, and paranormal abilities that augment accepted human abilities. Creativity is expressed as increased inner resources, spontaneity, openness (less defensiveness), and an enhanced capacity to transcend sensory and conceptual limits.

Healing events are recalled with vividness and continuity.

One's ordinary sense of self is altered. Self-awareness, body awareness and personal identity are weakened. Distortions of body image or diminishing body definition are reported. Although applied at treatment onset, personal will is replaced by impersonal intentionality, from gentle release to a complete surrender. Experiences include dissoci-

ation from one's ordinary identity, a non-ordinary sense of wholeness, decreased personal needs, enhanced feelings of interconnection to others, nature, the cosmos, etc. A non-personal, 'deeper' or 'higher' self, may emerge, endowing the healer with knowledge or abilities ordinarily considered ego-dystonic or transpersonal. Dissolution of the ordinary self is often accompanied by identification with forces and energies or discarnate entities.

Some healers explain experiences using known energies – electricity, magnetism – but these are used metaphorically to communicate concepts and experiences. There is greater use of beliefs in non-validated, quasi-realistic energies, for example qi, 'current', prana, or abstract energy such as light, or rays. The energy is said to originate from an interaction of the self and a source beyond the self.

Healers believe consciousness is a fundamental organismic awareness existing as an extended, non-local, distinguishable entity. Not limited to humans, it is possessed by and interconnects all living things. It is, therefore, capable of interacting with and influencing the physical world. Individual (local) consciousness is limited by personal identity and cultural factors. Setting these aside, it becomes possible to merge one's consciousness with that of another organism to acquire information from or influence the other. Individual consciousness is believed to be subsumed within higher, expansive orders of consciousness, ultimately interconnecting with a universal consciousness or intelligence. Belief in a spiritual (non-sensory) reality is common and it is frequently believed that the laws governing spiritual reality interact with those of physical reality.

Most healers report a state of hypoarousal, although two interviewees described hyperarousal. In the majority, heart and pulse rates decrease and respiration is self-regulated at first, becoming slower, deeper, and rhythmic. Initial effort associated with breathing lessens and respiration becomes more effortless. Muscle tension is relaxed.

With altered reality testing, non-ordinary physical sensations are experienced, including quasi-energy feelings, such as vibrations, oscillations, rhythmic reverberations, non-ordinary warmth or coldness.

Environmental modifications are unnecessary, although non-distracting surroundings are preferred. The healee's presence is desirable, although healing may occur remotely. Sensory stimulation is reduced by closing one's eyes, self-regulating attention, and initially restricting motor activity.

Self-regulative, meditative techniques including 'centering,' meditative prayers, and healing meditations are employed more often than prayers of petition, intercession, thankfulness, or forgiveness. 'Passes' or gestures are used, most often to detect healee 'energy' emanations or as symbolic gestures representing a transfer of energy.

Atypically heightened emotional responses are experienced. These are primarily positive, although negative emotions may occur. Healers report interpersonal warmth, inner harmony and tranquility, joy, exultation, and altruistic caring or love.

Attitudes of spontaneity, love, and empathy are most frequently advocated, accompanied by altruism and being receptive to the needs of the healee. Patience, hope, and determination to effect a beneficial outcome are also valued.

As indicated, personal or consciously-directed processes are lessened and may be surrendered, although not completely subordinated. Instead, conscious and subconscious processes operate integratively and synergistically. A resultant 'expanded' awareness facilitates increased access to subconscious materials, including sudden intuitions, flashes of information, the appearance of symbols or images seeming to spring from beyond the healer's ordinary self. Healers assert that awareness and discrimination of the healer's personal subconscious contents is necessary to differentiate between one's own and the healee's, acquired in empathic or sympathetic interactions. The consensus of interviewees suggests that subconscious processes are significant, support processes underlying faith and belief, and are associated with the onset and direction of healing.

Decreased investment of attention in the general environment causes the perceptual field to alter resulting in temporal and spatial distortions, heightened responsiveness to colors and qualities of objects, and changes in the ordinary salience of objects and events. United with altered sense of self and cognition, these factors lead to a reorientation of the generalized reality orientation (Shor 1972), which may be experienced as a major 'existential shift' (Ehrenwald 1978).

Environmental sensitivity increases relative to a single focus of attention: the healee. Decreased self-awareness and weakened personal identity through absorbed attention result in a waning of subject–object differentiation, and contribute toward a 'merging' with the healee or other entities, real or constructed. Physiognomic perceptions and empathic or sympathetic responses may result.

Time is frequently distorted and may be a major sign that ordinary consciousness was altered. Timelessness is reported most frequently, although there may be other temporal aberrations.

Paranormal phenomena are reported, whether directly or indirectly associated with healing. Telepathy and clairvoyant diagnoses are most frequent, the latter characterized mainly by visual and somesthetic imagery. Also reported are precognition, retrocognition, and perception of a viewed or felt energy field (or aura) around the healee. Mediumistic experiences were generally unrelated to healing types practiced by my participants.

Grey (1985) reported that some individuals develop healing ability following a Near Death Experience. An unexpectedly high number of interviewees (seven of 10) reported almost losing their lives, although only one described Near Death Experience features.

Altered meanings are common, most frequently associated with specific events, objects, or sensations involving interactions with physical reality. Neither common nor rare, intense mystical (or 'peak') experiences may occur.

Motor activity is reduced. When movement occurs, personal control and effort varies according to the depth of the healing state. Normal voluntary control and effort are present at times. At other times, movements feel automatic and non-ordinarily effortless (Green et al 1991).

Typology of Healers

LeShan developed a taxonomy of five healer types:

- *Type 1* alters consciousness, experiences a merging with the healee into a single entity within the 'Clairvoyant Reality' without a loss of individuality. There is a loving, caring focus with no effortful attempt to do anything to the healee. The only intention is to merge. This may be brief, but fills the entire perceptual field.
- *Type 2* perceives physical sensations, including flows of energy, usually in the hands. This signals readiness to heal. Conscious, personal effort is made. There is caring, but no attempt to merge with the healee.
- *Type 3* involves 'spirit' possession and physically invasive surgical procedures, such as those described by Puharich (1974).
- *Type 4* also involves spirit possession, but non-physical 'operations' are performed on the 'etheric body' (or aura), a conjectural field of energy surrounding the body.
- *Type 5* healing is a rare extension of type 1 in which major biological changes may occur. It is

associated with a third reality, the 'Transpsychic Reality' within which the healer feels interconnected with all-there-is, yet remains unique, a participant in a mutually interactive relationship in which the part affects the whole and vice versa. Paranormal information is acquired through merging as an outreach towards a greater, universal whole.

In his writings, LeShan tends to emphasize Type 1 healing, blending psychological processes with physical behaviors. Van Dragt only vaguely addresses typology as dichotomously passive or active types, similar to LeShan's Types 1 and 2.

In Cooperstein's (1990) analysis, healers' consciousness was plotted against beliefs central to healer's efforts (Fig. 14.3).

The arc connecting groups (Fig. 14.3) suggests that healing types are not distinct, falling along a continuum from those most dependent on ordinary (or near-ordinary) consciousness and relying upon realistic and quasi-realistic constructs, to those in which consciousness is extensively altered and metaphysical (spiritual, religious) beliefs are emphasized.

Using these coordinates, Cooperstein identifies six healing types:

1. Class I ($N = 4$) are individuals identifying themselves as a Magnetic Healer, Psychic Healer, a Transmitter of Universal Energy, and a practitioner of Laying-on of Hands:

   - They depend upon logic to explain their behaviors, maintain ordinary (or near-ordinary) consciousness and an ordinary sense of self
   - Although stressing reality-based constructs, quasi-realistic constructs are cited most often
   - Not averse to supporting the notion that subconscious operations play a role in the healing process, they emphasize rational processes
   - This group would be expected to rely upon physical (or focusing) devices to supplement or amplify their healing treatment and diagnosis, such as use of the hands to direct energy, dowsing devices, and crystals.

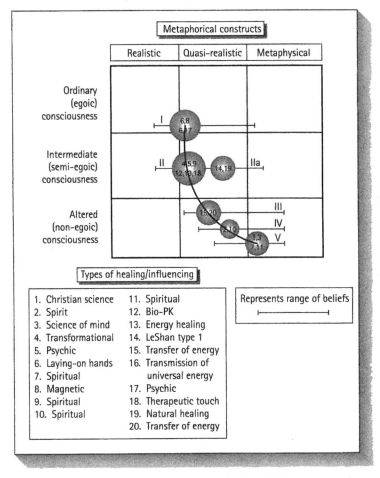

Figure 14.3 Distribution and taxonomic classification of 20 transpersonal healers based upon estimates of level of consciousness and the structure of metaphorical constructs derived from content analysis and interview materials.

2. Class II (*N* = 6) includes a Transformational Healer, Psychic Healer, Spiritual Healer, Energy Healer, and Therapeutic Touch Healer:

   - Although these individuals combine realistic, quasi-realistic, and metaphysical beliefs, they are less likely to rely upon physical objects, although they may use their hands to 'sense'
   - Consciousness is altered more extensively, to a moderate-to-extreme level, including sense of self
   - There is the desire to access unconscious processes for diagnosis and treatment

   - They report *transegoic threshold*, or *access level phenomena*, such as feeling a presence, or co-consciousness
   - Although weakened, reality testing is present and apposing conscious– subconscious processes are reported.

3. Class II A (*N* = 2) includes a LeShan Type 1 healer and a natural healer:

   - There are moderate-to-extreme alterations in consciousness, but emphasis is on non-reality-based (abstract, formless) and non-spiritual constructs (e.g. merging) while not using quasi-sensory imagery

- IIA healers appear to be a special case of Class II describing what seems to be a 'mythless' experience
- They attempt to suspend beliefs in physical and metaphysical metaphors and not depend upon mythic beliefs
- However, the constructs of merging and consciousness (as an extended, non-local entity) remain fundamental to their beliefs
- They are more dependent on physical and spiritual realities than Class II and more oriented to the healer's personal experience.

4. Class III (N = 2) are Transfer of Energy Healers:

- They identify fully with a quasi-realistic 'energy'
- Although that is primary, they may also identify with the healee. Their experience involves extensive, transegoic alteration of consciousness with a complete loss of self-awareness.

5. Class IV (N = 2) includes a Spirit Healer and Spiritual Healer:

- They undergo extensive, transegoic alterations of consciousness and emphasize realistic and quasi-realistic constructs, although expressed beliefs may run the gamut from reality-based to spiritual (non-reality-based)
- Spiritistic beliefs and mediumistic behaviors are highlighted and may be used to channel energy or receive spirit guidance for diagnosis or treatment.

6. Class V (N = 4) includes a Christian Science healer, a Science of Mind Healer, and two Spiritual Healers:

- Transegoic consciousness is induced and quasi-realistic (e.g. energy) and metaphysical (unstructured, non-reality-based) constructs are blended
- Although they combine quasi-realistic constructs (e.g. energy and mytho-historic beings) with non-reality-based constructs, this group induces the most unstructured, conceptually remote cognition among all groups.

Figure 14.4 is based upon an analysis of Therapeutic Touch (Krieger 1979), Spiritual Healing (Beard 1951), and LeShan's types using an ego operations-metaphorical construct grid to illustrate correspondences. LeShan's types correspond with four of the six types emerging from Cooperstein's research; LeShan's Type 5 is not represented and may be rare, comparable to *samadhi* or the attainment of 'cosmic consciousness'. Class V appears to approach this level.

Figure 14.5 represents the healing classes within a three-dimensional context, based on dimensions of metaphorical constructs, generalized reality orientation, and altered sense of self. Ordinary and 'cosmic consciousness' are used as points against which the healers' changes in consciousness are referenced.

Class I healers experience minimal changes in consciousness, emphasize empirically based constructs, and maintain an ordinary (or near-ordinary) sense of self. Continuing along the continuum, Classes II and IIA are intermediate in their use of metaphorical mediating constructs and increased alteration in the generalized reality orientation and sense of self. Classes III, IV, and V undergo the most radical changes, shifting away from conventional reality and consciousness towards non-egoic operations within an alternate reality.

A MODEL FOR HEALING AND CAVEAT: SHAMANIC CONSCIOUSNESS

The psychology of healing appears similar to processes used in shamanic practices as a 'unifying dialogue . . . between ordinary consciousness and the mythic imagination' (Larsen 1988, p. 171) and transpersonal healing (i.e. in Therapeutic Touch) as a 'deep level of one's being . . . where it is possible for one facet of an individual's personality to be in dialogue with another facet' (Krieger 1979, p. 70).

Shamans mobilize a *preparatory* set (or state) and establish conditions – rituals and ceremonies – under which intent is expected to manifest. The activities and symbols associated with helping

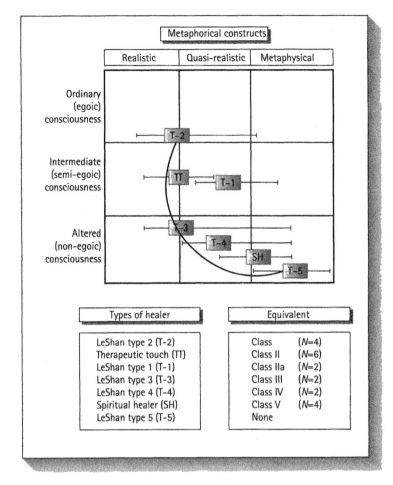

Figure 14.4 Comparative distribution of LeShan healing types, therapeutic touch, and spiritual healing based upon estimates of level of consciousness and the structure of metaphorical constructs.

spirits aid in identification with the spirits' powers to transcend the 'profane world' and enter 'sacred time' and a mythic reality.

Consciousness is altered intentionally. The shaman's ordinary sense of self is suspended as he or she enters an intense, mystical identification with transcendent spirits guiding travels through the projected, alternate realities constructed from the culture's mythology. These factors alter the shaman's metaphysical orientation. Through the assumption of an alternate identity, the shaman is said to acquire non-ordinary abilities.

In my research, I refer to the 'Shamanic Complex' as having a transpersonal, transcultural, psychological, and physiological infrastructure underlying the different methods, beliefs, and contexts within which a possibly *inherent biological tendency* is activated.

With the apparent correspondences to shamanism, we must guard against the tendency to project cultural, professional, and personal biases on alien practices and alleged anomalous resultant phenomena. Appelbaum (1993), for example, gave projective tests to healers and concluded that 'typical healers' test reality accurately, but are self-deluding, expansive and grandiose, tend to reject conventionality, and show 'sublime self confidence.' Implementing a Western psychoanalytic frame of reference, he attributes this to 'an infantile layer of the

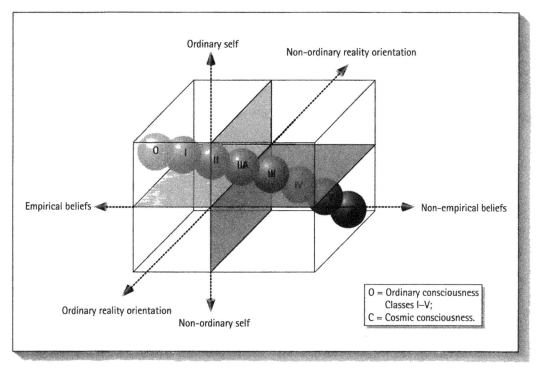

Figure 14.5 Conceptualized plot in three-dimensional space of six transpersonal healer classes as contrasted with ordinary and 'cosmic' consciousness.

mind' based upon a (presumably) symbiotic mother–child relationship.

However, in a contrasting anthropological study, Rorschach tests were administered to Apache shamans, non-shamans, and pseudo-shamans (Boyer et al 1964). The shamans' reality testing and approach toward ambiguous stimuli[2] was equivalent to non-shamans, but shamans showed an ease of regression, greater awareness, better tolerance of ambiguity, and a strong orientation towards theoretical thinking. Although indications suggested clinical hysteria (i.e. by Western standards), the authors found shamans to be less hysterical, demonstrating a mental stability superior to that of the other groups. Brown et al (1977) administered the Minnesota multiphasic personality inventory to Therapeutic Touch healers. In further disagreement with Appelbaum, subjects were 'remarkable for their normality,' although heterogeneous in individual patterns.

---

[2]See Cognition section in my research.

RESEARCH SUPPORT AND PROPOSALS FOR FUTURE STUDIES

The results of LeShan, Van Dragt, and Cooperstein have received some validation in the following studies:

- a phenomenological study of contemporary shamanic practices (Krycka 2000)
- a physiological study of the laying-on of hands (Maher et al 1996)
- a study of integrative counseling, psychotherapy, and healing (West 1997)
- a review of EEG studies related to healing (Charman 2000)
- a study of charismatic Christian healing (Davis 1990)
- research into brainmapping a bioenergy practitioner and client (Fahrion et al 1992)
- Russian physiological research into transformation of brain activity in altered states of consciousness (Koyokina 1998)
- a physiological study of therapeutic touch healers (Brown et al 1977).

Based upon these investigations, the following research is proposed, involving healers (or psychokinetic influencers) who demonstrated empirical experimental or clinical effects:

1. Collation of phenomenological information related to healing/influencing from various fields: for example cultural anthropology, parapsychology, mysticism, and nursing research.
2. Assessing healers personality variables, creativity, hypnotic susceptibility, absorption, ego-permissiveness, mental imagery, and mystical, parapsychological, and transpersonal experiences.
3. Criterion-based studies incorporating the aforementioned and assessing empirical healing/influencing effects in a standardized array of organic and non-organic materials.
4. Replications of earlier studies with measures of physiology. Neurophysiology, measured by EEG, isopotential mapping, and PET scans could assess cerebral processes involved, hemispheric synchronization, power spectra shifts, and the specific brain areas that change in the healers. Individuals designated fantasy-prone personalities counteract absorbed imagination through increased verbalizing (Wilson & Barber 1983), a process considered governed by left hemispheric activity (Gazzaniga, 1974). Braud (1975) claims that psi-conduciveness is associated with decreased left hemispheric activity. Comparative studies of increased and decreased left hemispheric activity among right-handed healers/influencers may provide insight into the facilitation and inhibition of effects. This has received some support from Koyokina's (1998) recent neurophysiological work in altered states of consciousness.
5. Descriptive information acquired during experiments should be recorded and taped debriefings held after healing/influencing for compilation and analysis.
6. Psychological assessments of healees are needed. Collation of related extant phenomenological explorations of transpersonal self-healing (e.g., Borg, 1994) should examine personal and transpersonal features of self-healing and receptivity to healing by healers.
7. The healing abilities of psychokinesis subjects and the psychokinetic abilities of healers should be compared. For example, see similarities of psychokinetic subjects presented by Heath (2000).
8. Concurrent physiological healer–healee physiological measurements before, during, and after healing are of extreme importance

COMMENTS

A considerable body of literature involving experimental investigations of transpersonal healing effects has accumulated over three decades, suggesting the existence of an anomalous healing/influencing process that may be potentiated by trained and 'intuitive' transpersonal healers, as well as naïve individuals, under controlled conditions. Despite promising ongoing research, many mainstream scientists refuse to consider the possible authenticity of this purported potential and dissent continues among the small group of researchers who at least suspect that it is a legitimate phenomenon. Within this small community, competing models, disagreements over the mechanisms of the process, and conflicting opinions over the development of effective programs for investigating it reflect a preparadigmatic phase of research. Multidimensional theory must be developed with the capability of integrating the seemingly discordant models (Krippner & Villoldo 1976).

The source of anomalous healing appears to lie within the human thrust towards holistic functioning; this mechanism must be examined if the operations of healing/influencing are to be understood. Too great a scientific preoccupation only with the control and measurement of empirical effects must be counterbalanced by providing equal attention to the investigation of the psychological and physiological processes of the healer and healee (or target materials). The interpersonal, or social/environmental climate within which positive and negative effects occur requires more intensive scrutiny and the physical medium(s), if any, through which these effects are mediated should be explored. Holistic research of this type requires that the healing/influencing setting, whether field or laboratory, should be treated as a complete system, a comprehensive process requiring the equal distribution of researchers' attention towards physical, psychological, and parapsychological aspects and not the control and measurement of physical effects alone.

Interdisciplinary collaboration between such fields as psychology, medicine, biology, physiology, physics, and anthropology is essential to avoid imposing a single theoretical or methodological prism upon a process that extends beyond ownership by any single discipline.

Increased understanding of the mechanisms underlying healing/influencing may ultimately challenge the established metaphysical underpinnings supporting currently held physicalistic concepts of human nature, consciousness, existence, and reality. The emergence and integration of an opposing reality paradigm would parallel, on a collective level, the transpersonal healer's solitary effort to resolve the inner tension established by the juxtaposition of two disparate realities.

The rising popular interest in non-traditional healing practices (McGuire 1989) and parapsychological phenomena (Greeley 1987) may signify a social reaction to the gap in meaning-orientation created by the limitations of, and disparity between sensory (scientific) and non-sensory (spiritual) paradigms. If this hypothesis is accurate, alternative or complementary healing practices may satisfy a psychosocial need for integrative, holistic paradigms and reconcile the physical–spiritual worldview dichotomy by offering symbols of integration and transcendence: a return to a fundamental, personal, direct experiencing of integrative meaning through the activation of an ancient transpersonal potential and, through this, re-alliance with transcendent orders of reality.

REFERENCES

Appelbaum S A 1993 The laying on of health: personality patterns of psychic healers. Bulletin of the Menninger Clinic 57: 33–40
Beard R 1951 Everyman's search. Arthur James, Worcestershire, UK
Borg E 1994 The experience of healing during non-ordinary states of consciousness: an heuristic investigation. Unpublished doctoral dissertation. Union Institute, Cincinnati, OH
Boyer L B, Klopfer B, Brawer F B, Kawai H 1964 Comparisons of the shamans and pseudoshamans of the Apaches of the Mescalero Indian reservation: a Rorschach study. Journal of Projective Techniques 28: 173–180
Brown C C, Fischer R, Wagman A M I, Horrom N, Marks P 1977 The EEG in meditation and therapeutic touch healing. Journal of Altered States of Conscious 3: 169–180
Braud W G 1975 Psi-conducive states. Journal of Communication 25: 142–152
Charman R A 2000 Placing healers, healees, and healing into a wider research context. Journal of Alternative and Complementary Medicine 6: 177–180
Cooperstein M A 1990 The myths of healing: a descriptive analysis and taxonomy of transpersonal healing experiences. Unpublished doctoral dissertation. Saybrook Institute, San Francisco, CA
Davis F S 1990 Charismatic Christian spiritual healing in two cultural contexts: an existential-phenomenological approach. Unpublished doctoral dissertation. Duquesne University, Pittsburgh, PA
Ehrenwald J 1978 Psi phenomena, hemispheric dominance and the existential shift. In: Shapin B, Coly R (eds) Psi and states of awareness. Parapsychology Foundation, New York
Eliade M 1974 Shamanism. Princeton/Bollingen, Princeton, NJ
Fahrion S L, Wirkus M, Pooley P 1992 EEG amplitude, brain mapping, and synchrony between a bioenergy practitioner and client during healing. Subtle Energies 3: 19–52
Gazzaniga M S 1974 The split brain in man. In: Ornstein R E (ed) The nature of human consciousness. Viking, New York
Greeley A 1987 The 'impossible': it's happening. Noetic Sciences Review, Sausalito, CA
Green E E, Parks P A, Guyer P M, Fahrion S L, Coyne L 1991 Anomalous electrostatic phenomena in exceptional subjects. Subtle Energies 2(3): 69–94
Grey M 1985 Return from death: an exploration of the near-death experience. Arkana, New York
Halifax J 1982 Shaman: the wounded healer. Thames and Hudson, London
Heath P 2000 The PK zone: a phenomenological study. Journal of Parapsychology 64: 53–72
Koyokina O I 1998 Transformation of brain activity in altered states of consciousness. Monterey Institute for the Study of Alternative Healing Arts Newsletter 20–21, Monterey, CA
Krippner S and Villoldo A 1976 The realms of healing. Celestial Arts, Millbrae, CA
Krieger D 1979 The therapeutic touch. Prentice-Hall, Englewood Cliffs, NJ
Krycka K C 2000 Shamanic practices and the treatment of life-threatening medical conditions. Journal of Transpersonal Psychology 32: 69–88
Larsen S 1988 The shaman's doorway. Station Hill, Barrytown, NY

LeShan L 1969 Toward a general theory of the paranormal. Psychological Monographs, No. 9. Parapsychology Foundation, New York

LeShan L 1975 The medium, the mystic, and the physicist. Ballantine, New York

Maher M, Vartanian I A, Chernigovskaya T, Reinsel R 1996. A physiological concomitant of the laying-on of hands: changes in healers' tactile sensitivity. Journal of the American Society of Psychical Research 90: 77–96

McGuire M B 1989 Healing ritual hits the suburbs. Psychology Today, New York

Puharich H K 1974 Psychic research and the healing process. In: Mitchell E D, White J (eds) Psychic exploration. Putnam's, New York

Royce J R 1978 How can we best advance the construction of theory in psychology? Canadian Psychological Review 19: 259–276

Shor R E 1972 Hypnosis and the concept of the generalized reality-orientation. In: Tart C T (ed) Altered states of consciousness. Anchor, Garden City, NY

Tart C T 1975 States of consciousness. Dutton, New York

Tilley J A 1989 A phenomenology the Christian healer's experience. Unpublished doctoral dissertation. Fuller Theological Seminary, Pasadena, CA

Van Dragt B 1980 Paranormal healing: a phenomenology of healer's experience. Unpublished doctoral dissertation. Fuller Theological Seminary, Pasadena, CA, vols 1–2

West W 1997 Integrating counseling, psychotherapy, and healing: an inquiry into counselors and psychotherapists whose work includes healing. British Journal of Guidance and Career 25: 291–311

Wilson S C, Barber T X 1983 The fantasy-prone personality: implications for understanding imagery, hypnosis, and parapsychological phenomena. In: Sheik A A (ed) Imagery: current theory, research, and application. John Wiley, New York

APPENDIX 1

A Comparison of Anomalous Healers' Phenomenological Qualities

Van Dragt (1980) N = 10	Tilley (1989) N = 10	Cooperstein (1990) N = 20
Fundamental qualities	Modal qualities	Experiential features
Altering one's state of consciousness.	[Suggestion of healing state] Use scriptural revelation for entering into and/or conducting healing.	Attention is self-regulated through the use of selective attention, or concentration, while rejecting irrelevant sensory input. Attention is withdrawn from the outer environment.
Being internally still or quiet.	'... often spent time alone with God before healing' (p. 14).	Inner verbalization (i.e. discursive thought) usually decreases and may reach a point of 'inner silence.' Motor activity is ordinarily reduced.
Centering one's self.	'... often spent time alone with God before healing' (p. 14).	Meditative self-regulation (or healing meditation) is the chief means of altering consciousness. Healers are vague in discriminating between centering and meditation. The terms are

Van Dragt (1980) N = 10	Tilley (1989) N = 10	Cooperstein (1990) N = 20
Fundamental qualities	**Modal qualities**	**Experiential features**
		often used interchangeably, although meditation is referred to most frequently.
Altering the focus of one's awareness to exclude or subdue one's own thoughts and other extraneous influences.	Not addressed.	Closing eyes. Selective attention, or concentration. Withdrawn attention from the outer environment. Inner verbalization (i.e. discursive thought) usually decreases and may reach a point of 'inner silence.'
Putting one's [personal] self in the background by becoming less conscious or aware of, or involved with, one's self or body.	Not addressed.	Alterations in ordinary sense of self. Emergence of deeper, higher, or non-self. Awareness of body image is decreased. Personal identity should be set aside in order to merge with the target of attention through transcendence of the self-object dichotomy.
Being [emotionally] balanced or secure in one's self.	Not addressed.	Emotional tranquility, balance.
Functioning by intent: intending fully what one is about in the healing [becoming absorbed; immersed].	Not addressed.	Selective attention or concentration. Absorption. Determination.
Keeping one's emotions in abeyance and not allowing them to interfere.	Not addressed.	Atypically heightened emotional responses. Primarily positive.
Maintaining an objective or impersonal perspective and letting go of expectations [surrender of personal volition implied].	Not addressed.	Ordinary, personal volition and non-ordinary, non-personal volition are present, although at different times. Personal control is decreased or surrendered. Cognition is expectational relative to the initial goal setting. Interviewees' responses suggest *dual* processes:

(Continues)

Van Dragt (1980) $N = 10$ Fundamental qualities	Tilley (1989) $N = 10$ Modal qualities	Cooperstein (1990) $N = 20$ Experiential features
		an active, subjective involvement apposing a process of passive, objective detachment and receptivity.
Maintaining a positive or trusting attitude or expectation toward the process.	Healer was to act in faith and perceive what God did.	Decreased effort.
Becoming a channel or conduit through which something beyond one's self – whether power or being – operates on, or flows toward the other.	Power effecting healing change originated not from healers, but from God: 'The supernatural invaded the natural realm'; surrender to the Holy Spirit; Healers aware of scripture during healing.	The sense that a different personality or motivating force has taken on the control relinquished by the healer.
Experiencing the source of healing as something beyond one's self.	God is the source by which supernatural healing takes place. Christian healing relies upon being open to Jesus and committing one's self to Him.	The sense that a different personality or motivating force has taken on the control relinquished by the healer and extraordinary abilities have been acquired. The locus of energy or power is an interaction of the self and a source beyond the self.
Being in relationship with, and receiving help from some being or force beyond one's self.	Healing considered an 'outpouring of the healers' own relationship with God.' (p. 14). Influenced and complemented by scriptural awareness while healing.	Experiencing the presence of a higher, or more transcendent force, power or intelligence.
Scanning or assessing the condition of the others' body and/or psyche by extrasensory means.	Not addressed.	Altered consciousness expands awareness and brings to awareness aspects of the healee's subconscious. Healers believe that they perceive the healee's physical symptoms as expressed through their own bodies.
Mentally asking questions about the other and receiving answers in an extrasensory mode.	Not addressed.	Flashes of information and non-ordinary somatic sensations.

Van Dragt (1980) $N = 10$	Tilley (1989) $N = 10$	Cooperstein (1990) $N = 20$
Fundamental qualities	Modal qualities	Experiential features
Receiving extrasensory information. Receiving extrasensory visual input.	Experience supernatural guidance at the beginning and throughout the healing event. The 'Holy Spirit . . . also provides supernatural guidance (sometimes referred to as Word of knowledge).'	Flashes of information, awareness, or images that seem to originate from beyond the self. Anomalous diagnostic experiences whether or not healee is present. Telepathic communication, clairvoyance (remote viewing), clairsentience. Visual and other images; occasionally intrapsychic perceptions of light. Clairvoyance (remote viewing).
Experiencing extrasensory temperature sensations. Sensing the other's feelings.	Not addressed. Not addressed.	Thermal changes. Increased empathy. Absorption within the healee's experience.
Experiencing the other's non-physical body.	Not addressed.	Not found.
Experiencing extrasensory abilities intermittently.	Not addressed.	Confirmed.
Interpreting extrasensory data according to internal or idiosyncratic criteria.	Distinguishing the demonic from the psychological in etiology.	Confirmed.
Focusing on the other.	Not addressed.	Environmental awareness sensitized and narrowed, directed toward specific feature (usually the healee). Perception of the general environment tends to be decreased.
Experiencing some sort of positive regard or caring for the other.	Not addressed.	General loving feeling: Experienced as originating from within Healer. Experienced as originating from source beyond Healer. Love, unconditional, selfless.
Typology not developed: Some healers *allow* to happen for the other whatever is to happen. Some healers *actively* seeking to bring about or alter	Typology not developed: [Types] A differentiation between healers ministering with God's help and God ministering with the healer's help. Willingness to give up control,	Six healer types identified.

(*Continues*)

Van Dragt (1980) *N* = 10	Tilley (1989) *N* = 10	Cooperstein (1990) *N* = 20
Fundamental qualities	**Modal qualities**	**Experiential features**
specific conditions in the other.	particularly intellectual control.	
Projecting, beaming, or channeling energy to the other, and doing this at least sometimes through one's hands.	Experience a flow of power, of the Holy Spirit.	Confirmed.
Experiencing sensations relating to the flow of energy.	Experience a flow of power, of the Holy Spirit.	Sensations of non-ordinary energy are frequently experienced during healing, usually localized in the hands or arms.
Influencing the condition of the other's physical, physiological, emotional, and/or mental state by means of one's thoughts.	Not addressed.	Mental imagery is important, but not essential. Visual images aid in the induction of the healing state, treatment, and the visualization of aims and goals.
Healing the other's psyche.	Not addressed.	Not addressed.
Finding the experiences in the other's past in which are responsible for current maladies.	Not addressed.	Implied but not addressed.
Working with the other's memories of traumatic experiences to effect change in the present.	Receive the 'word of knowledge from the Lord that they have dealt with specifically what to pray for, or may have revealed hidden traumas or sins in the Healee's past that may have been key to accomplishing the healing' (pp. 16–17).	Implied but not addressed.
Relaying information to the other.	Not addressed.	Confirmed.
Asking the healee questions.	Not addressed.	Confirmed.
Helping the other to be his or her own healer.	Not addressed.	Not addressed.
Healing remotely.	Not addressed.	Healee's presence is helpful, but not considered essential.
Acting in response to the other's need rather than according to one's own agenda.	Christian healing goals encompass 'restoration of functioning and wholeness in the physical, relational, emotional/psychological,	Decreased personal needs.

Van Dragt (1980) $N = 10$	Tilley (1989) $N = 10$	Cooperstein (1990) $N = 20$
Fundamental qualities	Modal qualities	Experiential features
	and spiritual dimensions of being' (p. 23). Establish openness to Jesus and commitment to Him.	
Healing the whole person.	Not addressed.	Not addressed.
Refusing to take responsibility for the other.	Not addressed.	Not addressed.
Experiencing time and space as altered.	Not addressed.	Temporal (timelessness) and spatial distortions.
Being ethical in one's approach.	Not addressed.	Not addressed.
Not addressed.	Increased effectiveness over time.	Confirmed.
Not addressed.	Some healers were motivated toward healing by feelings of inadequacy trying to help others.	Not confirmed.
Not addressed.	Healers frequently experienced some form of healing in their own lives.	Confirmed.
Not addressed.	Demonic influences were experienced as real phenomena and one source of problems requiring healing.	Not addressed.
Not addressed.	Healers did not endorse belief in redemptive, God-sent suffering.	Not addressed.
Not addressed.	Worship services [community] provided a vital [social support] context for healing ministry.	Modifications of the environment are usually unnecessary. Healers refer to these as aids rather than needs.
Not addressed.	Team [social; community] approach.	Other individuals, in addition to the healee, are not required.
Not addressed.	[Influence the healee's metaphysics, their view of the nature of reality]. Build attitude that God loved them and His will was to heal them. Attempt to maintain healing by helping the healee develop a system [of beliefs] as an enduring framework, including scripture or deepened relationship with Christ.	Not confirmed.
Not addressed.	Loose attachment to particular healing methods; openness to methological diversity.	Not addressed.

(Continues)

Van Dragt (1980) *N* = 10	Tilley (1989) *N* = 10	Cooperstein (1990) *N* = 20
Fundamental qualities	Modal qualities	Experiential features
Not addressed.	Healers' can grow in effectiveness.	Confirmed.
Not addressed.	Laying-on of hands.	Confirmed.
Not addressed.	Speaking in tongues. In this way, Healers could hear God speaking and providing a word of knowledge [guidance].	Not confirmed.
Not addressed.	Healing can occur with and without 'signs'.	Confirmed: 'signs' interpreted interpreted as immediate physical manifestations.
Not addressed.	[No judgment, blame, criticism] of themselves or the healee if nothing happened during session; healing may occur in the future.	Not addressed.
Not addressed.	Distinguish problems of a psychological origin versus demonic origin.	Not confirmed.
Not addressed.	Not addressed.	Enhanced feelings of affiliation, communion, or interconnection, to other individuals, nature, the cosmos, etc.
Not addressed.	Not addressed.	Non-ordinary sense of completeness, or wholeness.
Not addressed.	Not addressed.	Intense identification process. Healer may identify with healee and/or a variety of functional constructs (e.g., entities, powers, energies) attributed with the capability of transcending the limits of physical reality. Most transpersonal healers in this research identified with forces and quasi-realistic (e.g. likened to known) energies.
Not addressed.	Not addressed.	Enhanced awareness of, and increased sensitivity towards, inner events/ processes without complete exclusion of the external world.
Not addressed.	Not addressed.	Perception of two concurrent appositional modes of cognitive processing: ordinary (rational) and non-ordinary (nonrational).
Not addressed.	Not addressed.	Cognition is more non-analytical, non-critical, and expectational.
Not addressed.	Not addressed.	Rate of thinking may seem ordinary or increased.
Not addressed.	Not addressed.	Increased tolerance of ambiguity.
Not addressed.	Not addressed.	Verbal affirmations, non-imaginal beliefs, and mental imagery are the chief methods of realization, or 'making real' the healer's intent.

Van Dragt (1980) N = 10	Tilley (1989) N = 10	Cooperstein (1990) N = 20
Fundamental qualities	Modal qualities	Experiential features
Not addressed.	Not addressed.	While healing, visual images (1) increase in quantity and vividness, (2) tend to be more dynamic rather than static, (3) take forms that are predominantly realistic and/or quasi-realistic, and (4) are either selected by the healer and/or emerge spontaneously.
Not addressed.	Not addressed.	Selected images/symbols are chosen by the healer for induction or treatment.
Not addressed.	Not addressed.	Intuitions are experienced as hunches, or feelings, that prove to be accurate but which were not deduced through logical, analytical thinking.
Not addressed.	Not addressed.	Imagination is expressed in the combined use of imagery and belief constructs.
Not addressed.	Not addressed.	Creativity and healing are associated in terms of: Increased inner resources. Spontaneity. Openness (less defensiveness). Enhanced capacity to transcend sensory and conceptual limits.
Not addressed.	Not addressed.	Events experienced during healing are ordinarily recalled with vividness and continuity.
Not addressed.	Healing is a function of the working of the kingdom of God [transcendent reality] and as a fulfillment of the Great Commission.	Some healers perceived s/he entered one or more alternate, transcendent realities.
Not addressed.	Not addressed.	Healers believe consciousness is: A fundamental organismic awareness. Has 'thinghood' (Royce 1978); it is an entity rather than only a psychological construct. Has extensiveness. Has nonlocality. Is part of a ubiquitous network of animate and inanimate awareness nested within a limitless, universal consciousness, or intelligence.
Not addressed.	Not addressed.	Somatic reports: Heart and pulse rate tend to decrease during healing. Respiration slows. Body tonus relaxes. Alertness increases.
Not addressed.	Not addressed.	Healers may also experience: Nonordinary vibrations. Oscillations or rhythmic reverberations.

(Continues)

Van Dragt (1980) $N = 10$	Tilley (1989) $N = 10$	Cooperstein (1990) $N = 20$
Fundamental qualities	**Modal qualities**	**Experiential features**
Not addressed.	Not addressed.	About half the 20 healers used prayer in healing. They usually referred to meditative prayer. In meditative prayer the healer: Induces an alteration in ordinary consciousness. Acknowledges the presence of a higher, or more transcendent force, power or intelligence Attempts to merge his/her being/identity within that force or entity to effect interventions, or access abilities considered improbable or impossible in ordinary consciousness.
Not addressed.	Not addressed.	Hand passes or gestures are commonly used, most often to detect energy emanations, or symbolically, representing the transfer of energy to the healee.
Not addressed.	Not addressed.	Most important attitudes are: Love Trust Empathy Hopefulness Altruism Receptivity Patience Spontaneity Determination (regarding the welfare of other).
Not addressed.	Not addressed.	The subconscious: Conscious processes become less a focus of attention and are often surrendered during treatment, although not entirely subordinate. Conscious and subconscious processes operate in an integrative, synergistic manner. Increased access to pre- or subconscious materials resulting in intuitions (i.e., unconsciously processed flashes of information or awareness), or symbols, and images that may seem to originate from beyond the self. Plays a significant role in relation to faith and belief in healing. Involved in directing healing energy.
Not addressed.	Not addressed.	Awareness of the environment: Altered and decreased. Body boundaries altered relative to merging. Colors are more vivid and intense during and immediately after healing. Directed toward specific feature (usually the healee).

Van Dragt (1980) $N = 10$	Tilley (1989) $N = 10$	Cooperstein (1990) $N = 20$
Fundamental qualities	**Modal qualities**	**Experiential features**
Not addressed.	Not addressed.	Physiognomic perceptions. A naturally occurring developmentally early process of primitive perception involving intense unity (or merging) between the subject and an object mediated by the motor-affective reactivity of the organism.
Not addressed.	Not addressed.	Ordinary meanings are altered during healing.

15

Models, measurement descriptors and outcome measures in healing research

Seán ÓLaoire
Wayne B Jonas

This chapter discusses issues involved in selecting outcome measures in spiritual healing.

Do changes in consciousness have specific or general effects? Does mental healing act like a radio wave broadcast to a wide area, but only picked up by the properly tuned person? Or is it more like a pool of homeostasis into which meditators and their patients fuse? What is prayer for? Is it to increase cardiac output, reduce pain and anxiety, or enhance alignment with God? Knowing which outcomes to select for measurement and which are essential before beginning a study is a general principle of scientific inquiry. Lack of consensus on what prayer energy and consciousness is for presents a formidable challenge to the study of healing. Many spiritual leaders say that prayer is for improving one's relationship with God and should not be used to affect specific diseases. Many healing systems and the majority of patients pray or emit energy for improvement of specific problems. In part one of this chapter, Seán ÓLaoire, a Catholic priest, challenges us to think of new outcome measures for spiritual healing. He proposes one called the alignment scale and outlines its possible components. In an addendum Wayne Jonas describes a wide array of outcome measures already available to clinical researchers and the levels of the person they capture. He suggests that unless a clear rationale for selecting a specific outcome is developed, investigators should use sample measures from each level of this 'outcomes tree.' **WBJ**

PART I: MODELS OF HEALING AND THEIR IMPLICATIONS FOR RESEARCH

INTRODUCTION

In a hilarious scene in one of the Pink Panther movies, Inspector Clouseau (Peter Sellers), a klutzy, feckless detective, arrives at an Alpine inn laden with luggage. He manages, with great difficulty, to open the main door and come in from a snowstorm. Inside is a huge welcoming log fire, a recumbent German Shepherd dog, and an elderly, not easily impressed, unfriendly and altogether arrogant desk clerk. Sellers asks '*Does your dog bite?*' Without even lifting his gaze from his work, the clerk replies '*No, monsieur.*' Sellers deposits several bags on the floor, thus freeing up one hand, and reaches out to pat the dog, which promptly savages him. Alarmed and with a hint of betrayal in his voice, Sellers reprimands the clerk: '*I thought you said your dog doesn't bite?!*' Stiffly and with great dignity the clerk disengages himself temporarily from his tasks to haughtily declare '*That is not my dog.*'

Asking the wrong questions based on false models of reality and unproven expectations can only give irrelevant or even dangerous answers – in Alpine inns or in scientific research.

In the arena of human enquiry, the questions, the models, and the expectations have varied throughout history. To put it simplistically, there have been two main movements, each with twin poles. Within the first movement, 'homo religiosus', acknowledging the presence of a first cause, created a way of doing research which in its purest form became experimental mysticism, and in its corrupt form dogmatic, sectarian theology. In the Age of Enlightenment, a second movement swept dramatically center stage. In its purest form it is the rigorous but open-minded scientific method; in its corrupt form it is materialistic, reductionistic, close-minded scientism.

Prayer research should be careful not to be hijacked by the allegedly revealed dogma of any organized religion, nor sabotaged ·by the self-professed infallibility of scientism.

It is time to create a synthesis between their enlightened poles and abandon the war between their corrupt excesses. A new wedding is called for, a union of science and experiential mysticism. The practitioners will, I believe, be a blend of mystics and scientists – I will call them 'mysticists.' They will have the courage to radically review the two basic pillars of human enquiry: first, our models of reality, and second, our research methodologies. Obviously, these two pillars are inextricably interconnected, as hen and egg, in an ongoing cycle. But for the purpose of this chapter I will temporarily tease them asunder.

So the body of the chapter is divided into two sections. The first examines our models and their underlying assumptions. The second looks at design methodologies.

OUR MODELS AND THEIR UNDERLYING ASSUMPTIONS

Models of Spirituality

There are embedded models and postulates in all research. I propose that for the kind of research we are undertaking, there needs to be a new and more adequate cosmology. I believe it may contain, among many others, the following elements, as examples:

Higher forms do not emerge from lower forms by some kind of a fortuitous concatenation of accidental coincidence. Rather the evolution from matter to life to mind to soul to spirit was only possible because spirit was the origin and very essence of the evolutionary thrust to begin with. Higher forms, then, are the manifestation of pre-existing possibilities in the synthesizing of lower forms. A group of letters from the alphabet does not accidentally take on meaning because it falls together in a particular configuration, rather the grouping manifests a preassigned meaning.

Therefore trying to do prayer research without a mystical cosmology is like trying to do biological research without a theory of life.

The mystical literature speaks of four stages of the process:

1. First, it says that God never reveals teachings but only experiences of Herself. These are

unitive experiences in which all sense of self and time disappears. And these experiences are totally ineffable.

2. Stage two begins after the experience has ended. The blissed-out experiencer wants to try to maintain a link, so he comes up with symbols that somehow represent this ineffable event.

3. Stage three is the development of concepts in order to make mental sense of the symbols.

4. And stage four is the articulation in words (spoken or written) in order to share the concepts with others.

Models of the Human Person

Biology (the study of 'bio' – life) has a strange way of conducting its research. It kills and dissects in order to figure out how life works. Psychology (the study of the 'psyche,' or soul) has a stranger way of conducting its research. For most of the 20th century it totally ignored soul and purported to research the human condition while denying that soul even exists. One may as well try to study anthropology (the study of 'anthropos' – humans) while denying that humans exist.

The perennial philosophy claims that reality exists on two levels: the unseen, mystical, unmanifest level, and the seen, secular, manifest level. The latter is conceived, birthed, and sustained by the former. We have a special term in Gaelic for a place or experience that temporarily renders the divide diaphanous. We call it a *Caol Áit* ('thin place'). Those who hang out regularly in such energies claim that we are not just physical entities but spirits in spacesuits.

Since we have been doing research without an adequate understanding of 'human', we have most certainly not had operational definitions of what a fully-alive human might look like.

Models of Body

The Western medical model of body – a kind of a WYSIWYG notion – may well be very inadequate. Other systems have much more sophisticated models. For example, Hinduism teaches that we have seven levels of body, all vibrating at different frequencies and manifesting different levels of

energy. The chakra system operates as transforming stations to step up or step down the energy from one level to the next. Any research coming out of such a model is bound to ask different questions and create different scientific models of the phenomenological world.

Models of Illness

The Spindrift researchers claimed that the further an organism was from homeostasis, the more dramatic were the results of prayer interventions. They worked primarily with plants, which they could 'stress' by watering them with a saline solution. The more stressed the plants, the more astounding were the prayer effects – up to a point. Stressed beyond a certain point, the plants could not be restored to health. On the other hand trying, by prayer, to push the plants out of homeostasis proved a more difficult task.

Homeopathy reports the same phenomenon. Samuel Hahnemann, the founder, was a German allopathic physician who became disillusioned with Western medicine's efforts to treat disease by suppressing symptomology. He believed that illness existed on three levels. Unlike healing which (as in embryonic development) proceeds cephalo-caudally and proximo-distally, illness, he said, begins with physical symptoms and, as it progresses, goes inwards and upwards. Since symptoms are evidence of the body actually healing itself, the suppression of symptoms inevitably drives the illness into the next level – the emotional arena. The symptoms manifested here are a further attempt by the organism to heal itself, but again suppression means that the illness has nowhere to go but to the third and most serious level of all – the mental/spiritual level.

So, we need an adequate model of illness and wellness. I believe that illness is a composite of several sources:

1. Genetic predisposition – different families and different ethnic groups are more prone to different illnesses

2. Environment, by which I mean everything from our in-utero experience, to family and social, physical, emotional, and mental experiences

3. Personal lifestyle – diet, exercise, sleep patterns, behavior, etc.
4. Personal belief systems – prejudices, and what we hold about the existential, political, cultural, and social issues
5. Karma – the lessons we have come to learn in a particular lifetime
6. The bodhisattva dimension – there is a little of the bodhisattva in each one of us.

Perhaps a particular illness is our gift to the scientific community that it may exercise its ingenuity or to the extended family that it may exercise its compassion.

Any prayer that attempts to influence a disease caused by points one through four above, may well prove 'successful', but prayer that seeks to undo any illness occasioned by points five or six above is obviously 'kicking against the goad' and may be unsuccessful.

Models of Healing

In counseling clients who are wrestling with a life-threatening illness, I have developed a six-stage model of intercessory prayer:

1. The first stage is meditation, in order to try to determine the origins and purpose of the illness. Meditation is, I believe, one of the most powerful practices for bringing a person into alignment with mission and disidentifying with ego. If I am badly out of alignment, I may well be attempting, through my prayer, to push myself further away from homeostasis.
2. Stage two, once I have gotten into alignment, in so far as I am able, is to pray for the outcome which I think is indicated.
3. Stage three is to do all in my power to facilitate the emergence of that outcome (e.g. activate resources via professionals, family and friends, as well as interior abilities such as creative visualization and exterior behaviors such as adequate sleep, diet and exercise, etc.).
4. Stage four is to detach and work with the outcome, even if I believe it to be merely a temporary outcome.
5. Stage five is to go back to meditation and try to fine-tune my alignment and thinking about

the source and purpose of the illness, in the light of stages one through four.
6. Stage six is to consciously develop a personal cosmology that buoys me up and assures me that whatever the final outcome, I cannot fail, since I am a spirit in a spacesuit. My origin, my journey, and my destination are about God.

Doing prayer research with subjects who practice such a method and who hold such a cosmology would, if we were using appropriate instruments (for example the alignment scale, see later), yield very statistically significant results, I believe.

Models of 'Successful' Prayer

How does one judge the success of a ballpoint pen? If I attempt to use it to clean my ears and then report that it failed to clean them, but rather has smudged my outer ear and pierced my eardrum, then the ballpoint pen could be judged a total failure. Except, of course, it was not designed or intended for that job. What if I test its writing capacity instead?

We may have forced prayer to do things it was not intended to do, and then claimed it failed. It would surely be better to see what prayer actually does and take it from there. Our operational definition of successful intercessory prayer is at the core of the problem. The scientist in us wants to define 'successful prayer' as that which impacts a dependent variable in the desired direction; but the mystical literature always avers that successful prayer is that which aligns us with the ineffable ground of our being.

We may be forcing through a definition of success that is at variance with the purpose of the instrument. It is a modern-day version of the old 'God indulges the prayers of holy people by changing His intended outcome' model. We are simply substituting the word 'scientific' for the word 'holy.'

So we first need a model of how prayer works. I believe that prayer does *not* operate in any of the following manners:

1. It is not merely chatting about the inevitable – i.e. it's not that God, who is omnipotent, omniscient, omnipresent, and eternal, knows what I am going to ask for and has already

taken it into consideration and so my petitions are superfluous.

2. It is not a satellite-dish model, whereby I bounce my request off God and She redirects it to my intended target.

3. It is not an Abrahamic model, whereby I can bargain with God in the good, old-fashioned, Middle-Eastern fashion (e.g. Genesis 18:23–32).

4. It is not a discover-the-trick model, in which, like Moses, in a battle against the Amalekites, I try to figure out what the secret is (e.g. Exodus 17:8–13).

5. Prayer is not a hose turned on selected subjects by an experimenter-directed process, but rather a pool of cosmic compassion into which anybody (even someone in the control group) is free to plunge.

Hence, expectation and belief penetrate the artificial barriers of controlled, blinded studies. And we need to see expectation and belief as valuable allies rather than as contaminating, extraneous variables. Blindly-constructed blinded controlled studies may be part of the way in which we are failing to recognize how prayer really works. It may well be giving us lots of false negatives. Perhaps, instead, we may need to build expectation and beliefs into our methodologies.

Prayer may be more like a garden sprinkler system, in which all the water comes from one source (whatever name we choose to give this source), and resides within the system, but whose flow may be impeded or facilitated by the state of the pipes (our intentionality).

Is successful prayer then miraculous? Does God really change cosmic laws to gratify faith? Or is the universe perhaps so much more complex that what passes for a miracle is merely the manifestation of its deeper recesses? And do the very laws governing evolution themselves evolve, driven perhaps by consciousness (laserized through intention and amplified through the collective)?

DESIGN METHODOLOGIES

Two Ways in Which Science Has Been Done

There have always been two ways of doing good science. The first way is to look at a collection of data; try to identify some inherent pattern; formulate a hypothesis to explain the putative pattern; conduct an experiment to establish whether or not the hypothesis is correct; replicate the experiment, if it appears to be correct, in other laboratories; establish a principle or law; and then construct a model that can accommodate and explain all the data. This is a kind of bottom-up system. It is very powerful, though mistakes can enter in at any one of the stages.

The other way of doing good science is to start with an 'aha' experience, an insight; conduct a thought-experiment; and then set about looking for data that uphold the intuitive flash. Einstein, among others, was a master of this technique.

One method starts with pieces and finally constructs a model; the other method starts with a model and then casts about for the pieces ('I know they're around here somewhere!'). But whichever technique we favor, there is no gainsaying the fact that the two methods are inextricably interconnected. Even the most dyed-in-the-wool empiricist is operating out of presumed models which unconsciously bias his new searches; and even the most esoteric of thinkers has to learn to tie her shoelaces. Each of these two operates with some measure of faith. Kurt Gödel shocked the scientific community in 1931 by showing that any axiomatic system (even pure mathematics, the most rigorous of all the sciences), *ipso facto*, must contain at least one postulate which can neither be confirmed nor denied. Whether we like it or not, all scientific models are a house of cards. The extraordinary journey of Andrew Wiles in his 10 year reclusive battle to solve Fermat's enigma, showed just how susceptible any 'proof' is to the myriad of delicate logical connections that constitute the lower stories of the skyscraper of scientific models. Add to that the realization that all formulas, all equations, and all models are, at best, approximations of the phenomenological world, and it well behooves us to walk with humility. Science has put its foot in its mouth almost as frequently as has organized religion.

Failure to dream outside the box in both our intuitive models and our empirical methodologies will, inevitably, lead to stagnation. The dogma of science is no less stultifying than the dogma of religion.

I believe that we have been rather lax in our application of validity. Validity is meant to ensure that we are really measuring what we claim to be measuring. If I step on a weighing machine and watch it climb to 183, and then believe it shows that I am 6 feet tall, I have mistaken pounds for centimeters and weight for height.

By the same token we are in danger of merely measuring associated features when we think we are measuring the 'thing in itself.' For example, EEG equipment can show when I am dreaming, but it can say nothing about the content of my dream. Similarly, BP levels, respiration rate, heart rate may say something about the physiological correlates of meditation but can say nothing of the subjective spiritual experience of the meditator.

I believe that we may, in the past, have been primarily concerned with the correlates of meditation, of prayer and of intentionality, and mistaken the results for evidence of the Holy Grail.

A New Way of Doing Science

Is it time for a different kind of science – what Ken Wilber calls 'Deep Science'? In essence, all true science consists basically of just three parts:

- An injunction
- An apprehension
- A confirmation/falsification.

For example, if I want to establish scientifically how many legs a flea has, I must first look at the flea (the injunction); second, I must count the legs (the apprehension); and third, subject my findings to a test, by comparing my results with those of other researchers who have gone through the same process (the confirmation/-falsification).

Or if my research in is the mental domain rather than in the physical domain and I wish to solve a quadratic equation ($ax^2 + bx + c = 0$), then

$$x = \left(-b \pm \sqrt{b^2 - 4ac}\right) \div 2a$$

I go through the same three steps. First I slot the values of a, b and c into the formula (the injunction); then I calculate my answer (the apprehension); and, finally, I compare my result with those of others who have solved the same equation (confirmation/falsification.)

If my research is in neither the physical nor the mental realm but in the spiritual, I follow the same three steps. Over five millennia of practice has suggested what kinds of injunctions give what kinds of results that have been compared across spiritualities. This is exactly the same type of deep science we use in physical and psychological research.

Moreover, there are new techniques (such as Organic Inquiry, which comes out of the Institute of Transpersonal Psychology in Palo Alto) that make the outrageous claim that research should also be about transformation, and not merely about information. What if they are right?

Perhaps, we need the courage to have a two-pronged approach: intuitively creating models which we can subsequently test in order to give us the data, while, at the same time, garnering data which will lead to the creating of new models.

A Theory of Change

Any research that attempts to influence a dependent variable has to begin with a theory of change. What constitutes 'movement'? The spiritual literature is replete with such information. For example, in Christian mystical writings, it is held that the seeker, through prayer and meditation, moves through four distinct stages of development: the purgative (in which one is conscious of one's own inadequacies); the illuminative (in which one is more concerned with God's beauty than one's own sin); the dark night of the soul (in which God seems to have vanished in spite of one's best efforts to live a holy life); and, finally, the unitive stage (in which one merges with God).

Our research needs an adequate theory of change before we can meaningfully engage in rewarding experimentation. We would be well served by culling the great mystical literature (as distinct from the divisive, sectarian, dogmatic theologies) for such models. These are the experiential experts, and there is an extraordinary agreement among them, over several millennia, and across all spiritual traditions.

I am convinced that an instrument could be constructed, based on the distillation of these mystical traditions, which would be a far more suitable measure of the effectiveness of prayer. As a temporary name, I will call such an instrument the 'Alignment Scale.' Physiological and psychological improvement may sometimes be correlates of movement along this scale, but they are not core to it. I would predict that whereas prayer may or may not positively affect physical or emotional scales, it will *always* positively affect the alignment scale.

The Alignment Scale

A first stab at creating an alignment scale might look like the following (a simple Likert measure could be used for each section of each question):

+ 2	+ 1	0	− 1	− 2
Definitely true	Slightly true	Not sure	Slightly untrue	Definitely untrue

1. Irrespective of circumstances, I increasingly feel at peace with:
   a. My body
   b. My emotions
   c. My mind
   d. My core self
   e. My relationships
   f. My 'God'
   g. My work
   h. My life.
2. I *increasingly* try to live my life with mindfulness for:
   a. The planet
   b. All life forms
   c. Future generations.
3. I *increasingly* have experiences of being connected to the whole universe.
4. I *increasingly* experience life as purposeful rather than as a series of accidents.
5. I *increasingly* find it easier to forgive:
   a. Myself
   b. Others
   c. 'God'

6. *Increasingly* I am able to accept illness as a part of life:
   a. My illnesses
   b. The illnesses of others.
7. I *increasingly* feel compassion for
   a. Myself
   b. Others
   c. All life forms.
8. *Increasingly* I am able to directly experience life rather than to need to understand it and explain it.
9. I spend *more time* now than I used to in:
   a. Prayer
   b. Meditation.
10. *Increasingly* I believe that the purpose of prayer and meditation is not to bend 'God' to my will, but to bring myself into alignment with 'Him'.
11. I am *less and less* disturbed by the notion of death:
    a. Mine
    b. Others.

Descriptors

I want to suggest that in prayer research there may be (at least) two kinds of useful descriptors, namely demographics and belief systems.

Demographics

The following is a partial list of factors that may correlate with outcomes of prayer intervention:

- Age
- Gender
- Educational level
- Ethnicity
- Spiritual orientation (Jew, Christian, Muslim, etc.)
- Frequency of formal worship
- Marital status
- Does the subject have children, and if so, how many?
- Employed, and if so, occupation?
- Family income level
- Stress level of life and work
- Ability to manage stress
- Recent trauma
- Birth order, and number of children in family of origin.

Belief system

The following three items may correlate with the outcomes of a prayer intervention:

1. Do you believe in the power of 'prayer for others'?

   Yes   No   No opinion

2. Where do you believe God acts in your life?

   Inside   Outside   Both   Neither   No opinion

   (In my own research, both of these items, administered at pre-test, correlated very significantly with improvement)

3. Do you believe you were in the experimental (prayed-for) group or not?

   Yes   No   No opinion

   (In my own research, this item, administered at post-test, correlated very significantly with improvement, though it may merely have been a kind of retroactive prognosticator.)

From the models of spirituality, of the human person, of the body, of illness, of healing, and of successful prayer, outlined in the first section of the chapter, a large group of questions, could easily be constructed and scaled (e.g. a five-point Likert):

-2	-1	0	$+1$	$+2$
Strongly disagree	Some what	No opinion disagree	Some what agree	Strongly agree

Near Outcomes and Far Outcomes in Research

Now I want to distinguish between near-term and far-term outcomes, and between what I will call core issues (having to do with alignment outcomes) and correlated issues (having to do with physiological and psychological outcomes.) Most simply this can be done in a 2×2 matrix:

	Correlated issues	*Core issues*
Near-term outcomes	1. TV evangelism	3. Mainstream religion
Far-term outcomes	2. Mainstream science	4. Mysticism

1. Near-term correlated issues are the domain of TV evangelism (e.g. did the 'cripple' walk away without the wheelchair? TV evangelists insist on big, near-term outcomes. These make the headlines and 'prove' that prayer works.

2. Far-term correlated issues are central to mainstream science. It still has not grasped that physiology and psychology are not of the essence of the human being and insists on repeated, long-term measuring of these factors as the only indicators of a successful intervention.

3. Near-term core issues are the specialty of mainstream religion. These outcomes will be directly due to the intervention and be immediately obvious (e.g. a person may report that she spent 15 minutes of quiet time each day for a month or that he gained a greater knowledge of a scriptural tradition).

4. Far-term core issues bring us into the heart of mysticism. People in this place may say they have experienced a whole new level of inner peace, or made significant lifestyle changes, or acquired a higher degree of understanding of life's purpose. I believe that the most important of the far-outcome core-issue measures will be progress on the alignment scale.

However, more cosmologically-sophisticated models, ranging from that of Plotinus (in the 2nd century CE) to that of Ken Wilber (a contemporary philosopher), could easily be rendered scaleable and also be used as measures of far-outcome core issues, since they all have one thing in common – they provide empirical, testable stages for a theory of change as a result of engaging in prayer or meditation (or other spiritual practices.)

Far-term core issue outcomes tend to be more subjective but they may be no less important for all that. Remember the famous study to find what were the best prognosticators of a first heart attack? The experimenters were sure it would be obesity, smoking, lack of exercise, diabetes, high blood pressure. It proved to be none of the above but rather two very subjective measures, satisfaction in work, and with life.

One important contrast

'Interventionist' petitionary prayer by others will, I believe, affect both the near-term core issue and near-term correlated issue outcomes for the targeted subjects, while a practice of prayer or meditation by the subject is more likely to result in far-term core issue outcomes. In my own research those who prayed for others experienced more dramatic improvement, on all dependent variables, than those for whom they were praying. This distinction can easily be measured by follow-on post-testing at 1 month, 3 months, 6 months and 1 year intervals.

Following the Lead

Rather than force prayer to do our bidding (rather like using the ballpoint pen to clean one's ears) why not see what prayer does, left to its own devices? This may reveal its real strength rather than insist it be tested for a purpose for which it was not built and then pronounced a failure.

So how would it be if, during the pre-testing, the experimenter were to ask the recipient what he hopes will happen during the study, or, more manageably, to name three outcomes she would most like to have impacted by the received prayer? These idiosyncratic needs will then cluster, across subjects, and so could be measured on Likert scales, and correlated with outcome measures.

Moreover, it might be very informative to have the subjects keep a log during the study in which they record any changes they deem important in their physiology, psyche, relationships, creativity, spirituality etc. In the manner of the 'provings' of homeopathy, the intersection set of such changes may be a very accurate description of what prayer really does well.

By perusing: (a) the clusters of stated hoped-for results; (b) the subjects' logs; (c) the demographics; and (d) the belief systems, it will become obvious which factors influence the outcomes. Thus the outcomes 'hatch' themselves. This will allow the development of maturity models (i.e. models that can flush out and flesh out entire contexts and stages and mechanisms, and help determine what impacts a recipient's ability to benefit from the prayer).

The variables of implementation and effect are, then, of paramount importance. In particular:

1. Accurate measurement of the frequency and duration of the prayer. Did they pray each day for the specified amount of time?
2. Some measure of the quality of the prayer – perhaps two Likert scales at the end of each prayer period to assess the mindfulness of the session and its intensity.
3. A measurement of the effects of the prayer – the families of variables and contexts that were reported.
4. In particular, measuring the alignment factor will be vital.

I wrote earlier of the mystical stages of the spiritual journey with its theophanies. It seems appropriate to run a set of studies to distinguish between those who do/do not have these experiences. This at once allows validity to be established and also captures a baseline for the field. Furthermore it can be used in such a way that each subject becomes his or her own control. So it becomes both a between-group and within-group measure.

CONCLUSION

I remember, as a young boy, watching Ireland's *Telefís Scoile* ('school television') and seeing a physics teacher with a group of 10-year-olds. He had a very simple apparatus that consisted of a glass beaker three-quarters full of water, with a long pencil lolling inside and resting against the top rim. He asked the children *'What do you see here?'* All hands shot up and a chorus of voices begged to be chosen to answer. He picked one, and the child said *'I see a jug of water with a bent pencil in it!'* The teacher took the pencil out, and, of course, it was a straight pencil. The children all laughed. The teacher said: *'I want to teach a very important lesson today – the pencil only appears to be bent because water and air refract light differently.'* He then asked them to leave the lab and promised to call them back within 5 minutes. When they came back they found the same equipment in the very same configuration. Again the teacher asked *'What do you see here?'* Again the enthusiastic response of hands. He chose a different child who proudly announced *'I see a pencil lying inside a beaker of water and it seems to be bent but it's not. It's only because water refracts light in a different way from how air does!'* And he sat down very pleased with himself. Then the teacher took the pencil out of the water, and it was bent! In between sessions, he had broken the pencil at the waterline. The kids howled in delight. And I, watching at home, made a very important discovery that day. I realized that there are three different kinds of people in our world: those who see what *appears* to be, those who see what they *expect* to see and, finally, those who see what really *is*.

Scientism has seen what appears to be; sectarian religion has seen what it expected to see; now is the time to bring on the mysticists – those who have the courage to see what really is.

PART II: FINDING AND SELECTING OUTCOME MEASURES IN HEALING RESEACH

The first step was reducing the problem of human illness – with all its intricate physical, social, emotional, and cultural aspects – to the biological problem of disease. The second reductive step follows from the scientific investigation of diseases, here the findings of science become the accepted picture of disease, further over simplifying the problem.

> Eric Cassell, The Sorcerer's Broom, 1993, Hasting's Center Report 32, Vol. 23, p. 33.

We cannot afford to ignore feelings just because they present difficult scientific problems....Patients often seek medical care for the sympathy, reassurance, and validation provided; thus, these outcomes should be included when measuring the effectiveness of a clinical intervention.

> Donald A. Redelmeier, JAMA 1993;270:74

Disease Outcomes and Illness

Nowhere do the differences between science and healing come into sharper focus than in the selection of outcomes of disease to study. As expressed by Eric Cassell in the quote above, human illness is an experienced multi-dimensional complex with a multitude of potential outcomes to measure. Science, in its attempt to identify and isolate causal links between influ-

ences and physical disease, must select a primary outcome to measure from this multitude in any given study. Other outcomes, while perhaps important to patients, become secondary to the task of science. The dilemma is that the illness is a network of experience in several dimensions while each study picks one primary item to measure.

When a primary outcome is not characteristic of a disease (as in most chronic diseases) or directly influenced by a treatment (as in many spiritual or energy healing methods) then a wide array of outcomes may need to be measured. Premature selection of a single or a few outcomes then becomes a strategy error and leads to outcomes substitution, false negative data or false attribution of the effects of a treatment (Jonas and Linde, 2002). For the purposes of healing research outcome measures can be organized into groups or tiers, dependent on the degree of specificity desired from a measure for a particular population, disease or treatment. I call this tiered like organization 'The Outcomes Tree' off of which investigators can pick the outcome measures that best suit their goals.

The Outcomes Tree

The Outcomes Tree (OT) offers a method of organizing the type and selection of outcomes available in healing research so they are more easily and appropriately selected for the specific goals of a research project. The OT has four major tiers or types of outcome measures from the most general and flexible for use in various settings to those developed for highly specialized and targeted populations, conditions, treatments and purposes.

Outcome Categories: The Outcomes Tree has four outcome-measure categories arranged around the strength of affinity each measure has for a specific diagnostic taxonomy, practice model, and user. The four categories are: (1) individualized quality of life, (2) general health quality of life, (3) health status and functional measures, and, (4) disease specific outcome measures for a) conventional or b) complementary medical illness taxonomies. Outcome measures in each of these categories can be 1) internal, experientially derived, or 2) external, observationally derived. The following describe and list example measures from each category. More details on these and other measures can be found at the end of this chapter.

I. *Individual Quality of Life*: One tier of outcome type (OT, tier 1) involves patient-based quality of life measures. These measures are independent of practice model, disease classification, or intervention. These measures are selected and weighted by the patient and serve as subsequent markers for success. Examples in this category are Individual Quality of Life (IQoL, and SEIQoL) measurements, Goal Attainment Scaling (GAS), the Repertory Grid, and the Patient-Generated Index (PGI). The gold standard in this area is probably the comprehensive medical interview, provided it is not oriented towards making a diagnosis or providing an illness classification.

II. *General Health Status*: In the second tier of outcome types are the general and health related quality of life measures. These have at least two categories, global and summary. Examples of global measures are the EVGFP, the LADDER, the Physician GLOBAL, and the Duke Health Profile. Examples of summary health measures of such include the SF-36 and the SEIQoL (this measure has a structure allowing both individual QL or/and general health related OL assessment), the Sickness Impact Profile (SIP) and the SIC to Walk. These outcome measures are most useful for capturing overall health and disease or general health related outcomes and behaviors. They are often developed for measuring non-specific interventions such as across different health payment plans, different practice styles, specialties, delivery systems, and practices. Also interventions that address the common determinates of chronic disease (CDCD) as a unit (e.g. lifestyle therapies, health promotion programs, etc.) often use this tier of measurement tools. Some have been applied to more specific disease categories.

III. *Health Status and Functional Measures*: The third outcome type category involves intermediary health status measurements. These measures are often developed in the context of specific diagnostic conditions but then have been tested in other diagnostic conditions and capture some general health outcomes. Examples of these include activities of daily living, the POMS, the ESR, number of general mental health measures, and health behavior measurements related to the specific diseases. This OT tier includes functional and laboratory outcomes that measure cellular or organ function that have a broad impact on multiple health conditions such as biochemical tests for Phase I and Phase II hepatic detoxification functions, inflammatory cytokine and chemokine patterns, gene and protein array chips, hormone precursors such as DHEA, combination tests for assessing functional age, and tests such as the pupilary reaction test to environmental toxins.

IVa. *Disease Specific Measures:* The fourth outcome category involves disease or illness specific outcome measures. These are derived specifically to measure the effect of a particular intervention on a specific disease or illness classification. These include measures such as the HAQ, the MACTAR, the AIMS, the Beck Depression Inventory, other disease specific measures, health behavior measurements specific to illness categories, and laboratory disease specific outcomes such as blood pressure. This tier also includes more specific biological markers and laboratory tests such as liver function and kidney function tests, blood sugar level, and other tests that are more closely linked to specific clinical conditions.

IVb. *CAM Specific Measures:* Also within the disease specific measures category are outcome measures that are specific to complementary and alternative medicine systems. These include patterns of pulse diagnosis in Chinese medicine, electrodermal diagnostic measures, Gas Discharge Visualization, voice resonance patterns in bioacoustics, keynote symptoms or constitutional symptom patterns in classical homeopathy, and specific vitamin and mineral functional tests in nutritional and functional medicine.

Finally, outcome measures of interest in health care management are those measuring costs, social impact such as health care utilization, effects on practitioner–patient dynamics, number of office visits, cost of procedures, time required for procedures, convenience and/or suffering induced by interventions, etc.

Selection and Development of Outcome Measures

Appropriate matching of research goals with outcome measures depends upon a number of factors: 1) the model of health and disease under study as described in the first part of this chapter; 2) the type of diagnostic taxonomy present and its degree of clarity and measurement reliability and accuracy; 3) the goal of the healing intervention being studied; 4) the interest of the end user of the research (patient, practitioner, policy maker); and, 5) the source of the outcome measurement, that is, the information experts. When selecting outcome measures for comparison across healing systems and diagnostic categories or for measurement of illness and wellness and for patient-centered decision making, outcome measures drawn from the first two outcome tiers on the Outcomes Tree are most appropriate. When trying to identify the impact of a specific intervention on a certain disease classification for marker, outcome measures from tiers on the most disease specific part of The Outcomes Tree are most appropriate. No single outcome measure can capture the richness of health experience, therefore, strategies for outcome selection and synthesis are essential. Outcomes on the third & fourth parts of the Tree may be more sensitive and specific than those on the first & second parts and in many cases are easier to standardize. Outcomes drawn from the latter, more general part of the Tree, however, may allow for more, cross-system and general comparability, and often have more relevance for the patient and other users.

Of course other measures than those already available may require development that focus more specifically on healing. The Alignment Scale proposed by Seán ÓLaoire in the first part of this chapter is an example of one that may be appropriate for prayer studies. Physiological measures such as EEG, Heart Rate Variability and electromagnetic frequency measurement may be needed to more objectively assess when a bioenergy healer is genuine or when the process of healing has been effectively turned on. Cellular and physiological markers such as cytokine or gene and protein expression changes that reflect improved wellness may also be important for assessing when healing is taking place even when disease specific measures do not change.

Patient outcomes in complex chronic disease must be based on long-term evaluations in a variety of populations, should include patient preferences, and should be validated, not only statistically, but qualitatively to establish whether the outcomes selected in research have meaning to those on which they are subsequently applied. Ultimately, using core clinical and laboratory outcomes that have value across all health care systems will be required if direct comparison of disparate healing practices are going to be assessed using valid standardized tools.

Sources of Validated Outcomes Measures

There is a wide array of validated outcome measures available for the evaluation of healing practices. A number of excellent books and websites are available for selection of outcome measures. The following references are recommended for review when deciding on measures to use in the investigation of healing.

Websites:

http://www.outcomes-trust.org
http://www.leeds.ac.uk/nuffield/ infoservices/UKCH/oad.html
http://www.ahrq.gov/qual/qiix.htm

Summary Texts:

Bowling A (1991) (2nd edition) Measuring health: A review of quality of life measurement scales, Milton Keynes: Open University Press.

Bowling A (1995) Measuring disease, Milton Keynes: Open University Press.

McDowell I and Newall C (1987) Measuring health: a guide to rating scales and questionnaires, Oxford: Oxford University Press.

Wilkin D, Hallam L, and Doggett M (1992) Measures of need and outcome for primary health care, Oxford: Oxford University Press.

REFERENCE

Jonas W B and Linde K Conducting and evaluating clinical research in complementary and alternative medicine. In *Principles and Practice of Clinical Research*. Gallin J (ed.). New York: Academic Press. 2002; pp. 401–426.

16

A qualitative research perspective on healing

Once, when travelling on a ship, a young Italian came to me and said, 'I only believe in eternal matter.' I said, 'Your belief is not very different from my belief.' He was very surprised to hear a priest (he thought I was a priest) saying such a thing. He asked, 'What is your belief?' I said 'What you call eternal matter, I call eternal spirit. You call matter what I call spirit. What does it signify? It is only a difference in words. It is one Eternal.'

Inayat Khan (1974)

David Aldridge

This chapter describes the role of qualitative research design in the investigation of healing. It describes how qualitative methods are used in healing research and provides examples of such research.

Complex diseases and therapies are not easy to reduce into measurable and objective dimensions, especially when they deal with perception and subjective phenomena as in spiritual and energy healing and consciousness research. Reduction and measurement of the subjective may fail to capture the relevance of events and relationships for the patient. When this happens we have rigorous, but irrelevant research. Qualitative research, in which detailed 'thick' case descriptions are taken on a sample of the population, can serve several roles in research all directed toward assuring that the data collected is relevant to the populations studied. For example, prior to conducting a trial, qualitative research can help identify the most important outcomes. During a trial it can be used to check on perceptions and meanings among different subjects in the populations studied, and after a trial it can be used to provide a rich data set for understanding and conceptualizing variations of responses seen. Recently, sophisticated statistical programs have been developed to better quantify and analyze qualitative data sets. In this chapter, David Aldridge describes the role and methods of qualitative research used to study healing. **WBJ**

INTRODUCTION

Within recent years there has been a series of studies about the meaning of spirituality in health care delivery and intentional healing. In support of the demand to include spiritual concerns within integrated medical practices there has been a corresponding need for research that will underpin such a demand. One of the ways in which we can begin to understand intentional healing approaches and the concept of spiritual healing is through the broad spectrum of research approaches called qualitative research.

Health care is invariably defined in positivist terms as an object, a phenomenon, or a delivery system. Knowledge gained through scientific and experimental research is objective, quantifiable, stable, and measurable (at best measurable by instrumentation, reducing human error). In qualitative approaches, however, we have a shift in paradigm. Knowledge about health is considered to be a process, a lived experience, interpretative, changing, and subjective (at best gleaned through human interaction as personal relationship). Indeed, from this qualitative perspective we may be encouraged to think of the gerund form of the word 'health' as 'healthing.' In the same way, we can also consider what we do as professionals, and what our patients are involved in continually, as the 'relationship of healing'.

While being human is to err, the collection of data through human interaction is not in itself an error. Qualitative research is not a testing mode of enquiry but a discerning form requiring the collaborative involvement of those participating in that healing relationship. This emphasis on the verb, healing, rather than on the noun, health, goes some way to explain why qualitative approaches have found such resonance in nursing research, with its emphasis on nursing and caring as relational activities, rather than health care research, which is by definition nominal and objective.

If healing is a relationship, then we have to ask ourselves how we evaluate relationships. Would we take friendship, for example, and rate it on a 1–5 Likert scale? Or would we value our friendships for their various qualities? It is possible meaningfully to explain to another person what the value of a relationship is without quantifying it if we wish to demonstrate the nature of that friendship. So too for the relationship that is healing.

As the reader will have noticed, this is a major opposition between scientific paradigms and the first question often asked of qualitative research in medicine is 'Is it scientific?' The short reply to this is 'Yes, it is social science.' Medicine, being a social activity, is susceptible to being understood by a social science paradigm as much as it is by a natural science paradigm (Kleinman 1973, Mechanic 1968). To fulfil the functions of health caring adequately, we need both quantitative and qualitative approaches.

Social psychology, ethnography, and medical anthropology are acceptable scientific approaches for studying human behavior and qualitative research takes much of its methods from those fields. Indeed, suffering, distress, pain, and death are experiences relevant to understanding health care but elusive to measurement. Similarly, well-being, hope, faith, living a full life, and satisfaction are experiences central to health care but not immediately amenable to quantification. But they can be apprehended by understanding (Lewinsohn 1998) and these understandings are gleaned in relationship, the central activities of which are listening and telling stories. As stories are central to the therapeutic relationship, and a vital part of qualitative research, then I shall develop in some length within this chapter the concept of narrative (Aldridge 2000).

HEALTH CARE NARRATIVES: CONTEXT AND MEANING

In modern scientific terms, physicists, in their pursuit of understanding the nature of physical reality, have reached a stage where they have lost the concept of solid matter; they can't come up with the real identity of matter. So they are beginning to see things in more holistic terms, in terms of interrelationships rather than discrete, independent, concrete objects. (Dalai Lama 1999, p. 351)

Our lives are dynamic and performed in defining contexts that lend them meaning. The context of life in the cell will be the organ, the context for the organ will be the body, that of the body will be the 'environment'. This environment may indeed be the physical environment; it will also be a social environment, a broader ecological environment of nature, but also an environment of ideas. Thus meaning is central to understanding health care behavior.

Our lives gain their meaning in interaction and the interpretation of events. In this sense, identity is performed in various social arenas with a variety of purposive actors that lend meaning to what is performed. Culture is an ecological activity binding the meanings of individuals in relationships together, what Bateson refers to as an 'ecology of mind' (Bateson 1972). What we do as individuals is understood in the setting of our social activities and those settings are informed by the individuals that comprise them (Browner 1998, Hsu 2000, Voss et al 1999). Here too, the body, and the presentation of symptoms, is seen as an important non-verbal communication that has meaning within specific personal relationships that are located themselves within a social context. Symptoms are interpreted within relationships.

Spiritual meanings are linked to actions, and those actions have consequences that are performed as prayer, meditation, worship, and healing. What patients think about the causes of their illnesses influences what they do in terms of health care treatment and to whom they turn for the resolution of distress. For some people, rather than consider illness alone, they relate their personal identities to being healthy, one factor of which is spirituality. The maintenance and promotion of health – or becoming healthy – is an activity. As such it will be expressed bodily, a praxis aesthetic. Thus we would expect to see people not only having sets of beliefs about health but also actions related to those beliefs. Some of these may be dietary, some may involve exercise, some prayer or meditation. In more formal terms, patients may wish to engage in spiritual healing and contact a spiritual healer among the health care practitioners they consult. Indeed, some medical practitioners refer patients to spiritual healers.

What we have to ask, as health care practitioners, is, does the inclusion of spirituality bring advantages to understanding the people who come to us in distress? As soon as we talk about life being something which we can cherish and preserve, that compassion for others plays an important role in the way in which we choose to live with each other, that service to our communities is a vital activity for maintaining well-being, that hope is an important factor in recovery, then we have the basis for an argument that is spiritual as well as scientific. Essentially I am arguing for a plurality of research understanding in healing. How do we make meaningful connections that form the narratives we make as patients and practitioners, and how do those narratives inform each other?

Anecdotes: The Applied Language of Healing

Complementary medical approaches are often dismissed as relying upon anecdotal material, as though stories were unreliable. My argument is that stories are both reliable and rich in information. While we as medical scientists may try and dismiss anecdote, we rely upon it when we wish to explain particular cases to our colleagues away from the conference podium (Aldridge 1991a, 1991b). Even in scientific medicine, it has been the single case report that has been necessary to alert practitioners to the negative side-effects of current treatment.

While anecdotes may be considered as bad science, they are the everyday stuff of clinical practice. People tell us their stories and expect to be heard. Stories have a structure and are told in a style that informs us too. It is not solely the content of a story, but also how it is told that convinces us of its validity. While questionnaires gather information about populations and view the world from the perspective of the researcher, it is the interview that provides the condition for the patient to generate his or her meaningful story. The relationship is the context for the story and patients' stories may change according to the conditions in which they are related. This raises significant validity problems for questionnaire research. Anecdotes are the very stuff of social life and the fabric of communication in the healing encounter. As Miller writes: 'every time the experimental psychologist writes a research report in which anecdotal evidence has been assiduously avoided, the experimental scientist is generating anecdotal evidence for the consumption of his/her colleagues' (Miller 1998). The research report is itself an anecdotal report.

Stories play an important role in the healing process and testimony is an important consideration. Indeed, we have to trust each other in what we say. This is the basis of human communication in the human endeavor of understanding; it is the central plank of qualitative research. When it comes to questions of validity, then we have the concepts of trustworthiness in qualitative research. Testimonies are heard within groups that challenge veracity.

MULTIPLE PERSPECTIVES

What I shall be arguing for here is a multiple perspective for understanding health care delivery that is not solely based upon a positivist approach but also upon an interpretative approach. To take such a position is political in that it challenges the major paradigm of scientific research in medicine, a paradigm that is often transparent to those involved. Quite rightly, the qualitative paradigm is also seen as being critical – it challenges both the power and privilege of a dominant scientific ideology (Aldridge 1991a, 1991b, 1991c, 1992; Trethewey 1997).

An advantage of qualitative research is that it allows us to see how particular practices are being used. We can discover the meanings attached to activities as they are embedded in day-to-day living. The terms 'healing,' 'spirituality,' 'intentional' and 'energy' are subject to dictionary definition but also defined by their practice. Qualitative research helps us to understand how such terms are understood in practice and that is a political activity, as the feminist movement has reminded us. We have the right to call our experiences by what terms we wish

without a dominant group telling us how that term should be used. While many of us may question the use of the term 'energy' in healing, the word is used by both patients and healers alike, and we might be better directed to discovering its use in practice if we wish to understand it better. When we come to discuss the meaning of healing itself, what role spirituality has in health care, the nature of intentionality, then we are discussing the role of meaning in people's lives. One way to discover those meanings is to ask the participants. The rigor of the asking and the way those meanings are interpreted is the scientific method – the methodology – of qualitative research.

To understand the health implications of prayer, for example, we can discern the effect of prayer by experiment. However, I shall argue later in this chapter that the impact of prayer from a spiritual perspective is better understood in its subjective interpretation as a qualitative study. Both complement each other. If we successfully argue for a complementary medicine that is increasingly being called an integrative medicine, then surely we can have a congruent paradigm for health care research that is complementary and integrative.

A way of seeing how these differing perspectives can be applied to a common problem would be to study those patients who fail to complete a course of treatment – what is sometimes referred to as non-compliance. A positivist paradigm may hypothesize that compliance with the prescribed treatment regime is a matter of patient education. By designing a patient education program to raise an understanding of the treatment then compliance would be improved according to specific criteria for evaluation. We could design an experiment that would randomize identified non-complying patients to a taught education program, to a leaflet education program, and to no education. Their compliance with medication could then be measured by an assessor blind to the education program itself.

A qualitative approach would not initially set-up an experiment, nor would it try to measure anything. In this instance we would be interested in the experience of patients consulting a practitioner, listening to what the practitioners say, prescribe and advise, and then ask whether patients have complied with that advice. We would be asking where, when, with whom, and on what grounds the decision was made not to comply with medical advice. In this case the perspective of the non-complier is as important as that of the practitioner. Similarly, we may also question patients who complete a course of treatment and compare them with those who fail to complete. This would include interviews, observations in various settings such as the consulting room and the home, and possibly written material such as diaries. Once we knew the circumstances of non-complying, then we could design initiatives to investigate experimentally. Non-compliance may be located in the patient, it may be a located in the practitioner, or it may be an artifact of the relationship between the two. Unless we discern with whom and when, then our experimental work will be inevitably limited.

From a critical research perspective, we would be interested in how a clinic is so organized that that some groups fail to have their treatment needs met and some patterns of treatment response are endemic. This may mean a collaborative enquiry with a self-help patient group and entail some form of advocacy between the clinic and the group (Aldridge 1987d, Reason & Rowan 1981). This latter approach reflects the strong participatory action component of early social science research.

Qualitative research is an umbrella term. Some approaches lean toward an emphasis on analyzing texts and interviews (like content analysis and discourse analysis), while others rely upon descriptions of interaction that may use a variety of media and are based upon ethnography, ethnomethodology, symbolic interactionism, and phenomenology. Other methods set out to build theories. Other approaches may set out to discover a particular historical background and locate this within an ideological or political perspective – the assimilation of acupuncture within modern Western medicine, for example, contrasting its acceptance in various European states.

QUALITATIVE RESEARCH AS CONSTRUCTED MEANINGS IN CONTEXT

Qualitative research covers a variety of approaches. What characterizes these approaches is an emphasis on understanding the meaning of social activities as they occur in their natural contexts. These are interchangeably called field studies, ethnographies, naturalistic inquiries, and case studies. A central plank of these approaches is that we can discern the meaning of social behavior such as healing and prayer from the experiences that people have in particular contexts, and that these meanings themselves are constructed – constructed in the sense that people *make* sense of what they do. The difficulty these approaches face, from a perspective of positivist science, is that because sense is continually being made, and this sense may vary from context to context, there are no universally applicable laws of human behavior but a series of locally constructed meanings in specific contexts where cultures of healing exist.

Participant observation

Participant observation is a generic term for a qualitative approach where the researcher observes what is happening from an insider position. Rather than administering a set of pre-formed interviews, the participant observer works alongside the staff and patients asking what is going on and listening to what is spontaneously said. Lawton (1998) worked directly alongside patients, their families, and staff in a hospice to see what was happening. She observed 280 different patients in an intensive study of the dying patient and the dying process in an attempt to answer why some patients are admitted to hospital and others are not. She found that patients are admitted to hospices when bodies begin to disintegrate such that contemporary concepts of the hygienic, sanitized, bounded body become challenged. This builds on the original work of Glaser & Strauss, who studied the process of dying, that gave rise to qualitative research as grounded theory

(Glaser & Strauss 1967). What Lawton does is to challenge the homogenous concept of the hospice as a place for the dying patient and the dying process. She see the hospice as a place where marginalized cancer patients are referred when they experience difficult symptoms and their bodies deteriorate beyond a socially acceptable boundary. This reflects the challenging nature of qualitative research, its location in practice and personal experience.

Narrative Analysis

Researchers from a wide variety of disciplines have found narratives to be useful in explaining cross-level psychological phenomena (Mankowski & Rappaport 2000). Narratives with different sources and functions occur at group level and as individual levels of analysis. Research on narratives is particularly useful for understanding the relationship between social process and individual experience, especially in spiritually based communities (Aldridge 1986, 1987a, 1987b, 1987d). Narratives in spiritual settings appear to serve a variety of functions in community life. They define community and facilitate personal change (Aldridge 1987c). As such, local community narratives are vital psychological resources, particularly where dominant cultural narratives fail adequately to represent the lived experience of individuals.

In a family-based treatment approach for suicidal behavior (Aldridge 1998), what the patient tells as a story and the narratives of those involved with the patient generate important bases for treatment initiatives as well as providing an important source of research material. When analyzing family narratives of illness, it was possible to identify specific family features that led to suicidal behavior: a situation where a family was about to change (by someone leaving or joining), where the identified patient could only do wrong (even when he or she tried to put things right), and where that person had always been the 'sickly' member of the family. Personal narratives, while being individual, are also located within family narratives, which themselves are located within social contexts. However, these narratives are not accessible to a questionnaire approach; people have to tell them to a listener.

As we have seen earlier, the understanding of patients' stories is vital. Stories in the hospice offer the context for elucidating hidden meanings. Little et al (1998) investigated the illness narratives of patients who had undergone colectomy for colorectal cancer. They asked patients to tell the story of their illness from its first intimations, in their own words with minimal prompting. These interviews were then transcribed and analyzed using a grounded theory approach. From this observational material emerged two phases of subjective experience. An initial phase of disorientation and a sense of loss of control followed by an enduring adaptive phase where the patient constructs and reconstructs his experience through narrative. This last phase they call liminality: a dynamic process of adapting to the experience of being ill as expressed in a narrative account of a body that must accommodate the disease and the self.

Potts (1996) examined the role of spirituality in the cancer experiences of 16 African Americans living in the southern United States. Without any investigator-initiated mention of spirituality, participants referred to many categories of spiritual beliefs and practices that were relevant in their experiences with cancer. When spirituality was specifically explored, there was an even greater elaboration on the initial categories. Key findings included a belief in God as the source of healing, the value of prayer as an instrumental practice, a strategy termed 'turning it over to the Lord,' and locating the cancer experience within the context of a greater life narrative. The willingness of care providers to address spiritual and cultural dimensions of cancer enhances therapeutic relationships and the efficacy of psychosocial interventions.

Such narratives are not only important for understanding the process of a disease; they can also make an important contribution to understanding what helps in the process of recovery (Aldridge 1998, Garrett 1997, Spencer et al 1997). People of faith find meaning in their struggle. Black's study (Black 1999) of the spiritual narratives of 50 elderly African American women found that those women 'believed their hardship had meaning, because *they* interpreted it as a measure of their strength, imbued it with divine purpose, and foresaw a just end' (p. 372). If we are engaged in countering hopelessness as a precursor to failing health, then surely the narratives of these women, and the understandings that we can glean from them, are important factors for consideration in health care research.

Ethnographic Studies

Qualitative researchers are often engaged in fieldwork. They have to physically visit the people in the clinic, the home, the hospital ward, the street, or the village. The forms of documentation necessary for these studies will also vary. Anthropologists have pioneered these methods of learning about other cultures and we too are being challenged to learn about other cultures of healing. At the heart of these approaches is an emphasis on the researcher being a primary instrument in the research process for the collection of data and for analysing that data. The researcher is involved in the context in which she or he works; there is an expectation that the researcher will be sensitive to non-verbal communication and will be interpreting what she or he experiences. These will be referred to here as ethnographic studies.

For example, in a study of mental disorder in Zimbabwe (Patel et al 1995), 110 subjects were selected by general nurses in three clinics and by four traditional healers from their current clients. The subjects were interviewed using an interview schedule. Mental disorder most commonly presented with somatic symptoms, few patients denied that their mind or soul was the source of illness, and spiritual factors were frequently cited as causes of mental illness. Subjects who were selected by traditional healers reported a greater duration of illness and were more likely to provide a spiritual explanation for their illness. Most patients, however, showed a mixture of psychiatric symptoms that did not fall clearly into a single diagnostic group and patients with a spiritual model of illness were less likely to conform to criteria of 'caseness' and represented a unique category of psychological distress in Zimbabwe.

The significance of healing rituals is important for understanding how health care may best be implemented. An ethnographic study of a church-based healing clinic in Jamaica (Griffith 1983) shows how mixing spiritual, psychological, and conventional medical needs, with their heterodox beliefs and values, creates tension. While a new ritual format needed to be introduced, it is difficult to transform traditional formats of healing. Such an ethnographic qualitative perspective could be used to discern how complementary medicine approaches are used within modern healing cultures within health care clinics.

Ethnographic approaches have investigated interdisciplinary work (Sands 1990), experience of the intensive care unit from a patient's perspective (Rier 2000), the traditional health beliefs and practices of black women (Flaskerud & Rush 1989) the experience of caring for elderly parents in the home (Lewis et al 1995), pregnant adolescents' responses to the preparation for motherhood class curriculum (Lesser et al 1998), adapting to chronic diseases such as asthma (MacDonald 1996) and AIDS (Kotarba & Hurt 1995).

Phenomenology

While experience and interpretation are at the heart of all qualitative methods, there are also particular phenomenological approaches that look to the essence of a structure or an experience. The assumption that an essence of an experience exists is similar to the assumption by an ethnographer that culture exists. Prior beliefs are first identified and then temporarily set aside so that the phenomenon being studied may be seen in a new light. In a study of the phenomena of prayer we would want to know what constitutes the consciousness of praying, what the sensory experiences of prayer are, what our thoughts are, and what emotions are involved. Setting and context would also be central to this phenomenological understanding. In this way, we see that the lives of the mystics would provide documentary evidence of a phenomenological approach to understanding prayer and meditation.

DoRozario (1997) used a hermeneutic and phenomenological perspective to understand how individuals with disability and chronic illness survive and cope successfully with their lives in spite of overwhelming difficulties. The lived experience of 35 informants and 14 autobiographers who represented a wide range of people with disability and chronic illness was used as the basis for understanding the phenomenological world of chronic conditions. Five factors that facilitated coping and adaptation were identified: the combined elements of spiritual transformation, hope, personal control, positive social supports, and meaningful engagement in life enabled individuals to come to terms with their respective conditions The research identified processes by which people reconcile their outer forms of disability, decay, or suffering and discover an embodiment of their own inner resources and strengths.

Phenomenological studies are well suited to understanding the world of the sufferer. An interpretive phenomenological study, which began as a study of the meaning of being restrained, offers a glimpse into mental illness (Johnson 1998). Ten psychiatric patients were interviewed and the audiotaped interviews transcribed. The resulting texts were analyzed using a process methodology developed from Heideggerian hermeneutical phenomenology. Two major themes emerged, 'struggling' and 'why me?', revealing what it was like for the participants to live with a serious mental illness. As part of their struggling, patients asked the existential question 'Why me?', a question that is repeatedly heard when working with the dying. This study underscored how important it is for the nurse caring for a psychiatric patient to enter into, and try to understand, the world of patients with mental illnesses, emphasizing the practical application of research for practice. Similarly, Savage & Canody (1999) found that for patients with a life-sustaining device, then spirituality, humor and strong family relationships were essential to a positive outlook.

Grounded Theory

The strategy of research is inductive where theories are gleaned from experience. This is not theory testing but theory generation where existing theories are either lacking or fail to explain the phenomenon satisfactorily. Given that placebo, for example, is a concept in common use by practitioners, qualitative research would ask, and observe, those practitioners when they believed placebo to be occurring and ask what they understood a placebo practice to be. Similarly, they would ask patients about their understanding of what was happening. This breaks the cycle of abstract definitions being brokered among scientists and locates explanations in everyday practices. In this way, theories are generated that match the data gathered from experience. This has led to the approach known as grounded theory (Strauss & Corbin 1990). Grounded theory elucidates substantive theories applicable to understanding localized practices that have a high internal and content validity, rather than grand theories of medicine.

In Camp's study of coronary artery bypass grafting (Camp 1996), spiritual issues are extremely important. The operation is perceived by the patient as a life-threatening event and the study aimed to discover the spiritual needs of patients undergoing surgery and how these needs are met during hospitalization. Postoperative data were collected through interviews with 17 adults aged from 34 to 83 years. What emerged was that spiritual needs centered around having faith in their own decision-making, faith in the hospital staff (especially the nurses), and an overwhelming faith in God during a time of great stress, alongside feelings of being 'pulled apart' and fragmented. Consequently, patients needed to recover a sense of wholeness that included physical, psychological, and spiritual aspects of their experience.

RESEARCH IN HEALING

Medical professionals are becoming aware that there are aspects of health that do not fall within their range of knowledge. For those elements to be incorporated into practice, a realm of quantitative clinical evidence is being demanded that is quite inappropriate. I am not saying that spirituality and its influence on health care practices should be accepted simply because it is a good idea, rather that the means of gathering and displaying evidence should be discussed, particularly when we know that existential matters are important for human well-being. We do not need to validate such a position from scientific studies; we have some residual knowledge within our cultures of healing that we need not abdicate. Scientific medicine is but one pillar of the culture of healing; the aesthetic and the spiritual are two others.

Critics have often found the strict methodology of natural science wanting when applied to the study of human health care behavior (Aldridge & Pietroni 1987; Burkhardt & Kienle 1980, 1983), and this critique has stimulated calls for innovation in clinical medical research and therapy (Aldridge 1992, 1996; Reason & Rowan 1981). A significant factor in the desire for innovation is a growing awareness by doctors of the importance of a patient's social and cultural milieu, and a recognition that a patient's health beliefs and understanding of personal meanings should be incorporated into treatment. What we need in clinical research is a discipline that seeks to discover methods that express clinical changes as they occur in the individual rather than methods which reflect a group average. How clinical change occurs and is recognized will depend not only on the view of the researcher and clinician but also on the beliefs and understanding of the patient and his or her family (Aldridge 1998).

There is often a split in medical science between researchers and clinicians. Researchers see themselves as rational and rigorous in their thinking and tend to see clinicians as sentimental and biased, which in turn elicits comments from clinicians about inhuman treatment and reductionist thinking. We are faced with the problem of how to promote in clinical practice research that has scientific validity in terms of rigor, and, at the same time, a clinical validity for the patient and clinician.

The randomized trial appears to be theoretically relevant for the clinical researcher but has all too often randomized away what should be specifically relevant for the clinician and patient. A comparative trial of two chemotherapy regimes assumes that the treatment or control groups to which patients are randomly assigned contain evenly balanced populations. What is sought from such a trial is that one method works significantly better than another when comparing group averages. Yet as clinicians we want to know what method works best for individual patients. Our interest lies not in the group average but with those patients who do well with such treatment and those who do not respond so well. Furthermore, it is randomizing of patients with specific prognostic factors which obscures therapeutic effect. Rather than searching for a non-specific chemotherapy treatment of a particular cancer, we may be better advised to seek out those factors which allow us to deliver a specific treatment for recognized individuals with a particular cancer. This is not to argue against randomization exclusively, rather that we have randomized the patient rather than the treatment. As Weinstein says:

randomisation tends to obscure rather than illuminate, interactive effects between treatments and personal characteristics. Thus if Treatment A is best for one type of patient and Treatment B is best for another type, a randomised study would only be able to indicate which treatment performs best overall. If we wanted to discover the effect on subgroups, one would have to separate out the variable anyway. (Weinstein 1974)

We may well say the same of the non-specific use of prayer. We do not know the existing use of prayer by a patient in a group, nor those praying for her. Nor do we know what stage that person is in terms of suffering such that prayer will bring not only relief but a new understanding. Prayer is not like a medication; as yet no dose–response formula has been discovered.

Science and Medicine: What Science Does Not Know

Modern science implies that there is a common map of the territory of healing, with particular coordinates and given symbols for finding our way around, and that the map of scientific medicine is that map. We need to recognize that scientific medicine emphasizes one particular way of knowing among others. Scientific thinking maintains the myth that in order to know anything we must be scientists; however, people who live in vast desert areas are able find their way across the trackless terrain without any understanding of scientific geography. They also know the pattern of the weather without recourse to what we know as the science of meteorology.

In a similar way, people know about their own bodies and have understanding about their own lives without the benefit of anatomy or psychology. Furthermore, people know of their own God or connection to a higher power without the benefit of an elaborated theology. They may not confer the same meanings on their experiences of health and illness as we researchers do, yet it is toward an understanding of personal and idiosyncratic beliefs that we might most wisely be guiding our research endeavors. By understanding the stories people tell us of their healing and the insights this brings, we may begin truly to understand the efficacy of prayer. That health and the divine are brought together in such spiritualities is a challenge for renewal of our understanding in health care, not a ground for dismissal as invalid.

When we speak of scientific or experimental validity, we speak of a validity that has to be conferred by a person or group of people on the work or actions of another group. This is a 'political' process. With the obsession for 'objective truths' in the scientific community then other 'truths' are ignored. As clinicians we have many ways of knowing: by intuition, through experience, and by observation. If we disregard these 'knowings' then we promote the idea that there is an objective definitive external truth that exists as tablets of stone and that only we, the initiated, have access to it. This criticism applies also to the dogma of religion that refuses to consider what other evidence the world provides. Simply saying that the world is evil will not resolve the need for the necessary dialogue for transcending seemingly opposing views.

The people with whom clinicians work in the therapist/patient relationship are not experimental units. Nor are the measurements made on these people separate and independent sets of data. While at times it may be necessary to treat the data as independent of the person, we must be aware that this is what we are doing, otherwise, when we come to measure particular personal variables, we face many complications. The clinical measurements of blood status, weight, and temperature are important. However, they belong to a different realm of understanding than do issues of anxiety about the future, the experience of pain, the anticipation of personal and social losses, and existential feelings of abandonment. These defy comparative measurement. Yet if we are to investigate therapeutic approaches to chronic disease, we need to investigate these subjective and qualitative realms. While we may be able to make little change in blood status, we can take heed of emotional status and propose initiatives for treatment. The goal of therapy is not always to cure; it can also be to comfort and relieve. The involvement of the physician with the biologic dimension of disease has resulted in amnesia for the necessary understanding of suffering in the patient (Cassell 1991).

In the same way, we can achieve changes in existential states through prayer and meditation, the evidence for which can only be metaphorically expressed and humanly witnessed. Are we to impoverish our culture by denying that this happens and discounting what people tell us? What then are we to trust in our lives – dialogue with our friends or the displays of our machines? This is not an argument against technology. It is an argument for narrative and relationship in understanding what it is to be human; that is, the basis for qualitative research.

In terms of outcomes measurement, we face further difficulties. The people we see in our clinics do not live in isolation. Life is rather a messy laboratory and continually influences the subjects of our therapeutic and research endeavors. The way people respond in situations is sometimes determined by the way in which they have understood the meaning of that situation. The meaning of hair loss, weight loss, loss of potency, loss of libido, impending death and the nature of suffering will be differently perceived in varying cultures. To this balding, aging researcher, hair loss is a fact of life. My Greek neighbour says that if it happens to him it will be a disaster. When we deliver a powerful therapeutic agent then we are not treating an isolated example of a clinical entity but intervening in an ecology of responses and beliefs which are somatic, psychological, social, and spiritual.

In a similar way, what Western medicine understands as surgery, intubation, and medication, others may perceive as mutilation, invasion, and poisoning. Cultural differences regarding the integrity of the body will influence ethical issues such as abortion and body transplants. Treatment initiatives may be standardized in terms of the culture of the administrating researchers, but the perceptions of the subjects of the research and their families may be incongruous and various. Actually, we know from studies of treatment options in breast cancer that physicians beliefs also vary, and these beliefs influence the information the physicians give to their patients (Ganz 1992). If we return to the concepts of placebo and non-compliance, then it is surely a qualitative research paradigm that will encourage a practical understanding of the patient–practitioner relationship.

Difficulties in Researching Prayer and Spiritual Healing

We know that there are major difficulties with intentional healing research:

1. Achieving transcendence, an understanding of purpose and meaning as a performed identity, is an activity. It occurs in a relationship and that relationship is informed by culture. Research initiatives that concentrate on the healer fail to understand the activity of the patient, lose sight of the relationship, and ignore the cultural factors involved. (I am using 'culture' here to refer to the system of symbolic meanings that are available, not demographic data.) Losing this nesting of contexts fragments the healing endeavor emphasizing a passive patient who receives healing rather than an active patient participating in a common enterprise. A qualitative approach would emphasize the involvement of the patient and that healing is a relational activity.

2. Much research is carried out using a conventional medical science paradigm but the intention of that research is not always made clear. If the intention is to demonstrate the efficacy of spiritual healing approaches and prayer, then the methodology is clearly misguided. I suspect that much of this research is not being carried out for patients but as a strategy in the politics of establishing alternative healing initiatives within conventional medical approaches. Therefore we have healing groups promoting their own interest and adopting the methodological approach of randomized clinical trials considered to be suitable for acceptance rather than looking at what is necessary for discovering what is happening. This is not to say that the results of clinical randomized trials are not influential, rather that they are limited in their applicability as far as prayer and healing are to be understood if: (a) the patient is expected to be active; (b) there has to be a relationship with the healer; (c) there are no definite end-points in time; (d) healing can appear as differing phenomena; and (e) the prayer has to be non-specific and non-directional.[1]

3. Healing, like prayer, is not an homogenous practice and is not susceptible to standardization. Attempts at standardization would make it no longer prayer but superstitious incantation or magical hand-passes.

4. The ability to heal is seen in some traditions as a divine gift. It may not be available to all and even to those that have the gift not available all of the time. Ascertaining who has it, and when, is not easy. Healing is also considered in some traditions to be a secondary ability of spiritual development that can be systematically applied, but it is an advanced ability. This again proves to be a difficulty, as presumably there are more practitioners with lower abilities than advanced practitioners who are more reliable in their efficacy. And who in the world of healing practitioners is going to say that they are less advanced? Those who are advanced in such understandings will probably see no need to subject such knowledge to material worldly proof.

---

[1]The concept of 'Thy will be done' as an effective form of prayer, following Dossey (1993), ruins a one-tailed statistical test.

Indeed, we must return to the purpose of proof. We see already that spiritual healing is practiced and that medical practitioners refer to such healers. If the grounds of research are for payment or to institute professional practice then may be the results will be more elusive than when the purpose is the pursuit of human knowledge. One system of knowledge cannot be predicated on proofs from another system of knowledge.

CONCLUSION

It would be wrong to permit medicine to use the authority it has gained from scientific and technical proficiency ... as a cloak to gain authority over questions that most in society consider moral and religious. (Smolin 1995)

When people come to their practitioners they are asking about what will become of them. What will their future be like? Will there be a change? Some practitioners make a prognosis based on the interview that they have had with the patient. Sometimes this will be the dreaded answer to the question 'How long do I have to live?' But with each interview there is the question of when healing will take place. What can be expected in the near future, and is there any hope of a cure? The story of what happens is, in part, a clinical history. It is also no less than the narration of destiny, the unfolding of a person's life purpose (Larner 1998). When we talk with the dying, it is this sense of purpose, 'Was it all worthwhile?,' that is a critical moment in coping with the situation. The telling and listening, the *relating* of these stories, is the very stuff of qualitative research.

Narratives are the recounting of what happens in time. They are not simply located in the past but are also about real events that happen now and what expectations there are for the future. The teller of the narrative is an active agent, not merely passively experiencing his or her past but performing an identity with another person. That other person as doctor, priest, or healer, has the moral obligation through the therapeutic contract to listen and engage in the healing relationship. Narratives are told. This performance aspect is what gives a narrative vitality and

instructs us, as listeners, to what we must attend (Aldridge 1996). Narratives are not simply private accounts that we relate to ourselves, they have a public function and will vary according to who is listening and the way in which the listeners are reacting. Qualitative research has incorporated such narratives into its approach to understanding health care (Aldridge 1998, Hall 1998, Strauss & Corbin 1990, van Manen 1998).

Narratives bring a coherence and order to life stories. Stories make sense. Yet the scientific null hypothesis assumes, at the very core of its reasoning, that there is no such coherence (Larner 1998). Technology strives to domesticate time as *chronos*, to make time even and predictable. In an earlier book (Aldridge 1996), I wrote of time as *kairos*, uneven, biological, and decisive, in that the moment must be seized. This makes a mockery of fixed outcomes in that the time and logic of healing may have modes elusive to commercialized requirements of health care delivery. Peace of mind may occur but no cure. Forgiveness may take place but no change in survival time. Are we really to throw away such outcomes of peace of mind and forgiveness because they find no immediate material expression? Perhaps it is the very denial of those qualities that provokes the restlessness of people today as they seek an elusive state of health despite the material riches of Western cultures.

No material change may occur in spiritual healing, but the individual transcends his or her immediate situation. Furthermore, there are no personal stories in medical science but group probabilities. This is seriously at odds with the demands of the patient's encounter with the doctor, which is personal. People are subjective. They are indeed subjects, and subjects who need to relate a story to another person who understands them. To be treated as objects in a world of social events deprives them of meaning. It is this very lack of meaning that exacerbates suffering.

Becoming sick, being treated, achieving recovery, and becoming well are plots in the narrative of life. As such they are a reminder of our mortality. They are a historical relationship; meanings are linked together in time. Stories have a shape, they have purpose and they are bounded in time. Thus, we talk about a case history. It is for this reason that group studies fail to offer an essential understanding of what it is to fall ill and become well. Generalization loses individual intent and time is removed. The individual biographical historicity is lost in favor of the group. Purpose and intent are important in life; they are at the basis of hope. If that purpose is abandoned through hopelessness, then suicide and death are the outcome. In our healing endeavors we need to consider the circumstances in which healing occurs and how those circumstances are enabled. This is not the technological approach of cure but the ecological approach of providing the ground in which healing is achieved, whether it be an organic, psychological, social, or spiritual context. Those healing contexts will also be part of a biography, they have an historicity, and this must be included too in our research.

At the heart of much scientific thinking in the medical world is a desire for prediction, to base treatment strategies and outcomes on a group statistic of probability. This is quite rightly explained as the desire to provide the optimum treatment and to eliminate false treatment that harms. Such a statement too is based upon belief, a touching faith in statistical reasoning. Behind this thinking is an assumption that tomorrow will be the same as today, that the future is predicated on the past. What many of our patients hope, and the purpose of our endeavors in both practice and research, is that tomorrow will be new. Qualitative research methods are one way of discovering the new in the way in which we tell our stories together.

REFERENCES

Aldridge D 1986 Licence to heal. Crucible April–June: 58–66
Aldridge D 1987a A community approach to cancer in families. Journal of Maternal and Child Health 12: 182–185
Aldridge D 1987b Families, cancer and dying. Family Practice 4: 212–218
Aldridge D 1987c One body: a guide to healing in the Church. S.P.C.K., London
Aldridge D 1987d A team approach to terminal care: personal implications for patients and practitioners. Journal of the Royal College of General Practitioners 37: 364
Aldridge D 1991a Aesthetics and the individual in the practice of medical research: a discussion paper. Journal of the Royal Society of Medicine 84: 147–150
Aldridge D 1991b Healing and medicine. Journal of the Royal Society of Medicine 84: 516–518
Aldridge D 1991c Spirituality, healing and medicine. Journal of British General Practice 41: 425–427
Aldridge D 1992 The needs of individual patients in clinical research. Advances 8(4): 58–65
Aldridge D 1996 Music therapy research and practice in medicine: from out of the silence. Jessica Kingsley, London
Aldridge D 1998 Suicide: the tragedy of hopelessness. Jessica Kingsley, London
Aldridge D 2000 Spirituality, healing and medicine: return to the silence. Jessica Kingsley, London
Aldridge D, Pietroni P 1987 Research trials in general practice: towards a focus on clinical practice. Family Practice 4: 311–315
Bateson G 1972 Steps to an ecology of mind. Ballantine, New York

Black H 1999 Poverty and prayer: spiritual narratives of elderly African-American women. Review of Religious Research 40(4): 359–372
Browner C 1998 Varieties of reasoning in medical anthropology. Medical Authropology Quarterly 12(3): 356–362
Burkhardt R, Kienle G 1980 Controlled clinical trials and drug regulations. Controlled Clinical Trials 1: 151–164
Burkhardt R, Kienle G 1983 Basic problems in controlled trials. Journal of Medical Ethics 9: 80–84
Camp P 1996 Having faith: experiencing coronary artery bypass grafting. Journal of Cardiovascular Nursing 10(3): 55–64
Cassell E 1991 The nature of suffering and the goals of medicine. Oxford University Press, New York
Dalai Lama 1999 The path of tranquillity. Viking, New York
DoRozario L 1997 Spirituality in the lives of people with disability and chronic illness: a creative paradigm of wholeness and reconstitution. Disability and Rehabilitation 19(10): 427–434
Dossey L 1993 Healing words: the power of prayer and the practice of medicine. Harper Collins, New York
Flaskerud J, Rush C 1989 AIDS and traditional health beliefs and practices of black women. Nursing Research 38(4): 210–215
Ganz P 1992 Treatment options for breast cancer – beyond survival. New England Journal of Medicine 326: 1147–1149
Garrett C 1997 Recovery from anorexia nervosa: a sociological perspective. International Journal of Eating Disorder 21(3): 261–272

Glaser B, Strauss A 1967 The discovery of grounded theory: strategies for qualitative research. Aldine, Chicago

Griffith E 1983 The significance of ritual in a church-based healing model. American Journal of Psychiatry 140(5): 568–572

Hall B 1998 Patterns of spirituality in persons with advanced HIV disease. Research in Nursing and Health 21(2): 143–153

Hsu L 2000 Spirit (Shen), styles of knowing, and authority in contemporary Chinese medicine. Culture, Medicine and Psychiatry 24: 197–229

Johnson M 1998 Being mentally ill: a phenomenological inquiry. Archives Psychiatric Nursing 12(4): 195–201

Khan I 1974 The development of spiritual healing. Hunter House, Claremont, CA

Kleinman A 1973 Medicine's symbolic reality: on a central problem in the philosophy of medicine. Inquiry 16: 206–213

Kotarba J, Hurt D 1995 An ethnography of an AIDS hospice: toward a theory of organizational pastiche. Symbolic Interactaction 18(4): 413–438

Larner G 1998 Through a glass darkly. Theory and Psychology 8(4): 549–572

Lawton J 1998 Contemporary hospice care: the sequestration of the unbounded body and 'dirty dying'. Sociology of Health and Illness 20(2): 121–143

Lesser J, Anderson N, Koniak-Griffin D 1998 'Sometimes you don't feel ready to be an adult or a mom:' the experience of adolescent pregnancy. Journal of Child and Adolescent Psychiatric Nursing 11(1): 7–16

Lewinsohn R 1998 Medical theories, science, and the practice of medicine. Social Science and Medicine 46(10): 1261–1270

Lewis M, Curtis M, Lundy K 1995 'He calls me his angel of mercy:' the experience of caring for elderly parents in the home. Holistic Nursing Practice 9(4): 54–65

Little M, Jordens C, Paul K, Montgomery K, Philipson B 1998 Liminality: a major category of the experience of cancer illness. Social Science and Medicine 47(10): 1485–1494

MacDonald H 1996 'Mastering uncertainty:' mothering the child with asthma. Pediatric Nurse 22(1): 55–59

Mankowski E, Rappaport J 2000 Narrative concepts and analysis in spiritually-based communities. Journal of Community Psychology 28(5): 479–493

Mechanic D 1968 Medical sociology. Free Press, New York

Miller R 1998 Epistemology and psychotherapy data: the unspeakable, unbearable, horrible truth. Clinical Psychology: Science and Practice 5(2): 242–250

Patel V, Gwanzura F, Simunyu E, Lloyd K, Mann A 1995 The phenomenology and explanatory models of common mental disorder: a study in primary care in Harare, Zimbabwe. Psychological Medicine 25(6): 1191–1199

Potts R 1996 Spirituality and the experience of cancer in an African-American community: implications for psychosocial oncology. Journal of Psychosocial Oncology 14(1): 1–19

Reason P, Rowan J 1981 Human inquiry. John Wiley, Chichester

Rier D 2000 The missing voice of the critically ill: a medical sociologist's first-person account. Sociology of Health and Illness 22(1): 68–93

Sands R 1990 Ethnographic research: a qualitative research approach to study of the interdisciplinary team. Social Work Health Care 15(1): 115–129

Savage L, Canody C 1999 Life with a left ventricular assist device: the patient's perspective. American Journal of Critical Care 8(5): 340–343

Smolin D 1995 Praying for baby Rena: religious liberty, medical futility, and miracles. Seton Hall Law Review 25(3): 960–996

Spencer J, Davidson H, White V 1997 Helping clients develop hopes for the future. American Journal of Occupational Therapy 51(3): 191–198

Strauss A, Corbin J 1990 Basics of qualitative research: grounded theory procedures and techniques. Sage, Newbury Park, CA

Trethewey A 1997 Resistance, identity, and empowerment: a postmodern feminist analysis of clients in a human service organization. Community Monographs 64(4): 281–301

van Manen M 1998 Modalities of body experience in illness and health. Qualitative Health Research 8(1): 7–24

Voss R, Douville V, Little Soldier A, Twiss G 1999 Tribal and shamanic-based social work practice: a Lakota perspective. Social Work 44(3): 228–241

Weinstein M 1974 Allocation of subjects in medical experiments. New England Journal of Medicine 291: 1278–1285

17

Statistical issues in healing research

Jessica Utts

This chapter reviews basic statistical techniques and their assumptions and discusses their implications for healing research.

Statistical analysis is an essential component of modern research. It is used for quantitative description of observations, for comparison of the effects of healing interventions, and for inference about cause from those interventions. Failure to properly use statistical methods can make a bad study look good and deceive readers as to the significance of a finding. Modern statistical inference rests on certain assumptions about cause and effect and about how events are normally distributed. Not all healing systems share these assumptions, and recent data on mind–matter effects indicate that, at least where consciousness is involved, the normal assumptions of cause and effect may not be sufficient.

In this chapter, Jessica Utts outlines the basic rationale and methods used in proper statistical analysis and then presents several challenges that arise from research on consciousness and healing. New research design and analysis methods may be needed in order to address phenomena that do not follow the normal assumptions inherent in current statistical procedures. **WBJ**

INTRODUCTION

Randomized controlled clinical trials have advanced our understanding of medicine tremendously. Two key components of these studies are appropriate design and appropriate use of basic statistical methods to analyze the results. Both the design and analysis phases rely on certain assumptions about how nature operates, assumptions that are reasonable under our current understanding of biology and physics. However, mind–matter research over the past few decades calls some of these assumptions into question. The design and statistical analysis methods that require these assumptions, and subsequent results, are thus also called into question.

There are two consequences of questioning the standard assumptions underlying the design and analysis of clinical trials. One consequence is that some of the results of earlier clinical trials may not be as sound as previously thought. The second consequence is that future clinical trials may need to be designed differently to account for different conjectures about how nature operates.

This chapter begins with a review of standard statistical methods and study design used in medical research, including hypothesis testing, confidence intervals, power analysis, designing randomized experiments, and conducting observational studies. Next, a review of findings from mind–matter research is given, with emphasis on how these findings challenge the traditional assumptions used in statistical experiments and analyses. Finally, suggestions are given for incorporating the mind–matter research findings into the design and analysis of future clinical trials, especially those for distant healing and intentionality.

THE BENEFIT OF STATISTICAL METHODS

Statistical methods are used to make inferences about a population on the basis of a sample. For example a study led by the Steering Committee of the Physicians' Health Study Research Group (1988), to determine whether taking aspirin helps prevent heart attacks, recruited over 22 000 male physician volunteers. They were randomly assigned to take aspirin or a placebo, and heart attack rates were compared for the two groups. The placebo group had almost twice the rate of heart attacks as the aspirin group (17.13 per 1000 and 9.42 per 1000, respectively). Based on these *sample* results, inferences can be made that aspirin is beneficial for the *population* of males who are similar to those in the study.

Statistical methods are useful for two purposes:

- To establish the existence of a benefit due to a treatment, the difference between two drugs, non-chance psychic abilities, and so on – hypothesis testing is used to accomplish this
- To estimate the magnitude of these benefits, differences and abilities – confidence interval estimates are used to accomplish this.

Statistical methods are generally not needed:

- If no variability in outcomes is involved; for example, if everyone who took aspirin were prevented from having a heart attack, that fact would be obvious and statistical methods would not be needed
- If a causal explanation is already known, except perhaps to find the magnitude; if there had been an established causal mechanism for how aspirin prevents heart attacks, a statistical study would not have been needed to establish the relationship.

HYPOTHESIS TESTING

In this section a review of the steps taken in hypothesis testing is given, followed by an extended discussion of the aspirin and heart attack example and an example of a distant healing study. There are four steps required to test hypotheses using statistical methods:

Step 1: Determine two competing hypotheses

- *Null hypothesis:* no relationship, no effect, nothing interesting, status quo
- *Alternative hypothesis:* a relationship, ability, etc. exists in the population.

Step 2

Collect data in such a way that *if* the null hypothesis is right, you know approximately what to expect just by chance in the data. For instance, randomly assign people to take aspirin or a placebo. Expect about equal rates of heart attacks in the two groups if aspirin does not work.

Step 3

Using the collected data, find the *P* value by assuming the null hypothesis is true, and then asking how likely we would be to observe sample results as extreme as those seen (or more extreme) under that assumption. For example, suppose the truth (unknown, of course) is that aspirin does not prevent heart attacks. In a study, 11 000 men take aspirin and 11 000 men take a placebo, and the heart attack rate in the aspirin group is half what it is in the placebo group. The P value answers the question: How likely is it that *by chance alone* the one group would have only half (or fewer) as many heart attacks as the other group?

Step 4

Use the P value to make a decision – usually, if the P value is less than 0.05 (1/20), conclude that the alternative hypothesis is indeed true. In other words, rule out chance as an explanation for the unusual results. The rationale is that if there really were no effect, chance alone would be unlikely to have produced the observed results. Therefore there must be an effect.

When the P value is small enough to rule out chance differences as an explanation, and thus to believe the alternative hypothesis, the result is said to be *statistically significant*. Notice that this hypothesis testing method will fail for about 5% of the studies in which the null hypothesis is actually true. For those studies which do result in extreme data just by chance we will erroneously conclude that something beyond chance is responsible for the results when it is not. Unfortunately, there is no way to know when this has happened, which is one reason why replication of studies is so important before making firm conclusions.

Example: Hypothesis Testing for the Physicians' Health Study (Steering Committee of the Physicians' Health Study Research Group 1988)

The participants in this study were 22 071 healthy male physician volunteers. Half of them were randomly assigned to take aspirin, half to take placebo, for 5 years. Here are the four steps for carrying out a hypothesis test to see if aspirin helps prevent heart attacks:

Step 1

- Null hypothesis: risk of heart attack is the same after taking aspirin as after taking placebo
- Alternative hypothesis: risk of heart attack is different after taking aspirin than after taking placebo.

Step 2

The resulting data are shown in Table 17.1.

Based on the data in Table 17.1, the *relative risk* of having a heart attack taking aspirin versus placebo is 9.4/17.1 = 0.55. In other words, the rate of 9.4 heart attacks per 1000 individuals taking aspirin is only 55% of the rate of 17.1 heart attacks per 1000 individuals taking placebo, so the risk is almost halved.

Step 3

Is this likely if the null hypothesis is true? The appropriate statistical procedure in this case is called a chi-square test for homogeneity, the result is a P value of less than 0.00001. In other words, if heart attacks in the population are equally likely taking aspirin and taking a placebo, a relative risk as far from 1.0 (chance) as that observed (0.55) or farther would be observed less than once in every 100 000 studies. Thus, it is unlikely that this is the explanation for the results in this experiment.

Step 4

Conclude that the alternative hypothesis is true. The risk of heart attack is reduced when taking aspirin, at least for all men similar to those in this study.

Example: Distant Healing and AIDS

Sicher et al (1998) conducted a randomized double blind study of the effect of distant healing on advanced AIDS. The participants were 40 volunteers with advanced AIDS, and they were matched into pairs based on age and severity of their illness.

One member of each pair was randomly chosen to receive distant healing for 10 weeks (DH), and

Table 17.1 Results of the physician's health study on aspirin and heart attacks

	Heart attack	No heart attack	Total	Rate per 1000
Aspirin	104	10 933	11 037	9.4
Placebo	189	10 845	11 034	17.1
Total	293	21 778	22 071	13.3

the other member of the pair was assigned to a control group (C). The study was double blind, meaning that neither patients nor their physicians knew who received the healing treatment. Healers were given photographs only and never met the patients. Healers were throughout the United States, self-identified as healers, and were from a variety of healing traditions.

The following results were given in the abstract of the article:

At 6 months, a blind medical chart review found that treatment subjects acquired significantly fewer new AIDS-defining illnesses (0.1 versus 3.6 per patient, p-value = 0.04), had lower illness severity (severity scores 0.8 versus 2.65, p-value = 0.03), and required significantly fewer doctor visits (9.2 versus 13.0, p-value = 0.01), fewer hospitalizations (0.15 versus 0.6, p-value = 0.04), and fewer days of hospitalization (0.5 versus 3.4, p-value = 0.04). Treated subjects also showed significantly improved mood compared with controls (Profile of Mood State score – 26 versus 14, p-value = 0.02). There were no significant differences in CD4+ counts. (Sicher et al 1998, p. 356)

Notice that several separate hypothesis tests were completed. In each case, the null and alternative hypotheses were:

Null hypothesis. In the population of AIDS patients similar to the ones in this study, the mean value of [new AIDS defining illnesses, doctor visits, etc.] would be the same whether or not distant healers were assigned to care for the patients.

Alternative hypothesis. In the population of AIDS patients similar to the ones in this study, the mean value of [new AIDS defining illnesses, doctor visits, etc.] would be better [lower or higher depending on the context] if distant healers were assigned to care for the patients.

Conclusions. When the *P* value < 0.05, reject the null hypothesis and conclude that the alternative hypothesis is true. Notice that this conclusion holds for all of the stated comparisons except CD4+ counts.

The assignment of distant healing appears to have significant value for the population of all such patients, and not just those in this study. One issue that cannot be controlled is that any or all of the patients may have had other distant healers attending to them. Therefore, the results apply to the additional effect of the distant healing assigned by the experimenters to the DH group.

One technical issue. Some statisticians believe that multiple comparisons must be taken into account when assessing *P* values. The idea is that if all null hypotheses are true, by chance alone 0.05 or 1 in 20 will have a small enough *P* value to lead to rejecting the null hypothesis. Therefore, the overall probability of rejecting at least one null hypothesis if they are all true should be controlled, instead of controlling for this separately for each test.

My philosophy about multiple testing is that researchers should report the results of all tests they conduct, with corresponding *P* values. Where possible, confidence intervals (covered in the next section) should be provided as well. Readers can reach their own conclusions about multiple testing. In the study by Sicher et al the results appear to be even more convincing, not less so, because most of the hypotheses tested produced statistically signficant differences between the distant healing and control patients.

HOW CONFIDENCE INTERVALS WORK

Hypothesis tests allow us to reject chance as an explanation for data and to conclude that a relationship between two factors or a difference between two groups exists. However, hypothesis testing does not provide information about the magnitude of the relationship or difference. To estimate the magnitude, confidence intervals are used.

Assume there is an unknown and unmeasurable 'true' value of interest, called a *population parameter*. For example, we assume that there is a true but unknown relative risk of heart attack after taking aspirin compared with placebo for the population of all men similar to those in the study described above.

To compute a confidence interval for a population parameter, collect data for a sample of individuals who are representative of those in the population. Statistical methods have been developed that can then be used to estimate the unknown population parameter, and to create an interval of values that we are fairly confident covers it. It is standard to create a 95% confidence interval. The method used to create such intervals produces a correct interval 95% of the time, meaning that the interval actually captures its target (the population parameter) in 95% of all cases.

Example: Confidence Interval for the Physician's Health Study (Steering Committee of the Physians' Health Study Research Group 1988)

In the aspirin study, the relative risk for the sample of 22 071 men was 0.55. A 95% confidence interval for the relative risk for *all* men like these is 0.42 to 0.67. The heart attack risk when taking aspirin is likely to be between 42% and 67% of the risk when taking placebo. This is further indication that aspirin works, because the interval is not even close to the chance relative risk value of 1.0.

For most studies, both hypothesis testing and confidence intervals are used. Tests provide evidence of whether anything other than chance is at work, and confidence intervals are used to estimate the magnitude of observed effects.

THE POWER OF STATISTICAL TESTS

When designing a statistical study it is crucial to collect enough data to find convincing evidence for a relationship or difference if it truly exists in the population. The probability of finding a significant result when the alternative hypothesis is indeed true is called the *power* of a statistical test. Power depends on the magnitude of the true effect – the larger the effect the more likely that it will be convincingly detected.

Power also depends on the number of participants, which statisticians call the *sample size*. If the sample is too small, even a strong effect will not be convincingly detected. For example, if the aspirin study had used only 2200 participants instead of 22 000 but had still found a difference of the size found, the P value would not have been small enough to conclude that aspirin helped prevent heart attacks.

Example: Power for the Physicians' Health Study (Steering Committee of the Physicians' Health Study Research Group 1988)

Suppose the true population difference in rates of heart attacks when taking aspirin and placebo is the difference observed in the study, i.e. 9.4 heart attacks per 1000 versus 17.1 per 1000. Table 17.2 shows the power for the study based on different possible sample sizes. For example, with 100 participants in each group, the probability of finding a statistically significant reduction in heart attack rates would have only been about 0.19, or 19%. Even with 1000 participants in each group, the probability would only have been about 0.58, or 58%.

Power for Binomial Experiments and Two-Sample t-tests

To further illustrate the importance of taking a large enough sample, consider two common

Table 17.2 Power for possible sample sizes in the aspirin study

Sample size (each group)	100	1000	5000	10 000
Power	0.191	0.582	0.985	0.9999

statistical methods. First, consider a binomial experiment in which each trial (or participant) either succeeds or fails (e.g. lives or dies). Define P = probability of success for each trial or participant. Suppose the null hypothesis is that $P = 0.5$. For instance, an experiment might pair patients and give one a medication and the other a placebo. A *trial* is a pair of patients. A *success* is that the patient taking the medication has better results. By chance, the probability would be 0.5 of that occurring for each pair.

Table 17.3 provides the power for this binomial experiment for a variety of sample sizes, and for possible 'true' success probabilities of 0.52 and 0.60. For example, if there is really a 60% chance that the patient with the medication will do better than the patient with the placebo, and if 30 pairs of participants are used, then the probability is only 0.29 that the study will have a statistically significant result. That means there is a 71% chance that the study will fail to find a benefit for the treatment, despite the fact that in 60% of all possible pairs in the population it would beat the placebo. If the true probability of a 'success' in each trial is only 0.52, the results are much worse. Even with 5000 trials, the probability of rejecting the chance value of $P = 0.50$ is only 0.882.

Table 17.4 presents the power for a two-sample t-test, which is used to compare the means of two populations. Two situations are given for the 'truth' in terms of *effect size*. The effect size measures the difference between the population means of the treatment group and the control group in terms of number of standard deviations for the control group. For example, suppose a study is done to determine whether a medication helps reduce

blood pressure when compared with a placebo. Suppose in truth, on average, the medication reduces blood pressure by a tenth of a standard deviation. Table 17.4 indicates that a study with 30 patients under each condition (medication and placebo) would produce a statistically significant difference in blood pressure with probability of only 0.103. Even with 500 patients in each condition, the probability of detecting a difference would only be 0.474, or under 50%.

In summary, it is important to make sure a study has enough power to detect a relationship or difference if it actually exists. Before going to the expense of conducting a study, researchers should always do a power analysis. There are numerous statistical packages and websites that will calculate power for specified sample sizes and effect sizes. In addition to adequate sample size, it is important to design studies to maximize the relationship or effect that actually does exist. For instance, in distant healing studies it is wise to use patients with serious illnesses because they are most likely to benefit from treatment.

RANDOMIZED EXPERIMENTS AND DESIGN ISSUES

Randomized double blind experiments are the gold standard in medical research because they attempt to control for all factors that might explain a difference in outcomes except the factor being tested. For example, the study by the Physicians' Health Study Research Group divided the participants into similar groups, and treated them in similar ways except for the contents of the pill they took (aspirin or placebo). The

Table 17.3 Power for binomial experiment with 'chance' value of $P = 0.50$

Sample size	30	50	100	500	5000
Power if true $P = 0.52$	0.080	0.086	0.106	0.226	0.882
Power if true P = 0.60	0.29	0.41	0.64	0.998	1.000

Table 17.4 Power for a two-sample t-test

Sample size (each group)	30	50	100	500	5000
Power if effect size = 0.1	0.103	0.125	0.174	0.474	0.9996
Power if effect size = 0.3	0.31	0.44	0.68	0.999	1.000

study by Sicher et al (1998) matched AIDS patients who were similar and treated them in similar ways except that one person in each pair was assigned to receive distant healing and the other was not.

A number of elements are necessary for a well-designed experiment:

Placebos and Control Groups

Depending on the treatment, it is important to include either a placebo group or a control group in an experiment. A control group is a group of participants who are treated in the same way as those receiving the active treatment except that they do not receive an active treatment. For example, in a study designed to measure the effect of magnets to reduce pain, a control group might have pieces of metal of similar size and weight attached to them for the same amount of time. When the treatment is a medication, the control group should receive an identical medication that simply lacks the active ingredient(s) being tested. For instance, in the study by the Physicians Health Study Research Group, the pharmaceutical company that provided the aspirin also provided placebos that looked identical to the aspirin.

Control groups or placebos are important because comparisons can be made between the active treatment and the control, rather than the active treatment and nothing. Effects due to the special attention of being in an experiment, the expectation that a drug will work, and so on, should apply to both groups, so any remaining differences are attributable to the treatment.

Randomization

If possible, treatments (active versus placebo, treated versus control group, etc.) should be randomly assigned to participants. Random assignment is not the same thing as haphazard assignment, and should be done carefully, using computer routines or other methods specifically designed for this purpose. If the experimenters were to decide which participants received which treatment, they could obviously choose the healthier ones to receive the preferred treatment. If all treatments are given to all participants, the order should be randomly assigned. (This may become more of an issue with the ethical debate about using placebos.)

One benefit of random assignment is that it tends to balance out differences such as age, general health and so on, across treatment groups. Sometimes, especially in smaller studies, partial randomization is used but groups are adjusted to be similar in age, gender, etc.

If all treatments are used on all participants, random order is necessary to rule out learning, habituation, preferences, etc. as the cause of differences. For example, in a study to compare two sunscreen lotions, participants may be asked to apply one to each arm. If lotion A was always applied to the right arm and lotion B to the left arm, perhaps lotion A would wear off sooner because the right arm tends to be used more than the left by most people. Frequency of use of the arm would be a confounding variable. Instead, which lotion to apply to which arm should be randomly assigned for each participant.

Matched Pairs, Blocks, Repeated Measures

Matched pairs, blocks and repeated measures are all methods used to match treated and control (or placebo) participants one-for-one on extraneous but important variables such as age, sex, and health. Pairs of similar participants are created, then random assignment is done within each pair. The term 'block' is used when more than two participants are matched, for instance if there are three treatments and they are randomly assigned to triples of similar individuals. The term 'repeated measures' is used when the participants are each given multiple treatments.

Pairs and blocks are often used because, especially in small studies, it is possible that random assignment will leave the treatment groups unequal in terms of important factors such as age and health. Even in larger studies, pairing or blocking reduces extraneous variability and allows for more direct and efficient comparisons.

Blinding (Masking)

Participants, and if possible evaluators, should not be told who is receiving which treatment. 'Double blind' means neither group knows, while 'single blind' means only one group (participants or evaluators) is blind. Blinding helps to avoid self-fulfilling prophecies, expectations, and experimenter effects.

OBSERVATIONAL STUDIES

In observational studies, researchers measure but do not intervene. For example, *USA Today* reported on a study showing that elderly people who regularly prayed and attended church had lower blood pressure than those who did not (Davis 1998). Participants were obviously not randomly assigned to pray and attend church or not, they were simply observed to see whether they did so.

The problem with observational studies is that there are too many possible confounding variables for a cause and effect conclusion to be reached. A confounding variable is one that is related to the treatment and that is likely to have an effect on the outcome. For instance, when taking aspirin, drinking an extra glass of water could be a confounding variable if placebos were not used. Those taking aspirin would consume an extra glass of water each day, and that might help improve their health. In the prayer and blood pressure example, confounding variables are social support, ability to get out on Sundays and go to church (due to good health), possible depression, and so on. For example, people who are in general ill health may stay home on Sundays, and it could be the ill health rather than the lack of church attendance that caused the higher blood pressure.

RESEARCH RESULTS FROM PARAPSYCHOLOGY

In the past few decades the accumulating evidence has been overwhelming for non-chance results in experiments designed to test *anomalous cognition* (see, for example, Bem & Honorton 1994; Radin 1997a; Utts 1991, 1996; Palmer & Broughton 2000). Anomalous cognition is a generic term used in parapsychology for the ability to obtain information that could not have been obtained by normal means. It does not indicate a mechanism, and could be telepathy, clairvoyance, precognition or some other ability that has not yet been suggested. The most common types of studies in anomalous cognition have focused on two methods, called *remote viewing* and *ganzfeld* studies.

There is also accumulating evidence for anomalous interaction between living systems (see Radin 1997a, and sources therein), and for distant healing (see Astin et al 2000). These studies are sometimes called *DMILS* studies, an acronym for distant mental influence on living systems.

Recent successful experiments have also focused on *presentiment*, which is an apparent physiological 'presponse' to a stimulus that occurs *before* the stimulus is presented (see Radin 1997b, Bierman & Radin 1999, Bierman 2000). There is also evidence that the results of some double blind experiments in these areas depend on the experimenter, even though the experimenter should not be able to influence the results (e.g. Wiseman & Schlitz 1997).

Numerous studies have been done on the influence of humans on physical systems (Radin 1997a, Utts 1991). May et al (1995a, 1995b) have used these same studies to propose an alternative explanation. They have shown that humans may have an ability to augment decisions by gaining information from the future about the probable results of making a particular decision. They suggest that this 'decision augmentation' may be used routinely to help people make decisions about what actions to take, including how to know when a favorable sequence is about to be generated by a random number generator.

There are thousands of additional studies that could be cited, and dozens of possible explanations that have been proposed for their results. Given that we do not know what mechanism is operating in these experiments, I will use the generic term mind–matter research in the remainder of this chapter.

The studies quoted, and other mind–matter research studies, indicate that communication may be possible by unknown means, that time may not behave as we have assumed, and that humans may be able to interact with distant living and non-living systems. If these preliminary indications are correct, the assumptions upon which most medical (and other) research is based may not be accurate.

RETHINKING TRADITIONAL ASSUMPTIONS

Traditional design and analyses of medical studies are based on the following assumptions, all of which are in question based on the recent studies discussed in the previous section:

- The causal arrow of time is past → present → future
- Interactions/agreements between individuals are not possible without known means of communication
- Physical influence of individuals on living systems (or non-living systems) is only possible with direct physical contact
- The physical world (non-biological) stays constant, at least in a short timeframe.

If these assumptions are indeed erroneous, the implications for past and future medical research are enormous. Both the design and the analysis phases of experiments would need to be revised to accomodate the implications of a world that behaves differently from what has been previously assumed.

CHALLENGES IN THE DESIGN PHASE

Challenges to Randomization, Control Groups and Placebos

There are numerous challenges to the efficacy of random assignment to treatments and controls that emerge from the combined results of the mind–matter research:

1. Some participants may know when to sign up to get the desired treatment, based on information gained through anomalous means.
2. Experimenters may be able to influence the randomization device.

3. Randomization requires decisions by the experimenter, such as what computer program to use and when to activate it, and 'decision augmentation' could be used to help the experimenter make advantagous random assignments.
4. It is well-established that participants try to please experimenters. Experimenters could envision the desired outcome and communicate it to the participants, who in turn respond differently based on which treatment they are receiving.
5. Experimenters could directly influence the biology of participants, differently for different treatments.
6. In repeated measures, the order of outcomes could influence the order of random assignment (future outcome → past randomization).

Challenges to Double Blind

It may be impossible to conduct single or double blind experiments, based on the results of mind–matter research. For example:

1. Feedback about who received which treatment is eventually given, or results published. It could be that the future knowledge of who got which treatment affects past performance.
2. Information about who had which treatment is known by someone, even if coded (similar to coordinate remote viewing), so could be transmitted to participants or evaluators. For example, someone had to provide the aspirin or placebo tablets to the physicians.
3. Depending on the treatments, participants could 'know' which treatment they had, and communicate this information to the evaluator.
4. In single blind studies, either the participant or the evaluator already knows what treatment each participant has, and could communicate it to the other party.

CHALLENGES IN THE ANALYSIS PHASE

Two basic assumptions accompany almost all procedures for hypothesis testing and confidence intervals:

1. Observations are independent across participants. In other words, results for participants are uncorrelated with each other.
2. Each participant is considered to be representative of a larger population with a fixed mean, fixed variability, and so on. Generally it is the mean and not the variability that is compared for different treatments.

Challenges To Assumptions Commonly Used In Analyzing Experiments

Based on the mind–matter research results, the statistical models generally employed may be much too simplistic. For example:

1. Interconnected participants do not allow for independent observations. Perhaps a 'group mind' cooperation makes an entire experiment succeed or fail.
2. 'Reality' may not be fixed in time. Perhaps aspirin worked in the 1990s to prevent heart attacks, but a 'group habituation' lessens the effect over time.
3. The interesting effects may be in the change (variability) and patterns, and not in the mean. In that case, different questions need to be asked. For example, recent research has suggested that the position of the earth, measured by local sidereal time, may influence the amount of 'noise' in experimental results (Spottiswoode 1997).

CONCLUSIONS AND SUGGESTIONS FOR RESEARCH DESIGN

The results of the mind–matter research provide challenges to the methods currently used in medical research. In general, the challenges fall into three broad categories:

1. It may be impossible to hide information (no 'blind' experiments).
2. It may be impossible to randomly assign participants to treatment conditions.
3. It may be impossible to separate individual influences, such as the influence of the healer versus the desire of patients to be in the treated group, leading to decision to enter study at just the right time.

Challenges also present opportunities. The following recommendations are particularly relevant for studies to test distant healing and intentionality. Some of the recommendations are based on ordinary statistical principles, and some are the steps that the mind-matter research suggests can enhance the results of experiments:

- If 'decision augmentation' works, it is better to randomize at multiple decision points, to increase the chances that the random assignments will result in favorable outcomes.
- If experimenters can convey desired results, motivate everyone involved in the experiment to expect a positive outcome.
- Do not design experiments with small effect sizes and low power by adding a treatment that can only have a small incremental effect. For example, for studies of the efficacy of prayer, do not choose participants who are already part of a supportive religious community in which they probably already receive such attention.
- Based on past results of distant healing studies, the patients with the most severe illness tend to improve the most. For this and for ethical reasons, if distant healing works it is wise to use serious illnesses to test its efficacy.
- Design experiments in ways that will allow possible causes to be separated. For example, assign unmotivated participants as 'healers' as a control condition. (For ethical reasons, all patients could be treated by both these and motivated healers, in random order.)

More complex statistical models may be needed to accomodate new assumptions. Current assumptions of independence and fixed constants (such as relative risk, probability of a successful outcome, etc.) may need to be revised. For instance, in remote viewing and similar studies it is difficult to tell the difference between a fixed probability of success on each trial, and a perfect chance of success on certain trials, but only chance on other trials. New designs, models, and methods of analysis could help distinguish different possible mechanisms. As an example, see May et al (1995a, 1995b) for methods to distinguish between decision augmentation and remote influence in experiments designed to test remote influence.

A Final Note: Aspririn or Anomaly?

It may seem that the results of mind–matter research are so small that they make no difference, but in fact the effect sizes in some experimental paradigms are much larger than the effect size found in the study by the Physicians' Health Study Research Group, the study that has led millions of people to take aspirin to prevent heart attacks.

Ganzfeld studies, for example, have consistently shown that people can choose the correct answer about 33% of the time when presented with four choices, one of which was randomly selected as the correct answer (Utts 1991, Bem & Honorton 1994, Bem et al 2001). By chance, the correct answer should be selected about 25% of the time. In the Physicians' Health Study, the proportion of participants who had heart attacks after taking placebo and aspirin were respectively, 0.009423 and 0.017129.

The appropriate effect size measure for comparing two sample proportions p and q, or one sample proportion p to a fixed proportion q, is Cohen's h (Cohen 1988, p. 181):

$$h = 2 \times |\arcsin \sqrt{p} - \arcsin \sqrt{q}|$$

Cohen's h for the Physicians' Health Study is 0.0681, whereas Cohen's h for the ganzfeld studies, comparing a success rate of 0.33 to a chance rate of 0.25, is 0.1767. Therefore, the ganzfeld effect size is more than two and a half times the size of the effect that has led millions to take aspirin daily.

It may be argued that even one life saved by taking aspirin is important, whereas the mind–matter research is simply demonstrating an interesting anomaly. But the point made in this paper is that there are numerous mechanisms through which the results demonstrated by mind–matter research could be affecting medical studies. If the mind–matter effect size is large compared to the effects found in some medical studies, how can we rule out the idea that those effects are completely, or at least substantially, due to anomalies shown to exist in mind–matter research? For this reason, it is imperative that future research be directed toward understanding the mechanisms for the anomalies that have clearly been demonstrated in mind–matter research.

REFERENCES

Astin J A, Harkness E, Ernst E 2000 The efficacy of 'distant healing': a systematic review of randomized trials. Annals of Internal Medicine 132(11): 903–910

Bem D J, Honorton C 1994 Does psi exist? Replicable evidence for an anomalous process of information transfer. Psychological Bulletin 115: 4–18

Bem D J, Palmer J, Broughton R S 2001 Updating the ganzfeld database: a victim of its own success? Journal of Parapsychology 65: 207–218

Bierman D J 2000 Anomalous baseline effects in mainstream emotion research using psychophysiological variables. Proceedings of the Parapsychological Association 43rd Annual Convention. Parapsychological Association, Durham, NC, pp. 34–47

Bierman D J, Radin D I 1999 Anomalous unconscious emotional responses: evidence for a reversal of the arrow of time. In: Hameroff S R, Kaszniak A W, Chalmers D J (eds) Tuscon III: towards a science of consciousness. MIT Press, Cambridge

Cohen J 1988 Statistical power analysis for the behavioral sciences, 2nd edn. Lawrence Erlbaum Associates, Hillsdale, NJ

Davis R 1998 Prayer can lower blood pressure. USA Today August 11, 1998: 1D

May E C, Utts J M, Spottiswoode S J P 1995a Decision augmentation theory: toward a model of anomalous mental phenomena. Journal of Parapsychology 59(3): 195–220

May E C, Utts J M, Spottiswoode S J P, James C J 1995b Applications of decision augmentation theory. Journal of Parapsychology 59(3): 221–250

Palmer J, Broughton R S 2000 An updated meta-analysis of post-PRL ESP-ganzfeld experiments: the effect of standardness. Proceedings of the Parapsychological Association 43rd Annual Convention. Parapsychological Association, Durham, NC, pp. 224–240

Radin D 1997a The conscious universe: the scientific truth of psychic phenomena. HarperCollins, San Francisco

Radin D 1997b Unconscious perception of future emotion: an experiment in presentiment. Journal of Scientific Exploration 11(2): 163–180

Sicher F, Targ E, Moore 2nd D, Smith H S 1998 A randomized double blind study of the effect of distant healing in a population with advanced AIDS. Western Journal of Medicine 169: 356–363

Spottiswoode S J P 1997 Apparent association between effect size in anomalous cognition experiments and local sidereal time. Journal of Scientific Exploration 11(2): 109–122

Steering Committee of the Physicians' Health Study Research Group 1988 Preliminary report: findings from the aspirin component of the ongoing Physicians' Health Study. New England Journal of Medicine 318(4): 262–264

Utts J M 1991 Replication and meta-analysis in parapsychology (with discussion). Statistical Science 6(4): 363–403

Utts J M 1996 An assessment of the evidence for psychic functioning. Journal of Scientific Exploration 10(1): 3–30 [reprinted in Journal of Parapsychology 59: 289–320]

Wiseman R, Schlitz M 1997 Experimenter effects and the remote detection of staring. Journal of Parapsychology 61: 197–201

18

Randomized clinical trials

Jeffery A Dusek, Jane Sherwood

This chapter summarizes the goals of research design in randomized clinical trials of prayer and healing and current unresolved issues that arise in designing and executing such studies, including conducting multisite investigations.

Randomized clinical trials (RCTs) are considered the gold standard for determining if a treatment works and is safe and effective. As discussed in the previous chapters in this book, considerable preliminary work using other methods is needed before a properly conducted RCT can be constructed. Premature execution of an RCT risks presenting irrelevant or misleading evidence. Once prepared, conduct of a RCT is a complex task, especially in multisite studies, in order to assure that proper quality control is maintained. **WBJ**

INTRODUCTION

This chapter focuses on the practical issues associated with the design and conduct of double blind randomized controlled trials (RCTs) in evaluating the possible benefits of an intercessory prayer (IP) intervention. The purpose of this chapter is not to completely review the procedures required for conducting a standard RCT of pharmaceutical interventions – others have already done so (Friedman et al 1998). Rather, the goals of this chapter are to highlight the similarities and differences between RCTs of pharmaceutical interventions and RCTs of IP, identify the specific challenges that occur during the design of an IP clinical trial, as well as to review procedures necessary for the implementation of a multicenter RCT of IP. The chapter is organized chronologically with trial design specifics addressed prior to issues of trial implementation.

CURRENT STATUS OF IP RESEARCH

Research into the possible beneficial effects of IP in medical populations is a relatively new phenomenon in modern American medicine. Recently, several independent investigations have demonstrated beneficial effects of IP (or distant healing) in cardiac coronary care unit (CCU) (Byrd 1988, Harris et al 1999), AIDS (Sicher et al 1998), and infertile (Cha et al 2001) patient populations. However, others report no effect in chronic illness (Joyce & Whelldon 1965), leukemic children (Collipp 1969), psychological well-being (O'Laire 1997), major depression (Greyson 1997), rheumatoid arthritis (Matthews et al 2000), chronic pain (Abbot et al 2001), kidney dialysis (Matthews et al 2001), and cardiac (Krucoff et al 2001), and cardiac CCU patients (Aviles et al 2001). Importantly, two studies display negative effects of IP with increased alcohol abuse in chronic alcoholics (Walker et al 1997), and on the size and number of warts in a sample of healthy volunteers (Harkness et al 2000). Finally, results from an un-blinded study, in which participants were aware whether they were receiving distant healing or not, show improvement on health in a heterogeneous group of chronic illness patients (Wiesendanger et al 2001).

Physicians, statisticians as well as clergy have questioned the variable quality and specific methods used in these published single institution RCTs (Goldstein 2000, Hamm 2000, Hammerschmidt 2000, Hoover & Margolich 2000, Karis & Karis 2000, Pande 2000, Price 2000, Sandweiss 2000, Sloan & Bagiella 2000, Smith & Fisher 2000, Van der Does 2000, Waterhouse 2000). Still others question the ethical limitations or relevance of conducting such clinical trials at all (Cohen et al 2000, Halperin 2001). Although the reports of positive results are intriguing, the failure to make *a priori* decisions identifying a single primary end-point as well as statistical irregularities have severely limited the medical and scientific communities' acceptance of the reported beneficial effects of IP.

As systematically reviewed by three independent groups (Abbot 2000, Astin et al 2000, Roberts & Ahmed 2000), the published data from completed IP trials are equivocal. Nevertheless, all three reviews conclude that the overall positive trend justifies further investigation using established clinical trial methodology. Thus, as traditional medical practitioners and the American public become increasingly interested in the results of studies exploring the efficacy of IP, this additional scrutiny necessitates the careful planning, implementation, and conduct of RCTs evaluating the effects of IP.

It should be stated from the outset that, in our opinion, RCTs of IP are not designed to put God to the test. Nor are they able to determine whether God exists, whether God does or does not respond to IP, whether it is possible to evaluate the presence of God in a controlled clinical trial, or whether God would withhold treatment from any study group. Rather, we believe that well-designed and carefully implemented RCTs of IP can be used to examine the possible effects of a clearly defined IP intervention on a predefined end-point in a restricted patient population.

STUDY DESIGN

Study Personnel

Prior to evaluating the effects of any intervention (including IP) on the outcome after illness, study investigators need to establish a study protocol that includes: a specific objective and hypothesis; a validated and clearly defined primary end-point; a defined and described intervention; strict eligibility criteria; an appropriate informed consent process; a valid randomization process; procedures to preserve masking; valid sample size calculation; procedures to ensure and evaluate the accuracy of administration of study therapy; and a predefined statistical plan employing an intent-to-treat analysis. The study protocol serves as a guide for study personnel and establishes the procedures to be used in the trial.

The success of any RCT is based on having qualified and experienced individuals involved in the study. Requirements for a multicenter clinical trial include collaboration and cooperation between investigators at participating hospital centers, a data coordinating center (DCC), and the steering committee. Motivated and interactive principal investigators are necessary to supervise patient recruitment at each hospital center; the DCC develops the manual of operations and monitors data collection and management, whereas the steering committee oversees conduct of the entire trial. Ideally, the steering committee should be multidisciplinary and include at a minimum an established principal investigator, clinical trialists, co-investigators experienced with the chosen patient population, and a bio-statistician as well as a representative of the DCC. While assembling a multidisciplinary team may seem unwieldy, the heterogeneous makeup of the steering committee ensures inclusion of unique perspectives and allows diverse viewpoints to aid in the development of the study protocol and oversight of the trial.

Primary End-point

Regardless of the studied intervention (pharmaceutical or IP), selection of a clinically relevant and biologically plausible primary end-point should be required for an RCT. Ideally the choice of the end-point would be supported by the collection of preliminary data, but at very least must be validated prior to the start of the trial. The merits of choosing a single end-point are discussed below. To limit the effects of patient or investigator expectation, it is suggested that the end-point be objectively determined by review of clinical data or medical records and not based on subjective patient or investigator reports. As will be indicted in the blinding section below, all end-point data should be collected by study personnel blinded to the patient's treatment allocation.

The typical pharmaceutical RCT purports to examine the efficacy of a treatment (acting through specific mechanisms) on a 'biologically relevant' outcome in a particular patient population. One major difference between pharmaceutical and IP trials is that in the latter there is no empirical evidence identifying a precise mechanism, biologically plausible outcome, or even the

appropriate patient population. Thus, it is very difficult (some would say impossible) to select the proper outcome to measure without a known mechanism or considerable preliminary data to indicate what the specific effect may be. This lack of specificity has been especially problematic in IP research and has probably added to the inconsistency in published results.

Nevertheless, although selection of a biologically plausible end-point is currently impossible in an IP trial, it is possible to investigate the effect of IP on an outcome that is widely accepted to be clinically important in a specific study population.

Statistical Analysis

Design of any RCT requires development of a statistical analysis plan, including statement of hypothesis, projection of probable effect size, sample size calculation, choice of primary end-point, and statistical tests. Since there is limited information on mechanisms underlying the possible effects of IP, data from smaller pilot studies can assist investigators in hypothesis generation and provide expected effect size for the larger RCT. Additionally, data from either pilot studies or the published literature may be used as the basis for a realistic sample size calculation. Importantly, studies that do not enroll enough patients to detect differences between treatment arms are statistically 'underpowered'. Underpowered trials risk incorrectly accepting the null hypothesis (that there is no beneficial effect of an intervention) when a difference does exist (type II error). In addition to limiting the pursuit of an effective intervention, results from underpowered studies may hamper progress in promising areas of research.

Unless there is compelling evidence necessitating the inclusion of multiple end-points, use of a single, primary end-point is suggested for two reasons. First, the comparison of multiple end-points without correction to the overall P value, which has been used in previous IP trials, increases the risk of rejecting the null hypothesis (that there is no benefit of an intervention) when a difference does not exist (type I error). Second, appropriate correction for multiple comparisons reduces the likelihood that significance would be achieved for a given end-point. For example, if an investigator were to compare outcome on 20 different end-points, use of the Bonferonni technique (O'Brien 1984) would reduce the standard *P* value of 0.05 to 0.0025 (*P* value/number of outcomes or 0.05/20). Finally, well-designed clinical trials should also include a predefined analysis plan with a contingency for patients lost to follow-up, patient withdrawal as well as those who do not undergo the studied procedure. Use of intent-to-treat analysis is standard in well-designed pharmaceutical trials and must be employed in IP trials.

IP as a Clinical Intervention

There are numerous challenges to the use of IP as a clinical intervention in RCTs. First, although the majority of IP studies have not included a clear description of the IP intervention, it is vital to clearly define the intervention that is being tested. Some report the number of minutes intercessors provide the intervention (e.g. 30 minutes a week for 6 weeks), whereas others provide the number of days intercessors prayed for a given patient (e.g. 30 days). Other factors to be clarified are the onset and offset of IP. Is it necessary that the IP be initiated prior to the start of a medical procedure or can IP be initiated after the procedure has started? Does the length of IP vary according to when the patient may be discharged from the hospital or is a standard 'dose' provided to all patients regardless of their particular pattern of recovery? Is there a critical mass of necessary intercessors or is one intercessor enough? Other issues include the length (10 minutes *vs.* 1 hour) and frequency of IP administration (once a day *vs.* once a week), the merits of providing follow-up dosing and contingencies for providing IP when a procedure has been delayed by several hours or days. The lack of a clearly defined intervention has limited the generalizability of previous results because of non-uniformity of the IP intervention.

Second, the ideal amount and duration ('dose') of IP that should be provided is unknown because of the lack of biologic basis for the effect of IP. In pharmaceutical RCTs, patients are provided with a specific dose of an intervention for a specified length of time. Because the quality of the pharmaceutical is reliable (for the most part), these trials can examine whether larger doses are more efficacious or establish a dose–response curve. Is a dose of IP an accurate analogy or a reasonable assumption? It is clear that in each RCT the number of prayers (five intercessors) can provide IP for a given length of time (1 minute every day for 6 weeks). However, does the difficult (some would say impossible) task of quantifying the quality of the IP preclude the provision of IP as a dose? Perhaps not, for if the quality of the IP providers can be established by selecting experienced, committed, professional intercessors, the notion of dose may not be inconceivable.

Third, although few will disagree that RCTs of IP should use clearly defined intervention that matches the primary end-point, doing so can be challenging. As part of defining the studied IP, does the investigator allow intercessors to employ their usual methods of prayer or does she or he constrain intercessors by developing a specific prayer intervention for the study? Either choice is valid, but there are limitations to both choices. The limitation of allowing intercessors to use their usual methods of prayer is that the intervention may not be relevant to the primary end-point. For example, if the primary end-point is the patient's perception of pain after a medical procedure, prayers for 'acceptance of God's will' do not appear related to the end-point. For a typical clinical trial, patient mortality is classified as a negative event. However if the focus of IP was for 'Thy will be done,' death may be deemed 'Thy will' by some individuals, but unlikely to be defined as a success by the medical investigators.

Fourth, IP provided in a clinical trial may be different from IP usually provided by the intercessors, limiting generalizability of the results. Are there limitations to 'sterilizing' or reducing prayer to a single component, as opposed to the richness of the usual prayers employed by intercessors? Rather than limiting the intercessors to a study-directed prayer, one solution may be for the investigators to simply add a specific intention to the usual methods of the intercessors. In so doing, the duration and content of the intervention can be clearly defined without changing the established methods of the intercessors. Even with this consideration, the question remains that there might be reduced effectiveness of IP when strangers (rather than family and friends) pray for a patient.

Fifth, since it is impossible to attempt to limit prayer provided by family, friends, and others, a study of IP could only evaluate the effects of *additional* IP, not the effects of prayer in general. Because examining the effects of all prayer is not possible, investigators must distinguish between the study intervention or additional intercessory prayer offered by intercessors with non-study prayer, which is offered by the patient, family, friends, or others. Of course it would be unthinkable, not to mention impossible, to attempt to limit these non-study prayers. Thus, although the exact extent of the non-study prayer may never be obtained, it is important to ascertain from the patient their knowledge of such non-study IP to ensure that there are no differences in the amount of non-study being provided to the groups.

Finally, there must be established methods for the investigators to conduct quality assurance checks of the IP intervention. It would be an inconceivable to attempt to quantify the quality of an individual intercessor's prayers, but ensuring that the intervention was provided as directed in the study protocol is possible. As part of the quality assurance process as well as to retain blinding of hospital centers, in a multicenter trial the DCC may serve to relay information between hospital centers and the IP groups. To ensure adequate administration of the IP intervention, a clear method of contact (fax, telephone, and e-mail) with backup procedures should be in place before the start of the trial. Regardless of the specifics chosen, an established mechanism to document the IP intervention (e.g. use of prayer logs) must be included in IP trials to clearly document the extent of the intervention.

Data and Safety Monitoring

Because previous studies have not reported serious negative effects associated with IP, some might consider participation in a study of IP to be risk-free. However, by convening an independent data and safety monitoring board (DSMB) to review the clinical trial, the investigator establishes safeguards and protection for patients as well as a mechanism for independent review of the on-going trial. Typically, a DSMB is provided with results from interim analyses and makes recommendations to study investigators. For example, if study intervention were found to result in a higher event rate, a DSMB would probably recommend early termination of the study. Likewise if an intervention proved significantly more effacacious, then a DSMB may recommend early termination so that all patients would have access to the successful intervention. The advantage for the investigators is these recommendations are offered while the study is active and the investigators are still blinded. DSMB recommendations may provide valuable insight and even allow for important adjustments to the study of an IP intervention.

STUDY IMPLEMENTATION
Patient Recruitment

For any RCT it is vitally important to follow the guidelines of each participating institution's institutional review board in the identification and recruitment of patients into the study. Typically, hospitals require that each patient's primary care physician or the nurse caring for the patient provide permission before study personnel are allowed to approach a patient. Especially with the enrollment of aged patients, this process is thought to ensure that the patient is physically and mentally stable and able to provide informed consent. Additionally, the nurse caring for the patient can provide the researcher with pertinent information about the person's health concerns and support system.

When approaching eligible patients in hospital, it is necessary for the researcher to clearly explain the study as well as the requirements expected of each participant. Although many eligible patients will be interested in participating in an IP trial, recruiting patients for any study is challenging. Reasons for not participating in an IP trial may include: no interest in participating in any research study; no interest in prayer research, anxiety about being assigned to a non-prayer group; anxious, tired, stressed out by their illness and hospitalization; or would rather spend time with family or friends. As is the case with any trial, it is important to record the number of patients who accept or refuse to participate in the study – some studies even collect demographic information about eligible individuals who refuse to participate in a patient registry. In order to generalize the study results from the study sample to the larger population, specific information of patients enrolled in the trial is necessary.

Unlike a pharmaceutical RCT, many patients may not expect to be approached for participation in a clinical trial of IP. As such, it is necessary for study personnel to separate their personal religious beliefs and convictions from their role in the trial. By checking their personal religious and spiritual beliefs at the door study personnel limit the unconscious and conscious bias of their beliefs on the design and implementation of the study as well as on the recruitment of subjects and collection of study data.

Informed Consent

Eligible patients obtain information about a clinical trial from the study investigator as well as from a written consent form. The process of obtaining informed consent for an individual to participate in any clinical trial is extremely important. Along with informing patients about the study requirements, it is necessary to notify patients of the possible benefits and risks of the intervention from participating in the trial. Individuals must be fully informed that while their medical records may be reviewed for research purposes (depending on the trial), their confidentiality will be respected. Recently, two studies of IP were conducted without informing the patients that they were participants in the study (Cha et al 2001, Harris et al 1999). Although each investigator's IRB had reviewed the protocol and approved the study, neither written nor verbal informed consent was obtained from any of the research subjects. The lack of any informed consent raised ethical concerns in the medical community (Goldstein 2000).

Theoretically, it is possible that there is a scientific advantage to not obtaining informed consent (Cha et al 2001, Harris et al 1999). These investigators contend that by not obtaining informed consent, or even letting a subject know they are participants in a clinical trial, it is likely that all eligible patients will be involved in the study and thus limit study sample bias. The notion is that limiting study sample bias can lead to increased generalizability of the results. In addition, if subjects are not aware of their involvement in a research study of IP, they may experience less anxiety from study participation. Finally, because family and friends are unaware of the IP study, they may be less likely to pray for the subject and consequently limit the amount of non-study prayer.

Nevertheless, there are many ethical limitations for failing to obtain informed consent. First, although no studies have reported adverse events associated with IP, there still may be risks associated with the intervention. Second, it is a common occurrence in clinical trials for study personnel to review medical records for adverse events or when determining the incidence of the primary end-point (such as complications after a medical procedure). Clinical review of the patient's medical record does not compromise confidentiality, whereas unauthorized reviews for research purposes may. Third, in accordance with ever-increasing scientific standards, obtaining written informed consent may be necessary for IRB approval, for obtaining Federal funding and for publication in most medical journals (Belmont Report 1979). Fourth, by providing informed consent and actively participating in the study process, the patient has the satisfaction of knowing she or he has made a contribution to scientific knowledge about the effects of IP on health outcomes. Finally, the process of obtaining informed consent ensures that each patient's autonomy is fully protected throughout the process of his or her study involvement.

Randomization/Masking

Issues of randomization and masking are critical to all RCTs. Correct and appropriate use of randomization techniques removes potential bias in allocation of subjects to study groups. Specifically, use of a random number generator when developing a randomization table makes it is virtually impossible for any patient, investigator, or statistician accurately to predict to which group a given subject has been randomized. Use of unsophisticated randomization techniques may seriously limit the scientific acceptance of study results and potentially unmask study personnel as to the assignment of specific patients.

The double blind study is the gold standard of clinical trials (Friedman et al 1998). In a double blind clinical trial examining efficacy of pharmaceutical medication both the patient and the investigator following the patient's outcome are blinded to the patient's group assignment (Friedman et al 1998). Thus even though the investigator (or hospital pharmacy) provides the active intervention or placebo pill, the patient's treatment is unknown to patient and investigator. In addition, individuals collecting data from medical records and statisticians conducting the analyses remain blinded to a patient's treatment condition.

Although not uniform, it is common in many clinical trials of IP for the patient, study investigator, data collector, and statistician to be blinded to treatment, but for the intercessors providing IP to be informed of the names of patients randomized to receiving IP. In terms of definition, this type of trial still qualifies as a double blind RCT. However, because the intercessors are unblinded to patients' group assignment, it is vital for intercessors to have no contact with the hospital center personnel who are blinded to assignment. To retain masking, in a multicenter trial the DCC may serve as an intermediary between IP groups and hospital centers.

Another difference between a study of pharmaceuticals and a study of IP is that an IP intervention may be provided without the patient's awareness. As opposed to physically taking an active or placebo pill, participants in IP studies are provided with an unseen intervention. Although patient compliance in the trial is established, the disbursement of the intervention by the prayer groups must be monitored. Another important difference is that in the IP trial non-study intervention may be provided (by friends, family, church members) without the investigators' or subjects' awareness. Thus, as it would be impossible to test the effects of 'all' aspirin that a patient may take as part of their participation in a pharmaceutical trial, it is virtually impossible to test the efficacy of a consistent 'dose' of all IP (that which is provided as part of the study and that which is not) in the IP RCT. Rather, investigators are testing the efficacy of a dose of *additional* IP from study intercessors. Assessing patient awareness of non-study prayer during the trial (e.g. before and after the procedure) can provide the patients' perception of awareness of presence or absence of non-study IP.

CONCLUSIONS

As described in this chapter, there are numerous challenges to the design and conduct of a study of IP, as well as limitations to study conclusions. First, since there is no accepted scientific basis for the effect of IP, it is difficult to select a biologically plausible end-point for use in a clinical trial. Second, the timing, amount, and duration that IP should be provided are unknown because of the lack of biologic basis for the effect of IP. Third, since it is impossible to attempt to limit prayer provided by family, friends, and others, a study of IP can only evaluate the effects of additional IP, not the effects of prayer in general. Similarly, the intervention can only be described as the prayer provided by the intercessors, not as an effect or result of communicating with God. Fourth, the need to precisely document how and when the study IP is administered may result in changes from the intercessors' usual practice. IP provided in a clinical trial may be different from

IP usually provided by the intercessors, limiting generalizability of the results. Finally, IP trials are not designed to determine whether God exists, whether God does or does not respond to IP, whether it is possible to evaluate the presence of God in a controlled clinical trial, whether God would withhold treatment from any study group, or to put God to the test. IP trials focus only on the effects of additional IP on outcomes after a medical procedure or illness, not on the effects of any type of prayer. Based on these challenges to study design and implementation, it is not surprising that previous studies of IP are controversial. Additional well-designed and appropriately implemented clinical trials of IP are needed and may serve to limit the current controversy.

REFERENCES

Abbot N C 2000 Healing as a therapy for human disease: a systematic review. Journal of Alternative and Complementary Medicine 6: 159–169

Abbot N C, Harkness E F, Stevinson C, Marshall F P, Conn D A, Ernst E 2001 Spiritual healing as a therapy for chronic pain: a randomized, clinical trial. Pain 91: 79–89

Astin J A, Harkness E, Ernst E 2000 The efficacy of 'distant healing': a systematic review of randomized trials. Annals of Internal Medicine 132: 903–910

Aviles J M, Whelan S E, Hernke D A et al 2001 Intercessory prayer and cardiovascular disease progression in a coronary care unit population: a randomized controlled trial. Mayo Clinic Proceedings 76: 1192–1198

Belmont Report 1979 Ethical principles and guidelines for the protection of human subjects of research. Report of the National Commission for the Protection of Human Subjects of Biomedical and Behavioral Research. Accessed from the website of the Office for Human Right Protections/US Department of Health and Human Services http://ohrp.osophs.dhhs.gov/humansubjects/guidance/belmont.htm [accessed May 26, 2002]

Byrd R C 1988 Positive therapeutic effects of intercessory prayer in a coronary care unit population. Southern Medical Journal 81: 826–829

Cha K Y, Wirth D P, Lobo R A 2001 Does prayer influence the success of in vitro fertilization–embryo transfer: report of a masked, randomized trial. Journal of Reproductive Medicine 46: 781–787

Cohen C B, Wheeler S E, Scott D A, Edwards B S, Lusk P 2000 Prayer as therapy: a challenge to both religious belief and professional ethics. Anglican Working Group in Bioethics. Hastings Center Report 30: 40–47

Collipp P J 1969 The efficacy of prayer: a triple-blind study. Medical Times 987: 201–204

Friedman L M, Furberg C D, DeMets D L 1998 Fundamentals of clinical trials, 3rd edn. Springer-Verlag, New York

Goldstein J 2000 Waiving informed consent for research on spiritual matters. Archives of Internal Medicine 160: 1870–1871

Greyson B 1997 Distance healing of patients with major depression. Journal of Scientific Exploration 10: 447–465

Halperin E C 2001 Should academic medical centers conduct clinical trials of the efficacy of intercessory prayer? Academic Medicine 6: 791–797

Hamm R M 2000 No effect of intercessory prayer has been proven. Archives of Internal Medicine 160: 1872–1873

Hammerschmidt D E 2000 Ethical and practical problems in studying prayer. Archives of Internal Medicine 160: 1874

Harkness E F, Abbot N C, Ernst E 2000 No beneficial effects on warts from distant healing. American Journal of Medicine 108: 448–452

Harris W S, Gowda M, Kolb J W et al 1999 A randomized, controlled trial of the effects of remote intercessory prayer on outcomes in patients to the coronary care unit. Archives of Internal Medicine 159: 2273–2278

Hoover D R, Margolich J B 2000 Questions on the design and findings of a randomized, controlled trial of the effects of remote, intercessory prayer on outcomes in patients admitted to the coronary care unit. Archives of Internal Medicine 160: 1875–1876

Joyce C R B, Whelldon R M C 1965 The efficacy of prayer: a double-blind clinical trial. Journal of Chronic Disease 18: 367–377

Karis R, Karis D 2000 Intercessory prayer. Archives of Internal Medicine 160: 1870

Krucoff M W, Crater S W, Green C L et al 2001 Integrative noetic therapies as adjuncts to percutaneous intervention during unstable coronary syndromes: monitoring and actualization of noetic training (MANTRA) feasibility pilot. American Heart Journal 142(5): 760–769

Matthews D A, Marlowe S M, MacNutt F S 2000 Effects of intercessory prayer on patients with rheumatoid arthritis. Southern Medical Journal 93: 1177–1186

Matthews W J, Conti J M, Sireci S G 2001 The effects of intercessory prayer, positive visualization, and expectancy on the well-being of kidney dialysis patients. Alternative Therapies in Health and Medicine 7: 42–52

O'Brien P C 1984 Procedures for comparing samples with multiple end-points in clinical trials. Biometrics 40: 1079–87

O'Laoire S 1997 An experimental study of the effects of distant, intercessory prayer on self-esteem, anxiety, and depression. Alternative Therapies in Health and Medicine 3: 38–53

Pande P N 2000 Does prayer need testing? Archives of Internal Medicine 160: 1873–1874

Price J M 2000 Does prayer really set one apart? Archives of Internal Medicine 160: 1873

Roberts L, Ahmed I, Hall S 2000 Intercessory prayer for the alleviation of ill health. Cochrane Database Systemic Review 2: CD000368

Sandweiss D A 2000 P value out of control. Archives of Internal Medicine 160: 1872

Sicher F, Targ E, Moore D, Smith H 1998 A randomized double-blind study of the effect of distant healing in a population with advanced AIDS: report of a small scale study. Western Journal of Medicine 169: 356–363

Sloan R P, Bagiella E 2000 Data without a prayer. Archives of Internal Medicine 160: 1870

Smith J G, Fisher R 2000 The effect of remote intercessory prayer on clinical outcomes. Archives of Internal Medicine 160: 1876

Van der Does W 2000 A randomized, controlled trial of prayer. Archives of Internal Medicine 160: 1871–1872

Walker S R, Ronigan J S, Miller W R, Corner S, Kahlich L 1997 Intercessory prayer in the treatment of alcohol abuse and dependence: a pilot investigation. Alternative Therapies in Health and Medicine 3: 79–86

Waterhouse W C 2000 Is it prayer, or is it parity? Archives of Internal Medicine 160: 1875

Wiesendanger H, Werthmuller L, Reuter K, Walach H 2001 Chronically ill patients treated by spiritual healing improve in quality of life: results of a randomized waiting-list controlled study. Journal of Alternative and Complementary Medicine 7: 45–51

19

Outcomes research: costs and quality of life

Harald Walach

This chapter summarizes the goals, rationale and requirements for conducting longitudinal, observational trials of healing and the assessment of its impact on costs and quality of life.

Controlled trials, while needed to test assumptions about treatment effects, are not the real world of clinical practice. Even treatments proven safe and effective in clinical trials may not have significant impact when used in regular practice. For this reason, studies of clinical interventions, including those involving mental and spiritual healing, must be assessed in actual practice. This is done with observational and outcomes research that document the impact.

Outcomes research also has a role before initiating tests of safety and efficacy in randomized controlled trials (RCTs). As described in Chapter 18, one cannot conduct an RCT until a clearly described intervention is established and a reasonable primary outcome for the intervention is selected. In outcomes research, a wide array of end-points can be selected including biochemical, disease specific, and general, such as quality of life, mortality and costs. From such data, a reasonable set of primary outcomes for testing in RCTs can be selected. Thus, outcomes research has a role both before and after RCTs. In this chapter, Harald Walach describes the role of observational and outcomes research in mental and spiritual healing, together with its variations and limitations. **WBJ**

THE EPISTEMOLOGICAL ROLE OF OBSERVATION

Good and systematic observation is at the base of any scientific endeavor. We tend to forget, for instance, that the progress of astronomy was only possible because many observers patiently noted the position of stars, night after night, over generations. Most people have heard of Kepler and his laws describing the motion of the planets around the sun which heralded one of the biggest revolutions in the modern history of science. Not only did this achievement prove that it was possible to describe the universe by mathematical laws and that nature followed laws describable by numbers, but it foreshadowed the modern scientific enterprise whose mission it is to explain complex natural phenomena by understanding their underlying structure. While Kepler is well known, what is less well known is the fact that Kepler's achievement was only possible because he could build on the enormous amount of data which had been collected by his mentor and predecessor, the Danish astronomer Tycho Brahe, who had meticulously compiled lists of planet positions over years of patient and laborious observations. Kepler later published these observations as the famous Tabula Rudolphina, and they were the foundation on which his later fame was built (Oeser 1979a, 1979b). Thus, observation has a primary and important place as a first step in the scientific endeavor of understanding the world. It supplies us with the raw data from which more complex operations take their beginning, like the tentative formulation of theories, the hunch of a new phenomenon hitherto unthought of, or the new understanding of old phenomena including anomalistic results unaccounted for by prevailing theories (Laudan 1981, 1977) One such serendipitous observation which changed the progress of medicine was Edward Jenner's observation that dairymaids who had suffered from cowpox were less likely to contract smallpox; this led to the discovery of immunization and immunologic functions. This is a specifically interesting historical example, since in this observation two elements are brought together. The observation itself – dairymaids having a smaller likelihood of contracting smallpox – is quite a complex operation, involving a kind of intuitive comparison of normal and lowered incidence of disease. This observation is linked to a hypothetical structure: immunization. This again gives rise to a prospective test in a deductive step: inoculate healthy people with cowpox, or a small amount of smallpox, and susceptibility to the disease should decrease.

Epistemologically, then, observation fulfils an important role and has done so in many important scientific innovations. It provides the raw data and/or the anomalies which stifle theoretical understanding, the building or changing of theories, the stumbling details which inspire new and bold hypotheses, which in turn stimulate empirical research.

Observation and Comparison

Observation is never blind and naked. It is always, even in its most simple acts, a complex constructive process which involves internal or external comparison to explicit or implicit standards. This has been pointed out already by Gestalt psychologists (Koffka 1935, Wertheimer 1944) and is a well-founded result of modern brain research and cognitive science (Churchland 1986, Oeser & Seitelberge 1988, Roth 1997). Thus, Tycho Brahe was only able to compile his data because he had an inner or outer system of reference by which to order his observations. And Kepler was only capable of arriving at a comprehensive structure to map Brahe's data because he had some ideal standard (Copernicus's model) to which he could compare the empirical data. And Jenner was only able to arrive at a theory of immunization because he was able to conduct a comparison of incidence rates in dairymaids and normal population, even if he did it only implicitly at first. Thus comparison is always an explicit or implicit element of any observation.

The Manipulation of Comparison in Modern Methodology

In modern methodological wisdom comparison is always an *explicit* element. For example, in randomized controlled clinical trials (RCTs) a comparison group is built up artificially at random. In other types of studies, such as cohort or quasi-experimental studies, naturally existing groups are used as comparison standards. In other designs other forms of comparison are introduced, such as comparison with a previous state. RCTs are normally considered the gold standard of clinical research, the summit of scientific achievement, and the holy grail of methodological rigor. However, several authors have already pointed to limitations and problems with RCTs (Black 1996, Feinstein 1998, Kaptchuk 2000, Rochon et al 1999, Fogg & gross 2000). Most prominent among their limitations are the lack of representativeness of study populations, and hence a lack of external validity, a possible masking bias because of the blinding of studies, investigator bias, or bias due to the consent procedure, all of which hamper internal validity (Kaptchuk 2000). In what follows I do not want to reiterate these limitations of RCTs, rather I would like to point to other research options and to the circumstances under which they are appropriate, as well as to the reasons why they might be preferable for some questions. What will emerge from this discussion is a plea for a multidimensional research approach instead of methodological monoculture.

I start by pointing out a silent and unreflected presupposition of RCT methodology and discuss the ramifications, namely randomness itself. I will then describe examples, preconditions and limitations of other research strategies than RCTs.

THE ALLEGED GOLD STANDARD OF RESEARCH AND A POSSIBLY PROBLEMATIC ASSUMPTION

The invention of the randomized controlled trial (RCT) has been hailed as the single most important methodological innovation, since it allows for a control of bias (Fuchs et al 2000). By randomizing patients to groups a RCT ideally achieves a homogenous distribution of prognostic variables across groups and thus allows for a clearcut interpretation of results. If differences between groups can be observed, it is legitimate to conclude that a difference between groups after an intervention is not due to differences among groups before the intervention, but due to the intervention itself, if one is willing to follow the underlying reasoning set out by John Stuart Mill (for some bright arguments against this, see Royzman 2000). It is the closest possible adaption of an experiment of natural science to problems of medicine, and thus makes arguments for a causality between intervention and effect plausible, although this is a difficult and tricky field (Abel & Koch 1998) which I do not want to enlarge (Feinstein 1989). Apart from the possibility of a causal argument from a RCT, randomization is a precondition for applying the statistical models usually used for the quantitative assessment of the results.

There can be no doubt that the RCT is an extremely valuable research tool for certain questions. A placebo or sham controlled RCT is certainly the method of choice when specific efficacy of an intervention is at issue. It is the only method which can precisely answer the question: does intervention X have a specific effect for disease A (i.e. are the ingredients of intervention X more efficacious for treating A than the mere passage of time, the psychological effects of being treated and cared for, the suggestive effects of doctors' opinions, the expectations of improvement, or the methodological artifacts of measurement)? A comparative RCT, which uses a standard treatment as comparison, is the method of choice if one wants to answer the question: is treatment X more effective than or equally as effective as standard treatment Y (for people willing to apply and indifferent to both options)? The clause in parentheses here is the important part: the results of RCTs only apply to subjects who are willing to be treated under the preconditions of RCTs.

Preconditions of RCTs

Preconditions of RCTs are generally thought to be the following:

1. There is equipoise between the two treatment options. Treating physician and patient feel

that both treatment options are equally likely or unlikely to have a benefit.
2. There is no strong preference. Both physician and patient feel that both treatments are equally harmful or desirable.
3. There is too little knowledge about a treatment.
4. There are enough preliminary indications that a treatment might be effective.
5. There is a necessity to find a treatment for a condition, either because no treatment exists, or because existing options are not effective enough, or not effective for all patients, or because costs are too high, or because harm from existing treatments is unacceptable.

The above preconditions are pragmatic and ethical preconditions. However, there is also a methodological, even fundamental precondition which is rarely mentioned or reflected upon: the possibility of a truly random allocation and the independence of experimenter intentions, patient intentions, and outcome of the study. It is immediately obvious that the test of the effectiveness of healing, particularly at a distance, as in healing or prayer studies, by the RCT paradigm is a contradiction in terms. Should healing at a distance or the positive influence of a course of a disease by prayer be a possibility, then by the same token it is evident that an investigator or a patient, by strong wishing, praying, or using his or her own energies, could influence randomization or study results. Thus a positive result of a randomized blinded trial of healing would lead straight away into a paradox: if healing at a distance or prayer can be shown to be effective this would undermine the very foundations of the experimental paradigm, namely separability and randomness. Put differently, if patients randomly allocated to a treatment group profit from prayer or distant healing (i.e. from intentions and mental events occurring at a distance), why should it not be possible in the first place that researchers conducting the research influence the results? Why would it not be an option that patients have had an influence on the randomization code which allocated them to the group which would turn out improved? Investigating phenomena

such as healing or prayer by randomized trial methodology is an implicit challenge to the foundations of this very methodology. Of course these questions touch at the questions asked by parapsychologists and researchers into anomalies. Although this area is still highly controversial, there is some evidence at the horizon that intentional influences might be possible after all (Bem & Honorton 1994, Radin 1997, Radin & Nelson 1989, Schlitz & Braud 1997). Without going into details here it is obvious that, should healing and prayer prove effective, it cannot be by RCTs alone that these methods can be researched, since intentional effects cannot be restricted to areas of interest for the researcher. Apart from that, the pragmatic preconditions for RCTs mentioned above are frequently not met within healing research. They are violated in several ways:

Equipoise and preference

It is difficult to find medical conditions for which, and patients for whom, this precondition is met. Usually patients have a clear preference. Furthermore, patients who willingly choose a method such as healing or prayer as a treatment are unlikely to be the same as patients who have no definite opinion about healing and thus are in equipoise. The same is true for doctors.

Preliminary knowledge and lack of definite evidence

Healing and prayer as interventions have low a priori probability to be effective, if one abstracts from existing data. Thus, although evidence is accumulating, it is likely that we have indeed too little preliminary knowledge to be able to conduct RCTs. This is the place where observational studies come in as a methodological stepping-stone for other types of trials.

Conditions

Modern medicine has many effective strategies at hand, although there are many conditions for which no healing in the medical sense is possible, or only palliation is available. Randomized trials would have to be conducted in these fields, then, for example in patients with type A diabetes, or with chronic fatigue syndrome, or in terminal cancer patients, to name but a few, with a rather low a priori probability of effectiveness or small effect sizes, with the consequence of having to recruit huge numbers of patients. Or else one would have to restrict trials to patients with no treatment option left over. Thus, only a small proportion of patients for whom healing or prayer could be effective, if true, could be studied in RCTs.

Arguments for alternatives abound. Let us have a look at some of them.

THE SCOPE FOR OUTCOMES AND OBSERVATIONAL STUDIES

What Observational and Outcomes Studies Can and Cannot Do

The terms 'observational studies' and 'outcomes studies' are used in a loosely interchangeable way in this chapter. While 'observational study' denotes the generic class of these studies, 'outcomes studies' refers more to a specific group of studies which emphasize patient reported outcome (or else a specifically desired outcome) as the main parameter as opposed to doctor reported outcome or studies using some laboratory parameter as a surrogate end-point. When the outcome is documented in a well-defined, natural treatment group (i.e. a group of patients who chose that treatment themselves), and compared to another group of patients who naturally did not select that treatment, this type of study is normally called a cohort study. When rigid selection criteria are employed it is called a comprehensive cohort design. In the evaluation literature these studies are also sometimes called quasi-experimental studies, because they do not represent true experiments with random allocation (Cook & Campbell 1979). It is a common prejudice that these designs provide evidence of inferior quality. While evaluation researchers who had to navigate in socially and methodologically more complex space than their medical colleagues have

long ago dropped the dogma that only randomized studies can be trusted (Cook & Wittmann 1998, Rossi & Freeman 1982), it is now becoming acceptable even among researchers within the medical community that outcomes and observational studies can yield evidence of the same quality as RCTs, if well conducted (Abel & Koch 1998). Two recent studies have compared results of RCTs and observational cohort studies and concluded that not only did cohort studies have the same point estimates of effects as the randomized studies in most cases, but also had narrower confidence intervals because results of cohort studies normally come from larger studies with a more varied study population (Benson & Hartz 2000, Concato et al 2000).

Cohort studies can be conducted in natural groups of self-selected patients, thus they are a good research tool for complementary and alternative medical approaches such as healing. Here we normally find patients with a difficult and long history of ineffective, mostly conventional treatment, who are usually unwilling to be randomized, and who choose to be treated by spiritual healing. It is a methodological challenge to find a good comparison group or a cohort of patients willing to be observed just as closely as the healing group. And it takes considerable statistical expertise to statistically control for initial group differences, although methods do exist, such as the calculation of the propensity score (Rosenbaum & Rubin 1983, Rubin 1998). This method, basically, is a logistic regression which predicts group membership from prognostic variables. This so called propensity score is a quantitative index which gives the propensity or probability to be a member of one of the two natural groups just because one falls naturally into some of the prognostic categories. It can be used as a weight to adjust group comparisons. One of the preconditions, of course, is that the most important prognostic variables are known and measured. While a randomized trial relies on randomization to equalize the distribution of prognostically relevant variables in groups, at least in theory, and therefore it is not necessary to know or measure them all, in non-randomized studies it is of paramount importance to know any prognostic variables which might influence the outcome. With more obvious variables such duration of the disease, sex, age, clinical prognosis it is evident that they need to be documented. But what if personality is a potentially important prognostic variable, or level of stress, or number of live events, or the social network, coping styles, or even more outlandish ones such as the amount of time spent in meditation or prayer each day? It is therefore necessary for a non-randomized study to have thorough knowledge of potentially important variables and to have good measures for all of them. Conclusions based on such studies are more susceptible to threats to internal validity than RCTs. On the other hand, non-randomized trials can be conducted on a more varied patient population, thus making results more robust. Non-randomized trials normally do not answer questions of specificity, let alone causality, but have a more pragmatic tone. They can, however, answer questions of relative effectiveness, and such answers are normally more useful for practical decisions. This certainly is the bottom line of the methodological discussions within evaluation research over the last 40 years (Wittmann & Walach 2000). Studies such as this will certainly not be able to answer the question whether there is a specific element in healing or not. This can – if at all – only be achieved by masked randomized trials or randomized trials with more arms and some masking elements. But for all practical purposes it is the question whether this is at all a relevant question. What is interesting for purchasers, patients, and the public is the question of whether patients with a certain disease, a certain history, and with certain preferences will profit from this treatment over and against a comparison standard. It is certainly academically interesting to ask whether the factor operative in healing is specific or non-specific, causal or acausal, mechanistic or probabilistic, regular or stochastic, but it is possibly, and debatably, easier to study such questions in simple and repeatable laboratory models of healing, as in the DMILS setting (see Ch. 3), and leave the question of practical usefulness for pragmatic cohort studies or, where possible, pragmatic RCTs.

Observational Studies with Intraindividual Control

If possible, concurrent control groups are always preferable to historical controls. They control not only for the effects of the intervention in general, but also for secular trends. However, sometimes it is not possible to find a concurrent control group comparable to the treatment group, and sometimes it is not necessary. There are certain preconditions in which patients can be their own control, and where the comparison standard is the patient's previous status. Healing in particular is a kind of last resort for many patients. Such patients see healers after they have tried everything else (Binder & Wolf-Braun 1995, Walach et al 2000, Wiesendanger 1994). They have finally resolved to invest time, money, and effort in seeing a healer, and it might be exactly this intricate combination of desperation, effort, and point in time which is a cofactor in healing (Brown 2000). There will be no comparison group in the world, randomized or non-randomized, which will be able to map the status of this group. The only status which can be used is patients' status before they decided to see a healer. The effects of such a type of intervention can be documented in large and long-term single-group observational studies. If the condition of the patients studied is sufficiently stable, if the prognosis of the condition and its natural history is well known, if the status before the intervention took place is well documented, and particularly if the patient has tried everything else and this is well documented, there is no reason why a within-case comparison should not be highly informative. Provided the group is large enough, the medical condition stable (or progressing) and clinically relevant, changes which do not regress back to the initial stage but are lasting improvements would be impressive (Pincus 1997). Of course one would have to make plausible that the change observed is not otherwise explicable than by the intervention. In particular, the natural history of the disease, spontaneous remissions or fluctuations, concomitant treatments, and measurement errors are points for debate. The natural history has to be known in terms of clinical prognosis. The better the documentation is for both the treatment and the disease history, the easier it is to argue that lasting and strong changes are unlikely to be due to natural history, the more so when the observed group is large enough. If concomitant treatments are monitored, and if previous treatments are known to have been ineffective, the argument that concomitant treatment was the reason for improvement can be countered. Measurement errors can be avoided or minimized by using well known instruments with acceptable properties. Although disease specific measurement instruments are desirable, such instruments do not always exist. Apart from that it is advisable to also have generic instruments, for example generic quality-of-life or health status measurement instruments such as the SF (McHorney et al 1993, Ware et al 1998, Ware & Sherbourne 1992), the sickness impact profile, or the like. These instruments are normally used in a wide variety of clinical trials and it is easy to find reference data for patient groups from other types of trials.

Thus, under certain circumstances, observational studies with intraindividual, within-patient control can be feasible. Especially if patients are to be studied who naturally choose healing, and therefore external validity is to be maximized, this type of study might be the only possible one.

Also, under situations where an initial attempt at documenting possible effect sizes, applicability of a healing treatment to types of patients, predicting responders to treatment through baseline variables, or diagnosis is an issue, single-group observational studies can be very useful. It is a particularly unfortunate omission in many CAM trials that RCTs have been conducted without proper sample size estimations. Sample size estimations are more often based on theoretical considerations and would-be effect sizes than on real life data. This results in the bemourned status of badly powered trials which fail to detect effects between treatment and control, as documented in a recent review (Ezzo et al 2000). Documentation of effect sizes in a clinical practice is not a guarantee for significant results in a subsequent controlled trial, as in Dowson et al (1985), where a systematic observation has produced an effect

size which was substantially lower in a controlled trial conducted with the same practitioner and the same outcome measure. On the contrary, CAM suffers from what I have termed the efficacy paradox: while in uncontrolled, observed practice effects are quite large, trials often fail to detect these effects. Still the systematic documentation of effects in general practice is the only feasible way of arriving at least at meaningful estimates of effect sizes.

Wait-list Controlled Trials

A little explored compromise between a randomized trial and documentation in practice are wait-list controlled trials. In that variant of a RCT the control condition is a waiting group, but the allocation to this waiting condition is at random. There are at present to my knowledge two wait-list controlled trials of healing (Walach et al 2000, Dixon 1998). Both have shown beneficial effects for patients treated by healing. In our experience it is comparatively easy to convince patients who have decided to see a healer to enrol in a wait-list controlled trial. Patients, especially if they have had many encounters with doctors, are used to the fact that specialists have long waiting lists anyway. If a certain type of healing treatment is offered within a trial, it is possible to convince patients that treatment capacity is limited and that coin-tossing is the best way to decide who starts treatment first. In most cases this explanation will also be true, so that no ethical considerations arise. The natural limitation of wait-list controlled studies is the duration of the waiting period, which normally has to be limited to 6 months for pragmatic reasons. It is difficult to motivate patients for longer periods of waiting time. On the other hand, 6 months seems to be a minimal period to be able to document lasting and meaningful changes. By using a randomized wait-list controlled design it is possible to combine a well-conducted within-group comparison study (the waiting group) with a randomized comparison (the concurrent comparison of treated versus waiting group). It is obvious that this design can only control for secular trends and natural history, and in a limited way for concomitant treatments. It cannot control for expectation effects and thus cannot disentangle expectancy from true treatment effects. But this is a minor issue anyway, considered from the practical perspective of patients' and purchasers' needs. If one wants to disentangle expectancy effects, time effects and specific effects, one can conduct a four-armed trial, as we are planning to do, with two waiting and two treated groups, but one of them each knowing and not knowing in which group they are. By that method patients are either treated or not treated, no dummy treatment has to be employed and no placebo is used, and still specific and non-specific treatment effects can be disentangled.

The Complementarity of Methods

My contention with the above arguments would be that there is no hierarchy of research methods with a diamond on top of the pyramid, as often thought, but that research methodology is complementary. Rather than in a hierarchy, research methodology is ordered in a spectrum. Each method has its specific strengths and weaknesses, and there is no single study which is useful for

everything. Methods have to be applied in a flexible way, complementing each other's strengths and weaknesses. The term 'complementarity' here is used in direct analogy to its usage in the original sense (Walach & Römer 2000): if one opts for the strength of one method, say the internal validity of a blinded RCT, one usually trades this for the strength of another method, say the generalizability of a cohort study. Thus, the picture is only complete, if data stemming from different types of studies are taken together. This situation is depicted in Figure 19.1.

THE CHOICE OF OUTCOME MEASURES: RELEVANCE OF QUALITY OF LIFE AND COSTING PARAMETERS

Questions of design have to be discussed in the context of relevant outcome parameters. It has been a consensus over the last few years that whenever possible clinically relevant and meaningful outcome parameters should be used instead of laboratory or surrogate parameters. We can observe a shift in the medical literature toward patient-based, so-called soft or subjective

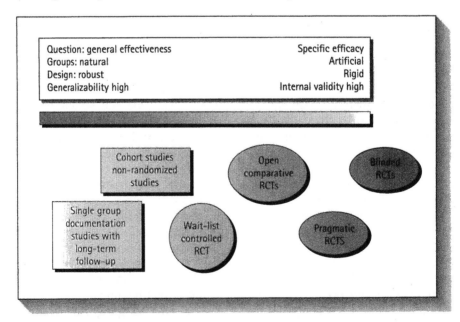

Figure 19.1 Spectrum of methods according to questions. Circles: randomized; squares: non-randomized.

outcome measures over recent years. This is because clinicians and researchers alike have become aware of the fact that clinical parameters are only part of a successful treatment, and that finally it is for the patient to decide whether a treatment did help or not. An especially striking example of the divergence between objective and subjective improvement has been reported recently by allergologists (Confino-Cohen et al 1999, Hyland 1999). In allergic patients it was observed that after a successful desensitization therapy, which normally gives nearly 100% protection against anaphylactic and systemic reactions, many patients still had debilitating beliefs and anticipated strong reactions. Patients with such beliefs had a lower quality of life than patients without such beliefs, although 'objectively' there was no reason for this lowered quality of life. Thus, Hyland (1999) observes that what really counts is not the clinical-immunological status, but the subjective one. In cancer patients it is a well known fact that subjective report correlates only little with objective status or doctor-based estimation of patients' well-being (Koller et al 1996). Instead, complaints of patients seem to be driven by patients' negative affect and experienced social stigma. Moreover, we know that it is subjective well-being which is prognostic for many hard outcomes such as survival, health status, or maintenance of remission from depression (George & Landerman 1984, MacLeod & Moore 2000, Idler & Kasl 1991). Such data and insights have shifted the general perception and made plausible that patient reported quality of life is of prime importance as an outcome measure. We have seen in our own study (Walach et al 2000), as well as in others (Dixon 1998, Brown 1995), that quality of life can be improved by distant healing. Thus, quality-of-life measures should be incorporated in every HER study, if not as the principal then at least as a secondary parameter, as is recommended for normal clinical trials (Fletcher 1995, Staquet et al 1998). Apart from conceptual problems with the notion of quality of life (Koch 2000, Lara-Munoz & Feinstein 1999, Moberg & Brusek 1978, Muthny et al 1990, Smith et al 1999), it is important to make some distinctions. There are at least three conceptually different constructs and several different ways of operationalizing them.

Quality of Life: Different Constructs

Quality of life is sometimes taken to be synonymous with functional status and life satisfaction. While most of the commonly used generic instruments which are supposed to measure health-related quality of life contain a scale of functional status, these two constructs are by no means interchangeable. A recent meta-analysis addressing this question (Smith et al 1999) found that quality of life is the broader construct with two main domains, psychological well-being and physical functioning. It is highly correlated with perceived health status ($r = 0.72$), but not identical with it. It is interesting to note that psychological health contributes more to quality of life ($r = 0.68$) than physical functioning ($r = 0.57$). These authors suggest visualizing quality of life as the weighted sum of $1.6 \times$ psychological well-being + physical functioning. A comparison of patients with different chronic diseases across measures shows that patients can have an acceptable quality of life although severely handicapped in functional status and vice versa (Patrick et al 2000). People have a remarkable capacity to adapt their inner standards in a way that allows them to be comparatively satisfied with their lives, even though they have a poor level of physical functioning. Psychological adaptivity and well-being are key moderators in the adaption process known as response shift (Carver & Scheier 2000, Schwartz & Sprangers 1999, Sprangers & Schwartz 1999). When people suffer from a severe chronic illness which handicaps their normal performance they start a series of cognitive appraisal and recalibration processes with the aim of adapting inner comparison standards to what is possible and 'normal' in the light of their new health status. This, in the end, may lead to a downregulation of inner standards, which might result in a paradoxically high quality-of-life score. We saw this in a sample of children with cancer in rehabilitation who had by far the highest score in a quality-of-life measure for children (Walach et al 1997). Therefore, it is necessary to decide what aspect of quality of life is important for a study. Measures at only one point in time and comparison with gauge or population data can be misleading because response-shift phenomena could change the actual picture. If response shift might be an issue, especially in patients with long-standing chronic and debilitating diseases, as are typical for HER, it is a good idea to take measures of physical functioning, since they are closer to a behavioral level of assessment, and to have multiple time points and long observation periods.

Different Operationalizations

There are basically three ways of operationalizing constructs of quality of life: generic, disease-specific, and individual. Generic measures try to find factors common to all diseases which are a component of quality of life and can be measured across diseases. Typically, they include such factors as physical functioning, social functioning, psychological well-being, role functioning, pain, vitality, sleep, and recreation, inner or social resources, to name but a few. Generic instruments such as the SF-36, the EuroQol, the sickness impact profile or the Nottingham health profile differ in which factors they include and how many items they use to measure them. But the basic measurement theory is the same, namely that subjects can be ordered in a multidimensional health space spanned by the factors, which are relevant for all subjects and all diseases. This concept of measurement results in very robust, generally valid and reliable, but rather insensitive measures. Usually one needs large numbers of patients and strong therapy effects in order to make these measures shift. They trade sensitivity and individual responsiveness for generality. Many studies have used these measures and there is a wealth of comparative data now. Moreover, most researchers know these scales. If it is possible to show a mean shift of 10 scale points in the SF36 scales, this is known to be a clinically relevant improvement (Lydick & Yawn 1998). In observational outcomes studies, with large numbers and long observation periods across a variety of diseases, these well-known generic measures provide a safe ground with good implicit comparison standards. There are many published reference data for various disease categories, which make it easy to compare one's own patient population, as well as to calibrate improvements and compare them to those of other trials. Although such historical controls are generally considered to be only weak, they nevertheless carry a strong suggestive element, if the improvement attained by a HER study is impressive enough.

In many diseases, quality of life is severely limited but does not show in a variety of scales; for example, women with candida vaginitis do usually not have pain, days off work, diminished physical functioning, or severely diminished psychological well-being, but they still feel that their quality of life is limited, and gynaecologists usually do not perceive the psychological and social stress involved. We have seen in an interview survey (Matter et al, study in progress) that most of the items on quality-of-life questionnaires would be irrelevant for these women. Likewise, in many diseases it is a specific set of symptoms or areas which shows limited quality of life. This so called disease-specific quality of life is generally thought to be a more specific measure. Whenever a study addresses a homogenous patient population it is a good idea to not only measure quality of life generically but also disease-specifically. A wide variety of instruments are now available; however, in many areas of interest it may still be necessary to construct one's own scale. Disease-specific measures are usually more responsive to change and thus are the variable of choice in a study with one or more homogenous diseases (Dahlöf et al 1997).

Disease-specific quality of life is half-way between a generic and a subjective measure. It has been argued that the only reasonable question to ask would be one that is highly generic and subjective at the same time, namely 'How is your quality of life?' (Lara-Munoz & Feinstein 1999). This is another variant of the argument raised some years ago by Joyce and colleagues that quality of life can only be measured individually (McGee et al 1991, O'Boyle et al 1992). They constructed a method, SEIQol, which basically consists in interviewing the patient about the most important domains of his or her life and then rating these as to their present quality. Thus, individualized standardized scores can be constructed which reflect very individual emphases and valuations. This is a time-consuming, albeit very valid, way of mapping quality of life and should be considered in research which is intensive and tries to combine qualitative and quantitative elements, or which can access only a few people and wants to maximize information from them. A related method is the so-called MYMOP – measure yourself medical outcome profile – which identifies areas of importance for a particular patient and measures this specific profile at follow-up visits (Paterson 1996). Individual-based evaluation methods have been used in psychosocial research for decades, starting with goal attainment scaling by Kiresuk & Sherman (1968), but they have never climbed the Olympus of clinical measures, since they are all subject to bias. In order to really make these measures valid one would have to use different people for constructing the profile, assessing it, and conducting the therapy, which usually involves high costs and a large effort, compared to its outcome. They will keep their place in evaluations of individual treatment programs, but are hardly useful in research addressing controversial issues such as HER.

Cost Parameters

In recent times the health technology assessment (HTA) movement has become an important interface between research and policy making. Recent HTA conferences have emphasized the importance of cost parameters for the evaluation of health technologies. One way of operationalizing costs is the use of preference-based measures of quality of life, which bring gains of quality of life in relation with the costs incurred (Kaplan 1998; Lalonde et al 1999a, 1999b). Existing instruments, however, such as the EuroQol (von der Schulenburg et al 1998, Brooks 1996, Dolan 1997), which incorporate such preference-based scales, are not without difficulties because people usually have difficulties understanding items based on standard-gamble or preference questions ('Imagine status X. When H means complete health, how many years of your life [or how much money] would you be willing to trade for coming from X to H'), because they involve complex cognitive operations which are difficult even for researchers in this area to comprehend. Since they are usually used in the context of an interview, it is difficult to incorporate that format in a questionnaire applicable to a large population. Recent validation studies have shown in patients with coronary heart disease that such preference based measures do not discriminate between healthy and ill subjects (Lalonde et al 1999a, 1999b). This is presumably due to the fact that subjective probability and valuation are quite different from objective ones. Thus, if the real probability of dying from surgery is, say, 0.25, and the alternative to death would be complete health, people rate the subjective probability of this event, death, much higher (namely 0.32) than the actual probability. Hence, although such preference-based measures are widely used, their psychometric properties are not well understood in the context of subjective health status.

However, there are other parameters which can be used for estimating costs such as days absent from work. Depending on the social system these data can normally be gleaned from insurance companies or from employers provided the recall period is not longer than 4 weeks, even from subjects themselves (Severens et al 2000). They approximate economic impact of an intervention, provided the database is large enough. Since there is normally a fund of statistical comparison data available both from public sources and as from insurance companies, they offer a good way of arriving at a meaningful comparison, even in one-arm observational studies. The presupposition, however, is that observation periods and numbers observed are large. There are certain diseases, for example fibromyalgia, chronic fatigue syndrome, or chronic low back pain, where work-absenteeism is high and where a clinical impact can easily be shown (if it is present). Other diseases, although subjectively handicapping, normally do not reflect in higher work-absenteeism, for example seasonal allergic rhinitis and migraine. Thus, it depends on the diseases studied and the number of patients available whether workdays-off is a suitable parameter. If it is, it can be gleaned validly by the help of insurers, and thus provide researchers with a good estimate of macro economic impact of a therapeutic measure. Should CAM methods such as healing prove that they are able to reduce workdays-off in patients with a relevant load of absenteeism, this would definitely be a strong argument in their favour. Since work-absenteeism is a parameter with strong epidemiologic trends, because it is subject to changes due to economic trends or changes in society at large, it is practically meaningless without a reference group. Thus, work-days off should always be calibrated on the respective reference groups of insured people in the same category of insurance level, age, and sex. This can normally be achieved by using published data of the insurance companies or national registers. These reference data can then be used to standardize own data, and thus shifts in work-absenteeism can be evaluated objectively and tested for their significance compared to the rest of the relevant population (Moebus et al 1998). In Germany this has proved to be a valuable parameter in discussions with purchasers.

If observational studies are large and conducted over a long period of time, with a sufficient number of patients to create enough variance in work-absenteeism, this can be a very strong, because objective and independent, measure.

SUMMARY

If one is very clear about the possibilities and limitations of observational studies and does not want to make claims about specific efficacy, but only pragmatic effectiveness, observational studies are a good option. They are easier to implement in practical terms, although they can be quite tricky from the point of view of statistical evaluation. They trade naturalness against rigidity, and thus they are at one end of the methodological spectrum. If one drops the idea of a methodological hierarchy with RCTs sitting on the top, but adopts a more spectrum-like or complementary model with certain methods adapted to specific questions, then observational studies become an important tool. They can be the method of choice in the study of very ill patients, in patients with strong preferences, in patients with a clear long-standing history, and whenever patient preference is a precondition to be honored. They are a necessary precondition for estimating effect size and thus are the forerunners of RCTs. Quality-of-life measures should be used to document effects in such studies, based on the research question studied. Costing parameters, especially work-absenteeism, could be an elegant way to demonstrate the economic impact of interventions in HER.

ACKNOWLEDGMENT

I am grateful to the Institut für Grenzgebiete der Psychologie, Freiburg, Germany, and Samueli Institute for Information Biology which currently sponsor this work.

REFERENCES

Abel U, Koch A 1998 The mythology of randomization. In: Abel U, Koch A (eds) Nonrandomized comparative clinical studies. Symposon Publishing, Düsseldorf, Germany, pp. 27–40

Bem D J, Honorton C 1995 Does PSI exist? Replicable evidence for an anomalous process of information transfer. Psychological Bulletin 115: 4–18

Benson K, Hartz A J 2000 A comparison of observational studies and randomized controlled trials. New England Journal of Medicine 342: 1878–1886

Binder M, Wolf-Braun B 1995 Geistheilung in Deutschland. Teil I: Ergebnisse einer Umfrage zum Selbstverständnis und zur Arbeitsweise Geistiger Heiler und Heilerinnen in Deutschland. Zeitschrift für Parapsychologie und Grenzgebiete der Psychologie 37: 145–177

Black N 1996 Why we need observational studies to evaluate the effectiveness of health care. British Medical Journal 312: 1215–1218

Brooks R 1996 EuroQol Group. EuroQol: the current state of play. Health Policy 37: 53–72

Brown C K 1995 Spiritual healing in a general practice: using a quality-of-life questionnaire to measure outcome. Complementary Therapies in Medicine 3: 230–233

Brown C K 2000 Methodological problems of clinical research into spiritual healing: the healer's perspective. Journal of Alternative and Complementary Medicine 6: 171–176

Carver C S, Scheier M F 2000 Scaling back goals and recalibration of the affect system are processes in normal adaptive self-regulation: understanding 'response shift' phenomena. Social Science and Medicine 50: 1715–1722

Churchland P S 1986 Neurophilosophy: toward a unified science of the mind-brain. MIT Press, Cambridge

Concato J, Shah N, Horwitz R I 2000 Randomized, controlled trials, observational studies, and the hierarchy of research designs. New England Journal of Medicine 342: 1887–1892

Confino-Cohen R, Melamed S, Goldberg A 1999 Debilitating beliefs, emotional distress and quality of life in patients given immunotherapy for insect sting allergy. Clinical and Experimental Allergy 29: 1626–1631

Cook T D, Campbell D T 1979 Quasi-experimentation design and analysis issues for field settings. Rand McNally, Chicago

Cook T D, Wittmann W W 1998 Lessons learned about evaluation in the United States and some possible implications for Europe. European Journal of Psychological Assessment 14: 97–115

Dahlöf C, Bouchard J, Cortelli P et al 1997 A multinational investigation of the impact of subcutaneous sumatriptan. II: Health-related quality of life. PharmacoEconomics 11: 24–34

Dixon M 1998 Does 'healing' benefit patients with chronic symptoms? A quasi-randomized trial in general practice. Journal of the Royal Society of Medicine 91: 183–188

Dolan P 1997 Modeling valuations for EuoQol health states. Medical Care 35: 1095–1108

Dowson D I, Lewith G T, Machin D 1985 The effects of acupuncture versus placebo in the treatment of headache. Pain 21: 35–42

Ezzo J, Berman B, Hadhazy V A, Jadad A R, Lao L, Singh B B 2000 Is acupuncture effective for the treatment of chronic pain? A systematic review. Pain 86: 217–225

Feinstein A R 1989 Epidemiologic analyses of causation: the unlearned scientific lessons of randomized trials. Journal of Epidemiology 42: 481–489

Feinstein A R 1998 Problems of randomized trials. In: Abel U, Koch A (eds) Nonrandomized comparative clinical studies. Symposion Publishing, Düsseldorf, Germany, pp. 1–13

Fletcher A 1995 Quality-of-life measurements in the evaluation of treatment: proposed guidelines. British Journal of Clinical Pharmacology 39: 217–222

Fogg L, Gross D 2000 Threats to validity in randomized clinical trials. Research in Nursing and Health 23: 79–87

Fuchs F D, Klag M J, Whelton P K 2000 The classics: a tribute to the fiftieth anniversary of the randomized clinical trial. Journal of Clinical Epidemiology 53: 335–342

George L K, Landerman R 1984 Health and subjective well-being: a replicated secondary data analysis. International Journal of Aging and Human Development 19: 133–156

Hyland M E 1999 The influence of beliefs on the quality of life of patients with allergic diseases [editorial]. Clinical and Experimental Allergy 29: 1591–1592

Idler E L, Kasl S 1991 Health perceptions and survival: do global evaluations of health status really predict mortality? Journal of Gerontology: Social Sciences 46: 55–65

Kaplan R M 1998 Profile versus utility based measures of outcome for clinical trials. In: Staquet M J, Hays R D, Fayers P M (eds) Quality of life assessment in clinical trials: methods and practice. Oxford University Press, Oxford, pp. 69–90

Kaptchuk T J 2000 The double-blind randomized controlled trial: gold standard or golden calf? Journal of Clinical Epidemiology 54: 541–549

Kiresuk T J, Sherman R E 1968 Goal attainment scaling: general method for evaluating comprehensive community mental health programs [abstract]. Community Mental Health Journal 4: 443–453

Koch T 2000 Life quality vs. 'quality of life': assumptions underlying prospective quality of life instruments in health care planning. Social Science and Medicine 51: 419–427

Koffka K 1935 Principles of Gestalt psychology. Harcourt-Brace, New York

Koller M, Kussmann J, Lorenz W et al 1996 Symptom reporting in cancer patients: the role of negative affect and experienced social stigma. Cancer 77: 983–995

Lalonde L, Clarke A E, Joseph L, Grover S A, Canadian Collaborative Cardiac Assessment Group 1999a Conventional and chained standard gambles in the assessment of coronary heart disease prevention and treatment. Medical Decision Making 19: 149–156

Lalonde L, Clarke A E, Joseph L, Mackenzie T, Grover S A, Canadian Collaborative Cardiac Assessment Group 1999b Comparing the psychometric properties of preference-based and nonpreference-based health-related quality of life in coronary heart disease. Quality of Life Research 8: 399–409

Lara-Munoz C, Feinstein A R 1999 How should quality of life be measured? Journal of Investigative Medicine 47: 17–24

Laudan L 1977 Progress and its problems: towards a theory of scientific growth. University of California Press, Berkeley, California

Laudan L 1981 Science and hypothesis. Reidel, Dordrecht, Netherlands

Lydick E, Yawn B P 1998 Clinical interpretation of health-related quality of life data. In: Staquet M J, Hays R D, Fayers P M (eds). Quality of life assessment in clinical trials: methods and practice. Oxford University Press, Oxford, pp. 299–314

McGee H M, O'Boyle C A, Hickey A, O'Malley K, Joyce C R B 1991 Assessing the quality of life of the individual: the SEIQol with a healthy and a gastroenterology unit population. Psychological Medicine 21: 749–759

McHorney C A, Ware J E, Raczek A E 1993 The MOS 36-item short form health survey (SF–36): II. Psychometric and clinical tests of validity in measuring physical and mental health constructs. Medical Care 31: 247–263

MacLeod A K, Moore R 2000 Positive thinking revisited: positive cognitions, well-being and mental health. Clinical Psychology and Psychotherapy 7: 1–10

Moberg D O, Brusek P M 1978 Spiritual well-being: a neglected subject in quality of life research [abstract]. Social Indicators Research 5: 303–323

Moebus S, Hirche H, Ose C, Jöckel K-H 1998 Results of an observational pilot study on the effects of non-conventional therapies: a pre/post comparison and cost outcome analysis. In: Abel U, Koch A (eds) Nonrandomized comparative clinical studies. Symposion Publishing, Düsseldorf, Germany, pp. 15–25

Muthny F A, Koch U, Stump S 1990 Quality of life in oncology patients. Psychotherapy and Psychosomatics 54: 145–160

O'Boyle C A, McGee H, Hlckey A, O'Malley K, Joyce C R B 1992 Individual quality of life in patients undergoing hip replacement. Lancet 339: 1088–1091

Oeser E 1979a Wissenschaftstheorie als Rekonstruktion der Wissenschaftsgeschichte. Band 1: Metrisierung, Hypothesenbildung, Theoriendynamik. Oldenbourg, Munich, Germany

Oeser E 1979b Wissenschaftstheorie als Rekonstruktion der Wissenschaftsgeschichte. Band 2: Experiment, Erklärung, Prognose. Oldenbourg, Munich, Germany

Oeser E, Seitelberger F 1988 Gehirn, Bewußtsein und Erkenntnis. Wissenschaftliche Buchgesellschaft, Darmstadt, Germany

Paterson C 1996 Measuring outcomes in primary care: a patient generated measure, MYMOP, compared with the SF–36 health survey. British Medical Journal 312: 1016–1020

Patrick D L, Kinne S, Engelberg R A, Pearlman R A 2000 Functional status and perceived quality of life in adults with and without chronic conditions. Journal of Clinical Epidemiology 53: 779–785

Pincus T 1997 Analyzing long-term outcomes of clincial care without randomized controlled clinical trials: the consecutive patient questionnaire database. Advances. The Journal of Mind-Body Health 13: 3–32

Radin D I 1997 The conscious universe: the scientific truth of psychic phenomena. Harper Collins, San Francisco

Radin D I, Nelson R D 1989 Evidence for consciousness-related anomalies in random physical systems. Foundations of Physics 19: 1499–1514

Rochon P A, Bins M Á, Litner J A et al 1999 Are randomized control trial outcomes influenced by the inclusion of a placebo group? A systematic review of nonsteroidal antiinflammatory drug trials for arthritis treatment. Journal of Clinical Epidemiology 52: 113–122

Rosenbaum P R, Rubin D B 1983 The central role of the propensity score in observational studies for causal effects. Biometrika 70: 41–55

Rossi P H, Freeman H E 1982 Evaluation: a systematic approach, 2nd edn. Sage, Beverly Hills

Roth G 1997 Das Gehirn und seine Wirklichkeit. Kognitive Neurobiologie und ihre philosophischen Konsequenzen. Suhrkamp, Frankfurt, Germany

Royzman E B 2000 Are experiments possible? The limitations of a posteriori control in experimental behavior analysis: the case of clinical process research. Theory and Psychology 10: 171–196

Rubin D B 1998 Estimation from nonrandomized treatment comparisons using subclassification on propensity scores. In: Abel U, Koch A (eds) Nonrandomized comparative clinical studies. Symposion Publishing, Düsseldorf, Germany, pp. 85–100

Schlitz M, Braud W 1997 Distant intentionality and healing: assessing the evidence. Alternative Therapies in Health and Medicine 3: 38–53

Schwartz C E, Sprangers M A G 1999 Methodological approaches for assessing response shift in longitudinal health-related quality-of-life research. Social Science and Medicine 48: 1531–1548

Severens J L, Mulder J, Laheij R J F, Verbeek A L M 2000 Precision and accuracy in measuring absence from work as a basis for calculating productivity costs in the Netherlands. Social Science and Medicine 51: 243–249

Smith K W, Avis N E, Assmann S F 1999 Distinguishing between quality of life and health status in quality of life research: a meta-analysis. Quality of Life Research 8: 447–459

Sprangers M A G, Schwartz C E 1999 Integrating response shift into health-related quality of life research: a theoretical model. Social Science and Medicine 48: 1507–1515

Staquet M J, Hays R D, Fayers P M (eds) 1998 Quality of life assessment in clinical trials: methods and practice. Oxford University Press, Oxford

Von der Schulenburg M, Claes C, Greiner W, Unger A 1998 Die deutsche Versoin des EuroQol-Fragebogens. Zeitschrift für Gesundheitswissenschaften 6: 3–20.

Walach H, Römer H 2000 Complementarity is a useful concept for consciousness studies: a reminder. Neuroendocrinology Letters 21: 221–232

Walach H, Koch V, Zabel S, Bengel J 1997 FALK – Fragebogen zur Erfassung der allgemeinen Lebensqualität bei Kindern. Validierung des Instrumentes. 7 Rehawissenschaftliches Kolloquium, Hamburg, pp. 255–256 [Abstract]

Walach H, Reuter K, Wiesendanger H, Werthmüller L 2000 Distant healing improves quality of life in chronically ill patients: results of a waiting-list controlled randomized study [abstract]. Forschende Komplementärmedizin 7: 54

Ware J E, Sherbourne D 1992 The MOS 36-item short form health survey (SF-36) I. Conceptual framework and item selection. Medical Care 30: 473–483

Ware J E, Gandek B, Kosinski M et al 1998 The equivalence of SF–36 summary health scores using standard and country-specific algorithms in 10 countries: results from the IQOLA project. Journal of Clinical Epidemiology 51: 1167–1170

Wertheimer M 1944 Gestalt theory. Social Research 11: 78–99

Wiesendanger H 1994 Das grosse Buch vom geistigen Heilen – Möglichkeiten, Grenzen, Gefahren. Scherz, Munich, Germany

Wittmann W W, Walach H 2000 Evaluating complementary medicine: lessons to be learned from evaluation research. In: Lewith G, Jonas W B, Walach H (eds) Research methodology for complementary and alternative medicine. Churchill Livingstone, London

20

Methods and issues of laboratory research

Garret Yount, Jerry Solfvin, Yifang Qian,

This chapter describes a rigorous, stepwise investigation of the effect of qigong on cellular function and growth in a standard laboratory model, and discusses methodological issues that arise when designing basic research in spiritual healing and energy medicine.

Can mental and spiritual healing be studied in the laboratory in a manner similar to other biomedical interventions? The summary of laboratory studies in Chapters 9 and 11 indicates this may be possible. Does laboratory research provide 'harder' and more 'objective' evidence of the value of these practices? Can laboratory research be done in parallel with clinical testing? While laboratory research does offer a measure of control not available in clinical studies, it is not without its challenges and variability. In addition, applicability to the clinical situation is always needed.

However, rigorous demonstration of mental, spiritual or bioenergy healing effects in the laboratory is important for demonstrating the reality of these effects and for studying their mechanisms. In this chapter, Garret Yount describes a clear and systematic project examining the effect of qigong on cellular models in the laboratory. It can serve as a model for other rigorous investigation of this type.   **WBJ**

INTRODUCTION

Since 1995, our research team at California Pacific Medical Center has endeavored to establish reliable *in vitro* models, easily replicated by independent laboratories, for evaluating the efficacy of distant healing modalities. Working closely with qigong practitioners in the United States and China, we began by adapting standard experimental protocols from molecular oncology to ask whether healing treatments can accelerate brain tumor cell death. Later studies used normal human brain cells as targets to assess the effect of qigong treatment on stimulating cell growth. We alternated trials comparing control treatment to simultaneous controls (sham/sham trials) with trials comparing qigong treatment to simultaneous controls (qigong/sham trials). During a study conducted in San Francisco, we accomplished four sham/sham trials alternated with four qigong/sham trials. These were followed by 29 trials (15 sham/sham and 14 qigong/sham), conducted in Beijing, China. Statistical analysis of the results revealed a small but significant change in cell growth in qigong/sham trials compared to sham/sham trials. Thus, experiments using this protocol suggest that changes in the growth of cultured human brain cells following qigong treatment can indeed be measured.

CELLS CULTURED UNDER STRESSFUL CONDITIONS ARE GOOD TARGETS

Prior work with psychoenergetic models indicated that unstable or *poised* systems are more susceptible to mental influence than stable systems (Pleass & Dey 1990, Tiller 1991). To explore this possibility, we conducted informal experiments with human glioma cells cultured at concentrations of growth serum that were either within the standard range used in cancer research or extremely low. The concentration of growth serum in the cell culture media is a critical determinant of the behavior of cultured cells including the responsiveness of cells to external stimuli, with low concentrations (0.1%) representing a stressed or relatively unstable condition. The qigong practitioners and psychic healers collaborating in the experiments delivered various forms of healing treatment to both groups of cells at the same time. Another group of cell culture plates was removed from the incubator at the same time and kept in a separate room during the treatment period to serve as a control group. The separate

room control plates also included both normal and extremely low growth serum concentrations. Two days after treatment, the number of living cells in each treatment group was assessed and some dramatic differences between the treated samples and the separate room controls were observed for the cells cultured at low serum concentration. No difference was observed between the two groups of cells cultured at the normal concentration of growth serum.

These data are consistent with the hypothesis that cells cultured under stressful conditions (low growth serum) are preferred targets for detecting the influence of qigong treatment. We therefore used this model system to design a pilot study.

PILOT STUDY WITH A QIGONG PRACTITIONER

We collected human glioma tumor cells in mitosis and cryogenically preserved them in aliquots. A fresh aliquot was thawed at the start of each trial to ensure uniformity in the genetic profile of the target cells throughout the study. Cell cultures typically include fractions of cells from all phases of the cell cycle; that is, they are asynchronous in relation to their cell cycle phase. Subtle cellular responses to therapeutic agents that are specific to a particular phase of the cell cycle can be undetectable in experiments utilizing asynchronous populations but revealed when synchronous populations are studied. We have adapted a mitotic selection protocol (Dewey et al 1970) that enables synchronization of human glioma cells in the G1 phase of the cell cycle, a phase during which the cells are highly susceptible to therapeutic agents (Yount et al 1996). We reasoned that this adapted protocol might enhance our ability to observe cellular responses following qigong treatment.

At the beginning of each experimental trial (three trials total), an aliquot was thawed and the cells were seeded into 54 independent culture plates in medium containing a low concentration (0.1%) of growth serum. The wells were randomly divided into three treatment groups and placed in the incubator according to random position assignment. All of the cells were allowed to progress through the cell cycle to the window of susceptibility (early G1 phase) in the cell cycle prior treatment.

The first treatment group (18 independent plates) was carried to a separate room where the practitioner was waiting. He was instructed to keep a distance of more than 20 cm from the cells. (It is interesting to note that many of the healers chose, when given these instructions, to sit or stand across the room, much further away from the target cells.) In this first pilot study, we asked the practitioner to maintain the 'intent to kill' the cells during a 20-minute treatment period. Simultaneously, a second group of 18 plates was kept outside of the incubator but in a separate room. Immediately after the first two groups of cells were returned to the incubator, the third group was brought in front of the practitioner while he sat calmly in his meditative state for 20 minutes and then the plates were returned to the incubator. This third treatment group was labeled 'neutral intentionality' because the healer was not asked to try to kill the cells. The following day, a scientist blinded to the experimental conditions assessed the growth rate of the cells in each individual well and did so every 7 days for 3 weeks. At the end of the 3-week period, the data were faxed to a scientist holding the blinding codes and the code was broken. The exact protocol was repeated a total of three times with the same practitioner.

Results of the Pilot Study Show High Degree of Variability

The number of cells in the 'neutral intentionality' group was significantly reduced compared to both of the other treatment groups when measured 3 weeks after treatment by the qigong practitioner ($P < 0.0001$). The low levels of growth serum in the culture medium caused the cell populations in the 'separate room control' treatment group to decline over the observation period but, remarkably, the cell populations in a majority of the culture plates in the 'neutral intentionality' group had died off almost completely by the third week of observation.

The cells in the 'intent to kill' treatment group died off more rapidly than those in the 'separate room control' group in the first trial but in the second and third trial the effect diminished. These data immediately raise the question: 'Why was there more cell death when the practitioner was not trying to kill the cells?' The answer given by some in the qigong community is that maintaining the 'intent to kill' is unnatural for a practitioner who has devoted a lifetime to healing, therefore, this experimental condition would interfere with the practitioner's natural healing *potency*. On the other hand, sitting in a calm meditative state, as was done in the 'neutral intentionality' treatment group, might allow a practitioner's natural healing influence to operate. The qigong practitioners felt that the reason the 'neutral intentionality' treatment group displayed the most robust response is that this experimental condition allowed the practitioner to behave naturally.

Assuming that a general healing influence could be exerted by a qigong practitioner maintaining a calm meditative state, the next question raised by the data is: 'Why did the cells die in response to healing?' Modern oncology offers an answer to this question. Cancer cells from tumor cell lines are thought to have outlived their natural lifespan; the term used in oncology is that the cells have become immortalized. Theoretically, healing a cancer cell would involve the eradication of this immortal characteristic and the result would be the long overdue natural death of the cell.

The high degree of variability in the response of the cells between trials limits the ability to draw conclusions from the pilot data. During the first trial, the degree of cell death observed in the cancer cell populations was significantly greater in both the 'intent to kill' and 'neutral intentionality' treatment groups as compared to the separate room control group, but this effect declined dramatically with each subsequent trial. The source of the variability may be related to waning interest or enthusiasm of the participants in the experiment. A similar decline effect has been described in the parapsychology literature for other experiments involving remote human influencers

(Dunne et al 1994). Numerous other sources of variability are possible, ranging from variation due to operations such as handling and processing of cell samples to more speculative possibilities such as a non-local adaptation response occurring within the genetically identical tumor cell population despite the physical separation of the cells into frozen aliquots.

Systematic Negative Controls: Minimizing Significant Systematic Errors

To address these issues of variability, we adopted the 'systematic negative control protocol' developed by Walleczek et al (1999) for the evaluation of weak electromagnetic field-induced effects on cultured cells (a model system with a similar potential for variability). According to Walleczek and colleagues, 'The systematic negative control protocol is defined as the conduct of sham treatment compared to simultaneous negative controls (i.e., sham/sham runs) alternated with, and equal in number to, real treatment compared with simultaneous negative controls (i.e., field/sham runs)' (Walleczek et al 1999). Systematic negative controls allow the quantitative assessment of potential systematic errors associated with the methodology used and therefore test the method's accuracy and reliability throughout the experimental series.

The information gained from these systematic negative controls proved to be critical for evaluation of a formal study we performed with four qigong practitioners in San Francisco: a subtle effect was seen, and the first question was whether some aspect of the experimental manipulations could have been the cause. Likewise, questions about the potential influence of variations in the weather or other physical parameters between treatment sessions were raised. The systematic inclusion of the sham/sham runs every time a qigong/sham run was conducted allowed us to answer these questions. If an unknown aspect of the experimental conditions had influenced the target cells, this should have been evident in both types of runs. But differences were seen only in qigong/sham runs. Application of the same statistical analysis to an independent set of data obtained through the same protocol except for the qigong treatment greatly increased our confidence that the effect was due to some aspect of the experimental intervention.

SAN FRANCISCO FORMAL STUDY

Culture of Target Cells and the Outcome Measure in San Francisco Study

Normal human astrocytes were grown to a large population size, aliquoted, and frozen viably for long-term storage. One hundred cells were plated into each of 12 cell culture plates, each labeled with a five-digit identifying code produced by a random number generator. The plates were placed into randomly assigned positions in an incubator. The outcome measure was cell growth assessed using the colony-forming efficiency assay. Colony-forming efficiency measures a cell's ability to duplicate itself again and again, forming a colony, under various treatment conditions. We purposefully seeded the cells sparsely into the plates so that any colonies that grew would not overlap and make accurate counting difficult. However, because human cells have difficulty growing in isolation (they do better with plenty of neighbors), these cells were growing under 'stressful' conditions. The methodology, first developed in the 1950s (Puck & Marcus 1956), was considered the gold standard assay in studies of *in vitro* sensitivity to therapeutic agents by the 1970s (Weisenthal & Lippman 1985). It remains a mainstay in the measurement of cell response *in vitro* (Gupta et al 1996).

Blinding Procedures: Prevention of Measurement Skewing

Each experimental trial consisted of two sessions conducted on the same day: either qigong/sham or sham/sham. Trials were conducted in five blinded steps, with blinding applied to each scientist having contact with the cell cultures, not just to the data collector. The blinding steps were as follows:

1. Scientist 1 prepared 12 cell cultures, labeled them with random identifying codes, and placed them into their randomly assigned positions in a cell culture incubator, blinded to the treatment conditions. This scientist then supplied the identifying codes to a biostatistician, who established randomized assignments to treatment boxes.

2. On the following day, scientist 2 transferred half of the culture plates (six independent samples) from the incubator (according to the plan supplied by the biostatistician) into positions randomly assigned in an opaque plastic box (box A). Scientist 2 then carried the box to the treatment room (about 15 meters away), immediately left the area, returned 30 minutes later to carry the box back, and placed the samples in their original positions in the incubator. This was repeated immediately for the second session of the trial, with the remaining half of the plates in box B. Scientist 2 was blinded to whether a treatment would occur.

3. Each session was either (a) a sham session, with the treatment room remaining empty, or (b) a qigong session, with a practitioner escorted into the room to conduct the qigong treatment. (Both the practitioner and the escort were blinded to the identifying codes on the plates.) Each trial was randomly assigned as qigong/sham or sham/sham. The qigong treatment on a qigong/sham trial was randomly assigned to either box A or box B.

4. After being returned to the incubator, all cell culture plates remained in position for 2 weeks to allow time for cells to divide and form colonies. Colonies were then counted by scientist 3, who remained blinded to the treatment conditions. Data were collected using only the random identifying codes.

5. The random codes were kept by an outside institute. Statistical analysis was conducted by a biostatistician blinded to what treatment each group had received. The data analysis was completed using only the code number of the group. The code was revealed after completion of the statistical analysis.

San Francisco Study: Trend Observation

A formal study was conducted in collaboration with four qigong practitioners in San Francisco. During a treatment session, a practitioner was escorted into the room and performed the same style of meditative practice that would be used to give a healing treatment to patients for 20 minutes. A distance of at least 20 cm was maintained from the box. Data analysis showed that more colonies had grown in the treated plates than in the sham plates. This increase in colony forming efficiency approached but did not reach statistical significance. The sham/sham trials did not show this trend. We used these results to calculate an appropriate sample size to test the reproducibility of the apparent trend.

BEIJING STUDY

Power Analysis for Formal Study in Beijing

A power analysis was conducted based upon the size of the average difference between the sham/sham and the qigong/sham trials. The effect size indicated that 28 more trials (14 sham/sham and 14 qigong/sham) would be needed to confirm the preliminary result. We moved the experiments to China through a collaboration with a laboratory in a major cancer research hospital in Beijing, China. Nine practitioners from four nearby traditional Chinese medical institutions participated in the study. We completed 29 trials (one more than required by the power analysis).

The colonies were permanently fixed to the plates at the end of each trial, and the plates were carried back to San Francisco.

Beijing Study: The Trend Confirmed

The results of the Beijing study were statistically significant. The trend seen in the San Francisco study was confirmed, that is, the astrocytes formed more colonies in the plates treated by qigong than in the sham plates. The dependent variable in this study was the ratio of the colony forming efficiency between box A and box B for a given trial. The colony forming efficiency for the six plates in each box were averaged to find the mean following standard and previously published methods (Gupta et al 1996, Yount et al 1996) and the ratio of the averages (A/B) computed, giving a single data point for each trial.

For each trial, box A was presented first and box B second. In order to rule out the possible effect of sequence on the results, the A/B colony forming efficiency ratios for all trials were tested against the null hypothesis of A/B colony forming efficiency ratio = 1, using the single mean t-test, two-tailed. For the eight trials conducted in San Francisco, the mean A/B colony forming efficiency ratio was 0.97, $t(7) = -0.95$, $P = 0.376$. Similarly, in Beijing, the 29 trials showed a mean A/B colony forming efficiency ratio of 0.97, $t(28) = -0.91$, $P = 0.373$. For all 37 trials, the mean A/B colony forming efficiency ratio was 0.971, $t(36) = -1.14$, $P = 0.263$. No significant difference occurred, therefore, between the colony forming efficiency of the boxes presented first or second. Next, the colony forming efficiency ratios for all qigong/sham trials in which the qigong treatment was applied to box B (second session) were inverted. In this way, the colony forming efficiency ratios for all qigong/sham trials would be in the same direction, with the directional research hypothesis that qi/sham colony forming efficiency ratio > 1.

Because some of the trials were conducted in San Francisco and some in Beijing, we next considered location as a blocking factor, that is, we determined whether the results differed from one location (block) to the other. A variation in the protocols used in the two locations was the involvement of different practitioners. A 2×2 factorial analysis of variance (ANOVA) was conducted, with the first factor being the blocking factor (SF $vs.$ Beijing) and the second factor being the type of trial (qigong/sham $vs.$ sham/sham). The blocking factor showed no significant difference in the results between locations (F[1,33] = 0.79, $P = 0.381$), and there was no significant block by trial type interaction (F[1,33] = 0.03, $P = 0.875$). Thus, the results did not differ significantly

between locations and could be pooled for an overall analysis.

Next, the colony forming efficiency ratios for sham/sham trials (SNCs) were tested against the null hypothesis of the colony forming efficiency ratio = 1 using the single mean t-test. The sham/sham trials did not differ significantly from chance expectation. The four San Francisco sham/sham trials resulted in a mean colony forming efficiency ratio of 0.972 (SD = 0.129), yielding $t(3) = -0.43$. The 15 Beijing sham/sham trials resulted in a mean colony forming efficiency ratio of 1.020 (SD = 0.183), which gives $t(14) = 0.43$. Combined, these 19 trials resulted in an overall mean colony forming efficiency ratio of 1.010 (SD = 0.171), yielding $t(18) = 0.26$. None of these values approaches statistical significance. The effect sizes are 0.21, 0.11, and 0.06 respectively. Because these trials were conducted under blind assessment, we can therefore be assured that no systematic errors influenced the outcome (see Table 20.1, sham/sham column).

The actual intervention trials, or qigong/sham trials, did show statistically significant deviations from chance expectation (colony forming efficiency ratio = 1) in the predicted direction. The four San Francisco qigong/sham trials resulted in a mean colony forming efficiency ratio of 1.042 (SD = 0.046) and yielded $t(3) = 1.84$. This trend did not reach statistical significance ($P = 0.082$, one-tailed) at the 5% level. The 14 Beijing qigong/sham trials resulted in a mean colony forming efficiency ratio of 1.111 (SD = 0.169), however, yielding $t(13) = 2.46$, $P = 0.014$, one-tailed (statistical significance at the 5% level). The combined data had a mean colony forming efficiency ratio of 1.096 (SD = 0.152), yielding $t(17) = 2.68$, $P = 0.008$, one-tailed (statistical significance at the 5% level). The effect sizes for the San Francisco and the Beijing qigong/sham trials were 0.92 and 0.66 respectively, and the overall effect size for the combined data was 0.63.

Overall, the qigong-treated samples showed about 10% greater colony forming efficiency than the simultaneous sham samples. Table 20.1 summarizes the mean colony forming efficiency ratios, t-tests, and effect sizes for the sham/sham and qigong/sham trials in the San Francisco

Table 20.1 Tests of null hypothesis that average colony-forming efficiency ratios = 1.0

Trial block	Statistics	Qigong/sham	Sham/sham
San Francisco	MN (SD)	1.042 (0.046)	0.972 (0.129)
	t	1.839	−0.427
	P	0.084	0.343
	Effect size (d)	0.920	0.214
Beijing	MN (SD)	1.111 (0.169)	1.020 (0.183)
	t	2.46	0.433
	P	0.014*	0.336
	Effect size (d)	0.658	0.112
All trials	MN (SD)	1.096 (0.152)	1.010 (0.171)
	t	2.675	0.264
	P	0.008**	0.398
	Effect size (d)	0.631	0.061

Note: One-tailed P values; $*P < 0.05$.; $**P < 0.01$.

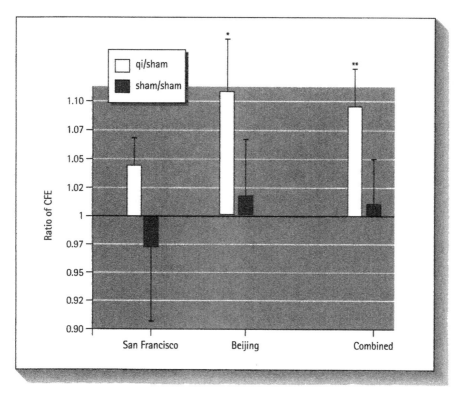

Figure 20.1 Means and error bars (1 SEM) for colony forming efficiency ratios of qigong/sham and sham/sham trials.

and Beijing studies separately and combined. Figure 20.1 displays the means and error bars (1 SEM).

To be certain of the analysis, we provided the data from all trials to a biostatistician, who was not aware of which trials were qigong/sham and which were sham/sham. He examined the data and conducted an analysis, utilizing a logarithmic transformation of the data and single mean, two-sided t-tests of the null hypothesis that the log mean is zero (i.e. ratio equals 1.0). After he had completed his analysis, the code was supplied to him. His independently produced results conformed to our original analysis. Sham/sham trials showed no statistically significant deviations from chance expectation ($t = 0.09$, $P = 0.47$ for Beijing trials) but qigong-treated samples did show a statistically significant advantage over sham treatment ($t = 2.33$, $P = 0.032$ for Beijing trials).

We explored other possible explanations for the effect. We used ANOVA to test whether position in incubator was confounded with qigong treatment (i.e. that the position was causing the effect rather than the qigong). We found no relation between position and colony counts ($P = 0.999$). We also used ANOVA to test whether the order in which the experimental runs were performed and the order in which the samples were analyzed affected plate counts. We found that these factors did not matter

($P > 0.05$). Of the variables analyzed, only qigong treatment was associated with the increase in colony formation.

CONCLUSION

The results found in the formal studies in San Francisco and Beijing are provocative and while they leave many questions unanswered about what aspects of the experimental intervention are influencing the cultured cells, they validate the *in vitro* protocol as a tool for the evaluation of distant healing modalities. The *in vitro* model is sensitive to subtle external influences and provides a well-controlled environment for quantifying objective measures. These measures can be easily replicated by independent laboratories to evaluate both the efficacy of distant healing and the treatment features that affect it.

REFERENCES

Dewey W C, Furman S C, Miller H H 1970 Comparison of lethality and chromosomal damage induced by X-rays in synchronized Chinese hamster cells *in vitro*. Radiation Research 43: 561–581

Dunne B J, Dobyns Y H, Nelson R D 1994 Series position effects in random event generator experiments. Journal of Scientific Exploration 8: 197–215

Gupta N, Lamborn K, Deen D F 1996 A statistical approach for analyzing clonogenic survival data. Radiation Research 145: 636–640

Pleass C M, Dey D 1990 Conditions that appear to favor extrasensory interactions between *Homo sapiens* and microbes. Journal of Scientific Exploration 4: 213–231

Puck T T, Marcus P I 1956 Action of X-rays on mammalian cells. Journal of Experimental Medicine 103: 653–666

Tiller W A 1991 Three profound psychoenergetic experiments. Lectures of the Qigong Institute, East West Academy of Healing Arts, vol. 10

Walleczek J, Shiu E C, Hahn G M 1999 Increase in radiation-induced HPRT gene mutation frequency after nonthermal exposure to nonionizing 60 Hz electromagnetic fields. Radiation Research 151: 489–497

Weisenthal L M, Lippman M E 1985 Clonogenic and nonclonogenic *in vitro* chemosensitivity assays. Cancer Treatment Reports 69: 615–632

Yount G L, Haas-Kogan D H, Vidair C A, Haas M, Dewey W C, Israel M A 1996 Cell cycle synchrony unmasks the influence of p53 function on radiosensitivity of human glioblastoma cells. Cancer Research 56: 500–506

21

Challenges for healing and intentionality research: causation and information

Edwin May

This chapter describes a testable model of healing intentionality research that can distinguish between causal and informational explanations.

Modern scientific methods are based on empirical observation and the assumption that events always occur in a cause and effect manner which is propagated locally and forward in time. Many mental and spiritual healing systems do not assume that this type of primary causation is the mechanism followed in these practices. Modern physics has demonstrated that non-local, space–time communication does occur in a microscopic world but not on the macroscopic level. However, it is known that observation, measurement, and the application of consciousness are key to the manifestation of non-local effects.

The experiments described and evaluated in this book provide data that point to non-causal mechanisms operating in the realm of consciousness and healing. The relationship of consciousness – the subject of mental and spiritual healing – to our perceptions of space and time, cause and effect and the exchange of information in biological systems is still a profound mystery. In this chapter, Ed May offers us an approach to empirically test different models of causation and informational interaction between mind and events. By testing models such as this, we can go beyond incomplete perceptions imposed by materialistic thinking and begin to understand the underlying principles of mental and spiritual healing in more fundamental and scientifically grounded ways. **WBJ**

INTRODUCTION

The most recent and authoritative review of the efficacy of distant healing (Astin et al 2000) provides a mixed assessment. Astin and colleagues concluded that there was sufficient evidence of some sort of intentionality-associated anomaly. However, the study pool was too heterogeneous for a formal meta-analysis. They found that 57% of the studies reviewed (23 studies involving 2774 patients) reported statistically significant effects, more than 10 times the number of significant studies expected by chance. An overall effect size of ES = 0.40 ($P < 0.001$) could be computed for 16 of the 23 studies across three categories of distant healing, therapeutic touch, and prayer. Astin et al also reported a 'fail-safe N' of 63 studies, i.e. the number of studies with statistical outcomes averaging zero ($Z = 0$) to reduce the observed result above the significance level of 0.05.

Let us assume from this database that some extra-chance phenomenon is occurring. The explanatory possibilities then fall into two general categories:

1. Error
   a. statistical 'fluke'
   b. protocol issues (e.g., improper randomization, poor controls)
   c. incorrect analyses

2. Other mechanisms
   a. distant influence: the intention of the healer reaches into the patient's physiology and influences it appropriately
   b. self-healing: the patient senses, perhaps through telepathy or some other psi perceptual process, that she/he is the recipient of good intentions and self-regulates accordingly
   c. divine intervention: the patient is the recipient of a deity's good intentions, and by some method, including 2a or 2b above, is healed
   d. information: healing *per se* does not occur, but rather experimenters use their psi abilities to sort patients into control and treatment groups such that healing is mimicked

3. Non-mechanistic: healing is a miraculous manifestation of consciousness.

It is beyond the scope of the paper to examine each of these possibilities. Instead, we will focus on a comparison between explanations based on distant influence *vs.* informational processes (2a and 2d above).

POSSIBLE MECHANISMS

If we wish to answer the question 'Can distant healing actually produce positive health benefits?', then we must proceed beyond the observed effects in clinical studies and pursue the mechanism question more deeply. Many experiments involving anomalous effects at a distance can be interpreted equally well either as intention 'forcing' the world to align to one's will, or as psi-mediated judicious selection of data. Fortunately, there exists a set of protocols that is capable in almost all experimental circumstances of determining which of these two mechanisms best fits the observed data (May et al 1995a).

In distant healing studies there are a number of possible outcome measures depending upon the study design. For example, in a between-groups protocol, the dependent variable is compared between a control and a treatment group. In a within-group design, the dependent variable is compared in a given group before and after treatment. Regardless of the measure, if the outcome is evaluated statistically (i.e. the effects are observed in control groups or in baselines as well as in treatment groups or conditions), then, as we will demonstrate, informational processes can mimic healing outcomes when actual healing has not occurred.

Research parapsychology has demonstrated a clear correlation between human intention and the statistical behavior of truly random number generators (Radin & Nelson 1989). Thus, a possible mechanism that must be considered in between-group distant healing designs is that an individual (for example an experimenter) uses psi to interact with the randomization mechanism or procedure in such a way as to sort healthier patients into the treatment group and less healthy patients into the control group. The net effect of this sorting would be to mimic genuine healing.

In within-group designs, the psi-mediated informational processes arise not in the sorting of patients but in selecting which patients participate in the study in the first place. In this case, using psi, experimenters tend to select patients who would have spontaneously improved over the course of the study even with no healing taking place, and they tend not to select patients who would not improve.

In the next sections we will outline a formal model of how this may occur, provide examples from the psi literature, and suggest protocols for healing studies that may isolate which of the competing hypotheses best fits the observed results.

DECISION AUGMENTATION THEORY

Background

A quantitative theory for treating psi-mediated data selection has been developed. This is called decision augmentation theory (DAT). May et al (1995a) formalized an idea that had its origin in much earlier psi research (Stanford et al 1975). It was Stanford's insight that an organism may use psi to select a path to a more desirable future among all possible less desirable futures. May et al extended the idea in that if psi is one way we can obtain information about the environment, then it would be most peculiar if that information was not integrated into the normal decision process. For example, suppose you had to decide when to cross the road? Inputs to that decision could include the following:

- *Real-time information.* The cars are speeding by – do not cross the road.
- *Past experience.* There is a car approaching, but you know from experience you cannot run fast enough to dash across before it comes – so you do not cross the road.
- *Intuition.* You cannot overtly hear, see, smell, or feel a car coming from around the bend in an otherwise clear road, yet you intuitively decide not to cross and in doing so avoid getting hit.

The above list of 'normal' factors that figure in decision-making can be extended through DAT by adding psi information as an additional input to augment the decision toward a favorable outcome. This simple idea has been applied to a large database of random number generator experiments and to a biologically oriented psi experiment (May et al 1995b).

Theoretical Outline

One goal of experimental science is to determine 'reality' as accurately as possible. No measurement is perfect, so the goal is to reduce sources of errors. All measurements contain two sources of errors: the first random and the second systematic. Random errors arise after many repeated measures. For example, suppose we wished to assess the efficacy of a drug. Suppose further that the outcome measure is the number of bacteria per milliliter of blood. The statistical spread of results after many independent measures is called random error.

The second source of error is called systematic. In our example, a systematic error would arise if the graduated cylinder in which we measured blood volume was marked slightly wrong. That is, what we believe was 1 ml is actually 0.9 ml. Therefore every measure of the number of bacteria per ml of blood will be slightly larger, and incorrect.

Another way to think about a systematic error is to ask whether nature is influenced or changed in some way, or not. Suppose in our example that the drug did *not* reduce the bacteria count, but a systematic error caused us to underestimate the blood volume. Then we might incorrectly conclude that the drug did reduce the bacteria count and nature was changed, when in fact it was unchanged.

It is beyond the scope of this chapter to delve into measurement theory, but suffice it to say that one goal of the experimental sciences is to reduce these two sources of errors as much as possible. Figure 21.1 shows an example of two measurement distributions, one with a systematic error and one without a systematic error. These are called *biased* and *unbiased* sampling distributions, respectively.

When measurements do not contain systematic errors, they can provide an accurate approximation of reality. However, if measurements contain an unknown systematic error, they become increasingly inaccurate and misleading depending upon the magnitude of the systematic error.

To fairly and comprehensively assess the efficacy of what appears to be distant healing, we must identify and understand the potential sources of systematic errors. If we believe our measurements are free of systematic error but in actuality they are not, then a case can be made that distant healing, conceived as an influence like a conventional medical intervention, may not be occurring at all. In the worst case, our measurements may have been flawed because of say, the use of 'dirty test tubes.' In a more subtle case, which is where DAT comes in, is the possibility that our measurements have been contaminated by psi-mediated systematic errors.

Figure 21.2 shows the situation under an influence hypothesis. The right curve represents the behavior of the natural system that has been changed (e.g. patients are healed) and our measurements contain no systematic error. The left curve represents mean chance expectation (MCE), i.e., what we would expect in the absence of an influence (e.g. patients are not healed).

As in Figure 21.1, these curves are also sampling distributions, but by construct they do not contain any systematic errors. As a result, they are good approximations of what is called the parent distribution or the inherent behavior of the natural system in question.

It is beyond the scope of this chapter to provide a complete mathematical derivation of the DAT formalism based on the assumptions shown in Figures 21.1 and 21.2; however, these assumptions lead to vastly different predictions in a variety of experimental circumstances.

Here, we outline how these ideas translate into a workable protocol to help determine whether our measures contain psi-mediated systematic errors and healing is mimicked, or our measures are free of systematic errors and healing is genuine. In other words, we will propose a

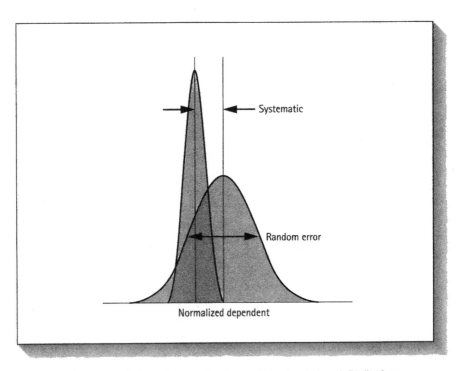

Figure 21.1 Schematic example of an unbiased and biased distribution.

methodology to answer the question we asked at the beginning of the chapter, namely 'Can distant healing actually produce positive ealth benefits?'

Region of Validity for DAT

Most models have a region in which they are valid. Galilean relativity, for example, is valid only at low velocities whereas Einstein's special relativity is needed when velocities are near to the speed of light. Similarly, quantum theory is valid for very small particles such as atoms or molecules and is not required for larger chunks of matter such as bowling balls and people.

Decision augmentation theory (DAT) is valid when the outcome of a series of measurements, each resulting from a single decision, are within a few standard deviations from chance. Most medical, biological, social, and psychological research results fall into this region. Another way of looking at this is to ask whether the observed effects also occur in the control group, just less often. If the answer is 'yes,' then DAT is applica-ble. If the observed effect never happens in the control group, then DAT is not applicable.

DAT and Influence Predictions

Because we are working in a statistical regime, we assume that the dependent variable may be converted to a standard normal deviant or Z score. We further assume that an independent variable, n, is defined in the protocol that counts the number of observations taken together. For instance, this variable might be the number of patients who are the recipients of a single healing session all at the same time, the number of binary bits obtained with a single button press in a random number generator experiment, the number of test tubes subjected to psi effort in one session, or the number of independent decision points in a given session.

Figure 21.3 presents mathematical models for mean chance expectation (i.e., nothing going on), for influence (i.e. causal force), and for DAT (i.e. psi-mediated sorting).

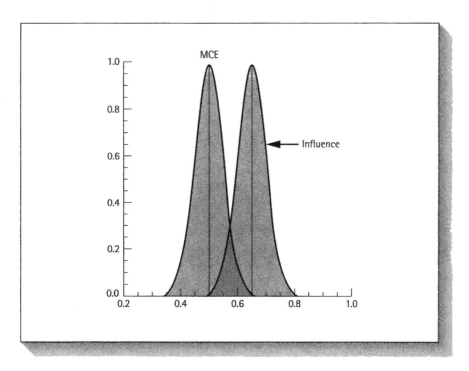

Figure 21.2 Probability of the dependent variable. MCE, mean chance expectation.

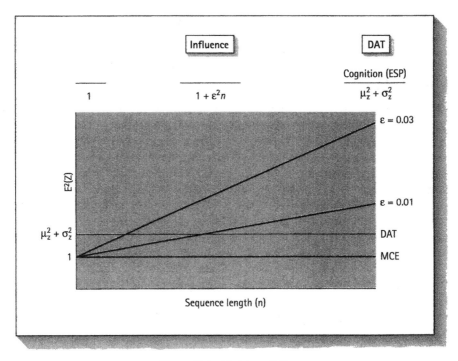

Figure 21.3 Model predictions.

Figure 21.3 plots the expected value of Z^2 against the number of samples in a given observation, which we call the sequence length. Here μ_z and σ_z are the mean and standard deviation of the distorted sampling distribution and ε is a hypothesized force-like effect size. The curves in Figure 21.3 show what is expected for a simple regression analysis of Z^2 versus n for a number of different sessions. The curves labeled with values of ε represent the best-fit lines to a causal or a force-like phenomenon.

The analysis of any set of data now becomes quite straightforward. Place all of the experimental trials on a Z^2 versus n scatter plot and simply conduct a least squares fit to a straight line (i.e. single regression analysis). If the slope is statistically positive, then a force-like mechanism is the best fit to the data; if the slope is not significantly positive, yet the intercept is significantly greater than 1, then an informational model (i.e. DAT) is the best fit to the data. Mean chance expectation is confirmed if the slope and intercept are not significantly different from 0 and 1, respectively. The next two sections apply the DAT analysis to the

psi random number generator database and to a biological psychokinesis experiment.

Application to the Random Number Generator Database

The basic claim of the psi random number generator (RNG) database is that there is a persistent and significant correlation between the output of true random number generator devices and human intention (Radin & Nelson 1989). In these types of experiments, a physical binary random number generator is constructed which generates a sequence of 1s and 0s, using either an electronic noise or a radioactive source as the basis of randomness. Usually the subject in these experiments is instructed to 'cause' more 1s than are expected to appear in a specified number of random bits (i.e., n in the above description).[1] The dependent variable is related to the number of 1s

---

[1]There are many variations on this theme. We have chosen this simple description for clarity.

observed in the *n*-bit sequence generated by the device. The *Z* score is constructed as:

$$Z = \frac{(\text{no. of 1s} - 0.5n)}{0.5\sqrt{n}}$$

This relation assumes a binary generator where the probability of observing a 1 is 0.5. May et al (1995b) analyzed 128 published studies from 1969 through 1989 according to the method outlined above. Figure 21.4 shows the result of this analysis.

From Figure 21.4 we can reject a force model. The line labeled DAT and the dashed lines surrounding it represent the best-fit line to the data and the one standard error bars associated with the slope. The single error bar in the center of the sequence-length axis is the standard error for the intercept, which is many (i.e. 6.4) standard errors away from MCE. The sloping and labeled dotted lines represent where the best-fit line would have been for two different values of the force-like strength parameter.

To understand what this means in terms of selection rather than force, consider a simple example. Suppose we used a fair coin flipper and

proceeded to generate 10 000 independent coin flips, and we then wrote down on a long piece of paper the result of each flip (e.g. HTTHTH-HTHTH . . . and so on). Now we ask you (the subject) to examine this long record and 'decide' where to draw a red line so that the next 100 coin flips beyond your line contained an excess of heads. Even for a fair and truly random coin flipper, you would have no difficulty in accomplishing that task because of the nature of truly random binary sequences, which tend to drift towards slightly more positive or negative regions at times. In the real world of RNG experiments, DAT hypothesizes that research participants use their psi abilities to peek into the future to decide when to start counting so as to have a large number of 1s in the next *n* bits. In other words, research participants become psi-mediated statistical opportunists rather than agents of force.

Application to a Biological System

In 1987, we provided a grant to Dr William Braud, then of the Mind Science Foundation in

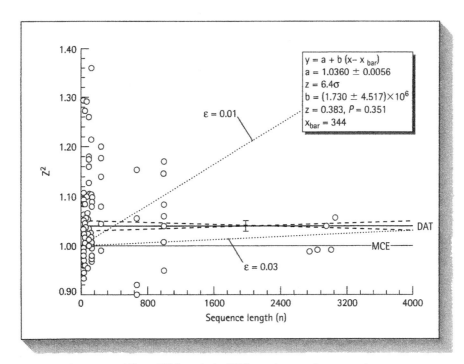

Figure 21.4 Binary RNG analysis. RNG, random number generator.

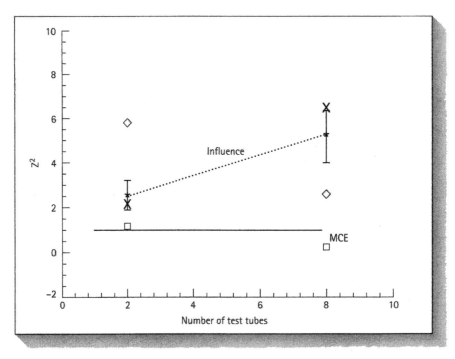

Figure 21.5 DAT analysis of Braud's hemolysis experiment (Braud 1990).

San Antonio, Texas,[2] to test the DAT hypothesis in a biological system. Braud (1990) conducted a carefully designed experiment on the hemolysis rate (the rate of red blood cell destruction in a saline solution) as a function of a healer's intention to slow the rate.

Research participants were asked to slow the hemolysis rate of red blood cells contained in either two or eight test tubes, and they were blind to the number of test tubes (n in the above model).

Figure 21.5 shows a DAT analysis of the results. The horizontal line represents $Z^2 = 1$ (i.e., MCE). The stars and their associated one standard-error bars represent the observed data. The open squares represent the experimental controls. Note that for the controls, the standard errors are smaller than the symbol. The xs represent the force-like prediction, and the open diamonds represent the DAT prediction. As in

Figure 21.3 above, the sloping dashed line represents the force-like model.

In this case, it is very clear from the results shown in Figure 21.5, that the force hypothesis is a significantly better fit to the data than is the DAT hypothesis. In other words, Braud's results suggest that the participants used their mental intention ability to 'reach in and shield' the blood from the destructive influence of the saline solution.

Of relevance to this observation is our extensive interaction with Russian psi researchers, who have conducted many more studies involving biological systems than European or American psi researchers (May & Vilenskaya 1992, Vilenskaya & May 1993). Predominantly, the Russian's opinion is that intentional force is impossible on inanimate systems but possible on biological ones. The RNG experiments and the hemolysis experiment appear to support their views. However, we should keep in mind that there were 128 independent studies in the RNG database and only one hemolysis experiment of this type.

---

[2]At that time the author was director of the research section of what became known as the US government program called STAR GATE.

DISCUSSION AND CONCLUSION

It is clear from the RNG analysis that humans seem to be able to make psi-mediated decisions that optimize the statistical outcome of electro-mechanically, electrically, and radioactive-based binary random number generators without exhibiting force-like influence on the devices. In addition, Radin & May (1986) found that DAT could be observed using pseudorandom computer-based generators without any evidence that the computer was influenced.

Therefore, as we said at the outset, it is possible that what appears to be intentional healing at a distance may be DAT instead. This possibility arises because the healing results all appear to be in the statistical regime – the region in which the DAT model is applicable.

The DAT model may seem pessimistic because it implies that genuine interventions do not occur in cases of apparent distant healing, but it does provide us with a simple way to create protocols that can distinguish between the two hypotheses (influence vs. selection). One of these designs has been hinted in the body of this paper: namely, ask subjects to attempt to heal two different numbers of patients at a time, but keep them blind as to the number. For example, in some sessions healers would work all at once on four patients and in other sessions on 16 patients all at once. If a statistical outcome measure can be converted to a Z score, then the DAT hypothesis predicts the same result for both groups but the healing hypothesis predicts that the outcome (i.e. Z^2) of the group of 16 patients will be four times larger.

May et al (1995a) suggested a second approach to determine which mechanism better describes the data. This method is based upon the number of decision points in an experimental session. The more decision points there are, the more opportunities there are for DAT to appear. A healing study could also incorporate this concept in the experimental design.

However, regardless of the details of the study protocol, it is possible to determine whether healing involves a genuine distant influence, or if it simply reflects favorable sorting of patients.

REFERENCES

Astin J A, Harkness E, Ernst E 2000 The efficacy of 'distant healing': a systematic review of randomized trials. Annals of Internal Medicine 132(11): 903–910
Braud W G 1990 Distant mental influence of the rate of hemolysis of human red blood cells. Journal of the American Society for Psychical Research 84: 1–24
May E C, Vilenskaya L 1992 Overview of current parapsychology research in the former Soviet Union. Subtle Energies 3(3): 45–67
May E C, Utts J M, Spottiswoode S J P 1995a Decision augmentation theory: toward a model of anomalous mental phenomena. Journal of Parapsychology 59: 195–220
May E C, Spottiswoode S J P, Utts J M, James C L 1995b Applications of decision augmentation theory. Journal of Parapsychology 59: 221–250

Radin D I, May E C 1986 Testing the intuitive data sorting model with pseudorandom number generators: a proposed method. Proceedings of presented papers: the Parpsychological Association 29th Annual Convention. Parapsychological Association, Dunham, NC, pp. 539–554
Radin D I, Nelson R D 1989 Evidence for consciousness-related anomalies in random physical systems. Foundations of Physics 19: 1499–1514
Stanford R G, Zenhausern R, Taylor A, Dwyer M A 1975 Psychokinesis as psi-mediated instrumental response. Journal of the American Society for Psychical Research 69: 127–133
Vilenskaya L, May E C 1993 Anomalous mental phenomena research in Russia and the former Soviet Union: a follow up. Subtle Energies 4(3): 231–250

22

Challenges for healing and intentionality research: social dynamics involved in entering the mainstream

David Hufford

This chapter gives an overview of the challenges faced for any attempts to rigorously investigate spiritual healing by the social dynamics of the scientific process.

While modern science is based on empirical observation and theoretical testing, it is also a social process, applied by humans with all their biases and errors in judgment and interpretation. Maintaining open intellectual curiosity and a fair system for the exchange of ideas and information is key for the scientific process to reach its maximum potential. When dealing with concepts and observations that challenge some of our most deeply held assumptions about the nature of the universe, it can become difficult to remain open, objective, and rational. This is especially true when those concepts and observations draw into question the accuracy of deeply held personal perceptions and experiences.

In this chapter, David Hufford gives us an overview of how the scientific community can handle the challenge to study mental energetic and spiritual healing. By acknowledging that these social factors can either impede or enhance knowledge and understanding, we are challenged to explicitly attend to them in order to uphold the true spirit of scientific. **WBJ**

INTRODUCTION

This chapter aims to focus on the challenges preventing the entry of healing research into mainstream science. Before beginning my description and analysis I first examine a conceptual issue that is inextricable from many of the barriers and that makes discussion difficult. The issue is the question 'What are we talking about?' This is not a criticism but a legitimate challenge: the topic is diverse; most healing advocates feel that there is a unity of some sort here, but there is no single term that refers to the entire topic collectively.

DEFINING THE TOPIC

The relationship of spirituality, bioenergy healing, and mainstream science is a product of their histories, and the present outlook of each reflects a very different view of those histories. In the conventional view, modern medical science has retained all that was most effective during the ascent from pre-scientific superstition, while the obsolete ideas it discarded drifted downward and were preserved in the lower layers of culture (Brown 1975, Cobb 1958, Glymour & Stalker 1983), and complementary and alternative medicine (CAM) healing in general, and spiritual healing in particular, are seen as composed primarily of those mistaken and obsolete ideas. On the other hand many spiritual healing advocates see the history of conventional medicine as a progressive narrowing, in which much of value was ignored, discarded, or, in the case of non-Western cultures, never known. A part of what the conventional view sees as obsolete, healing advocates see as repositories of forgotten wisdom and knowledge (Fulder 1982, Grossinger 1982, Kaslof 1978, Martin 1981, Hastings et al 1981, Kourenoff 1971, Mehl 1981, Otto & Knight 1979, Scarpa 1981, Shealy 1975, Stuart 1975, Wallnofer & von Rottauscher 1965). From these diametrically opposed views of history arise the current barriers that prevent healing research from entering the scientific mainstream.

Subjects dealt with in this book include particular kinds of practice: intention, religious and spiritual practices in general, prayer of several kinds, direct mental influence, mind–matter interactions, 'energy,' external qigong, and music therapy, as well as a variety of methodological topics bearing on the study of these practices. These define the domain. They are good descrip-tions of current practice and language use. But note the relationships among these categories: they overlap extensively (for example, 'energy' and qigong); and some are potential explanations for others (for example, direct mental influence and prayer). Also, some are inherently spiritual, such as prayer, while others, such as music therapy, may sometimes be spiritual and at other times not – or at least the attribution of spirituality would be different for different people. Music therapy has already substantially penetrated conventional medical practice, while most of the other topics have not. The common thread is the absence of obvious, known biological pathways through which the reported effects of these practices could operate. That comprises a negative definition which is socially appropriate, because it is this absence that causes mainstream science to be uniformly skeptical and to place obstacles in the path of research and practice in these modalities. In that sense this large category is strategically important for spiritual healing research advocates. But we need to be aware that this may not be a unified category at all in terms of mechanisms or kinds of effects. Even the discernment of spiritual dimensions in each modality cannot assure us that they are deeply similar. For many people there is a spiritual aspect to architecture, to giving birth, to botany, to all of human life. Spirituality itself can be a straightforward conceptual category, but it does not automatically unite the various practices dealt with here unless one holds a theory of spiritual mechanisms that explains them all. Some healing advocates do and some do not, but most mainstream scientists would find such an overarching spiritual connection to be a major obstacle to acceptance as science. Science can, at least in theory, handle tangible outcomes of spiritual behavior. But science consistently rejects spiritual forces and mechanisms as topics for systematic research. (This does not mean that scientists in general reject the existence of spiritual mechanisms, only that they do not consider them appropriate to scientific analysis and theorizing.) I will discuss the reasons for this below.

Despite the challenge it poses to conventional science, this conceptual diversity of the topic of healing is what many of us would expect. And the work of understanding these varied modalities and distinctions is part of the job of research. But if this diverse category is what we are talking about, what should we call it? This is no idle question. The development of umbrella terms for CAMs coincided with their growing salience in our society. The terminological development, beginning in the late 1960s with wholistic healing, then holistic healing, to alternative medicine, to CAM, and recently integrative medicine, has both reflected and facilitated the topic's influence. We need a handy term for our own discourse, but we need also to think of the effect of such terms on the field's progress with regard to science and the public. Meanwhile, this chapter simply uses the term 'healing', a word with spiritual roots that is not much heard in conventional medicine. The term derives from the Indo-European root *kailo* meaning uninjured or of good omen, giving rise to such modern words as health, holiness, and hallowed (Morris 1978).

THE IMPORTANCE OF BARRIERS

Box 22.1 outlines some of the consequences of the barriers to research on healing found in conventional mainstream science.

I begin with the assumption that healing research and practice exist as a fairly widespread activity, that mainstream science is a recognizable category (albeit with fuzzy boundaries), and that barriers to the entry of healing into mainstream science must exist because: (1) healing practitioners often seek access to mainstream science audiences, settings, and resources; and (2)

Box 22.1 The importance of barriers: consequences of mainstream barriers to healing

- Bias against:
  publication
  funding
  promotion and tenure
- Legal and regulatory obstacles to practice, rooted in the research base and peer review
- The risk of torturous warping as the price of mainstream entry
  Think co-option. 'All those that pass muster are welcome'.

---

such healing efforts have not resulted in acceptance by the mainstream science community. Under current configurations of 'science' in the US, failure to gain acceptance within mainstream science presents major difficulties in doing good research, including bias against publication that impedes communication, bias against funding that impedes research activities, and bias in promotion and tenure that turns young academic scientists away from research in healing. Barriers also include legal and regulatory obstacles to practice that are rooted in the publication, research, and faculty development problems just noted. Crucially, they include the risk of torturous warping of theory and practice as the price of entry to the mainstream (see, for example, the ways in which acupuncture and osteopathy have changed almost beyond recognition as the cost of entry to even marginal acceptance by the medical mainstream). The case of parapsychology shows that this warping can even affect disciplines that seek admission and fail, illustrating the remarkable power of the institutions of science in our society.

SOURCES OF BARRIERS INTERNAL (WHOLLY OR PARTIALLY) TO MAINSTREAM SCIENCE

Sources of barriers discussed in this section are summarized in Box 22.2.

The Anomalous Nature of Healing, by Definition

The most fundamental barrier separating healing from mainstream science lies simply in the nature of healing practices: healing observations appear anomalous in the Kuhnian (Kuhn 1970) sense with respect to conventional paradigms because they lack an apparent biological mechanism. The power of this obstacle is enormous. We often speak of CAM in general as calling for a revolution in medical paradigms, but many important aspects of CAM do not involve true anomalies. For example, neither botanical medicine nor whole food diets involve any observation or interpretation that is actually outside the

---

Box 22.2 Sources of barriers discussed in this section are summarized in Box 22.2.

- The anomalous nature of healing, by definition
- The popular origins of current interest in HEALING *vs.* normal science processes
- History:
  lack of academic infrastructure
  healing as a unified entity
  religion
  vitalism
  parapsychology
  the phrenology–snake oil problem
- Concepts:
  philosophical
  theoretical
  prior plausibility
  methodological
  machine registry
  placebo
  ethical (paternalism)
- The guild interests of conventional science:
  competition for:
  authority
  patients
  status and prestige

---

paradigm of conventional medicine. In fact, botanical medicine was a large part of conventional medicine into the early 20th century; for example, *Echinacea* was widely used as an anti-infective agent until the advent of sulfa drugs in the 1930s. The resistance to plant medicines arose through the convenience of pure extracts and, later synthetics, together with a tendency to think of single causes. But no medical researcher would have declared synergism in complex compounds an impossibility. In whole foods Sylvester Graham initiated the claim that low fiber diets are harmful in the 1830s (Whorton 1988), but it was not until the work of Burkitt 140 years later (Burkitt et al 1972) that the high fiber diet began to penetrate conventional medicine. Yet no 20th-century physician would ever have said that it was impossible in theory for diet to affect health. In this case too, it was not anomalies that were the problem; the obstacle was all of the social and economic incentives for an interventionist medicine based on prescription controlled drugs. Healing, in contrast, encounters all the same resistance found by other CAM modalities, but the reports of spiritual healing really are anomalous in a Kuhnian sense. This is the most basic

obstacle and the source of most other obstacles encountered by healing.

The Popular Origins of Interest in and Demand for Healing

Because mainstream science and medicine have blocked the entry of healing, researchers and practitioners have had to develop their own channels and funding sources. Findings have often been published in popular magazines and books, private funding and new foundations have developed, and Congress has become involved. The foundation for such publication and funding and for the interest of Congress is the interest and the experience of ordinary people. CAM in general, and healing in particular, are grass-roots movements. This is a part of their strength, but it does not sit well with conventional scientists who see it as failure to go through proper channels crucial to scientific progress, channels that have been blocked by conventional peer review process. Going outside those channels, however, is stigmatized as a failure to meet high standards – Catch 22. To quote debunker Wallace Sampson, publication outside conventional scientific journals means: 'Disaffected commentators can now find their articles published after tying their imaginations to long tethers and following trails of thought less encumbered by brambles of rigorous methodology' (Sampson 1997, p. 4). The involvement of legislators is seen as the pernicious intrusion of politics into science. The enormous role of politics in conventional science is ignored, also on peer review grounds: as long as legislation and regulation follow from the advice of conventional experts (as, for example, the role of the FDA) it is legitimate. When those experts are absent it is assumed that legislators and the public are incapable of making sound judgments in science and medicine-related areas on their own.

The History of Healing is a Source of Many Current Obstacles

Healing has a long history of association with ideas and practices that have been rejected during the past two centuries of development in modern medicine. The most important of these associations impeding healing's entry into mainstream science is its obvious connection to religion. Spirituality is a personal orientation to the transcendent, which to almost all humans has meant to the world of spirits: God(s), angels, souls, Jinn, etc. Religion is the institutional aspect of this orientation. Therefore, not all spirituality is religious, but religions are inherently spiritual. In contemporary healing research non-institutional spiritual practices tend to be emphasized, but institutionally supported religious healing clearly fits any reasonable definition of our topic; for example, such healing practices as Catholic prayers to saints and touching their relics, or the Protestant use of anointing and laying on of hands, and the enormous variety of other healing practices found throughout the religions of the world. Therefore, although the spirituality–religion distinction is important and clear, the two are inextricably linked.

This link is a source of several barriers. First, religious doctrines are notoriously metaphysical, and religious beliefs are heavily dependent on faith. While it is often granted that religious systems have an internally consistent logic, their metaphysical base makes it impossible to systematically link that logic to other beliefs or hypotheses in a direct manner. Most religious understandings of faith remove any need for observational evidence. It was on this basis that Enlightenment skeptic philosopher David Hume argued that one can never have rational grounds for a belief in miracles – by which he meant any spiritual cause for an event in the world (Hume 1963). This was a central move in the development of the split between religion and science that has characterized the Enlightenment project. The contemporary consequence of this is the view of spiritual healing as non-rational, and therefore, presumably, not scientifically investigable.

This connection to religions brings a wide variety of additional barriers: internal to science, there is the Enlightenment science/religion split which will be discussed below; internal to religion itself are the exclusive claims of particular religions that reject the healing practices of others (as in Protestant Christian rejection of Catholic prayers to saints, or general Christian distinctions between the prayers of believers and those of others). To a conservative Christian, healing theory may seem to be heresy, especially the heresy of indifferentism – the idea that all religions are equally good. While many healing investigators may assume that this is true, most traditional believers reject the idea very vigorously.

Magic

Within spirituality and religion an additional complexity and source of barriers lies in attitudes toward magic. 'Magic' refers to the production of effects in the natural world through the influence of the supernatural, that is, spiritual causality. In anthropology magic has been contrasted to religion in terms of 'instrumentality,' so that magical practices seem intended to coerce spirits, while religion – more worshipful in focus – pleads with spirits. But the Protestant Reformation, as it rejected medieval Catholic thought, went further, increasingly construing as magic any spiritual practice intended to achieve a tangible result in the natural world (Thomas 1971). Spiritual practices intended to produce effects, including physical healing, therefore, were increasingly stigmatized within religious teachings. Researchers need to be sensitive to these concerns.

The religious rejection of magic parallels the academic tendency in science to interpret magical practices as primitive science, i.e. bad science. In this view magic is the part of religion that overlaps science and attempts things to which it is poorly suited. More modern religion, then, should be less magical, compete less with science. That would mean abandoning its efforts to affect the world directly by spiritual means, a view that is in direct conflict with any spiritually-based healing ideas except as those that can be symbolically mediated and limited to psychological and behavioral effects. This use of magic is a negative criterion found in much contemporary rhetoric against spiritual and energy healing, but perhaps its clearest statement is found in George R. Price's article 'Science and the supernatural' in *Science* (Price 1955). The article is a rejection of the claims of parapsychology by a scientist who admits, 'I myself believed in ESP about 15 years ago.' Price recovered from his belief, he explained, when he became familiar with Hume's argument that it is always more likely that people are lying than that natural law is being broken. For Price all paranormal effects (as for Hume all spiritual effects) break natural law. This is in itself a very large claim, and often repeated, though one that is quite dubious. Nonetheless, it has become so pervasive that even many believers in such things as the supernatural efficacy of intercessory prayer accept the idea that these effects contradict some scientific knowledge or method.

Price illustrates the role of magic in his rejection of parapsychology when he states the following rule: 'The essential characteristic of magic is that phenomena occur that can most easily be explained in terms of action by invisible intelligent beings. The essence of science is mechanism. The essence of magic is animism . . . . Whenever we can imagine any sort of detailed explanation without introducing incorporeal intelligences we should . . . regard the phenomenon open-mindedly.' Otherwise we should not.

Price's rule would appear to permit such healing effects as therapeutic touch which can be imagined as operating directly through some as yet unknown force, but it would exclude intercessory prayer as requiring invisible intelligences. That is because intercessory prayer studies involve the same problem that Price describes in distant ESP tests when one asks how the percipient finds the cards in the first place? To Price it seemed that some other intelligence would have to carry out numerous intervening steps in parapsychology experiments. Similarly, at a CAM conference in Boston (Complementary and Alternative Medicine: The Scientific and Pluralistic Challenge. Hastings Center Alternative Medicine Project, Harvard School of Public Health, Boston, December 1999), Relman asked concerning the recent Harris et al intercessory prayer study (1999),

'How do the prayers get to the right patients without even their full names?' Even with their last names, social security numbers and addresses, the problem seems to remain unless one opts either for fraud or for an invisible intelligence (although many researchers have suggested a variety of subtle alternative concepts). The former would be the skeptic's choice, the latter the believer's. In fact, it seems that many skeptics do not make such fine distinctions as Price, and reject as magical even those practices such as healing touch that in theory might involve truly novel energies without requiring spiritual aspects.

Parapsychology

The role of 'non-local effects' and 'subtle energies' in healing inevitably links it to parapsychology and to its antecedents such as mesmerism. This link itself yields barriers to mainstream entry, and further complicates the relationship of healing to religion.

Healing has been associated not only with spirituality and religion, but also with several other areas now viewed as obsolete and/or disreputable by mainstream science. Its association with mesmerism is one of these, since the ideas of animal magnetism and the use of trance have healing connections. In the 18th century the Swiss physician Franz Anton Mesmer learned to induce trance and immediately began to use it both for healing and to investigate what would later be called the 'paranormal.' Mesmer explained his observations in terms of a force which he called 'animal magnetism.' This hypothetical energy is conceptually close to many ideas of energy in healing, and Mesmer's method of transmitting this energy with his hands has an appearance similar to several healing modalities. Unfortunately Mesmer's theory and his healing practices remain well known in conventional circles today principally as a prime example of 'fringe science' and charlatanry. In 1784 a committee established by the French government declared Mesmerism worthless. But while this made mesmerism decidedly 'alternative' it did not make it unpopular. Mesmer's student De Puysegur carried out widely noted experiments that suggested the mesmeric state was conducive to psychic powers, and by the time Poyen introduced mesmerism to the US in 1838 the idea of mesmeric healing was well established. By 1843 there were more than 200 'magnetic healers' (i.e. mesmerists) practicing in Boston. Conventional science split off the idea of hypnotism from mesmerism, but even that move has not rescued hypnosis from marginal status, despite substantial medical potential in such areas as pain control. Mesmerism and magnetic healing have continued to exert a strong influence, at least in popular ideas of healing (Fuller 1989), and this connection has brought continued stigma to the topic from the conventional science view.

Almost equally problematic is the fact that healing and parapsychology as a field are historically and conceptually linked, and parapsychology has never achieved mainstream acceptance, partly for the same reasons that have prevented the entry of healing. Modern parapsychology developed initially from the spiritualist movement in Britain and the United States. Beginning with the efforts of transcendentalists such as Emerson and Thoreau, many 19th-century intellectuals felt that the science of their day had made traditional European religions hopelessly outmoded. Yet they still sought spirituality. One stimulus in these developments was the first English translation of the Hindu scriptures, the Upanishads. Since that time this strand of intellectual tradition, actually the beginnings of current 'New Age' thought, has been fascinated with Asian philosophy for a combination of spiritual and philosophical alternatives to Western scientific views (Melton 1990), a connection clearly evident in CAM. Spiritualism was advocated as a thoroughly empirical kind of religion, complete with experiment and belief based on evidence, and many important scientists joined the movement. However, spiritualism offers great scope for fraud, and disrepute was not long in coming. With the establishment of the British Society for Psychical Research in 1882 (and in 1885 the initial establishment of the parallel American organization), 'psychic science' began gradually to replace spiritualism with a less religious and more scientific orientation. Despite this shift and the work launched by J. B. Rhine in the 1930s at Duke University which led parapsychology to become a field devoted to great methodological rigor, and even despite efforts of intellectual leaders such as anthropologist Margaret Mead to gain entry for parapsychology to the American Association for the Advancement of Science, parapsychology has remained a thoroughly marginalized field. Given parapsychology's lack of funding and university infrastructure, it is remarkable that American parapsychology has managed to continue as a field. However, its marginalization has produced barriers for healing. Because the forces apparently involved in healing are not understood in conventional terms, they are not clearly distinguishable from those involved in parapsychological research (although some, or all, may actually be very different). As a consequence healing suffers from the stigma of parapsychology in the eyes of conventional scientists as well as in those of many religious people. This has equal impact on those who seek to use parapsychological data and theories to advance healing and on those who seek to avoid the parapsychology connection.

Vitalism

An emphasis on various kinds of 'energy' is almost universal in CAM and it is crucial in mediating the concepts of harmony, balance and integration. This element places these systems within the tradition that in Western thought has been called vitalism:

In general, vitalism is the belief that the activities of living organisms are due to a VITAL FORCE . . . that is different from other physical forces in the universe. Other names have been used for this living force or principle: DEMIURGE; ELAN VITAL; ENTELECHY; NOUS (PLATO); PSYCHE (ARISTOTLE). Vitalism . . . contend(s) that there is an ultimate, radical, and real dichotomy between living (organic) and nonliving (inorganic) phenomena . . . . Usually this force is regarded as being nonphysical, invisible, intangible, and . . . possessing a unity of its own that can exist independently of the physical bodies to which it gives life. (Angeles 1981, p. 314)

Vital force has been seen as the power behind emergent evolution, consciousness, self-regulation, and the innate healing capabilities of living creatures. Thus this concept provides links among a great variety of specific theories of healing and general physical and metaphysical theories. It is also one reason that CAM and religious beliefs have such a strong affinity. However, it is also the case that vitalism was explicitly discarded in the development of modern medicine and biology. As philosopher Simon Blackburn puts it: 'The consensus among philosophers and biologists is that it [vitalism] offers no explanatory advantage that the life sciences need' (Blackburn 1994, p. 395). The perceived obsolescence of vitalism, coupled with vitalism's strong apparent connection with CAM in general and healing in particular, gives healing an archaic look in the eyes of conventional scientists.

If these historical links to healing were simply mistaken, like the tendency of superficial skeptics to link all of CAM healing to phrenology and snake oil, the solution would be simple even if hard to accomplish: show that the links are mistaken. But the links just described, from religion through parapsychology, are not mistaken, rather they are misinterpreted. To some extent, rehabilitating healing in the eyes of conventional scientists will involve rehabilitating the conventional views of religion, parapsychology and quite possibly vitalism. That is no small challenge!

One final historical issue is worth noting here. Because healing has been thoroughly marginalized it has not developed the kind of academic infrastructure that has been so fruitful for mainstream science and medicine. History and philosophy of science, bioethics, medical sociology, and anthropology, such fields are a basic part of the infrastructure of conventional work. But while healing researchers often employ concepts and materials from such fields, most scholars in those fields have never paid any substantial attention to healing as a set of important modern practices. In general these fields are expected to provide a critical attitude toward the biases of the scientist and physician, but regarding CAM healing most of these scholars have simply replicated the biases

of the mainstream, when indeed they have acknowledged its existence. These fields serve solidly as a part of the social foundation of mainstream science and medicine. This is a two-fold challenge. Healing needs to develop a solid infrastructure of scholarship in order for theory and practice to grow in a thoughtful manner; and healing needs to counter the negative stereotypes typically purveyed by most scholars currently interested in health matters.

Concepts from Which Barriers to Healing Flow

These are summarized in Box 22.3.

Philosophical and Theoretical Concepts

Rationality is perhaps the most important of the philosophical concepts related to barriers to healing, and this is intimately connected with the theoretical issue of prior theoretical plausibility. A perfect example of this was provided on November 10, 1999, at a conference on CAM held in Philadelphia where Dr Marcia Angell, editor of the *New England Journal of Medicine*, participated in a panel that addressed questions of editorial bias against CAM. Disclaiming bias against good scientific studies of CAM, Angell stated that in order to be good a study must offer a plausible biological mechanism for effects reported. Otherwise, the study would not be believable. Therapeutic touch, homeopathy, moxibustion, and intercessory prayer, she said, are 'preposterous' and 'impossible' because they lack a plausible biological mechanism, and studies of these

---

Box 22.3 Concepts from which barriers to healing flow

- Philosophical
  rationalities
- Theoretical
  prior plausibility
- Methodological
  machine registry
  (the subjectivity problem)
- Ethical
  (paternalism)
- Placebo

practices are only being published for social and political reasons (Hufford 2001). These remarks extended views previously expressed in print. Similar comments were made by some of the other editors on the panel under the heading 'prior theoretical plausibility.' (Technically this is an inappropriate use of Bayesian reasoning, because a null prior probability does not compute in Bayes theorem (Murphy 1981, pp. 157–158); strategically, however, this use neatly removes challenging observations from consideration.) Each of these examples is notable for apparently involving 'energies' that cannot be registered by machines but that seem to have important effects on humans.

The theoretical plausibility criterion implies the following, each of which has often been explicitly stated by critics of CAM and implied by anthropologists studying apparently irrational beliefs, and all of which are related: (1) existing conventional scientific knowledge is an adequate measure of whether an unconventional claim is true. Therefore (2), if a practice lacks theoretical plausibility there is no reason to think that it may work; and (3) empirical evidence of an event that is not theoretically plausible can be rejected out of hand. (4) Acceptance of theoretically implausible claims would require the abandonment of current scientific knowledge.

Individually and as a group these ideas support expert paternalism and suggest that a process of free inquiry open to diverse views is unnecessary and counterproductive in science, except within narrow bounds internal to conventional science. In CAM this suggests that the patient's autonomous right to refuse conventional treatment and to use legal alternatives is merely the right to be wrong (Hufford 2001).

Rationality becomes an issue for two reasons. The first is that many conventional scientists share the view recently stated by Dennett & Rorty (2000) that science is rationality, that what is not scientific is not rational. This does not make literature or music irrational, but it does make knowledge claims that are not supported by conventional science irrational. Second, a central criterion of contemporary scientific method is reliance on observations that are what philoso-

phers call 'public.' That is, they can be made repeatedly by anyone with proper technique. The assurance of this public nature in modern science is the availability of mechanical instruments to record the observable facts. In October 2000 I participated in the Boston University Colloquium on Philosophy of Science and was somewhat surprised to find that even some fairly liberal philosophers of science still hold that influences that can only be registered by living systems and not by instruments (if there are such – a hotly contested point) do not count for science. And further, that thinking that relied on observations about such influences were not only not science but either not rational or used a 'different rationality' than science. If the rationality of healing research were, in fact, qualitatively different from that of mainstream science, this would constitute an insuperable obstacle. I am convinced that this claim about rationality is not correct, but this perception is widespread so that even those who would be scandalized by Angell's statements cited earlier actually hold views that are implicitly similar.

Methodological concepts

This issue of observation is a central methodological obstacle for healing. We may call this the 'machine registry' barrier. It arises from current notions about subjectivity and objectivity. This is a topic on which many healing researchers and practitioners disagree markedly with conventional scientists. Interestingly it is an issue on which a great many in modern society are changing their views. Pure 'objectivity' is increasingly being recognized as an impossibility, and subject–object boundaries are being reconsidered. In some ways this is helpful to healing researchers, but it also raises substantially the guard of conventional thinkers. For many scientists the interest in spiritual healing is another indication of the postmodern rejection of objectivity, a trend which they see as threatening rationality altogether.

Bioethics concepts

In medical ethics in recent decades the idea of patient autonomy has displaced paternalism.

The moral obligation of the doctor to serve the best interests of the patient has been increasingly understood as a process that must be governed by the views of patients concerning their best interests rather than the views of medical experts. But this is primarily when the decisions in question are those arising within conventional medicine, such as when to discontinue interventions to extend the life of a dying patient. When decisions cross into CAM terrain paternalism suddenly resurfaces and bioethicists begin to speak of 'autonomy run wild.'

One might reasonably expect that since spiritual healing is at least not directly dangerous from a medical point of view (granting the possibility of conflict with medical advice) it would not be resisted with as great vigor as, for example, botanical medicine in which there are some life-threatening risks. But for many critics spiritual healing does its harm by being 'corrosive of rationality,' along with all sorts of other stigmatized ideas, undercutting the ability of patients and the public to reason effectively and, concomitantly, to understand and accept the authoritative knowledge of science and medicine. In ethical terms these critics assert that acceptance of spiritual healing does break the 'do no harm' obligation for this reason (Scientific Review of Alternative Medicine 1997).

Placebo

Placebo deserves its own place here, since its current wildly varying usages defy categorization. Many healing researchers value the placebo response reasonably enough as a force for healing. The problem arises with the equivocal ways the term and concept are employed in general discourse. In its narrow meaning placebo effect essentially refers to the effect of one's expectation. If you expect a pill to make you feel better it is likely to make you feel better, not only because of the activity – if any – of its contents, but also because you expect it to. A lot is known about this basic response including that it varies among people, seems partly a heritable trait, washes out over a predictable span of time, and can, at least in part, be blocked by endorphin antagonists

such as naloxone. Under this meaning, explaining spiritual healing as placebo effect means that all the modalities could just as well be replaced by sugar pills given with a persuasive lie. The equivocal use of the term that includes very different and more powerful effects in CAM discussions results in confusion and apparent self-contradiction. Two *New York Times* (Blakeslee 1998, Talbot 2000) stories on placebo, in which every 'gee whiz' kind of result, including classical conditioning, was simply labeled placebo, illustrate some of these hazards. More recently, a meta-analysis of studies with both placebo and no-treatment arms has suggested that for most conditions the placebo is weak or non-existent (Hrobjartson & Gotzsche 2001). Advocates and critics of healing research alike display great ambivalence about placebo, alternately embracing and rejecting it depending on both its rhetorical use and the mechanisms called upon to explain it.

The Guild Interests of Mainstream Science and Medicine are Naturally to Protect the Status Quo

The claims and aspirations of spiritual healing are in competition with those already in the mainstream for cultural authority, funding, patients, prestige, and status. They also challenge the deeply personal emotional investment of mainstream scientists and doctors which is most often expressed in terms of commitment to the public good. This is a major source of paternalism. When this investment is challenged the response is often severe and couched in terms of protecting the public.

This rhetorical situation always arises in the case for powerful institutions and one need not reject the legitimacy of an institution to recognize it. But legitimate or not, these interests always constitute bias. Hammer has described the biasing influence of such interests very well:

Science is inherently a social process in which judgments are made about the validity and value of information in the context of the inherent human bias. While the tools of rigorous scientific methodology are designed to minimize judgment errors and bias, scientists are not themselves anymore rational and objective than any other human group (Collins, Hufford, etc.). Trust, a common world view, the ability to communicate, a cooperative intention and a willingness to change based on agreed upon rules are all necessary for the proper application of scientific methods. When these common values are shared . . . (i.e.) Under conditions of (Kuhn's) normal science, research methods increase objectivity and reduce bias. When a common 'paradigm' or world view is not shared, or when distrust and miscommunication exist between groups, then the value of scientific methodology for managing judgment errors and bias is ineffective (Berger, Feyerabend). Under these conditions, research methods often become tools whereby political power, social bias and judgment error confound and decrease objectivity. (M. Hammer, unpublished report, 2000)

This is the situation that exists between mainstream science/medicine and spiritual healing, and it may well be the most important underlying source of barriers to the entry of healing research to the scientific and medical mainstream.

SOURCES OF BARRIERS PARTIALLY EXTERNAL TO MAINSTREAM SCIENCE

Ironically, while spiritual healing's association with religion stigmatizes it in the eyes of some conventional scientists, religious believers comprise an additional challenge to spiritual healing. This is true in the public at large and also within science since various religious commitments are actually quite common among scientists and health care providers.

For example, O'Mathuna wrote a negative assessment of therapeutic touch in Micozzi's *Physician's Guide to Alternative Medicine* (O'Mathuna 1999). Although negative, he gave credence to adverse effects reportedly caused by therapeutic touch such as pain, nausea, and anxiety. In his article he makes no reference to spiritual issues. However, he also wrote 'The subtle allure of therapeutic touch' in the *Journal of Christian Nursing* (O'Mathuna 1998), published by the Nurses Christian Fellowship. Here he asserted that it is wrong to assume 'that if TT heals, it must be pleasing to God' . . . (this is called utilitarianism. The end justifies the means. 'While

God wants all people to have good health, the means by which health is obtained are also important to him . . . . We cannot assume that all healing from other sources ultimately pleases God . . . . Performing acts with good intentions and good results is not as important as the source of the power behind those acts. The Evil One has great powers at his disposal. TT introduces practitioner and patient to a spiritual realm forbidden by God.'

These religious attitudes are an understandable source of resistance among conservative Christians. Scientists are also human beings and their religious commitments – devout, atheist or agnostic – influence their judgments. But in the scientific literature the rhetoric of objectivity renders these commitments tacit and covert. In turn the invisibility of these barriers makes them all the more powerful.

MECHANISMS BARRING ENTRY
Peer Review Problems

In conventional science publication, funding, promotion and tenure are the backbone of the scientific process, and they are governed by peer review. Peer review is supposed to guarantee that decisions in these areas are made by true experts. Peer review has a natural built-in seniority system which in theory enhances the expertise of reviewers and gives a more unbiased view because senior scientists might be expected to be more secure. This works moderately well in mainstream science, especially with the most conventional work. In newer areas this process has an inertia, a bias toward what has been around a while, that can be a problem. In unconventional areas such as healing the peer review system is an absolute stopper. In the first issue of the *Scientific Review of Alternative Medicine* (Sampson 1997), the editor, Sampson said of preexisting CAM journals that 'at least one . . . claims that its articles are peer-reviewed,' but they are really devoted to 'articles and theories that are outside the borders of science and objective reality' (Sampson 1997, p. 4). Until the advent of his new journal, Sampson said, 'there has been no truly scientific, peer-reviewed journal specializing in [CAM] ACM.' Or, as he put it in an interview when asked about peer-reviewed work in a CAM publication, 'they may be their peers, but they aren't our peers.'

Rhetoric

The assertion of grave risk

Assertions of harm while denying possible good are standard, and Sloan and his colleagues have now twice stated that even the use of religious belief to comfort the desperately ill involves the risk of great harm (Sloan et al 1999, 2000).

The allegation of fraud and the devastation of science

The assertion of fraud is related to the assertion of grave risk. If a practice is fraudulent then it is by definition ineffective, therefore the risk:benefit ratio in such an instance is always unfavorable: the risk is always greater than possible benefit. Fraud and harm are also linked historically in the idea of quacks victimizing and harming innocent though gullible people. In spiritual healing modalities in particular, popular depictions such as that in Sinclair Lewis's novel *Elmer Gantry* suggest grave harm as the likely consequence of the quest for healing outside the domain of medicine. Angell's comments about claims to have achieved 'impossible' results, as quoted above, provide the rationale for assumptions of fraud; the view is the same as that offered by Hume 250 years ago: 'that it is always more likely that people are lying than that natural law is being broken' (Hume 1963).

This leads to a somewhat more subtle rhetorical challenge: that accepting the validity of spiritual healing would devastate science because it would contradict basic knowledge. An excellent example is found in Maddox's editorial accompanying Benveniste's 1988 paper in *Nature* on the biological effects of infinitessimal dilutions of anti-IgE antibodies (Davenas et al, 1988). The editorial was entitled 'When to believe the unbelievable.' Referring to the possibility of such dilute solutions having the reported effect as 'supernatural', he said that

Benveniste's observations 'strike at the roots of two centuries of observation and rationalization of physical phenomena . . . that a substantial part of our intellectual heritage should be thrown away' (Maddox 1988, p. 787). Actually there is nothing supernatural in the basic homeopathic ideas that may explain Benveniste's observations, and even if it were a 'supernatural' effect it would not in any obvious way contradict current scientific knowledge. It would be different, but it would not contradict. The assertion of contradiction without any careful effort to demonstrate that the alleged contradiction exists is a common rhetorical means for urging resistance to observations of healing. The tendency of skeptics to use spiritual cause as a stigmatizing interpretation of unconventional observational claims (as in Price's rejection of parapsychology as magical, noted above, and Maddox's characterization of homeopathy as supernatural) suggests how powerful this rhetorical device becomes when the observations are explicitly connected with spirituality.

Lumping

The tendency of conventional skeptics to view all spiritual healing modalities as pretty much the same is another important challenge. We might label this the 'lumping' challenge. Ultimately all healing topics may prove to involve similar or related mechanisms, or they may not. But certainly they each involve different protocols and different research questions, and the research on each proceeds at different rates. Therefore, the conventional assumption that criticism of any one aspect of spiritual healing research applies to all impedes the individual progress of specific areas of research.

HOW SHOULD HEALING RESEARCHERS RESPOND TO MAINSTREAM BARRIERS?

First, always fear co-option! Acceptance as mainstream science would solve many of the current problems of spiritual healing research. However, it seems unlikely that all of healing, regardless of the quality of research, will be admitted to the mainstream any time soon for the reasons discussed above. Admission without unacceptable distortion of healing would require major conceptual and structural changes in science institutions. Gradual change in this direction, following a Kuhnian (1970) model (opponents do not change their minds – they retire or die) is most likely. Appropriate entry of a few aspects of healing, assuming the integrity of the portions admitted – that is, avoiding the torturous warping noted above – will be good, because it will, first, advance the incremental change, second, familiarize conventional scientists with healing colleagues as solid researchers, and third, give those on the 'outside' friends 'inside.' This is already happening to some extent.

For those aspects of healing not admitted to science in the near term it seems desirable to develop alternative structures for supporting and disseminating research. Already there is substantial progress in the area of publishing. Granting the undesirability of ghettoizing healing, simply waiting for entry is not practical. We might even grant that some separations will be warranted long term. There are several models. Within the mainstream there is the separation of mental health from other aspects of NIH and there is the distinction between public health and medicine. There are also fields outside of science proper that are recognized as contributing to science and that

receive support. Examples are bioethics, medical anthropology, and medical sociology. Obviously, as these examples show, neither status nor funding is evenly distributed across these divisions, but they do illustrate that entry is not an all-or-nothing proposition and that various kinds of support can develop well before entry.

Solid, systematic research that is scrupulously rigorous is the most important response for healing research to mainstream barriers. (However, it is clear that this alone will not bring about a paradigm change. The example of parapsychology is especially instructive here.) Equally important is the development of innovative methods and designs that avoid distorting the practices under investigation. And finally, it is necessary for the healing research community to be bold and innovative in responding the current cultural situation in which the public is as enthusiastic for this research as conventional science and medicine are resistant. That background is fraught with both opportunities and risks. Currently, as these topics acquire a certain cachet and a clear economic value because of growing public demand, the field is acquiring many new friends and influential figures are offering themselves as leaders. Finally, we should always keep in mind that newfound popularity brings a whole new set of risks to those long accustomed to being unpopular!

REFERENCES

Angeles P 1981 A dictionary of philosophy. Barnes and Noble, New York

Blackburn S 1994 The Oxford dictionary of philosophy. Oxford University Press, Oxford

Blakeslee S 1998 Placebos prove so powerful even the experts are surprised. New York Times, October 13, 1998: F1, F4

Brown H 1975 Cancer quackery: what can you do about it? Nursing 75: 24–26

Burkitt D P, Walker A R P, Painter N S 1972 Effect of dietary fibre on stools and transit-times, and its role in the causation of disease. Lancet 2: 1408–1412

Cobb B 1958 Why do people detour to quacks? In: Jaco E G (ed) Patients, physicians and illness. Free Press, New York

Davenas E, Beauvais J, Amara M et al 1988 Human basophil degranulation triggered by very dilute antiserum against IgE. Science 333: 816–818

Dennett D, Rorty R 2000 Science. In: The Connection, Christopher Leiden's Summer Philosophy Series, National Public Radio, Boston, June 2000

Fulder S 1982 The tao of medicine: ginseng, oriental remedies, and the pharmacology of harmony. Destiny Books, New York

Fuller R C 1989 Alternative medicine and American religious life. Oxford University Press, New York

Glymour C, Stalker D 1983 Engineers, cranks, physicians and magicians. New England Journal of Medicine 308: 960–964

Grossinger R 1982 Planet medicine: from stone age shamanism to post-industrial healing, rev. edn. Shambhala Publications, Boston

Harris W S, Gowda M 1999 A randomized, controlled trial of the effects of remote, intercessory prayer on outcomes in patients admitted to the coronary care unit. Archives of Internal Medicine 159: 2273–2278

Hastings A C, Fadiman J, Gordon J (eds) 1981 Health for the whole person: the complete guide to holistic medicine. Westview Press, Boulder, Colorado

Hrobjartsson A, Gotzsche P C 2001 Is the placebo powerless? An analysis of clinical trials comparing placebo with no treatment. New England Journal of Medicine 344: 1594–1602

Hufford D 2001 Complementary and alternative medicine and cultural diversity: ethics and epistemology converge. In: Callahan D (ed) Complementary and alternative medicine: the scientific and pluralistic challenge. Georgetown University Press and the Hastings Center, Washington, DC

Hume D 1963 An enquiry concerning human understanding. Section X, Parts I–II. In: Alston W P (ed) Religious belief and philosophical thought. Harcourt, Brace and World, New York, pp. 408–419

Kaslof L J (ed) 1978 Wholistic dimensions in healing: a resource guide. Doubleday, Garden City, New York

Kourenoff P M 1971 Russian folk medicine. Translated and edited by G St George Pyramid Books, New York

Kuhn T 1970 The structure of scientific revolutions, 2nd edn. University of Chicago Press, Chicago

Maddox J 1988 When to believe the unbelievable. Nature 333: 787

Martin M 1981 Native American medicine: thoughts for posttraditional healers. Journal of the American Medical Association 245: 141–143

Mehl L E 1981 Mind and matter: foundations for holistic health. Mindbody Press, Berkeley, California, vol. 1

Melton J G 1990 New age encyclopedia. Gale Research, Detroit

Morris W (ed) 1978 The American heritage dictionary of the English language. Houghton Mifflin, Boston

Murphy E A 1981 Skepsis, dogma, and belief: uses and abuses in medicine. Johns Hopkins University Press, Baltimore

O'Mathuna D P 1998 The subtle allure of therapeutic touch. Journal of Christian Nursing 15: 4–13

O'Mathuna D P 1999 Therapeutic touch and wound healing. In: Micozzi M S (ed) Physician's guide to alternative medicine. American Health Consultants, Atlanta, GA

Otto H A, Knight J W 1979 Dimensions in wholistic healing: new frontiers in the treatment of the whole person. Nelson-Hall, Chicago

Price G R 1955 Science and the supernatural. Science 12: 359–367

Sampson W 1997 Why a new alternative medicine journal? Scientific Review of Alternative Medicine 1: 4–6

Scarpa A 1981 Pre-scientific medicines: their extent and value. Social Science and Medicine 15A: 317–326

Shealy N C 1975 Occult medicine can save your life. Dial Press, New York

Sloan R P, Bagiella E, Powell T 1999 Religion, spirituality and medicine. Lancet 353: 664–667

Sloan R P, Bagiella E et al 2000 Should physicians prescribe religious activities? New England Journal of Medicine 342: 1913–1916

Stuart M R 1975 Alternative medicine: herbalism. Nursing Times: 1528–1531

Talbot M 2000 The placebo prescription. New York Times Magazine, January 9, 2000, pp. 34–39, 44, 58–61

Thomas K 1971 Religion and the decline of magic. Charles Scribner, New York

Wallnofer H, von Rottauscher A 1965 Chinese folk medicine. Translated by M Palmedo. Bell Publishing, New York

Whorton J C 1988 Patient heal thyself: popular health reform movements as unorthodox medicine. In: Gevitz N (ed) Other healers: unorthodox medicine in America. Johns Hopkins University Press, Baltimore

Annotated bibliography of clinical research on healing

Appendix 1

Annotated bibliography of controlled clinical trials with quality scores

Cindy C Crawford and Wayne B Jonas

Independent quality assessment of internal, external and model validity were done on all randomized controlled trial studies of humans suffering from a clinical condition using the comprehensive likelihood of validity evaluations (LOVE) scale (Jonas, 2000). The results of this scale are reported in the Annotated Bibliography section below. The table that follows summarizes the quality criteria used in the LOVE scale. The Jadad scale, which is also used below to score studies, is a scoring system that has three items adding up to a maximum score of five points: 0, 1, or 2 points can be given for randomization (explicit statement that allocation was randomized and description of an adequate generation of the random sequence); 0, 1, or 2 points for double blinding (explicit statement that patients and evaluators were blinded and that treatments were indistinguishable); 0 or 1 point for the description of dropouts and withdrawals (numbers and reasons in all compared groups given separately). This scale was developed by A. R. Jadad in 1996 and used extensively in both conventional and CAM research.

1. Jonas, WB and Linde, K. Conducting and evaluating clinical research in complementary and alternatifve medicine. In Principles and Practice of Clinical Research. Gallin, J (ed.) New York: Academic Press. 2002.

THE LIKELIHOOD OF VALIDITY EVALUATION GUIDELINES

W B Jonas, K Linde

DIMENSION	MAIN CRITERIA
Internal validity (IU) How likely is it that the effects reported are due to the independent variable (the treatment)?	**Randomization** (Was subject assignment to treatment groups done randomly and in a concealed manner?) **Baseline comparability** (Were gender, age, and prognostic factors balanced?) **Change of intervention** (Was there loss to follow-up, contamination, poor compliance?) **Blinding** (Did the patients, practitioners, evaluators, analysts know who got the treatment?) **Outcomes** (Was the objectivity, reliability, and sensitivity of the outcome assessed?) **Analysis** (Was the number treated large? Were P values significant? Were multiple outcomes measured and analyzed?)
External validity (qv) How likely is it that the observed effects would occur outside the study and in different settings?	**Generalizability** (Was there a range of patients as would be seen in practice or were there multiple or narrow inclusions and exclusions? Was the study done at several sites with similar results?) **Reproducibility** (Was what was done clear? Were confidence intervals reported? Was the treatment transferable to other practitioners?) **Clinical significance** (Was the effect size big enough to make a difference? Is the condition in need of this type of treatment? Were any preferences determined? Was adherence good?) **Therapeutic interference** (Was there flexibility in varying the treatment? Was feedback on the outcomes available? Is the treatment feasible in most (or your) practice settings?) **Outcomes** (Were the outcomes clinically relevant? Were the outcomes checked for importance with the patients? Were any important outcomes missing?)
Model validity (MV) How likely is it that the study accurately reflects the system under investigation?	**Representativeness/accuracy** (Were the therapists well trained and experienced? Was the treatment strategy adequate? Was the treatment clearly described?) **Informed consent** (Was the informed consent comprehensive? Was it effective – did patients understand it? Did it generate expectations different from practice?)

Methodology matching
(Were the goals of the study clear and limited?
Did the investigators select the correct research method to achieve the goals?)

Model congruity
(Were the patients classified, was the treatment determined and were the outcomes assessed according to the system of the practice being assessed?)

Context/meaning
(Did the patients/practitioners believe in the therapy?
How well was the intervention adapted to the culture, family, meaning of the patient?)
Each subitem was scored with a 0 (no) or 1 (yes). Total scores were summed and the percent of the maximum score was calculated (0–100%).

ANNOTATED BIBLIOGRAPHIES

Therapeutic Touch Reduces Anxiety in the Institutionalized Elderly

Objective: To determine the effects of therapeutic touch on state anxiety in a sample of institutionalized elderly.

Design: A double blind, sham-controlled, three group randomized controlled trial.

Setting: The research was conducted in privacy, in the subjects' rooms at two small rural and two large urban long-term care facilities.

Patients: A total of 105 institutionalized elderly, cognitively capable of participating, were used in the study. These patients in institutions are known to experience significant levels of state anxiety, and it is known that institutionalization itself increases anxiety.

Intervention: Patients were randomly assigned to either therapeutic touch (TT) in the form of a back rub from the primary investigator, who centered and made an effort to transfer energy, a control which involved a back rub from the primary investigator who also made a conscious effort *not* to center or transfer energy, or another control which involved a back rub from an experienced registered mental health nurse who had no knowledge of TT.

Main outcome measures: Anxiety levels in the institutionalized elderly were measured using an English Y–1 form of the Spielberger state-trait anxiety inventory (STAI), which had been modified to compensate for the special changes associated with aging. Possible scores on the STAI range from 20 to 80. The data were collected over a 2-week period.

Main results: The anxiety level of subjects who received TT in the form of a back rub was found to be significantly lower (mean score 27.09) than the anxiety level of subjects who received a back rub without TT, mean score 36.53 and 32.54 in control 2 and 1, respectively ($P = 0.001$). No significant difference was determined between the two control groups.

Conclusions: The results suggest that this non-invasive intervention (therapeutic touch) has potential for reducing anxiety in this population.

Reference: Simington J A, Laing G P 1993 Effects of therapeutic touch on anxiety in the institutionalized elderly. Clinical Nursing Research 2(1): 438–445

Quality scores: IV: 73.1   EV: 55.2   MV: 66.7   JADAD: 5

Therapeutic Touch Reduces Tension Headache Pain

Objective: To determine the effects of therapeutic touch on tension headache pain.

Design: Randomized, placebo controlled trial.

Setting: Not described.

Patients: Sixty volunteer subjects with tension headaches, age ranging from 18 to 59 years, with a mean age of 30 years, were used. They were recruited from the student health clinic at a mid-western university, the general student and staff population of the university, and the public at large via radio, newspaper, and bulletin board announcements; 75% of subjects were women; 70% were college students, and the remainder were white-collar workers. All but five subjects were white.

Intervention: Subjects were randomly divided into treatment and placebo groups, using a random numbers table. Intervention involved laying-on of hands through touching with the intent to help or heal the headaches for 5-minute intervals; the placebo touch involved a nurse with no intent to help or heal, who counted back from 100 while touching the patient.

Main outcome measures: The McGill–Melzack pain questionnaire was filled out by the subjects before, immediately afterward, and 4 hours post TT to measure headache pain levels.

Main results: A total of 90% of the subjects exposed to TT experienced a sustained reduction in headache pain, $P < 0.0001$ (before–after paired) compared with only 50% of the subjects exposed to the placebo touch. An average of 70% pain reduction was sustained over the 4 hours following TT, twice the average pain reduction following the placebo touch, $P < 0.01$ (unpaired between group). No *t*-statistics were reported with the P values.

Conclusions: Study results indicated that TT may have potential beyond a placebo effect in the treatment of tension headache pain.

Reference: Keller E, Bzdek V M 1986 Effects of therapeutic touch on tension headache pain. Nursing Research 35(2): 101–105

Quality scores: IV: 61.5   EV: 34.5   MV: 58.3   JADAD: 3

Paranormal Healing has No Significant Effect on Hypertension in a Small Trial

Objective: To see whether paranormal healing by laying-on of hands might reduce blood pressure in essential hypertension and whether such an effect might be due to a paranormal, psychological, or placebo factor.

Design: A prospective randomized, double blind, three group controlled trial.

Setting: Clinical laboratory.

Patients: A total of 115 patients who had a systolic blood pressure of 140 mmHg or above or a diastolic pressure of 90 mmHg or above (World Health Organization criteria for hypertension), or both, who responded to an advertisement in several national newspapers.

Intervention: Patients were in one of the three treatment groups: paranormal healing by laying-on of hands ($n = 40$), during which verbal communication was allowed; paranormal healing at a distance ($n = 37$), and no paranormal healing (controls; $n = 38$). Healing at a distance and no paranormal healing was investigated double blind. Treatment was given as a 20-minute session one morning a week for 15 weeks.

Main outcome measures: Blood pressure readings taken before and after each session to measure hypertension. The mean value of the last two readings of at least three recordings by automatic oscillometry was used for data analysis.

Main results: Systolic and diastolic blood pressures were significantly reduced in all three groups at week 15 (mean reduction (95% CI) 17.1 (14.0–20.2)/8.3 (6.6–10.0) mmHg). The mean falls in systolic blood pressure for healing by laying-on of hands was 19.3 (95% CI 13.7–24.9), for healing at a distance 17.5 (12.5–22.5), and for the control 14.2 (8.3–20.1) mmHg, and the corresponding falls in diastolic blood pressure were 9.4 (6.1–12.7), 8.6 (5.9–11.3), and 6.7 (4.0–9.4) mmHg, respectively. Only successive reductions in diastolic blood pressures among the groups from week to week were significantly different. Each week diastolic pressure was consistently lower (average 1.9 mmHg) after healing at a distance compared with control, but on paired comparison these differences were not significant.

Conclusions: No treatment was consistently better than another. The data cannot be taken as evidence of a paranormal effect on blood pressure; however, paranormal healing is safe. Probably the fall in blood pressure in all three groups was either caused by the psychosocial factors or was a placebo effect of the trial itself. Week to week variations among the groups could have accounted for any differences noted.

Reference: Beutler J J, Attevelt J T, Schouten S A, Faber J A, Mees E J, Geijskes G G 1988 Paranormal healing and hypertension. British Medical Journal 296: 1491–1494

Quality scores: IV: 80.8   EV: 55.2   MV: 55.3   JADAD: 5

Intercessory Prayer Improved Hospital Course in a Coronary Care Unit Population in a Large Trial

Objective: To answer the questions: (a) Does intercessory prayer to the Judeo-Christian God have any effect on the patient's medical condition and recovery while in the hospital? And (b) How are these effects characterized, if present?

Design: A prospective randomized, controlled, double blind trial.

Setting: The coronary care unit at San Francisco General Hospital.

Patients: A total of 393 patients admitted to the CCU were randomized to an intercessory prayer group (192 patients) or to a control group (201 patients).

Intervention: After randomization to a group, each patient was assigned to 3–7 intercessors, born again Christians with an active Christian life as manifested by daily devotional prayer and active Christian fellowship with a local church. The patient's first name, diagnosis, and general condition, along with pertinent updates in their condition, were given to the intercessors. The intercessory prayer was done outside of the hospital daily until the patient was discharged from the hospital. Under the direction of a coordinator, each intercessor was asked to pray daily for a rapid recovery and for prevention of complications and death, in addition to other areas of prayer they believed to be beneficial to the patient.

Main outcomes: Information on each patient, in a blinded manner, was collected during the study and at follow-up. Results of scoring the post-entry hospital course used a good, intermediate and bad scoring system which compared the conditions in patients exposed to intercessory prayer compared to the controls. Data were collated and entered into a PDP-11 computer for analysis, using the BMDP statistical package. The data were analyzed with an unpaired t-test for the interval data and a chi-square test for categorical data. A stepwise logistic regression was used for the multivariate analysis.

Main results: There was a significant difference ($P < 0.0001$) between the two groups based on events that occurred after entry into the study. Fewer patients in the prayer group required ventilatory support, antibiotics, or diuretics. In the prayer group, 85% were considered to have a good hospital course, no new diagnoses or problems were recorded for the patient after entry vs. 73% in the control group. An intermediate grade, if there were higher levels of morbidity and a moderate risk of death, was given in 1% of the prayer group vs. 5% of the controls. A bad hospital course, the course of patients who had the highest morbidity and risk of death or who died during the study, was observed in 14% of the prayer group vs. 22% of the controls. An analysis of these data gave a P value of < 0.01.

Conclusion: It was impossible to make sure that the controls were not praying or being prayed for. Therefore 'pure' groups were not attained in this study. However, based on these data, there seemed to be an effect in favor of supplemental prayer, and that effect was beneficial.

Reference: Byrd R C 1988 Positive therapeutic effects of intercessory prayer in a coronary care unit population. Southern Medical Journal 81(7): 826–829

Quality scores: IV: 73.1   EV: 65.5   MV: 66.7   JADAD: 5

Forty-four Patients with Chronic Symptoms Reported Feeling Better After Seeing a Spiritual Healer

Objective: To determine if spiritual healers can influence the course of an illness by 'spiritual' or non-physical means.

Design: Observation of consecutive subjects.

Setting: The Central London Healing Group used a room in a medical school, once a week from November 1986 to February 1988.

Patients: The primary author referred patients to this healing group and collected data on 44 patients who attended over 20 weeks. Seventeen of them suffered from pains in the musculoskeletal system and 11 had psychological problems; two had malignant disease.

Intervention: The healer asked the patient to maintain an open mind during the intervention. Healers began at the head or shoulders, then moved their hands all over the patient's body, including the painful area where the trouble was. The patients were told to relax and that they might feel very sleepy.

Main outcome measures: Age, sex, number of visits, treatment, complaints, and verbal responses to the healing encounter made by the patient and healer were compared.

Main results: The responses expected by the healers and those that occurred were remarkably consistent and did not differ by age or sex of the patient or healer. More visits conferred greater benefit, and more women responded. Benefits felt by the patient agreed with those experienced by the healer, suggesting that the relationship between them is part of healing. Of the 44 patients, 35 felt considerably better for attending.

Conclusion: The development of a therapeutic relationship takes time and, in this study, more benefit was felt by those who came several times. A sympathetic healer and the laying-on of hands in a relaxed atmosphere are excellent therapies for stress, fear, and loneliness.

Reference: Cohen J 1989 Spiritual healing in a medical context. The Practitioner 233: 1056–1057

Quality scores: Not applicable. Not a controlled trial.

'Healing' Improved Symptoms and Well-Being in Chronically Ill Patients Compared to 'No Healing'

Objective: To examine the effects of a healer seeing chronically ill patients.

Design: A quasi-randomized, controlled trial.

Setting: A semirural practice in mid-Devon, England, with seven physicians, covering a population of 12 000 patients with a Jarman index of −1.3. The trial took place between September 1994 and September 1996.

Patients: Fifty-seven patients had been referred by any of the seven partners to the healer by the research nurse. Patients were included if they had a condition that had lasted at least 6 months and had been unresponsive to previous treatments, conventional or otherwise (including healing).

They had to be older than 18 years of age and willing to see a healer.

Intervention: Study patients received 10 weekly 40-minute healing sessions, while their parallel controls had their healing deferred for 12 weeks (increased to 24 weeks for the 12 control patients in the second half of the study). The healing session included a discussion between healer and patient concerning symptoms and general well-being. The main part of the treatment involved the healer applying her hands close to the patient and slowly moving them over the entire body while visualizing the passage of white light passing through her and into the patient. Each session was accompanied by relaxing music. Control patients continued to receive conventional care from their GP.

Main outcome measures: Assessment was done at the beginning, 3 months and 6 months with all patients to determine severity of symptoms. Patients scored their symptoms on a scale from 0 (no symptoms) to 10 (unbearable). Any alterations in symptoms were quantified by comparing different symptom scores at different times. Patients scored themselves for anxiety and depression on the hospital anxiety and depression (HAD) scale. General functional ability was self-assessed by means of the Nottingham health profile. The percentage of natural killer cells (CD16 and CD56) was measured by standard assay methods along with total white cell and lymphocyte counts.

Main results: Two weeks after completion of sessions, 81% of the 27 study patients thought their symptoms had improved and 15 thought they had improved substantially. Study patients scored better than controls on both measures of symptoms ($P < 0.05$, $P < 0.01$), on anxiety and depression ratings ($P < 0.01$, $P < 0.05$) and on general function measured by the Nottingham health profile ($P < 0.01$). Treatment differences were evident 3 months later for one of the measures of symptom change ($P < 0.05$) and for both anxiety and depression ratings ($P < 0.01$; $P < 0.05$). The percentages of natural killer cells did not change significantly in either group.

Conclusion: For many chronically ill patients, healing appeared to be an effective treatment whatever its mechanism of working. No one reported any adverse effects and the treatment was relatively inexpensive.

Reference: Dixon M 1998 Does 'healing' benefit patients with chronic symptoms? A quasi-randomized trial in general practice. Journal of the Royal Society of Medicine 91: 183–188

Quality score: IV: 69.2   EV: 69.0   MV: 41.7   JADAD: 2

Therapeutic Touch Decreased Pain in Patients with Osteoarthritis of the Knee in a Small Trial

Objective: To determine if therapeutic touch is effective in the treatment of osteoarthritis of the knee.

Design: A single blinded, randomized control trial.

Setting: A family practice center with a community hospital family practice residency program in Pennsylvania from August 1995 to November 1995.

Patients: The patients ($n = 25$) were between the ages of 40 and 80 years, had been given a diagnosis of osteoarthritis of at least one knee, had not had knee replacement, and had no other connective tissue disease.

Intervention: The patients were randomized to therapeutic touch, mock therapeutic touch, or standard care. The patients were assigned a rating of mild, moderate, or severe osteoarthritis, according to their responses on an osteoarthritis of the knee questionnaire form and a rheumatologist's reading of the bilateral knee radiograph. The questionnaire and radiograph readings were equally weighted in describing the severity of the arthritis. All groups continued to receive their usual care throughout the study period. In addition, the treatment group received a TT treatment once a week for 6 weeks, and the placebo group received a mock treatment at the same rate, for identical amounts of time.

Main outcome measures: Pain and its impact, general well-being, and health status were measured, as well as a qualitative measurement of an improvement using an in-depth interview. The subjects completed two visual analog scales before and after each weekly treatment and the Stanford health assessment questionnaire (HAQ), and the West Haven–Yale multidimensional pain inventory (MPI). Repeated measures analysis on the scales were performed.

Main results: The treatment group had significantly decreased pain, $P = 0.0002$ for treatment vs. placebo, with the treatment average being 2.14 (SD 0.196) on pain severity scale and the placebo average being 3.27 (SD 0.173) vs. control average being 3.06 (0.183) as compared with treatment; improved function as compared with the placebo and control groups, such as with general activity level with treatment averaging 3.53 (0.161) vs. 2.74 (0.120) in placebo group, $P = 0.001$, and vs. control 2.50 (0.147), $P = 0.0005$. The qualitative depth interview confirmed this result.

Conclusion: Despite the small numbers, significant differences were found for improvement in function and pain for patients receiving therapeutic touch. A larger study is needed to confirm these results.

Reference: Gordon A, Merenstein J H, D'Amico F, Hudgens D 1998 The effects of therapeutic touch on patients with osteoarthritis of the knee. Journal of Family Practice 47(4): 271–277

Quality score: IV: 73.1   EV: 51.7   MV: 58.3   JADAD: 3

Added Prayers Reduced Mortality in a Small Group of Children with Leukemia

Objective: To determine the efficacy of prayer in leukemic children.

Design: A triple blind study.

Setting: The Meadowbrook Hospital in New York.

Participants: Eighteen leukemic children participated in the study. Ten families agreed to pray daily for the 10 children, while the rest (eight children) were not prayed for and served as a control. Doctors provided basic information.

Intervention: The names of the children were randomly selected and sent to friends in Washington who had agreed to organize a prayer group. They enlisted 10 families in their Protestant church to pray daily for the children, but they were not told that this was a study on the efficacy of prayer. Physicians treating these leukemic children supplied the name, age, date of diagnosis, and later, the date each child expired. Doctors did not know this was a prayer study.

Main outcome measures: At monthly intervals, the parents and physicians independently answered a questionnaire, which asked whether the illness, the child's adjustment, and the family's adjustment was better, unchanged, or worse.

Main results: Parents proved consistently more optimistic than doctors in response to all three questions concerned with attitudes toward the illness progress, child's adjustment, and the family's adjustment. After 15 months of prayer, of the 10 children with leukemia in the prayer group, seven were still alive; of eight in the control group, only two were alive. These groups are statistically significant.

Conclusions: Any future study design might be improved if patients are paired with respect to all variables known to influence survival and then randomly divided into two groups. In the particular group of 18 children, it was not possible to identify other variables which could be paired. Also, a larger sample size would increase the ability to generalize the results.

Reference: Collipp P J 1969 The efficacy of prayer: a triple-blind study. Medical Times 97(5): 201–204

Quality score: IV: 57.7   EV: 58.6   MV: 58.3   JADAD: 4

Therapeutic Touch Reduced Anxiety Levels of Hospitalized Patients over Controls

Objective: To determine the effect of therapeutic touch on the anxiety level of hospitalized patients.

Design: Blinded, matched cohort study.

Setting: A cardiovascular unit of a large medical center in New York City, in patients' rooms.

Patients: Ninety hospitalized volunteer men and women between the ages of 21 and 65 years.

Intervention: Three matched intervention groups were formed; each subject received an individual 5-minute period of intervention by therapeutic touch, casual touch, or no touch.

Main outcome measures: The dependent variable, state anxiety, was measured by the self-evaluation questionnaire. Subjects were administered this tool pre and post intervention.

Main Results: A comparison of the pre and post-test mean scores for the therapeutic touch group, using a correlated t ratio, revealed a highly significant difference ($t = -4.88$, $P < 0.001$) for reported state anxiety. After controlling for pre-treatment differences in state anxiety, therapeutic touch group was found to have significantly lower scores that the casual touch group according to anxiety, $F = 9.65$, $P < 0.01$. When comparing the therapeutic touch group with the no touch group on anxiety, therapeutic touch was found to have significantly lower scores on anxiety than the no touch group ($F = 7.21$, $P < 0.01$).

Conclusions: Therapeutic touch seemed to be highly effective for patients with anxiety compared to patients receiving sham therapeutic touch.

Reference: Heidt P 1981 Effect of therapeutic touch on anxiety level of hospitalized patients. Nursing Research 30(1): 32–37

Quality score: IV: 61.50   EV: 44.80   MV: 58.30   JADAD:1

Remote, Intercessory Prayer Improved Hospital Course of Patients in a Coronary Care Unit in a Large Trial

Objective: To determine whether remote intercessory prayer for hospitalized cardiac patients will reduce overall adverse events and length of stay.

Design: Randomized, double blind trial.

Setting: Private, university associated hospital.

Patients: A total of 990 consecutive patients who were newly admitted to the coronary care unit (CCU).

Intervention: At time of admission, patients were randomized to receive remote intercessory prayer (prayer group) or not (usual care group). The first names of patients in the prayer group were given to a team of outside intercessors who prayed for them daily for 4 weeks. Patients were unaware that they were being prayed for, and the intercessors did not know and never met the patients.

Main outcome measures: The medical course from CCU admission to hospital discharge was summarized in a CCU course score derived from a blinded, retrospective chart review.

Main results: Compared with the usual care group ($n = 524$), the prayer group ($n = 466$) had lower mean ± SEM weighted (6.35 ± 0.26 *vs.* 7.13 ± 0.27; $P = 0.04$) and unweighted (2.7 ± 0.1 *vs.* 3.0 ± 0.1; $P = 0.04$) CCU course scores. Lengths of CCU and hospital stays were not different.

Conclusions: Remote, intercessory prayer was associated with lower CCU course scores. This result suggests that prayer may be an effective adjunct to standard medical care.

Reference: Harris W S, Gowda M, Kolb J W et al 1999 A randomized, controlled trial of the effects of remote, intercessory prayer on outcomes in patients admitted to the coronary care unit. Archives of Internal Medicine 159: 2273–2278

Quality scores: IV: 69.2   EV: 48.3   MV: 50.0   JADAD: 5

Distance Healing Did Not Improve Major Depression over Standard Treatment in a Small Trial

Objective: To determine the effect of distance healing on patients being treated for psychiatric disorders.

Design: Randomized, double blind, prospective experimental protocol.

Setting: The inpatient psychiatric unit at the University of Connecticut Health Center.

Patients: Adult patients ($n = 40$) admitted to an inpatient psychiatric unit for major depression, aged 19–81 years, were randomly assigned either to an experimental distant healing group or to a standard care only control group.

Intervention: All subjects received standard treatment for depression; in addition, experimental subjects received distance healing daily for 6 weeks by volunteers trained in LeShan's meditation techniques. In these daily sessions, healers attempted to induce through meditation a particular altered state of consciousness for which they had been trained, described as 'nonlocal mind.' While in that state, they included the subject in their minds in a non-directive manner, excluding any other mental content or focus in a state of deep, intense compassion.

Main outcome measures: Outcome was measured weekly for 6 weeks and then biweekly for 6 more weeks using the Hamilton rating scale for depression (HRSD), brief psychiatric rating scale (BPRS), global assessment of function (GAF), and a visual analog scale for depression.

Main results: A non-significant trend was found for experimental subjects showing greater improvement than control subjects in depression, general psychopathology, and overall subjective distress. Among experimental subjects, favorable outcomes were significantly correlated with number of healing sessions received and with healers' ratings of the 'strength' of the healing sessions. The ANOVA on HRSD scores for the two groups over the 12-week study period did not suggest a significant difference between the two groups ($F = 0.61$, d.f. = 130). An ANOVA for BPRS scores over the 12-week period did not suggest a significant difference between the two groups ($t = 2.80$, d.f. = 130). The ANOVA for the GAF scores over the 12-week study period did not suggest a significant difference between groups ($F = 0.00$, d.f. = 130). The ANOVA conducted for the VAS scores did not suggest a significant difference between the two groups for the 12-week study ($F = 0.59$, d.f. = 130).

Conclusions: Subjects who received distance healing were rated as having less depression, and rated themselves as having less overall distress, but none of these were significantly different than the control subjects.

Reference: Greyson B 1996 Distance healing of patients with major depression. Journal of Scientific Exploration 10(4): 447–465

Quality scores: IV: 88.5   EV: 58.6   MV: 66.7   JADAD: 5

No Advantage of Prayer on Chronic Disease in a Small Study

Objective: To determine the efficacy of prayer on patients suffering from chronic disease.

Design: Double blind, block-randomized, controlled clinical trial.

Setting: Two outpatient clinics at a London hospital.

Patients: Forty-eight patients suffering from chronic stationary or progressively deteriorating psychological or rheumatic disease.

Intervention: The names of patients receiving 'treatment,' who were not told they were taking part in a trial, were sent to the leader of a prayer-group. The six prayer groups consisted of five groups organized by the Guild of Health and one by the Friends' Spiritual Healing Fellowship. The prayer groups agreed to expect no further news of the patients for whom they prayed until the termination of the trial. Each group was asked to submit details of its membership and to outline its own method of intercession. Approximately 5 minutes were spent per day on each patient by each group member, using a method of silent meditation. Those that did not receive this 'treatment' were controls.

Main outcome measures: Physicians examined patients at the start and end of the trial, and completed an evaluation form. At the end of 6 months, reminders were sent to the physicians, who, at various times, re-examined the patient concerned, and completed the second evaluation form. Patient's clinical state and attitude to the illness were the main variables used. Clinical state contained 5 points, 0 being 'very poor' and 5 being 'very good.' Attitude state scale was verbal: two terms (stoical; positive and cooperative) were scored plus; one (non-committal) as 0; and two (apprehensive; critical and complaining) as negative.

Main results: The results in clinical state of six individuals was judged better at the second evaluation and 26 were worse or unchanged. The observed improvement rates in the two groups may be compared with those expected. The treated group showed five improvements in 16 cases: 31% improvement, against the 57% expected. The control group had only one improvement, a rate of 6%, against 13% expected. Five out of the next six definite results showed an advantage to the control. The end result of the continued series shows no significant differences. The results for attitude states are similar, but give rather less information.

Conclusion: In view of the small sample involved, it is not surprising that no advantage to either group was demonstrated. The methods used in this trial need more testing, just as its conclusions require confirmation.

Reference: Joyce C R B, Welldon R M C, Litt B 1965 The objective efficacy of prayer: a double-blind clinical trial. Journal of Chronic Disease 18: 367–377

Quality scores: IV: 65.4   EV: 41.4   MV: 50.0   JADAD: 4

Distant Healing Improved Outcomes in Patients with Advanced AIDS

Objective: To determine if distant healing (DH), including prayer and 'psychic healing,' affects the health of patients with advanced AIDS.

Design: Small randomized, controlled, double blind study.

Setting: A San Francisco Bay area clinic, in addition to visits to the subjects' own homes.

Patients: Forty subjects with advanced AIDS were recruited by distributing fliers at clinics and AIDS-related events and through advertisements in both gay and mainstream newspapers in the San Francisco Bay area. A wide range of sociodemographic populations were selected. All subjects selected had to meet the criteria of the Centers for Disease Control AIDS category C-3 and to be taking *Pneumocystis carinii* pneumonia prophylaxis.

Intervention: Subjects were pair-matched for age, CD4+ count, and number of AIDS-defining illnesses and randomly assigned to either 10 weeks of DH treatment or a control group. DH treatment was performed by self-identified healers representing many different healing and spiritual traditions, located all over the United States. Subjects and healers never met.

Main outcome measures: Subjects were assessed by psychometric testing and blood was drawn at enrollment, at the end of the 10-week treatment intervention, and at follow-up 12–14 weeks later. Measurements taken were CD4+ count, psychological distress as measured by the profile of mood states (POMS), physical symptoms as measured by the Wahler physical symptom inventory (WPSI), and quality of life as measured by the medical outcomes survey (MOS) for HIV. Doctor visits, hospitalizations, and any new illnesses were also reported.

Main results: At 6 months, a blind medical chart review found that treatment subjects acquired significantly fewer new AIDS-defining illnesses (0.1 *vs.* 0.6 per patient, $P = 0.04$), had lower illness severity (0.8 *vs.* 2.65, $P = 0.03$), and required significantly fewer doctor visits (9.2 *vs.* 13.0, $P = 0.01$), fewer hospitalizations (0.15 *vs.* 0.6, $P = 0.04$), and fewer days of hospitalization (0.5 *vs.* 3.4, $P = 0.04$). Treated subjects also showed significantly improved mood compared with controls (measured by POMS). There were no significant differences in CD4+ counts. Differences on the WPSI and MOS were not significant between groups.

Conclusions: These data support the possibility of a distant healing effect in AIDS and suggest the value of further research.

Reference: Sicher F, Targ E, Moore II D, Smith H S 1998 A randomized double-blind study of the effect of distant healing in a population with advanced AIDS: report of a small scale study. Western Journal of Medicine 169(6): 356–363

Quality scores: IV: 84.6   EV: 62.0   MV: 66.7   JADAD: 5

Therapeutic Touch of Little Help in Relieving Postoperative Pain in a Small Trial

Objective: To determine the effects of therapeutic touch on pain experienced by postoperative patients.

Design: Block-randomized controlled trial, single blind, three group design.

Setting: A major North American urban medical center.

Patients: A total of 108 patients scheduled for major elective abdominal or pelvic surgery. Subjects were primarily Caucasian (74 women, 34 men), and ranged in age from 23 to 79 years.

Intervention: The experimental intervention, therapeutic touch (TT), consisted of a standardized 5-minute procedure in which the nurse assumed a meditative state of awareness and made the conscious intent to therapeutically assist the patient. She moved her hands, at a distance of 2–4 inches, over the patient from head to feet attuning to the condition of the patient. The mock therapeutic touch (MTT) intervention served as a single-blind placebo control intervention. It consisted of a standardized 5-minute procedure in which a nurse, with no experience with TT, made the conscious intent to mimic the physical movements of a nurse doing TT, with no attempt to assume any meditative state and no attempt to assist the subject. The standard intervention (SI) served as a standard control intervention against which to assay the effects of TT. It consisted of a standardized 5-minute intervention in which the nurse administered an intramuscular injection of PRN narcotic analgesic prescribed by the patient's physician for postoperative pain relief.

Main outcome measures: Pain visual analogue scale was used to measure pain before and 1 hour following the interventions.

Main results: A substantial reduction in pain from pre-intervention to post-intervention scores occurred in the SI group (mean decrease being 42%), as would be expected as a result of medication. A reduction also occurred in the TT group (mean decrease of 13%), whereas there was no reduction in the MTT scores. The difference between the TT and MTT means was 8.98 ($0.05 < P < 0.06$), indicating that TT is more effective than MTT, but this did not reach statistical significance. The difference between the TT and SI means was significant, 16.11 ($P < 0.001$) indicating that SI is much more effective than TT.

Conclusions: The hypothesis, that therapeutic touch would significantly decrease postoperative pain compared to the placebo control intervention, was not supported. Secondary analyses suggest that therapeutic touch may decrease patient's need for analgesic medication. Implications for further research and practice are suggested.

Reference: Meehan T C 1993 Therapeutic touch and postoperative pain: a Rogerian research study. Nursing Science Quarterly 6(2): 69–78

Quality scores: IV: 84.6   EV: 41.4   MV: 66.7   JADAD: 3

Healing by the Laying-On of Hands Raised Hemoglobin Levels

Objective: To determine the effects of laying-on of hands for changes in hemoglobin values.

Design: Small, non-randomized controlled trial.

Setting: Experiments took place during the summer of 1973, with all subjects living at the study site during the time they were either in the experimental or the control group.

Patients: Forty-six subjects with various illnesses were in the experimental group, 29 subjects in the control group, and one healer. It was not stated how subjects were recruited.

Intervention: Blood samples of all subjects were drawn upon arrival and labeled as 'pre-test' and separated according to whether the subjects were part of the control or experimental group. Next, healing by laying-on of hands took place for as much time as needed. Finally, blood samples were drawn again.

Main outcome measures: Pre and post-test hemoglobin values from the ill subjects were studied, using an AOHb-Meter, American Optical Corporation, to see if there were any changes due to the laying-on of hands.

Main results: The healer's hemoglobin value remained the same; however, the hemoglobin value of the healees did change after treatment. In the experimental group, the post-test mean hemoglobin values exceed the pre-treatment hemoglobin values (mean difference = 1.71, $t = 7.43$ (45 d.f.), $P < 0.001$). In the control group, there was no significant difference between the means of the pre and post-test hemoglobin values (mean difference = 0.12, $t = 1.71$ (28 d.f.), not significant). And the post-test mean hemoglobin values of the experimental group exceed the post-test mean hemoglobin values of the control group (mean difference for experimental = 14.6, where mean difference for control = 13.3, $t = 3.06$ (73 d.f.), $P < 0.01$). This was not due to any changes in temperature of the healer's hands or the environment.

Conclusions: Hemoglobin may be an indicator of physical change in 'healing' by the 'laying-on' of hands.

Reference: Krieger D 1976 Healing by the 'laying-on' of hands as a facilitator of bioenergetic change: the response of in-vivo human hemoglobin. Psychoenergetic Systems 1: 121–129

Quality scores: IV: 50.0   EV: 37.9   MV: 50.0   JADAD: 0

Non-Contact Therapeutic Touch Reduced Anxiety in a Small Study of Hospitalized Patients

Objective: To determine the effect of therapeutic touch without physical contact on state anxiety of hospitalized cardiovascular patients.

Design: Small randomized controlled trial.

Setting: A cardiovascular unit of a medical center in New York City.

Subjects: A total of 60 subjects, 37 men and 23 women, hospitalized in a cardiovascular unit of a medical center; age range of subjects was 36–81 years. The experimental and control groups were similar in ethnicity, sex, religion, medical diagnosis, surgery, number of hospitalizations, number of days in hospital, practice of meditation/relaxation, position during treatment, and number of days after surgery.

Intervention: Prior to random assignment to either experimental or control group, subjects received an explanation of the study. Subjects were randomly assigned to non-contact therapeutic touch (NCTT), or non-contact (NC). NC was defined as an intervention that mimics the movements of the nurse during TT but during which there is no attempt to center, no intention to assist the subject, and no direction of energy, as with the other interventions. All subjects received identical instructions before, during, and after intervention. Sessions lasted 5 minutes and hands were 4–6 inches from the subject's body.

Main outcome measures: The STAI self-evaluation questionnaire was used to measure state anxiety before and after intervention in both groups.

Main results: Subjects treated with non-contact therapeutic touch demonstrated a significantly greater decrease in state anxiety, from a mean of 38.55 (SD 10.85) score on pre-test to 31.79 (SD 10.57) at post-test, $P < 0.0005$, than subjects treated with a mimic control intervention, mean at pre-test 36.31 (SD 10.29) to post-test being 34.30 (SD 11.34), $P = 0.082$. The correlation between pre-test and post-test scores were 0.768 in the experimental group and 0.861 in the control group, indicating at the $P < 0.0005$ level that the experimental group scores decreased more than the control group scores.

Conclusions: There is a greater decrease in state anxiety scores in subjects treated with NCTT than those treated with NC. The results from this study for the effectiveness of NCTT were virtually identical to the other study using physical contact TT (Heidt 1981).

Reference: Quinn J F 1984 Therapeutic touch as energy exchange: testing the theory. Advances in Nursing Science 6(2): 42–49

Quality scores: IV: 65.4   EV: 48.3   MV: 66.7   JADAD: 3

Therapeutic Touch Reduced Anxiety but not Physiological Measures in Preoperative Patients

Objective: To determine the effect of therapeutic touch (TT), without eye or facial contact, on anxiety level of preoperative patients.

Design: Large randomized, blinded controlled trial.

Setting: A small private medical center in South Carolina.

Patients: A total of 153 subjects, 38 women and 115 men, hospitalized, awaiting open-heart surgery on the following day, ages 29–83 years, predominantly white Protestant men who had completed at least 12 years of education.

Intervention: On each data collection day, all treated subjects received the same treatment (TT or mock therapeutic touch (MTT)), while only one subject was randomly assigned to no treatment (NT). Subjects would turn on their sides while the investigator moved her hands above the surface of their skin for 5 minutes. TT group received TT during these 5 minutes, MTT received no intent to heal while moving the hands for 5 minutes, and NT subjects just lay for 5 minutes on their side.

Main outcome measures: The self-evaluation questionnaire, state-trait anxiety inventory, (STAI) was utilized to measure state anxiety pre and post intervention in all groups. Blood pressure was measured with a new Tycos R Aneroid sphygmomanometer and a Littman 2125 stethoscope. Heart rate was measured by counting the radial pulse for 1 full minute.

Main results: Changes in each of the post-test physiological measures occurred in the expected direction. The largest differences occurred in the TT group, the second largest in the MTT group, and the least in the NT group. Changes in post-test STAI scores were largest in the TT group, a decrease of 2.44 points with SD of 5.28, and smallest in the MTT group, a mean difference of 0.62 (SD 6.75). There were, however, no significant differences among the groups on post-test or retention anxiety, systolic blood pressure, or heart rate. Diastolic blood pressure did significantly change, $P < 0.02$, with TT group being significantly better than the NT group, $P = 0.007$.

Conclusions: All of the post-test measures did change in the predicted direction, i.e. the largest changes occurred in the TT group, and there was a significant difference in the diastolic pressure in the TT group. Further research is needed.

Reference: Quinn J F 1989 Therapeutic touch as energy exchange: replication and extension. Nursing Science Quarterly 2(2): 79–87

Quality scores: IV: 76.9   EV: 34.5   MV: 41.7   JADAD: 4

Therapeutic Touch Reduced Pain and Anxiety in Burn Patients

Objective: To determine whether therapeutic touch versus sham therapeutic touch could produce greater pain relief as an adjunct to narcotic analgesia, a greater reduction in anxiety, and alterations in plasma T-lymphocyte concentrations among burn patients.

Design: Randomized, blinded controlled trial.

Setting: A university burn center in the south-eastern United States.

Subjects: A total of 99 men and women between the ages of 15 and 68 hospitalized for severe burns.

Interventions: The TT practitioner began by centering or becoming relaxed and focused on assisting the subject. Using hands held with palms facing the subject, 2–5 inches from the subject's body, the TT practitioner assessed the energy field and implemented techniques such as clearing, directing, or balancing the energy flow, based on the assessment. Treatment length varied from 5 to 20 minutes, depending on the practitioner's subjective judgment of the state of the subject's energy field. The research assistants who administered the sham did not center and did not assess or attempt to therapeutically manipulate the subject's energy field, but counted backwards from 100 by serial sevens as they made random mimic TT movements for a random length of time, not to exceed 20 minutes. All sham group patients were given the illusion that they were receiving a therapeutic treatment. All patients received the treatment once a day for 5 days.

Main outcome measures: The McGill pain questionnaire, visual analogue scales for pain, anxiety and satisfaction with therapy, and an effectiveness of therapy form. Blood was drawn on days 1 and 6 for lymphocyte subset analysis.

Main results: Subjects who received TT reported significantly greater reduction in pain on the McGill pain questionnaire pain rating index (PRI) ($P = 0.004$) and number of words chosen (NWC) ($P = 0.005$) and greater reduction in anxiety on the visual analogue scale for anxiety ($P = 0.031$) than did those who received sham TT. Lymphocyte subset analyses on blood from 11 subjects showed a decreasing total CD8+ lymphocyte concentration for the TT group. There was no statistically significant difference between groups on medication usage ($P = 0.356$).

Conclusions: Subjects who received TT reported a significantly greater reduction in pain on the McGill PRI and NWC after receiving 5 days of therapy than did those who received the sham treatment. Because there was no statistically significant difference in the amount of analgesic medication taken per 24 hours between TT and sham group subjects, the greater pain relief reported by the TT subjects suggests that the combination of TT and analgesic medication was able to produce a more complete pain relief than analgesic medication alone.

Reference: Turner J G, Clark A J, Gauthier D K, Williams M B 1998 The effect of therapeutic touch on pain and anxiety in burn patients. Journal of Advanced Nursing 28 (1): 10–20

Quality scores: IV: 80.8   EV: 41.4   MV: 66.7   JADAD: 4

Mixed Effects of Remote Mental Healing on Cardiovascular Parameters

Objective: To determine whether or not spiritual mind treatments and other forms of mental healing have a significant effect upon the recovery of patients.

Design: Quasi-randomized, double blinded controlled trial.

Setting: Date 1976, setting not stated.

Patients: Ninety-six hypertensive patients between the ages of 16 and 60. Eight healers were selected on the basis of their reputation.

Intervention: The patients were assigned to the program at the rate of four per week, two to the control and the other two to the eight healers for treatment within the next week. This procedure was followed until 96 patients were allocated to the program and each healer had treated six patients. The general healing treatment used by the healers involved (a) a relaxation step, (b) attunement with a higher power or infinite being, (c) a visualization and/or affirmation of the patient being in a state of perfect health, and (d) expression of thanks to God or to the source of all power and energy. Each healer who participated in the program was asked to make a tape which described in detail his or her exact thoughts and feelings during the healing treatments.

Main outcome measures: Pre- and post-treatment data were taken from the medical records. Improvement was judged by changes in the diastolic blood pressure, systolic blood pressure, heart rate, and weight.

Main results: There was a significant improvement in the systolic blood pressure of the healer-treated group (12.94 units change) compared with the control group (8.22 units change), $P = 0.014$. There were no significant differences in the changes of diastolic blood pressure (average drop for the control group was 5.5 units and was 5.75 units for the healer-treated group ($P = 0.87$)). There were no significant differences in the changes of pulse (average change for the control group was −5.05 beats per minute compared with −3.5 beats per minute for the healer-treated group, $P = 0.055$), and no difference in weight of the two groups (average change for the healer-treated group was 2.56 pounds compared to a change of 1.42 pounds for the control group, $P = 0.1384$). Four of the healers had a 92.3% improvement in their treated group of patients compared with 73.7% improvement for the control group.

Conclusions: Four of the eight healers who participated in the study were effective in improving the health of their patients over and above that which could be expected. Although there were differences between the post-treatment readings for the diastolic blood pressure, pulse and weight of the control group and the healer-treated group of patients, the variation was not large enough to be considered statistically significant. Further research with larger sample sizes is needed in this area.

Reference: Miller R N 1982 Study on the effectiveness of remote mental healing. Medical Hypotheses 8: 481–490

Quality scores: IV: 65.4   EV: 48.3   MV: 41.7   JADAD: 5

Distant Intercessory Prayer is more Effective for those who Pray than those being Prayed for on Self-Esteem, Anxiety, and Depression

Objective: To determine the effects of distant intercessory prayer on self-esteem, anxiety, and depression for people being prayed for and people doing the praying.

Design: Large randomized, controlled, double blind study.

Setting: San Francisco Bay area.

Participants: A total of 496 volunteers; those who prayed (agents, $n = 90$) and those who were prayed for (subjects, $n = 406$). All participants were aged 18 years and over. The subjects were not chosen because of any condition or pathology. Those who volunteered to be agents were not known to be 'healers' in any medical, psychological, or religious sense.

Intervention: Agents were randomly assigned to either a directed or non-directed prayer group. Photos and names of subjects were used as a focus. Subjects were randomly assigned to three groups: those prayed for by non-directed agents, a control group, and those prayed for by directed agents. Prayer was offered for 15 minutes daily for 12 weeks. Each subject was prayed for by three agents.

Main outcome measures: The state-trait anxiety inventory (STAI), the Coopersmith self-esteem inventory (CSEI), the profile of mood states (POMS), the Beck depression inventory (BDI), demographic information, informed consent and a prayer log.

Main results: At pre-test, differences on five objective measures were dramatic ($P < 0.0001$). As a group the agents had higher self-esteem, lower state-anxiety, lower trait-anxiety, lower depression levels, and lower total mood disturbance levels than the subjects. All 406 subjects improved significantly ($P < 0.01$ to $P < 0.0001$) on all objective and subjective measures. For the subjects, the two methods of prayer did not show a difference. There were no significant differences between the experimental condition and the control condition. All 90 agents improved significantly on 10 measures ($P < 0.05$ to $P < 0.0001$). For the agents, the two methods of prayer did not show a difference.

Conclusions: No differences in outcome were found between the control and the experimental conditions. No significant differences were found between directed and non-directed groups on any of the measures among agents or subjects. Agents scored significantly better than subjects both in pre-testing and post-testing. It seems, then, as if praying is more effective than being prayed for.

Reference: O'Laoire S 1997 An experimental study of the effects of distant, intercessory prayer on self-esteem, anxiety, and depression. Alternative Therapies 3(6): 38–53

Quality scores: IV: 73.1   EV: 44.8   MV: 41.7   JADAD: 4

Promising but Inconclusive Evidence Exists for the Efficacy of Distant Healing in a Systematic Review

Objective: To conduct a systematic review examining the data for or against the efficacy of spiritual healing as a treatment for any medical condition.

Data sources: Studies were identified through an electronic search of MEDLINE, PSYCH LIT, EMBASE, CISCOM and the Cochrane Library databases from their inception to the end of 1999, as well as contacting researchers in the field.

Study selection: Studies that had random assignment; placebo or adequate control; publication in peer-reviewed journals; clinical (rather than experimental) investigations; and use of human subjects were included in the review.

Data extraction: Two investigators independently extracted data on study design, sample size, type of intervention, type of control, direction and nature of the outcome(s).

Main results: A total of 21 trials involving 2062 patients met the inclusion criteria and were analyzed. Among the trials, six examined prayer as the spiritual healing intervention, 10 assessed the healing technique known as non- contact therapeutic touch, and five examined other forms of spiritual and/or distance healing. Of the 21 studies, 11 (52%) had statistically significant treatment effects, nine showed no effect, and one trial showed a negative effect. Roughly equal numbers of positive and negative findings were seen across each of the three categories.

Conclusions: Methodological limitations from a number of the studies makes it difficult to draw definitive conclusions for the potential efficacy of these approaches. However, given that approximately 52% of the trials reviewed showed a positive treatment effect, it is believed that the evidence thus far is interesting enough to conduct further research.

Reference: Astin J A, Harkness E, Ernst E 2000 The efficacy of 'distant healing': a systematic review of randomized trials. Annals of Internal Medicine 132: 903–910

Quality scores: Not applicable.

Therapeutic Touch Research Needs Improvement

Objective: To perform an integrative research review and meta-analysis of therapeutic touch research.

Data sources: Bibliography maintained by the Nurse Healers-Professional Associates International; MEDLINE, CINAHL, and Psychlit databases; dissertation and master's theses.

Study selection: Thirty-eight research articles were included in the analysis. All dissertations and research articles were analyzed.

Data extraction: Data on 32 substantive characteristics of the sample, the therapeutic touch procedure, and the

article/dissertation were extracted following Moody's method for an integrative research review. The meta-analysis used studies that reported means and standard deviations of the treatment and control groups.

Data synthesis: The research questions were as follows: (1) What are the substantive characteristics of the sample, the therapeutic touch practice, and the article/dissertation in research studies from 1975 to 1997? (2) What does the research demonstrate regarding the efficacy of therapeutic touch as an intervention? (3) Based on the results of the review and meta-analysis, what are the gaps, trends, and outcomes of the therapeutic touch research studies?

Conclusions: Most studies are described incompletely, and the therapeutic touch practices vary across the studies. A meta-analysis was performed on 13 studies. The average effect size in these studies was 0.39, which is described as moderate.

Reference: Winstead-Fry P, Kijek J 1999 An integrative review and meta-analysis of therapeutic touch research. Alternative Therapies 5(6): 58–67

Quality scores: Not applicable.

Qigong Therapy Improves Pain in Late-Stage Complex Regional Pain Syndrome in a Small Trial

Objective: To determine the effect of qigong on treatment-resistant patients with late-stage complex regional pain syndrome type I.

Design: Block-random placebo-controlled clinical trial, small scale ($n = 26$).

Setting: The Pain Management Center at New Jersey Medical School.

Patients: Twenty-six adult patients (aged 18–65 years) with complex regional pain syndrome type I.

Intervention: The experimental group received qi emission and qigong instruction (including home exercise) by a qigong master. The control group received similar instructions from a sham master. The experimental protocol included six 40-minute qigong sessions over 3 weeks, with reevaluation at 6 and 10 weeks.

Main outcome measures: A comprehensive medical history, physical exam, psychological evaluation, necessary diagnostic testing, symptom check list 90, and the Carleton University responsiveness to suggestion scale. Thermography, swelling, discoloration, muscle wasting, range of motion, pain intensity rating, medication usage, behavior assessment (activity level and domestic disability), frequency of pain awakening, mood assessment, and anxiety assessment were all assessed.

Main results: Twenty-two subjects completed the protocol. Among the genuine qigong group, 82% reported less pain by the end of the first training session compared to 45% of control patients. By the last training session, 91% of qigong patients reported decreased pain compared to 36% of control patients. Even though anxiety was reduced in both groups over time, the reduction was significantly greater in the experimental group, $F = 6.23$, $P < 0.01$.

Conclusions: By using a credible placebo to control for non-specific treatment effects, it was found that qigong training resulted in a short-term reduction in pain for those suffering from late-stage CRPS-1, and a long-term reduction in anxiety. These positive findings were not related to pre-experimental differences between groups in hypnotizability. Future studies of qigong should control for possible confounding influences and use clinical disorders more responsive to psychological intervention.

Reference: Wu W, Bandilla E, Ciccone D S et al 1999 Effects of qigong on late-stage complex regional pain syndrome. Alternative Therapies 5(1): 45–54

Quality scores: IV: 76.9   EV: 51.7   MV: 75.0   JADAD: 2

Qigong and Therapeutic Touch had Mixed Effects on Muscle Tension by EMG

Objective: To measure effect of qigong therapy along with the relaxation effect of therapeutic touch (TT) relative to patient belief and expectancy using a multisite surface electromyographic (sEMG) assessment procedure.

Design: Double blind pilot study, $n = 45$, where subjects were monitored for 25 minutes, divided into 5 minute segments: (1) unrecorded baseline; (2) recorded baseline/control; (3) treatment one; (4) recorded baseline/control; (5) treatment 2. Subjects were randomly assigned either qigong therapy or TT for treatment one, and received the other therapy for treatment two.

Setting: Subjects were seated comfortably with eyes closed. An experienced practitioner administered the particular therapy through an opening in a doorway, 5 feet behind the subject. A non-healer stood at the opening during control segments. All subjects were blinded to the actual treatment.

Patients: Forty-five subjects were divided into three groups: (1) students/patients of a qigong master; (2) students/patients of a TT practitioner; (3) non-believers/skeptics of complementary therapies. Group one subjects were informed they would only receive qigong therapy; group 2, TT; group 3, assessment of neuromuscular activity.

Intervention: A traditional ABAC experimental design was used with each subject evaluated for one 20-minute session that included four 5-minute segments. Treatment sessions consisted of qigong and a modified form of TT intervention for all three groups.

Main outcome measures: Responses during tests were measured using multisite surface electromyographic (sEMG) electrodes placed on the frontalis, cervical (C4), thoracic (T6), and lumbosacral (L3) paraspinal areas.

Main results: Data from 44 subjects were analyzed. The lumbar site showed significantly greater effects than the others ($P < 0.0001$). A strong trend ($P < 0.09$) was found between treatment group and treatment, showing increased neuromuscular activity for group one (qigong), decreased activity for group 2 (TT), and no change for group 3 (control). Group 1 showed statistically significant muscle energizing ($P < 0.024$) when comparing baseline with qigong therapy. Modest drops in muscle energy occurred when group 1 received TT, as it did when group

2 received TT or qigong. Group 3 remained constant with both therapies.

Conclusions: Several confounding factors make these results preliminary and non-generalizable. For example, the subjects in groups 1 and 2 were familiar with one of the therapies and were expecting it. Further research is needed in this area.

Reference: Wirth D P, Cram J R, Chang R J 1997 Multisite electromyographic analysis of therapeutic touch and qigong therapy. Journal of Alternative and Complementary Medicine 3: 109–118

Quality scores: IV: 65.4   EV: 27.6   MV: 50.0   JADAD: 3

Therapeutic Touch Reduced and Improved Distress and Mood Indicators in Women

Objective: To evaluate the effects of therapeutic touch (TT) on biochemical indicators and mood in women.

Design: Randomized control trial.

Setting: A laboratory room, where controls completed questionnaires and the experimental group, in a separate room, was instructed to remove their shoes and lie on a hospital bed. Soft music was played on a tape player while TT was administered by a trained energy healer.

Participants: Forty-one healthy female volunteers who ranged in age from 30 to 64 years of age.

Intervention: Participants were randomly assigned to either an experimental group who received TT ($n = 22$) or to a control group who did not receive TT ($n = 19$). The TT steps followed by the practitioner involved centering, assessment, unruffling, directing and modulating energy, and stopping when the energy balance has been restored. The participants are then allowed to rest 5–10 minutes and then fill out their questionnaires.

Main outcome measures: Pre-test and post-test urine samples were collected to test nitric oxide (NO) levels. The profile of mood states (POMS) and the state-trait anxiety inventory (STAI) were administered across three consecutive monthly sessions.

Main results: Results show that mood disturbance in the experimental group decreased significantly over the course of the three sessions, while the control group increased in mood disturbance over time ($P < 0.01$). Specifically, experimental group participants showed significant reductions in tension ($P < 0.05$), confusion ($P < 0.01$), and anxiety ($P < 0.01$), and a significant increase in vigor across sessions ($P < 0.05$). Analyses of the biochemical data, through the collection of urine samples, indicated that TT produced a significant decrease in levels of nitric oxide in the experimental group by the third TT session ($P < 0.05$).

Conclusions: The positive findings of reductions in mood disturbance and decreased levels of nitric oxide across experimental sessions observed in this pilot study suggest that further research in this area is warranted.

Reference: Lafreniere K D, Mutus B, Cameron S et al 1999 Effects of therapeutic touch on biochemical and mood indicators in women. Journal of Alternative and Complementary Medicine 5(4): 367–370

Quality scores: IV: 42.3   EV: 41.4   MV: 50.0   JADAD: 1

Attentive Touch Improves Sleep, but No Other Parameters in Elderly Persons with Dementia

Objective: To test the efficacy of 'attentive touch' (focused touching or stroking of the hands, arms, shoulder, upper back, feet and legs) as a way to improve care for nursing home residents with dementia and to increase family visitation and satisfaction.

Design: Randomized, controlled, large scale ($n = 130$) study.

Setting: Eleven New York State nursing homes, over a 6 month period during the fall of 1997 and spring 1998.

Patients: A total of 130 nursing home residents diagnosed with dementia.

Intervention: The intervention group's family members used attentive touch on their relative for 15 minutes two times a week, with at least one other attentive touch session done by a family or staff member. One of the control group's family members spent at least 15 minutes two times a week in conversation with their relative, with at least one more conversation session done by a family or staff member. The second control group's family members visited their relative as usual, with no attentive touch or conversation protocol.

Main outcome measures: Relaxation level, agitation, depression, sleep disturbances, pre- and post-test data collected from families.

Main results: Significant results were found only in improved sleep patterns and a decrease in disorientation for the patient. The improved sleep patterns can have a profoundly positive impact on the entire nursing home community. Unfortunately, there were not enough completed pre- and post-tests on family members to determine the affect of attentive touch on family members.

Conclusions: It was found that attentive touch was correlated to improved sleeping patterns of residents with dementia and to reduced disorientation. Because of the difficulty in gathering sufficient pre- and post-tests of family members, the study did not determine the effect of attentive touch on families.

Reference: Foundation for Long-term Care 1998 Keeping in touch: attentive touch for nursing home residents with dementia. Foundation for Long-term Care, 150 State St., Albany, NY 12207

Quality scores: IV: 38.5   EV: 41.4   MV: 58.3   JADAD: 1

Therapeutic Touch Exceeds Casual Touch for Reducing Stress of Hospitalized Children

Objective: To compare the effectiveness of therapeutic touch and casual touch for stress reduction of hospitalized children aged 2 weeks to 2 years old.

Design: Controlled observational study ($n = 30$).

Setting: A private, 490-bed medical center in the mid-west region of the United States.

Patients: Children hospitalized for injury, acute illness or surgery were included in the study. Stress experiences included painful and non-painful procedures; being forcibly held, departure of parents, and being awakened from sleep. The population was selected from admissions to a 30-bed pediatric unit during a 5-month period until a sample of 30 was obtained.

Intervention: Data were gathered during the 6 a.m. to 2 p.m. time period. This is the time when the majority of care and most procedures, such as drawing blood, physician examinations, and invasive or surgical procedures, are performed. For the therapeutic touch intervention, the healer centered herself, assessed the child's energy flow, mobilized non-flowing energy fields, and directed energy through the hands to the client. Subjects receiving casual touch remained recumbent in the crib during intervention. The subject was comforted by the researcher by being stroked or patted on the head, upper torso or arms for 6 minutes.

Main outcome measures: Stress reduction was assessed via physiological measures, including pulse, galvanic skin response (GSR), and peripheral skin temperature (PST). An ANOVA was used to measure the effectiveness of the interventions at 3 and 6-minute intervals.

Main results: The ANOVA completed on the 3-minute scores demonstrate a significant difference in means between the group treated with TT compared with the group treated with casual touch at 3 minutes, $F = 26.98$, d.f.(1,29), $P < 0.05$, with the TT group having reduced stresses. The computed $F = 26.94$ at 6 minutes demonstrated at the $P < 0.05$, that still there remained a reduction in stress in the TT group as compared to the casual touch group at that time.

Conclusion: Therapeutic touch reduced the time needed to calm children after stressful experiences. This is very helpful; while it more quickly reduces the child's stress it will provide a longer time for comfort and in turn possibly less time for hospital stay.

Reference: Kramer N A 1990 Comparison of therapeutic touch and casual touch in stress reduction of hospitalized children. Pediatric Nursing 16(5): 483–485

Quality scores: IV: 42.3   EV: 34.5   MV: 41.7   JADAD: 0

Mental Healing for Chronically Ill Patients is more Effective for 'Positive' Thinkers

Objective: To determine if a healer could influence any patient in person and at a distance by a 'spiritual energetic' method, which involves a 'reconnection with the fundamental source of life.'

Design: Before–after intervention outcome study with psychological interviews and tests, as well as physical examinations.

Setting: January to July 1955, on four successive days each month, at the Freiburg Institute for Border Areas of Psychology and Mental Hygiene.

Patients: A total of 650 patients, who came voluntarily. The majority of the patients were suffering from chronic illnesses and had come to the mental healer because other methods of treatment had failed. Their illnesses covered an extremely wide range of both organic and functional maladies.

Intervention: The healer met with the patients and gave a lecture on what he did and what he believed in and then performed his energy work with the patients individually. During the period after treatment, patients held aluminum foil, which had previously 'charged' after leaving his presence, where he would continue to influence their diseases at a distance.

Main outcome measures: Patients were initially given psychological interviews and tests, as well as physical examinations both before and after treatment. The sociological structure of patient categories, their expectations and attitudes, were also recorded. The Z-test, the color pyramid test, and a perception-diagnosis experiment with the Exner disk were all performed to see if they were the same pre and post intervention.

Main results: During a 14-month follow-up period, subjective improvement and temporary improvement was reported by 61% of the patients. The influence of Trampler produced the main subjective changes in the condition of the patients, as objective improvements were stated in only 11%.

Conclusions: Subjective improvement stems largely from the patient's attitudes toward the healing and the healer. If you believe and think positively, positive reactions may occur, but if not, you may not notice any changes in your health. The negative group displayed a higher level of intelligence and stronger critical capacity, but also more self-confidence and a tense, not very relaxed personality structure as compared with the positive group. So, it seems that confrontation with a healer is not the only factor involved, and that the patient's predisposition can play a major role in the process. There is not enough evidence, however, to firmly state this is a factor in the healing process.

Reference: Strauch I 1963 Medical aspects of 'mental' healing. International Journal for Parapsychology 5: 135–166

Quality scores: Not applicable.

Reiki and LeShan Reduced Postoperative Pain after Surgical Removal of Impacted Third Molar Teeth in a Small Crossover Study

Objective: To examine the effect of Reiki and LeShan healing in combination on pain experienced after unilateral operative extraction of the lower third molar.

Design: A small scale ($n = 21$) randomized, double blind crossover trial.

Setting: A dental clinic, where surgery was performed between 9 a.m. and 12 noon each day.

Patients: Initially, 28 subjects from a dental clinic population volunteered for participation in the study. After exclusion of subjects for various reasons, 21 volunteers remained. Patients all had bilateral, asymptomatic, impacted lower third molar teeth with an equal anticipated degree of

difficulty of extraction for each side. The subjects included 12 women and nine men, aged 19–28, who were otherwise in good health.

Intervention: The patients were randomly assigned to the treatment or control condition prior to the first operation. For the second operation, patients crossed over to the opposite condition. All preoperative and postoperative conditions were identical for the treatment and control groups for both operations, with the exception that the treatment group received Reiki and LeShan healing postoperatively from a distance, in a separate building several miles from the subject, beginning at exactly 3 hours postoperatively. The LeShan and Reiki healers would begin by performing healing at a distance for 15–20 minutes utilizing a picture of the subject. They would alternate at each hour for a duration of 6 hours, with LeShan healers getting the even postop hours and Reiki healers performing at odd hours.

Main outcome measures: Patients assessed their pain intensity using a 100 mm visual analogue scale (VAS) for postoperative hours 3 through 9, and pain relief using a five-point pain relief (PAR) scale for hours 4 through 9. ANOVA was used to analyze the data, which took into consideration the effect of patient, treatment, period, sequence, and hour.

Main results: The five-factor analysis of variance utilized for the pain intensity data showed that there was no significant difference between the first operation and the second operation, i.e. no period effect ($F = 1.07$; d.f. = 1; $P > 0.30$) and also that there was no significant sequence effect ($F = 0.96$; d.f. = 1; $P > 0.34$). There was a significant effect between the treatment and control conditions ($F = 21.74$; d.f. = 1; $P < 0.0001$). The statistically significant difference between the treatment and control groups in both the level of pain intensity and the degree of pain relief was experienced for postoperative hours 4–9.

Conclusions: A combination of Reiki and LeShan healing may significantly reduce postoperative pain following the extraction of impacted lower third molar teeth.

Reference: Wirth D P, Brenlan D R, Levine R J, Rodriguez C M 1993 The effect of complementary healing therapy on postoperative pain after surgical removal of impacted third molar teeth. Complementary Therapies in Medicine 1: 133–138

Quality scores: IV: 46.2   EV: 27.6   MV: 41.7   JADAD: 3

Intercessory Prayer Did Not Improve Alcohol Abuse and Dependence Treatment in a Small Study

Objective: To conduct a pilot study on the effect of intercessory prayer on patients entering alcohol abuse or dependence treatment.

Design: A small scale ($n = 40$), randomized, double blind, control trial.

Setting: The University of New Mexico's Center on Alcoholism, Substance Abuse and Addictions.

Patients: Forty patients admitted to a public substance abuse treatment facility for treatment of alcohol problems, who agreed to participate. Twenty-two patients were assigned to the prayer intervention group and 18 to the group with no added prayer.

Intervention: In addition to their standard treatment, the patients were randomized to receive or not receive intercessory prayer by outside volunteers, who had at least 5 years experience. The standard treatment of the program includes detoxification, rehabilitation, group and individual counseling, medication, and psychiatric evaluation and intervention.

Main outcome measures: Alcohol breath tests and urine drug screens were obtained at each assessment point. Assessments were conducted at baseline, 3 months, and 6 months.

Main results: No differences were found between the prayer intervention and non-intervention groups on alcohol consumption. Compared with a normative group of patients treated at the same facility, the prayer study group experienced a delay in drinking reduction. Those who reported at baseline that a family member or friend was already praying for them were found to be drinking significantly more at 6 months than were those unaware of anyone praying for them. Greater frequency of prayer by the participants themselves was associated with less drinking, but only at months 2 and 3.

Conclusion: Intercessory prayer did not demonstrate clinical benefit in the treatment of alcohol abuse and dependence under these study conditions. Prayer may be a complex phenomenon with many interacting variables.

Reference: Walker S R, Tonigan J S, Miller W R, Comer S, Kahlich L 1997 Intercessory prayer in the treatment of alcohol abuse and dependence: a pilot investigation. Alternative Therapies 3(6): 79–86

Quality scores: IV: 73.1   EV: 27.6   MV: 58.3   JADAD: 5

No Effect of Therapeutic vs. Physical Touch for Reducing Stress Response Measures

Objective: To determine if people exposed to a stressful stimulus would become more relaxed being exposed to therapeutic touch or to physical touch.

Design: A small ($n = 60$), randomized, double blind controlled study.

Setting: A laboratory room, consisting of the data-collecting equipment, clock, table, chair, researcher, movie screen, projector, and the nurse who administered either therapeutic or physical touch. To eliminate changes in skin temperature due to environment, room temperature was kept at 70–74° F.

Participants: Sixty healthy volunteer female college students, none of whom were suffering from a physical or emotional illness or taking any medication. The age range was 19–53 years with a mean of 27 years.

Intervention: The film *Subincision* served as the stressful stimulus for the students. This film is a 13-minute silent film, which records a tribal ceremony, including a sequence of operations performed with a sharp stone on the genitals of adolescent boys. Electrodes were attached to the subjects while they sat for 5 minutes as the data-collection equipment was adjusted and baseline recordings obtained.

After baseline measurements, the film started and the nurse entered the room and lightly placed her hands on the subject's abdomen and lower back. The experimental group received therapeutic touch; the control group received physical touch.

Main outcome measures: The physiological response was measured by skin conductance level (SCL), electromyography level (EMG), and skin temperature, which are representative of central, autonomic, and peripheral nervous system functions.

Main results: For both groups, there were significant changes between baseline and the stressor point for the SCL measurement ($t = 5.02$, $P = 0.001$ for treatment and $t = -0.77$, $P = 0.001$ for control). For the EMG response a similar pattern occurred. The therapeutic touch group increased an average of 2.34 microvolts ($t = 5.02$, $P = 0.001$); the physical touch group elevated 2.08 microvolts ($t = 5.61$, $P = 0.001$). Thus, the results from the SCL and EMG readings showed an increased physiological stress response to the film. The mean hand temperature did not change significantly between baseline and stressor point for either group. The therapeutic touch group, a mean change of 0.63°F ($t = 1.19$, $P = 0.24$) while in the physical touch group the mean fell by –0.27°F ($t = 0.77$, $P = 0.45$).

Conclusion: There was no significant difference in the psychophysiological measures between groups when treated by therapeutic touch.

Reference: Randolph G L 1984 Therapeutic and physical touch: physiological response to stressful stimuli. Nursing Research 33(1): 33–36

Quality scores: IV: 56.7   EV: 34.5   MV: 41.7   JADAD: 3

Variable Effects on Stress-Induced Immunosuppression from Therapeutic Touch in a Small Trial

Objective: To determine the effectiveness of therapeutic touch in reducing the adverse immunological effects of stress in a sample of highly stressed students.

Design: Experimental, randomized controlled pilot study.

Setting: A large urban medical university in a southern coastal city.

Subjects: Twenty healthy medical and nursing students who are taking professsional board examinations. These students were among those who scored one standard deviation above the mean on the SSTAI given during final examination periods 5–6 months before the time they were to take the board exam. This was to assure that anxious people were among the sample.

Intervention: All students completed each tool and contributed a blood sample according to the study. Therapeutic touch students received three therapeutic touch appointments, at least 24 hours apart, at the same time of day, the week prior to the exams. The control students did not attend any therapeutic touch sessions but did participate in everything else as the therapeutic touch group.

Main outcome measures: Self-evaluation questionnaire form Y, the SSTAI, was used to measure state and trait anxiety, which ranges from 20 (no anxiety) to 80 (maximum anxiety). The profile of moods (POMS) factors scale, the impact of events scale, demographic data and health habits questionnaire were used. T-lymphocyte function (CD25) and immunoglobulin levels were measured.

Main results: Subjects who received therapeutic touch and subjects who did not had significantly different levels of IgA, mean of 5 (SD 10) for experimental (mean of −5 (SD 12) for control, $P = 0.05$,) and IgM, mean of 10 (SD 21) for experimental (mean of −7 (SD 10) for control, $P = 0.05$); CD25 ($P = 0.46$) and IgG ($P = 0.06$) levels differed in the expected direction between the two groups, but the differences were not statistically significant. Apoptosis was significantly different between the two groups, mean of −0.3 (SD 2) in experimental group vs. (mean of −3 (SD 4) in control, $P = 0.05$).

Conclusions: Differences between groups after treatment were found to be significant for IgM and IgA, but not for IgG or for immunoglobulin subclasses. The hypothesis is somewhat supported from these results. SSTAI scores indicated that both groups were stressed before the study began. No significant difference between the groups occurred after treatments, but the results did change in the expected direction. The small sample size requires cautious interpretation of the results. A power analysis suggests sample sizes of 90 subjects per group are required to confirm the conclusions.

Reference: Olson M, Sneed N, LaVia M, Virella G, Bonadonna R, Michel Y 1997 Stress-induced immunosuppression and therapeutic touch. Alternative Therapies 3(2): 68–74

Quality scores: IV: 65.4   EV: 31.0   MV: 58.3   JADAD: 3

State Anxiety Reduction by Therapeutic Touch Not Significant in a Small Study

Objective: To determine the effectiveness of the use of therapeutic touch in reducing subject anxiety in situations complicated by high levels of state anxiety.

Design: Small, randomized controlled trial, four-group, repeated-measures experimental design.

Setting: A quiet room where the subjects sat on stools during the intervention.

Subjects: Forty professional caregivers/students who were enrolled in the nursing or health-related program of a university. All reported being in good health.

Intervention: Subjects were first categorized by anxiety level and were then randomly assigned to either an intervention of therapeutic touch or a comparison group. All sessions occurred before a big exam, paper or presentation, when anxiety should be evident. All subjects had appointments to sit quietly in a room for 15 minutes during intervention or no intervention.

Main outcome measures: The outcome measured was the reduction of state anxiety. Three self-report measures of anxiety were used: the Spielberger's state/trait anxiety inventory (SSTAI), the profile of mood states (POMS) scale, and visual analogue scales (VAS).

Main results: The reduction in anxiety in the high-anxiety group was greater for those who had received therapeutic touch than for those who did not, but this did not reach statistical significance. However, the sample size necessary to find the statistically significant differences may not have been attained. It was determined that a sample size of 76 in each of the two high-anxiety groups would be needed to have statistical significance in this study.

Conclusions: Data gathered in this study are consistent with that of studies done in the past, showing that perceived anxiety seems to decrease after therapeutic touch in highly anxious subjects. By looking at highly anxious subjects vs. the less anxious subjects, it is apparent that there is little or no value in continuing to study TT for low-anxiety subjects. Therapeutic touch appears to be more effective for those who feel highly anxious.

Reference: Olson M, Sneed N 1995 Anxiety and therapeutic touch. Issues in Mental Health Nursing 16(2): 97–108

Quality scores: IV: 57.7   EV: 44.8   MV: 66.7   JADAD: 2

Non-Contact Therapeutic Touch Produces a Lower Level of Arousal than a Mimic

Objective: To investigate the effect of therapeutic touch without contact (NCTT) upon autonomic and CNS parameters.

Design: Randomized, blinded controlled, small scale ($n = 12$) crossover trial.

Setting: A retreat center in Northern California where subjects were seated facing a wall with their back toward the experimenter.

Participants: Twelve subjects, six men and six women, ranging in age from 21 to 52 years. The subjects were all community members or visitors of a yoga retreat center located in Northern California. They had 2–12 years of meditation experience with an average of 5.1 years. Ten of the subjects reported being healthy with no major medical problems, one complained of recurrent migraine headaches over the past several years, and one reported low back pain for the past 6 months at the time of the study.

Intervention: Each subject was monitored for one evaluation session. The session was divided into four segments: (1) baseline; (2) mimic or NCTT; (3) baseline; and (4) mimic or NCTT. The subjects were randomly assigned to receive either mimic or NCTT during segment 2. If mimic was received in segment 2, NCTT was received in segment 4. Each segment lasted 5–7 minutes with a total session time per subject of 20–28 minutes. The subjects sat for approximately 30 minutes meditating with their eyes closed. Once the sensors were attached, subjects were monitored for a 5 minute unrecorded pre-baseline period allowing them to become comfortable with the equipment and acclimated to the environment.

Main outcome measures: The impact of NCTT was assessed by multisite electromyographic EMG recordings located at the frontalis, cervical 4 paraspinals, thoracic 6 paraspinals, and lumbosacral 3 paraspinals. Autonomic indicators of physiological activity were also monitored and included hand and head temperature, heart rate, and end tidal CO_2 levels.

Main results: The results demonstrated that all of the autonomic indicators showed a general trend toward lower levels of arousal over time. The data also showed that three of the four muscle regions monitored – C4, T6, and L3 paraspinals – indicated a significant reduction in energy during and following the NCTT treatment sessions for a majority of the subjects. The C4 EMG showed a significant NCTT treatment effect ($F = 10.31$, d.f. = 1, $P < 0.009$), while the T6 EMG ($F = 13.49$, d.f. = 1, $P < 0.004$) and L3 EMG ($F = 4.74$, d.f. = 1, $P < 0.05$) also demonstrated significance. The TT procedure was associated with large to moderate decreases in EMG activation levels, while mimic showed slight increases in surface EMG activity. When the treatment effects of mimic minus baseline $vs.$ TT minus baseline were compared, significant treatment effects were found; C4 EMG ($F = 9.39$; d.f. = 1; $P < 0.01$), T6 EMG ($F = 10.37$; d.f. = 1; $P < 0.009$), and the L3 EMG ($F = 6.02$; d.f. = 1; $P < 0.03$).

Conclusions: The results of the study support three findings. First, that NCTT significantly alters the physiology of the individual treated. Second, that these changes were evident in the relaxation or normalization phase. And third, that the overall effects of either the meditation practice or habituation to the experimental setting made it more difficult to attribute changes in physiology to the NCTT treatment.

Reference: Wirth D P, Cram J R 1993 Multi-site electromyographic analysis of non-contact therapeutic touch. International Journal of Psychosomatic Research 40(1–4): 47–55

Quality scores: not applicable

Therapeutic Touch and Relaxation Therapy Reduced Anxiety in a Small Trial

Objective: To examine the effects of two non-invasive procedures on anxiety.

Design: Small, randomized controlled trial ($n = 31$).

Setting: An adult inpatient psychiatric VA hospital.

Participants: Thirty-one patients at an adult inpatient psychiatric VA hospital were included in the study. Ages ranged from 29 to 69 years, with a mean age of 43. Of the sample chosen, nine subjects were assigned to a placebo therapeutic touch (TT) condition, 10 to the TT intervention, and 12 to the relaxation therapy (RT) condition.

Intervention: Each subject completed a self-report anxiety measure and was rated for amount of motor activity before and after each of two 15-minute treatment sessions involving therapeutic touch, placebo therapeutic touch, or relaxation therapy in a 24-hour period.

Main outcome measures: Experienced anxiety was measured with the state-trait anxiety inventory (STAI), form Y-1 state anxiety, the frequency of extraneous physical movement over a 30-second period was collected during rest periods before and after each intervention, and a 10-item questionnaire to assess the subjects' confidence or belief in the treatment experienced.

Main results: Multivariate analysis of variance showed that relaxation therapy provided significant reduction of anxiety on the self-report measure (23% reduction). The nursing intervention of therapeutic touch also resulted in significant reductions of reported anxiety (26% reduction). The control group showed small but non-significant effects (7.7% decrease in anxiety). The TT and RT groups showed significant reductions in the STAI scores after treatment (TT: $F (1,9) = 43.87$, $P < 0.001$; RT: $F(1,11) = 13.3$, $P < 0.01$). The control group showed a small but non-significant change ($F (1,8) = 1.45$, $P > 0.05$). The only group to show a significant change in motor activity after treatment was the RT group ($F (1,11) = 25.63$, $P < 0.001$).

Conclusions: The results suggest that both relaxation and therapeutic touch are effective palliatives to experienced anxiety.

Reference: Gagne D, Toye R C 1994 The effects of therapeutic touch and relaxation therapy in reducing anxiety. Archives of Psychiatric Nursing 8(3): 184–189

Quality scores: IV: 53.8   EV: 44.8   MV: 75.0   JADAD: 3

Therapeutic Touch Improves Elderly Subjects' Sleep in a Small Observational Study

Objective: To determine if therapeutic touch improves residents' sleep patterns in a nursing home.

Design: Single subject, controlled design ($n = 6$) study.

Setting: Nursing home.

Patients: Six female nursing home residents who were mentally alert, socially responsive and functionally independent agreed to participate. Their ages ranged from 75 to 96 years with an average age of 85 years.

Intervention: The study was carried out for 9 days for three residents and 12 days for the other three residents. The first 3 days were used to establish a baseline of how well each resident slept. No therapeutic touch was done during this time. On the second 3 days, each resident received the therapeutic touch procedure at bedtime. On days 7, 8, and 9, the patients filled out questionnaires and for the residents who completed days 10, 11, and 12, the nurse talked to each resident for 10 minutes at bedtime, but no therapeutic touch was involved.

Main outcome measures: Visser's (1979) sleep quality questionnaire was completed each morning.

Main results: When sleep quality scores were graphed, five of the six residents were shown to experience significantly better sleep as a result of the therapeutic touch. Sleep quality scores for these five residents on days 4, 5, and 6 (the mornings after TT) were higher than any other days. On days when there was no TT, the sleep quality returned to baseline. And for the days when the nurse just talked with the residents before bed instead of TT, there was no improvement in the quality of their sleep from baseline. No statistical analyses were done.

Conclusions: Overall, therapeutic touch was effective in enhancing the sleep quality of this group of nursing home residents. It is a technique that should be added to the nursing measures used to help the elderly to sleep.

Reference: Braun C, Layton J, Braun J 1986 Therapeutic touch improves residents' sleep. American Health Care Association Journal 12(1): 48–49

Quality scores: Not applicable.

Reiki and Soft Music were Accompanied by Reduced Pain from Cancer in a Small Observational Trial

Objective: To explore the usefulness of Reiki as an adjuvant to opioid therapy in the management of pain.

Design: Pilot, intervention outcome study, non-randomized, non-controlled.

Setting: At a Reiki therapist's office, patients lie on a massage table fully clothed. Lights are dimmed, and a candle is lit; soft music plays in the background. The environment stays consistent throughout the entire 20 sessions.

Participants: Twenty people were recruited (18 women and two men) who ranged in age from 23 to 62 years (mean 44 years). All participants were currently experiencing pain from cancer, at least scoring a 3 on a visual analogue scale (VAS) (0–10) or a 2 on a Likert scale (0–5), at 55 sites on their bodies. Ten had pain in their upper body, and four in their lower body. The remaining six had pain in both the upper and lower parts of their body.

Intervention: Participants were given one treatment by the Reiki therapist in the office.

Main outcome measures: A pain VAS ranging from 0 to 10 and a Likert scale ranging from 0 to 5 were completed immediately before and after the Reiki treatment.

Main results: Seventeen participants on the VAS scale and 18 participants on the Likert scale reported a reduction in their pain following treatment (P = 0.001 and 0.0002, respectively). A comparison of the before and after scores using a paired t-test showed a mean decrease in pain scores for the VAS scale of 2.25 and for the Likert scale of 1.25 (P < 0.0001 for each test). Overall, 85% of the participants experienced pain reduction following Reiki treatment, 95% confidence interval (CI) ± 15.6%.

Conclusions: The results of this trial are difficult to interpret. The lack of a placebo control group does not allow us to rule out the possibility of a placebo effect. Also, from this trial it was not possible to determine its long-term benefit or the interaction between Reiki and other forms of pain management. The music played during the intervention may have also confounded the findings.

Reference: Olson K, Hanson J 1997 Using Reiki to manage pain: a preliminary report. Cancer Prevention and Control 1(2): 108–113

Quality scores: IV: 50.0   EV: 38.0   MV: 58.3   JADAD: 1

Changes in Certain Electrical Conductance Measures associated with Reiki Hands-On Healing

Objective: To evaluate the therapeutic effects of Reiki treatment on electrodermal conductance.

Design: Observational study (n = 5).

Setting: Reiki therapists' rooms.

Participants: Five patients with multiple sclerosis, lupus, fibromyalgia, or thyroid goiter.

Intervention: Patients were given 11 1-hour Reiki sessions using four different Reiki level two practitioners and one Reiki master, over 9 weeks. These Reiki practitioners systematically placed their hands over holding points of neurovascular regions on the cranium, neurolymphatic points on the trunk, and minor chakra points on the limbs. During this time period, patients received no other treatments. All participants initially received three consecutive Reiki sessions that were followed by one Reiki session per week for 8 weeks.

Main outcome measures: Changes in electrical skin resistance measurements at acupuncture/conductance points using the life information system TEN (LISTEN) device.

Main Results: Out of the 40 skin points measured per session, only three showed significant differences before and after Reiki treatment. These three skin points correlate with acupuncture/conductance meridians of Spleen One, SP1, adrenal glands, THI, and the cervical, thoracic region of the spine, NE2. Prior to Reiki treatment, the mean conductance measurements at these three points were below the normal range of 45.0–55.0 relative units, indicating a chronic illness and depletion of chi. The left side NE2 point statistically changed from 24% below normal to normal after the third Reiki session (P < 0.004). The right side NE2 point also improved into the normal range by the last Reiki session (P < 0.003), and both NE2 points were within the normal range by completion of the study at 45.0 ± 2.0 units. SP1, originally 16% below normal at 42.0 ± 6.0 units, reached the normal range of 48.0 ± 6.0 units after the third Reiki session (P < 0.005) and maintained normal electrical conductance throughout the study. The rise in conductance, an indication of greater electrical permeability statistically increased at NE2, SP1, and THI with Reiki, P < 0.01, P < 0.056, and P < 0.025, respectively.

Conclusion: This study demonstrates a method for quantifying subtle energy improvements after treatment with techniques of hands-on healing not easily measured by conventional testing. Further study in this area with a larger sample size is warranted.

Reference: Brewitt B, Vittetoe T, Hartwell B 1997 The efficacy of Reiki hands-on healing: improvements in spleen and nervous system function as quantified by electrodermal screening. Alternative Therapies 3(4): 89

Quality scores: Not applicable.

No Effect of Therapeutic Touch and Intercessory Prayer on Insulin Use in a Small Study

Objective: To examine the effect of non-contact therapeutic touch (NCTT) therapy and intercessory prayer (IP) on patient determined insulin dosage.

Design: Randomized, double blind, crossover design, small scale (n = 16) study.

Setting: An outpatient clinic where subjects sat in a recliner in one room and the healers present in an adjoining room, with a door equipped with a one-way mirror measuring 2 feet × 3 feet so that the healer could have a clear view of the subject.

Participants: Sixteen type I diabetes mellitus patients were included in this study. The patients were normotensive, non-ketotic, and in good health with an age range of 25–48 years (mean 37 years). There were 12 women and 4 men, all of whom were long-term diabetics utilizing a multiple-dose insulin regimen and on a regular diet.

Intervention: The patients were examined and treated daily by NCTT and IP healers from a distance of 4 feet, where the healer was on the other side of a one-way mirror, for a duration of 2 weeks. Each patient underwent two separate sessions – one in the treatment condition and one in the control condition – with the patients crossing over to the opposite condition for the second session.

Main outcome measures: Capillary blood glucose data, insulin dose and type, significant changes in food intake or activity, and any other event or thoughts which they felt were noteworthy.

Main results: The results indicated that while 11 of the 16 patients (69%) in the treatment group showed a reduction in insulin dose levels as compared to the control group, the difference in insulin dosage did not reach significance ($F = 2.35$; d.f. = 1; $P > 0.12$).

Conclusions: Various methodological considerations may have been important contributing factors to the non-significant results obtained. The 4 foot distance and mirrored glass barrier separating healer and patient could be confounding the results; the treatment and control sessions may have been too short to notice changes; the experimental instructions advising patients to adjust their caloric intake and energy expenditure prior to adjusting their insulin dose could have been a wrong idea; and the use of healthy long-term insulin dependent diabetes mellitus IDDM patients with a stable insulin dose who did not exhibit any diabetic sequelae could have been the wrong population to examine.

Reference: Wirth D P, Mitchell B J 1994 Complementary healing therapy for patients with type I diabetes mellitus. Journal of Scientific Exploration 8(3): 367–377

Quality scores: IV: 76.9   EV: 44.8   MV: 58.3   JADAD: 5

Psychophysiological Changes Occurred with a Hawaiian Healer and Client during Healing Sessions

Objective: To investigate whether within and between subject physiological changes might occur during a healing experience that would differentiate healing from baseline and control conditions.

Design: Clinical observational study ($n = 2$).

Setting: A quiet, dimly lit EEG laboratory, where the healer and client were seated next to each other.

Subjects: The subjects were a middle-aged Hawaiian couple, one being the healer and the other the client, involved in ancient Hawaiian healing arts for approximately 20 years. The healer practices a form of spiritual healing that involves the detection of putative energy blockages and the sending of *mana* or life-force to release the client's blockages.

Intervention: Nineteen active EEG scalp electrodes were applied to the healer and to the client according to the international 10–20 electrode system with conductive electrode paste. The protocol for the healer consisted of a 2-minute reading period followed by a 4-minute eyes closed baseline. Then another 2-minute reading period followed by a 4-minute meditation period occurred. After another 2 minutes of reading, a 12-minute healing session occurred. After the healing session, another baseline was recorded. The client's experimental protocol differed only in that instead of a meditation control period, there was a relaxation period. At the conclusion of the experiment both subjects, the healer and the client, filled out an assessment of the depth of their states of relaxation or meditation and the intensity of their healing session.

Main outcome measures: Simultaneous measurements of EEG absolute power and coherence, heart rate, skin conductance, and hand temperature were performed on the two subjects during the five periods.

Main results and conclusions: Each subject demonstrated significant physiological changes during healing that allowed differentiation of healing from their control and baseline conditions. Both EEG and somatic physiological measures indicated that the healer became more aroused during healing and the client more relaxed. The healer had a drop in frontal to occipital interhemispheric coherence during healing as well as increased heart rate and skin conductance. The client had a drop in frontal beta power and a drop in skin conductance. The client also exhibited a strong trend toward increased parietal interhemispheric alpha band coherence during healing. No meaningful increase in covariance of EEG or other physiological measures occurred between the subjects during healing.

Reference: Bearden T S 1995 Simultaneous psychophysiological assessments of a Hawaiian healer and client during healing. Subtle Energies 6(3): 241–266

Quality scores: Not applicable.

An Inadequate Study of Temperature Change Using a Subtle Energies Device

Objective: To determine if a subtle energy device, the Cayce Radial Appliance, could improve circulation in the extremities.

Design: A randomized, double blind, placebo controlled experiment.

Setting: Both in the laboratory and in the privacy of the subjects' own homes.

Participants: The subjects were volunteers who identified themselves as having cold hands or feet. The hands or feet had to be below 80° F, measured at the thumb and big toe. There were four men and 26 women; the mean age was 48.9.

Intervention: Baseline temperatures were taken initially and then subjects were hooked up to the Radial appliances, where half were turned into placebo devices with unconnected wires inside. Lab sessions 1, 4, and 16 consisted of 30 minutes baseline, and 60 minutes treatment. Home sessions 2–3, and 5–15 consisted of

60 minutes attached to appliance (no measurements). Temperature measurements were taken every 10 minutes during sessions 1, 4, and 16.

Main outcome measures: A digital thermometer to record the temperatures of the thumbs and big toes on hands and feet, which was taped to the skin for calibration.

Main results: Skin temperature turned out to be a difficult variable to work with, due to the wide variability in temperature apparently unrelated to the experimental situation. The strongest results were observed in the fourth session. During session baseline, differences between hand and foot temperatures of the experimental group were significantly greater than those of the control group (t [13, 11] = 2.49, P = 0.02). The 16th session did not yield significant differences between the experimental and control groups. However, in the experimental group, there was a correlation of r (9) = − 0.56 (P = 0.07) of hand temperature increase with the number of days it took to complete the 16 sessions. In contrast, in a clinical follow-up study with five subjects and no control, all subjects had a substantial increase in hand temperature following three sessions on the appliance. In this follow-up, use of the appliance was closely supervised, whereas in the blind study most of the appliance sessions were conducted in the privacy of the subjects' homes.

Conclusions: The results of the two studies indicate that the use of the Radial Appliance may not warm the hands.

Reference: Richards D G, McMillin D L, Nelson C D, Mein E A 1996 Improvement of circulation using the radial appliance. Subtle Energies and Energy Medicine 7(1): 71–85

Quality scores: Not applicable.

Remote Influence by a Ritual Healing Technique Calms Patients

Objective: To determine if remote calming effects of a traditional healing ritual can be objectively measured using indicators of electrodermal activity, heart rate and blood volume.

Design: Randomized, controlled trial, two experiments, DMILS.

Setting: The healer sat with a doll created by the patient, mementoes, pictures, and an autobiographical sketch provided by the patient, in one room, and the patient was located in another building in an isolated room.

Participants: The first, third and fourth authors were the subjects in the initial experiment, the experimenter, the healer, and the patient.

Intervention: A total of 14 sessions were conducted in the initial study and 16 sessions were conducted in the replication. In both experiments, the authors exchanged roles as experimenter, healer and patient. Healers were instructed to try to calm the remote patient using a set of traditional ritual magic strategies, or to exert no influence (as a control). The patient created a doll in his or her likeness and provided mementoes, pictures and an autobiographical sketch. The healer used these materials to form a sympathetic connection with the patient who was

located in another building in an isolated room. Each session consisted of five calming and five control epochs of 1 minute each. The order of the epochs was randomly selected by a pseudorandom number generator.

Main outcome measures: Electrodermal activity, heart rate, and blood volume.

Main results: The combined results of both experiments showed significant effects for changes in blood volume (P = 0.00002), heart rate (P = 0.001) and electrodermal activity (P = 0.013) associated with the ritual healing sessions compared to no ritual healing sessions. It did take 25–30 seconds for the effect to be present and the actual relaxing effect only lasted about 20 seconds.

Conclusions: Traditional magic healing rituals caused significant relaxation of the vascular system and arousal of electrodermal activity. These rituals appear to be helpful in focusing mental intention in laboratory investigations of direct mental interactions with living systems.

Reference: Rebman J M, Wezelman R, Radin D I, Stevens P, Hapke R A, Gaughan K Z 1995 Remote influence of human physiology by a ritual healing technique. Subtle Energies 6(2): 111–134

Quality scores: Not applicable.

EEG Amplitude, Brain Mapping, and Possible Synchrony in and between a Bioenergy Practitioner and Client during Healing

Objective: To evaluate brain electrical changes occurring separately in, and simultaneously between, a bioenergy practitioner and client during relaxation, meditation, and healing.

Design: A controlled, single-case study.

Setting: A Neurosearch-24 24-channel digitizing EEG computer was used in a laboratory setting to register EEG recordings of bioenergy practitioner and client. Earclip electrodes were applied to the client and healer's earlobes. The main electrode array was then applied to the healer according to the standard 10–20 International System montage using an Electrocap and Electro-Gel. Three Beckman gold cup electrodes were then applied to selected parietal and occipital regions of the client (P3, P4, and O1) with Ten20 Conductive EEG paste. Impedances were tested until satisfactory, with electrodes referred to linked ears.

Participant: A 39-year old woman with polycystic kidney disease for 23 years who had been on hemodialysis for the past year. She had been diagnosed with cancer of the appendix, which resulted in surgery and caused further complications. The bioenergy practitioner was a 52-year old man with an international reputation.

Intervention: The client and healer participated in several mutual tasks. Instructions for the first task, the self-relaxation period, were for both participants to relax without meditating; during the second task both were asked to meditate. During the third period, both were asked to think about healing a third person not present. Finally, both were asked to participate in a healing process with regard to the client who was present, where the healer would attempt to heal the illness of the client present.

Main outcome measures: A Neurosearch-24, 24 channel digitizing EEG computer was used to register EEG recordings of bioenergy practitioner and client during the four experimental conditions. The participants were also asked to rate their own experiences.

Main results: Brain maps of the bioenergy practitioner across conditions indicated the presence of a strong right hemispheric activation pattern compared to the left. High amplitude alpha rhythms were observed in the left and right occiputs, and high amplitude beta and gamma rhythms were also present in the right occiput and in other areas of the right hemisphere during all conditions, but especially during relaxation and meditation. Healing at a distance and healing (client present) were associated with high frequency, high amplitude beta and gamma rhythms localized in the right frontal area, together with low amplitude left occipital and central theta rhythm. Intra- and interpersonal synchrony between bipolar electrode pairs was determined for each condition. Beta, alpha, theta, and gamma synchrony in the bioenergy practitioner was higher and less variable than that in the client in all conditions, and was highest during healing, especially in alpha frequencies between left occipital areas of bioenergy practitioner and client.

Conclusions: The results provide confirmation of reports by healers of a state of consciousness during the healing process that is different from that seen during relaxation and meditation.

Reference: Fahrion S L, Wirkus M, Pooley P 1992 EEG amplitude, brain mapping, and synchrony in and between a bioenergy practitioner and client during healing. Subtle Energies 3(1): 19–52

Quality scores: Not applicable.

Small Study Reports Reduced Anxiety associated with Time and Therapeutic Touch in Post-Hurricane Hugo Subjects

Objective: To determine the effect of therapeutic touch on people stressed by a hurricane or its after-effects.

Design: Non-randomized, controlled intervention study with repeated sessions ($n = 23$).

Setting: Subjects were seated in a comfortable chair, and attached to the Hewlett-Packard model HP component monitoring system by means of three standard electrocardiograph electrodes placed on either side of the chest over the diaphragm and at the right shoulder.

Participants: Twenty-three people affiliated with the university who either worked during the hurricane itself or suffered loss in the form of injury, property damage, or power outages for extended periods of time participated and signed consent agreements. Ages ranged from 18 to 60 years. Twenty-two were women; one was male. Only 18 returned for a second session, and eight people returned for a third session (control session). The drop out rate reached 65% because subjects were busy reconstructing after the damages.

Methods: Sessions 1 and 2 were identical, separated by 3–7 days. Therapeutic touch was administered to the subjects by two experienced practitioners. Treatment sessions

ranged from 6.8 to 20 minutes. Session 3 was a control session in which the same procedures were followed with the exception that no therapeutic touch was done and the subject and healer just sat quietly for 20 minutes in the room.

Main outcome measures: Physiological measures such as heart rate, blood pressure, skin temperature, and respiratory rate. A Hewlett-Packard model HP component monitoring system was used to monitor all physiological parameters except skin temperature. Psychological instruments consisted of two visual analogue scales (VASs). Data were collected before, during, and after each session to track anxiety.

Main results: Findings indicate that stressed people report themselves to be less stressed following therapeutic touch ($P < 0.05$). Time of therapeutic touch intervention varied significantly between the two healers. The decrease in state anxiety was significantly correlated with session length for each session, session 1, $r = 0.4754$, $P < 0.02$, session 2 $r = 0.4626$, $P < 0.03$. Physiological outcomes of TT reflected relaxation trends. These changes, however, were not significantly different between treatment and control groups.

Conclusions: Results from this study showed a decrease in perceived stress following therapeutic touch in a population of stressed individuals.

Reference: Olson M, Sneed N 1992 Therapeutic touch and post-hurricane Hugo stress. Journal of Holistic Nursing 10(2): 17

Quality scores: Not applicable.

Music and Suggestion Reduce Short-term Pain in Patients with Cancer

Objective: To determine the effects of listening to relaxing music with positive suggestion of reducing pain on self-reported pain in patients with cancer who were receiving scheduled pain medication.

Setting: Mid-Western hospital.

Design: Randomized, controlled trial with pre and post tests ($n = 40$).

Participants: Forty patients who were admitted to one of four acute care mid-western hospitals with the diagnosis of cancer and chronic pain.

Intervention: Subjects were asked to lie down on their beds, and the McGill pain questionnaire (MPQ) and visual analogue scale (VAS) were administered. Next, the lights in the room were dimmed. Subjects in the experimental group then received 30 minutes of their preferred type of relaxing music via headphones. Patients controlled the intensity level of the music themselves. After 30 minutes, the MPQ and VAS were re-administered. The control subjects received the same procedure except they did not receive music via headphones.

Main outcome measures: Pre- and post-test VAS scores and MPQ indices, along with descriptive statistics were collected and computed.

Main results: There were no significant differences between groups on the demographic characteristics. There were statistically significant differences between the two groups post treatment for each on the MPQ pain indices ($P < 0.05$) except for the present pain intensity (PPI), $P = 0.056$. Those subjects who received music with positive suggestion of pain reduction had significantly lower scores on the MPQ as compared to those subjects who did not receive music with positive suggestion. There were significant interaction effects between the two groups by time on scores from the VAS ($P > 0.02$), and the affective component of the MPQ ($P < 0.001$). Follow-up of the main effects of these interactions indicated significance for the music group, $F = 12.69$, $P < 0.001$.

Conclusion: Results of this study indicate that listening to music with positive suggestion of pain reduction has an effect on cancer patients' pain. Given the initial effectiveness of music, its availability, and low risks, future research is needed to help identify the specific parameters of its usefulness.

Reference: Zimmerman L, Pozehl B, Duncan K, Schmitz R 1989 Effects of music in patients who had chronic cancer pain. Western Journal of Nursing Research 11(3): 298–309

Quality scores: IV: 65.4   EV: 48.3   MV: 75.0   JADAD: 3

Music is Associated with Decreased Cancer-Related Pain in a Small Study

Objective: To evaluate to what extent the therapeutic use of music would decrease pain in patients with cancer who were receiving scheduled analgesics.

Design: Randomized controlled crossover design trial ($n = 15$).

Setting: The Wasatch Front, Utah area, where patients were solicited from oncologists, oncology nurses, hospitals, and homecare agencies. The study was conducted in each subject's home setting.

Patients: Fifteen outpatients with cancer, experiencing cancer-related pain, 12 women and three men, all English speaking and all over the age of 18. The age ranged from 20 to 87 years old.

Intervention: Subjects were randomly assigned to listen to their preference of seven types (classical, jazz, folk, rock, country, and Western) of relaxing music or a control (a 60-cycle hum) for 45 minutes twice daily for 3 days. They then crossed over into the alternate group for the next 3 days.

Main outcome measures: Pain, the dependent variable, and mood, which was proposed as an intervening variable, were measured by visual analogue scales. The McGill pain questionnaire (MPQ) was also used to obtain entry data on pain.

Main results: There was an inconsistent relationship between pain and mood. The effect of the music on pain varied by individual; 75% had at least some response and 47% had a moderate or good response. Multivariate analysis of variance indicated a statistically significant decrease in pain from using either music or sound, but there was no effect on mood. Although the mean percentage of change in pain for music was twice that for sound, the results did not differ statistically.

Conclusions: The findings support the use of music as an independent nursing intervention to relieve pain, but more research with larger sample size is needed.

Reference: Beck S L 1991 The therapeutic use of music for cancer-related pain. Oncology Nursing Forum 18(8): 1327–1337

Quality scores: IV: 53.8   EV: 44.8   MV: 75.0   JADAD: 3

Belief and Expectancy Improved the Effects of a Spiritual Healing Encounter

Objective: To assess the impact of healer and patient expectations on mental and physical health parameters following a spiritual healing session.

Design: Observational study with pre- and post-test questionnaires.

Setting: A Northern California suburb of Marin County utilizing an American-born spiritual healer trained in the Philippines.

Participants: Forty-eight individuals, six cancer cases, five chronic physical pain cases, two AIDS cases and a host of other biological disorders, who received spiritual healing treatment during the spring of 1986. Participants were divided into two groups: (1) the high expectancy group and (2) the low expectancy group, based on their responses to a pre-test.

Intervention: Patients initially filled out a questionnaire. The patient then entered the healing room and received a 15–30 minute spiritual healing laying-on of hands treatment. After the session was finished, the healer completed the 'healer's questionnaire' which contained questions pertaining to duration of treatment, healer expectancy and the patient's condition. The questionnaires were collected once a week by the researcher. This procedure continued for a 2-month period.

Main outcome measures: A pre- and post-test questionnaire was utilized to gather data about the participants: demographic variables were collected on the participants to obtain a patient profile, and a mental health and physical health measure was constructed to evaluate the levels of improvement for each patient.

Main results: There was a statistically significant difference between the pre-treatment and post-treatment scores for all dependent variables at the $P < 0.005$ level. The data also demonstrated a significant difference between the high versus low expectancy groups for both patient and healer expectancy at the $P < 0.05$ level. This implies that patients with a high level of expectancy demonstrated a greater improvement in their condition and that high healer expectancy corresponded with improved patient condition more so than low healer expectancy. Of the 90% of patients who reported that their condition had improved, all attributed the improvement to the spiritual healing treatment.

Conclusion: The results of this study suggest that spiritual healing can significantly affect a wide range of psychological and physiological variables as assessed by comprehensive mental and physical health measures. The data obtained indicated that high expectancy of healing for both patient and healer were positively correlated with subsequent improvement in the patients' physical as well as psychological condition.

Reference: Wirth D P 1995 The significance of belief and expectancy within the spiritual healing encounter. Social Science Medicine 41(2): 249–260

Quality scores: Not applicable.

Pain Reduction but no Physical Effects from a Bioenergy Healing Technique compared to Sham

Objective: To examine the physical and psychological effects of a bioenergy healing technique upon chronic pain.

Design: Randomized, double blind (participants blind to treatment and physicians blind to the intervention assignment of participants), placebo controlled trial.

Setting: Physical examinations and treatment sessions were held at a physician's private practice office after regular office hours.

Participants: Forty-seven individuals with one of three long-term and chronic disorders, arthritis, headaches, or low back pain, recruited through advertisements placed in three local newspapers. There were 35 women and 12 men. The average age was 49.23 years, with a range of 26–71 years. Patients were randomly assigned to either a treatment group or an attention placebo control group.

Intervention: An experimental treatment or an attention placebo procedure (which appeared identical to the experimental treatment from the participant's viewpoint) was administered. Once all treatment sessions and physical exams were completed for the entire study, participants were debriefed as to group assignment. The bioenergy treatments (the experimental treatment) began with an attunement of the treaters to the individual participant. The treatment protocol consisted of hand movements and points of mental concentration that were performed in a prescribed order without touching the participant's physical body. A sense of energy flow was established by the healer as he attempted to balance the energy centers of the patient. The placebo control was identical except that the treater pretended to be performing the treatment. They actually used several techniques to block any potential energy flow so as to not treat the patient.

Main outcome measures: After the session was completed, a home pain diary was distributed for the following week for patients to record their progress due to treatment. The McGill pain home recording form was used to measure effects due to the treatment.

Main results: The McGill pain questionnaire demonstrated that the treatment group had significantly decreased severity of the sensory and affective aspects of pain while the attention placebo control group did not, $F = 4.87$, $P < 0.05$ for the affective scale of the McGill and for the sensory scale, $F = 5.88$, $P < 0.05$. No effects were seen for any physical outcome measures.

Conclusion: There was a lack of predicted findings for the majority of physical outcome variables. The experimental treatment did, however, significantly reduce the severity of sensory and affective aspects of the pain experience to a greater degree than the attention placebo treatment. In addition, the severity of evaluative and miscellaneous aspects of pain, as well as weekly pain severity ratings, demonstrated strong trends in the predicted direction of severity reduction for the treatment condition.

Reference: Redner R, Briner B, Snellman L 1991 Effects of a bioenergy healing technique on chronic pain. Subtle Energies 2(3): 43–68

Quality scores: IV: 73.1   EV: 51.7   MV: 66.7   JADAD: 4

Distant Healing did not Affect Skin Warts

Objective: To assess the efficacy of distant healing on common skin warts.

Design: Randomized, blinded controlled trial.

Setting: All healers were based around London, approximately 150 miles from the Exeter area where the patients lived.

Participants: Ninety-one volunteers aged 16 and older were recruited by press advertisements inviting people with skin warts to participate. Forty-five participants were randomly assigned to the distant healing and 46 to the control group. There were four withdrawals in the distant healing group and three in the control. The baseline characteristics were all similar between groups.

Intervention: The treatment group received 6 weeks of distant healing by one of 10 experienced healers; the control group received a similar preliminary assessment but no distant healing.

Main outcome measures: Number of warts and their mean size at the end of treatment period was compared with that from before treatment. Secondary outcomes were the change in hospital anxiety and depression scale and patients' subjective experiences.

Main results: The mean number and size of warts per person did not change significantly during the study. The number of warts increased by 0.2 in the healing group and decreased by 1.1 in the control group (difference = −1.3; 95% CI = − 1.0 to 3.6, $P = 0.25$). Six patients in the distant healing group and eight in the control group reported a subjective improvement ($P = 0.63$). There were no significant between-group differences in the depression and anxiety scores.

Conclusions: Distant healing from experienced healers had no therapeutic effect on the number or size of patients' warts.

Reference: Harkness E F, Abbot N C, Ernst E 2000 A randomized trial of distant healing for skin warts. American Journal of Medicine 108(6): 444–452

Quality scores: IV: 80.8   EV: 58.6   MV: 58.3   JADAD: 5

Non-Contact Therapeutic Touch Increases the Well-Being in Cancer Patients in a Small Trial

Objective: To determine the effect of three non-contact therapeutic touch treatments on the well-being of patients with terminal cancer.

Design: Randomized controlled trial that tracked assessment of change over 4 days ($n = 20$).

Setting: A palliative care unit of a university-affiliated hospital where the patients received treatment while lying in bed.

Participants: Twenty people with terminal cancer. Patients were French-speaking, and between the ages of 38 and 68 years old. After the patients signed the consent form, they were randomly assigned to either an experimental ($n = 10$) or to a control ($n = 10$) group. The main cancer site of these patients was the lung.

Intervention: The therapeutic touch group received treatment for 15–20 minutes, while lying in their beds. The control group was asked to lie down comfortably on their backs and to just relax for 15–20 minutes. There was an investigator present during the control that positioned herself in the patient's energy field, but that investigator counted subtractions mentally during that time so as to prevent any centering or intent to influence the patient. All interventions took place 1 hour after a regularly prescribed analgesic was administered. The patients received this treatment on days 2, 3, and 4. On day 1, they filled out questionnaires. After days 2 and 4, they filled out the well-being scales.

Main outcomes: The well-being scale, which evaluates pain, nausea, depression, anxiety, shortness of breath, activity, appetite, relaxation, and inner peace. This is a 10-point scale ranging from low sensation of well-being to high sensation of well-being. In addition to these questions, there is also a general well-being item, which is compared to the rest and provides validity to the estimates.

Main results: A significant difference was found in the mean progression of sensation of well-being between the experimental group and the control group, $t = -3.73$; $P = 0.0015$. The experimental group showed a mean increase of 1.70 (SD = 1.28) in sensation of well-being, whereas the control group showed a decrease of 0.31 (SD = 1.12). Sensation of well-being for only the experimental group improved significantly over time, $F = 17.56$, d.f. (1, 9), $P < 0.025$.

Conclusions: Patients with terminal cancer receiving therapeutic touch treatments have a higher sensation of well-being than do those simply resting, and these sensations of well-being increased following three therapeutic touch interventions. It must be noted, however, that the sample size for this study was very small.

Reference: Giasson M, Bouchard L 1998 Effect of therapeutic touch on the well-being of persons with terminal cancer. Journal of Holistic Nursing 16(3): 383–398

Quality scores: IV: 61.5   EV: 58.6   MV: 66.7   JADAD: 2

The Combination of Dialogue and Therapeutic Touch Lowered State Anxiety Preoperatively for Breast Cancer Patients

Objective: To determine the efficacy of dialogue and therapeutic touch (TT) on pre- and postoperative anxiety and mood and postoperative pain from breast cancer surgery.

Design: Randomized, double blind controlled experimental study.

Setting: The Mid-Atlantic region, where treatment and dialogue took place in the privacy of the participant's own homes.

Participants: Thirty-one English-speaking women diagnosed with breast cancer with no previous history of cancer. These participants were recruited via telephone from surgeon's referrals before their surgery. They were randomized to experimental ($n = 14$) and control ($n = 17$) treatments. Their age ranged from 31 to 84 years old.

Intervention: Women assigned to the experimental group were given a 10-minute session of therapeutic touch followed by a 20-minute session where dialogue occurred between the patient and nurse about feelings or questions concerning breast cancer. Relaxing background music was played during this whole time. The control group was instructed to sit quietly with their eyes closed for 10-minutes while this same music played and then a 20-minute dialogue occurred just as in the experimental group. This took place preoperatively and postoperatively.

Main outcome measures: The self-evaluation questionnaires, state-trait anxiety inventory, forms Y-1 and Y-2 (STAI, Y-1, Y-2) were used to measure anxiety. The affects balance scale (ABC) was used to measure mood. The visual analog scale-pain (VAS-Pain) was used to measure pain related to surgery.

Results: Preoperatively, women in the experimental group had statistically significantly lower state anxiety following the preoperative treatment session than women in the control group after controlling for trait anxiety ($F(1,28) = 8.15$, $P = 0.008$). No significant differences existed between the two groups in mood. Postoperatively, there was no statistically significant associations between the treatment groups and the combined expressions of anxiety, mood, and pain after controlling for trait anxiety (Wilks 1 (3, 25) = 0.95, $P = 0.72$).

Conclusion: The combination of dialogue and TT was associated with a lower preoperative pattern of state anxiety than dialogue and quiet time. The fact that there was no difference found between the experimental and control group for preoperative and postoperative mood and postoperative pain, together with relatively positive mood and low pain scores, indicate that the combinations of dialogue and TT and dialogue and quiet time were equally effective, non-invasive nursing modalities for the women in this study.

Reference: Samarel N, Fawcett J, Davis M M, Ryan FM 1998 Effects of dialogue and therapeutic touch on preoperative and postoperative experiences of breast cancer surgery: an exploratory study. Oncology Nursing Forum 25(8): 1369–1376

Quality scores: IV: 81.0   EV: 52.0   MV: 66.7   JADAD: 5

Therapeutic Touch and Progressive Muscle Relaxation Improved Functional Ability in Elders with Degenerative Arthritis

Objective: To determine whether therapeutic touch given to elders with degenerative arthritis improved functional ability.

Design: A randomized, two-group longitudinal design, where subjects served as their own controls.

Setting: An upper Mid-west city of approximately 60 000 people, with surrounding rural farming communities. Treatments were given in the private practice offices of the practitioners or in the homes of patients who were unable to travel.

Participants: A sample of 108 subjects were recruited and entered into the study from local churches, housing complexes, a recreational center, and meal sites for seniors. Subjects were between the ages of 51 to 90, non-institutionalized, had been diagnosed with degenerative arthritis for at least 6 months, and experiencing chronic pain for the last 6 months. A total of 82 participants completed the study. Forty-five subjects received therapeutic touch (TT) and 37 received progressive muscle relaxation (PMR).

Intervention: Subjects were randomly assigned to receive TT or PMR treatments. Subjects served as their own control for 4 weeks while receiving their routine care, then received six treatments at 1-week intervals of either TT or PMR by trained nurses in each practice.

Main outcome measures: Measurements of functional ability were made using the arthritis impact measurement scale, version 2 (AIMS2). The AIMS2 was self-administered twice during the baseline period and after the first, third, and sixth treatments.

Results: For the TT group, mean scores improved between baseline and post-sixth treatment on all 11 subscales; hand function ($t(45) = 2.81$, $P = 0.007$), pain ($t(45) = 3.02$, $P = 0.004$), tension ($t(45) = 2.56, P = 0.014$), mood ($t(45) = 4.67$, $P < 0.001$), and satisfaction ($t(45) = 2.78$, $P = 0.008$). The mean scores for the walking and bending approached significance ($t(45) = 1.75$, $P = 0.086$). For the PMR group, significant differences were found for the walking and bending ($t(32) = 2.1, P = 0.044$), pain ($t(32) = 4.25, P < 0.001$), tension ($t(32) = 2.32$, $P = 0.027$), mood ($t(32) = 2.82$, $P = 0.008$), and satisfaction ($t(30) = 2.87, P = 0.007$) subscales. The mobility subscale scores for the TT group were lower (meaning better function) than the PMR scores at all three measurement times. Improvement in the mobility subscale scores for the TT group occurred from treatment one to treatment three, with a slight loss of improvement at treatment six. The mobility scores in the PMR group did not appear to differ between treatments one and three, and improved only slightly by treatment six.

Conclusion: Both therapeutic touch and PMR were effective treatments to improve functional ability of participants with degenerative arthritis. Therapeutic touch was more effective than PMR and should be offered to persons with arthritis pain.

Reference: Peck S D 1998 The efficacy of therapeutic touch for improving functional ability in elders with degenerative arthritis. Nursing Science Quarterly 11(3): 123–132

Quality scores: IV: 69.2   EV: 52.0   MV: 66.7   JADAD: 3

Local but not Distant Intercessory Prayer Improved Clinical Outcomes among Rheumatoid Arthritis Patients in a Small Study

Objective: To determine if in-person intercessory prayer by a healing team will improve clinical outcomes among

patients with rheumatoid arthritis and if supplemental distant prayer offers additional effects on the long-term outcome of the patients.

Design: Controlled cohort study, $n = 40$.

Setting: The Arthritis/Pain Treatment Center in Clearwater, Fla., a private rheumatology practice.

Patients: Forty patients (mean age, 62 years; all white, 82% women). All patients had class II or III rheumatoid arthritis and took stable doses of antirheumatic medications.

Intervention: All patients received 3 days of 6 hours of education and 6 hours of direct-contact intercessory prayer. This was done in two time intervals. The first half of patients received prayer while the second half were on the waiting list as a control until the first half completed their 3 months. The second half then received the same treatment. Then 19 were randomly selected to receive 6 months of daily, supplemental intercessory prayer by individuals located elsewhere.

Main outcome measures: Repeated measures ANOVA and multivariate linear regression models of the 10 principal medical outcome variables (tender joints, swollen joints, grip strength, ESR, CRP, patient's pain, global functioning, and fatigue ratings, and AIMS and MGAQ scores) were fit providing estimates of the average change in outcome over time.

Main results: Multivariate analysis of the entire sample showed significant overall improvement after intervention at 12 months when compared with preintervention baseline ($P < 0.0001$). Univariate analysis showed that patients increased mean grip strength (244.3 *vs.* 278.8 mmHg, $P = 0.039$), and had significant reductions in mean number of tender joints (16.8 *vs.* 5.7, $P < 0.0001$), swollen joints (9.8 *vs.* 3.1, $P < 0.0001$), patient-rated pain (4.5 *vs.* 3.1 cm, $P = 0.004$), patient-rated fatigue (4.5 *vs.* 3.1 cm, $P = 0.007$), and level of functional impairment (AIMS scores, 121.2 *vs.* 107.7, $P = 0.0002$; MHAQ scores, 36.2 *vs.* 32.9, $P = 0.012$). Neither multivariate nor univariate analysis showed a statistically significant overall improvement after intervention in the 10 outcome variables for the group receiving supplemental experimental, distant intercessory prayer.

Conclusions: Patients with long-standing, moderately severe rheumatoid arthritis showed significant short-term and long-term physical benefits from in-person intercessory prayer, but no additional benefits from supplementary distant prayer occurred.

Reference: Matthews D A, Marlowe S M, MacNutt F S 2000 Effects of intercessory prayer on patients with rheumatoid arthritis. Southern Medical Journal 93(12): 1177–1186

Quality scores: IV: 65.0   EV: 58.6   MV: 75.0   JADAD: 1

Spiritual Healing as a Therapy did not Improve Chronic Pain in Patients

Objective: To determine if healing performed by experienced healers would reduce pain significantly more than simulated healing or no healing.

Design: Randomized, controlled, blinded study ($n = 120$).

Setting: The clinical laboratory of the Department of Complementary Medicine at the University of Exeter. The laboratory was furnished to resemble the kind of environment in which healers treat their clients. For part II of the study, healers sat in a wooden cabinet with a one-way mirror through which they could see the patients but the patients could not see them.

Patients: A total of 120 patients who had been experiencing chronic pain for at least 6 months. Intensity of pain was rated > 25 on the visual analogue scale (VAS), and age ranged between 18 and 75 years. None had experience with a healer.

Intervention: Part I of this study consisted of face to face healing or simulated healing by a non-healer which mimicked the healer except used no intention to heal, but counted backwards from 1000 by fives. Part II consisted of the same healers as in Part I, except this time the patients received distant healing or no healing. All patients were first randomized to Part I or Part II of the study and then further to treatment and control conditions. All patients were allocated to 8-weekly 30-minute treatment sessions from the same individual over a period of 10 weeks.

Main outcome measures: Primary outcome measure was the inter-group difference of total pain rating index (PRIT) score of the McGill pain questionnaire (MPQ) at week 8. Secondary outcome measures consisted of the VASs for pain intensity, the SF-36 quality of life scale, the hospital anxiety and depression (HAD) scale, the MYMOP (measure yourself medical outcomes profile), which is a recently developed individualized instrument which allows patients to choose two symptoms which bother them the most. They also specify an activity of daily living that is difficult, and a question about general well-being. Patients completed scales prior to study, at baseline, and at the 4th week and the 8th week (end of the trial).

Main results: The MPQ, PRIT score in part I decreased from 32.8 (95% CI 28.5–37.0) at baseline to 23.3 (16.8–29.7) units after eight sessions in the healing group; and from 33.1 (27.2–38.9) to 26.1 (19.3–32.9) units in the simulated healing group. In part II, the PRIT score decreased from 29.6 (24.8–34.4) at baseline to 24.0 (18.7–29.4) units in the distant healing group and from 31.0 (25.8–36.2) to 21.0 (15.7–26.2) units in the no healing group. There were no significant differences between the healing and control groups in either part for the outcome measures, except for the physical function component of the SF-36 which showed a greater improvement in the healing group in part I.

Conclusions: The findings suggest that healing does not have a specific effect on chronic pain over and above non-specific factors.

Reference: Abbot N C, Harkness E F, Stevinson C, Marshall F P, Conn D A, Ernst E 2001 Spiritual healing as a therapy for chronic pain: a randomized, clinical trial. Pain 91: 79–89

Quality scores: IV: 96.0   EV: 59.0   MV: 75.0   JADAD: 5

Spiritual Healing Improves Quality of Life for Chronically Ill Patients

Objective: To determine whether distant healing improves quality of life substantially for patients with chronic illness.

Design: Randomized, waiting-list controlled study (*n* = 120).

Setting: Not stated.

Patients: A total of 119 patients with a chronic illness, where nothing much more could be done by conventional treatment to alleviate the illness. These patients had all had their illnesses for at least 1 year, and to were resistant to any previous medical treatment. Patients had a mean age of 44.6 years, 68% were women, 51% were married, 60% were living together with a partner, 83% were religious, and 60% regularly or at least sometimes practiced their religion. All patients were open to spiritual healing, confident, and faithful.

Intervention: Patients were either randomized to the treatment group or the 5-month waiting list control. The patients in the treatment group were distributed into one of three treatment modalities of distant healing: Anonymous distant healing (*n* = 30), in which patients did not know who was treating them and when and where treated simultaneously by three or four healers who did not have contact with the patients; amulet distant healing (*n* = 10), in which the patients were given an amulet laden with healing energy, which was worn at night, by one healer who specialized in this technique and patients knew the healer but had no contact with the healer; and contact distant healing (*n* = 20), in which patients knew who was treating them and were able to make phone contact or see the healer if necessary, but personal contacts were restricted to an initial meeting and the healing took place at a distance. Patients saw a physician at the end of the study.

Main outcome measures: SF36 health survey questionnaire, along with items asking for expectations and health locus of control items were filled in by the patients while waiting to see the physician (patients of the treatment group) or at home (waiting list group). Patients kept a journal where they recorded their experiences.

Main results: The treatment group experienced improvement on all scales. In some, the improvement was substantial (emotional role-functioning, pain, mental health) whereas the control group reported either only slight improvements or aggravations. The pre-treatment–post-treatment difference of the sum of all SF36 items showed an improvement of 10.18 in the treated group, while the control group stayed virtually the same. This difference was significant ($t = -3.61$; d.f. 117; $P = 0.00045$). There was no statistically significant differences among the treatment modalities (anonymous, amulet, and contact distant healing), although patients of the contact group showed the greatest improvement (12 pts difference), patients in the amulet group medium improvement (10 pts), and the anonymous group the least improvement (8 pts).

Conclusions: This study of distant healing showed that patients suffering from various types of chronic diseases can experience a statistically significant and clinically relevant improvement in quality of life as measured by the SF36 health questionnaire after a 5-month treatment period with distant healing.

Reference: Wiesendanger H, Werthmuller L, Reuter K, Walach H 2001 Chronically ill patients treated by spiritual healing improve in quality of life: results of a randomized waiting-list controlled study. Journal of Alternative and Complementary Medicine 7(1): 45–51

Quality scores: IV: 77.0   EV: 79.0   MV: 83.0   JADAD: 3

Neither Intercessory Prayer nor Positive Visualization is Capable of Improving the Psychological Well-being of Patients with End-stage Renal Disease

Objective: To determine the effect of intercessory prayer and positive visualization on self-reported and medical measures of well-being for patients undergoing kidney dialysis as well as to assess the extent that any effect on psychological or physiological well-being is attributable to expectancy or actual treatment.

Design: A two by three, randomized, blinded (expectancy × treatment) factorial design.

Setting: An outpatient hemodialysis center at the University of Miami School of Medicine/Jackson Memorial Hospital in Miami, Florida.

Participants: Ninety-five adult patients diagnosed with end-stage renal disease (ESRD) and receiving hemodialysis treatment for a mean of 36 months. The mean age of the subjects was 49 years, 58% being male. There were six intercessors, all of whom were middle-aged Catholic women who had prayed together for many years. Six on-site pre-doctoral psychology interns served as the positive visualization group.

Intervention: Patients were randomly assigned to one of six treatment conditions. The intercessors prayed for the patients' emotional and physical healing using two specific and scripted prayers. The positive visualization group visualized patients' medical and psychological conditions improving, while being guided by audiotape. Each group did this individually for 5 days a week for 5 minutes, not to exceed 15 minutes. They joined together in their prayer group or positive visualization group once weekly during the 6-week period for the same amount of time to pray or visualize the patients' improved health.

Main outcome measures: Ten outcome measures typically used in evaluating patients with ESRD: KT/V, albumin, systolic blood pressure, diastolic blood pressure, interdialytic weight gain, serum level of inorganic phosphorus, hematocrit, number of hospitalizations since the study began, number of new medical problems since the study began, and a self-reported response to the question, 'Have you been feeling better, the same, or worse since the study began?' The self-reported measures used in the study were the SF-36 health status questionnaire, the Beck depression inventory (BDI), and the belief in prayer/positive visualization questionnarie (developed by the authors to assess belief). These measures were all used in a baseline assessment (five weeks prior to intervention), and a post-test assessment (2 weeks after the intervention).

Results: Patients who expected to receive intercessory prayer reported feeling significantly better than did those who expected to receive positive visualization ($F = 5.42$, $P < 0.02$). There was no indication of a treatment effect for those subjects who received intercessory prayer or positive visualization when compared to those subjects who received no treatment.

Conclusions: There was no significant main effect for expectancy or treatment on any of the medical or psychological dependent variables, even though it did provide general support for expectancy. This study failed to provide convincing evidence to support intercessory prayer or positive visualization as capable for improving the psychological and/or physiological well-being of patients with ESRD.

Reference: Matthews W J, Conti J M, Sireci S G 2001 The effects of intercessory prayer, positive visualization, and expectancy on the well-being of kidney dialysis patients. Alternative Therapies 7(5): 42–52

Quality scores: IV: 88.46   EV: 62.07   MV: 83.33   JADAD: 4

Noetic Phenomena in Coronary Patients Undergoing Percutaneous Coronary Intervention (PCI) Appears Feasible and Demonstrates Some Therapeutic Benefit

Objective: To examine the feasibility of applying four noetic therapies, stress relaxation, imagery, touch therapy, and prayer, to patients suffering from acute coronary disease.

Design: Prospective, randomized controlled pilot study where prayer and standard therapy were the only interventions double blinded.

Setting: A coronary care unit in a hospital between April 1997 through April 1998.

Participants: A total of 150 coronary care unit patients enrolled in the study, 120 received one of the four noetic therapies while 30 received standard therapy. Baseline characteristics were balanced between the groups.

Intervention: For those patients who were assigned to any of the three hands-on noetic trainings, a practitioner trained in that area worked with the patient before PCI. Prayer and standard therapy patients remained double blind to their assignment. There were seven kinds of prayer groups praying at various times. There were over 196 religious ones praying.

Main outcome measures: The Duke University religion (DUREL) index and the Spielberg state-trait anxiety inventory were filled out by patients upon enrollment to determine anxiety levels and religiosity. Index hospitalization end-points included post PCI ischemia, death, myocardial infarction, heart failure, and urgent revascularization. Mortality was followed for 6 months post hospitalization.

Main results: Results were not statistically significant for any of the outcome comparisons but there was a 25–30% reduction in adverse outcomes in patients treated with any noetic therapy compared with standard therapy. The lowest absolute complication rates were in patients receiving prayer. For the patients who scored high in spiritual belief questionnaire and high levels of anxiety, noetic therapies appeared to have the greater reduction in complication rates compared with standard therapy.

Conclusions: No outcomes differences between standard therapy and noetic therapy were significant; however, index hospitalization data suggested a therapeutic benefit with noetic therapies. Intercessory prayer showed the lowest complication rates of all the noetic therapies used. Mortality differences must be investigated further in future clinical trials.

Reference: Krucoff M W, Crater S W, Green C L et al 2001 Integrative noetic therapies as adjuncts to percutaneous intervention during unstable coronary syndromes: monitoring and actualization of noetic training (MANTRA) feasibility pilot. American Heart Journal 142: (in press).

Quality scores: IV: 80.8   EV: 51.7   MV: 58.3   JADAD: 5

Prayer Influences the Success of In Vitro *Fertilization–Embryo Transfer*

Objective: To determine if intercessory prayer (IP) can influence pregnancy rates in women being treated with *in vitro* fertilization–embryo transfer (IVF-ET).

Design: Prospective, double blind randomized clinical trial where patients were not aware of the study.

Setting: An IVF-ET program at Cha Hospital, Seoul, Korea. IP was performed by prayer groups in the US, Canada and Australia.

Participants: The patients consisted of 219 women aged 26–46 years who were treated with IVF-ET over a 4-month period. The patients were randomized to an IP group and a no IP group.

Intervention: All patients were treated with the same protocol that used a GnRH agonist and gonadotropins until at least three follicles were mature. ET was carried out 3 days after retrieval. In addition, patients assigned to IP were prayed for by prayer groups in different countries. They had only pictures of the patients and no information about them.

Main outcome measures: Clinical pregnancy rates in the two groups.

Main results: The IP group had a higher pregnancy rate as compared to the no IP group rate (50% *vs.* 26%, $P = 0.0013$). The IP group showed a higher implantation rate (16.3% *vs.* 8%, $P = 0.0005$).

Conclusions: A statistically significant difference was observed for the effect of IP on the outcome of IVF-ET, though this data should only be looked at as preliminary as more study is needed to verify.

Reference: Cha K Y, Wirth D P, Lobo R A 2001 Does prayer influence the success of *in vitro* fertilization: embryo transfer? Report of a masked, randomized trial. Journal of Reproductive Medicine 46(9): 781–787

Quality scores: IV: 69.2   EV: 48.3   MV: 58.3   JADAD: 5

No Significant Benefit from Intercessory Prayer for Cardiovascular Disease Progression Post Hospitalization

Objective: To determine if intercessory prayer (IP) is effective in cardiovascular disease progression.

Design: Randomized, controlled, double blind clinical trial.

Setting: The Mayo Clinic Rochester (MCR) between July 4, 1997 and October 21, 1999.

Participants: A total of 799 patients were eligible and were aged 18 years or older admitted to the Saint Mary's Hospital CCU and discharged alive with a cardiovascular diagnosis. Patients were randomized to either IP group or control (C) group upon discharge.

Intervention: All patients received standard cardiovascular care as prescribed. IP treatment was administered by five volunteer group intercessors, and consisted of prayer at least once a week for 26 weeks. Intercessors only had access to patients' first name, age, gender, diagnosis, and general condition.

Main outcome measures: Death, cardiac arrest, coronary revascularization, cardiovascular re-hospitalization, or emergency department visit due to cardiovascular disease.

Main results: Event rates for each component of cardiovascular disease progression were non-significantly different between groups (IP *vs.* C) as follows: death 8.1% *vs.* 9.0%; revascularization 3.9% *vs.* 6.1%; rehospitalization 18.5% *vs.* 20.3%; emergency department 8.4% *vs.* 8.2%; and cardiac arrest 0.3% *vs.* 0.3% (all $P > 0.05$). Analysis of event-free survival time showed a small benefit of prayer in the low-risk group ($P = 0.062$) as compared to the high-risk group ($P = 0.706$).

Conclusions: This study demonstrates no significant effect of IP for cardiovascular disease patients. It may be beneficial to the low-risk patents.

Reference: Aviles J M, Whelan E, Hernke D A et al 2001 A study of intercessory prayer and cardiovascular disease progression in a coronary care unit population. Mayo Clin Proc 76: 1192–1198

Quality scores: IV: 88.5%   EV: 69.0%   MV: 83.3%   JADAD: 5

Spiritual Healing Seems Harmless to Patients with Chronic Idiopathic Pain

Objective: To determine the efficacy of spiritual healing for patients with chronic idiopathic pain syndrome.

Design: Randomized control clinical trial.

Setting: An outpatient pain clinic.

Patients: Twenty-four patients suffering from idiopathic pain syndrome who had experienced numerous unsuccessful treatment attempts. The mean age was 51 years; half of them were women. The mean duration of chronic pain for patients was 12.7 years.

Intervention: Patients were randomized to either a spiritual healing group or a control group. Spiritual healing was received three to eight times from the same female healing practitioner for 40 minutes each time. The control group received no active therapy during the test period. This was conducted for 28 months.

Main outcomes: Patients filled out questionnaires at baseline, 2 weeks and 1 year. These included the pain database outline by the International Association of the Study of Pain (IASP), the visual analogue scale (VAS), and a basic history questionnaire. Psychological self-reporting tests included the Hopkins symptom checklist SCL-90, the Middlesex Hospital questionnaire, (MHQ), the coping strategy questionnaire, and a former Finnish health locus of control scale (HLC).

Main results: There was a slight decrease in analgesic drug intake and improvement in sleep patterns in patients treated with spiritual healing. Attitudes toward spiritual healing improved. There was a decrease in feelings of hopelessness ($P < 0.05$), and an increased acceptance of psychological factors as reasons for pain ($P < 0.05$). Most other variables were unaffected by treatment.

Conclusions: Spiritual healing seems harmless and was shown to be subjectively helpful to some patients suffering from idiopathic chronic pain syndrome, even though no medical changes were seen.

Reference: Sundblom D M, Haikonen S, Niemi-Pynttäri J, Tigerstedt I 1994 Effect of spiritual healing on chronic idiopathic pain: a medical and psychological study. Clinical Journal of Pain 10: 296–303

Quality scores: IV: 65.4   EV: 69.0   MV: 66.7   JADAD: 2

Remote, Retroactive Intercessory Prayer is Associated with a Shorter Stay in Hospital for Patients Diagnosed with Bloodstream Infection

Objective: To examine the effectiveness of remote, retroactive intercessory prayer performed for a group of bloodstream infected patients.

Design: Randomized, blinded controlled trial, $n = 3393$.

Setting: University Hospital at Rabin Medical Center, Beilinson Campus in Israel.

Participants: A total of 3393 adult patients whose bloodstream infection was detected at the hospital in 1990–1996.

Intervention: In July 2000, patients were randomized to either an intervention group or a control group. A short remote, retroactive intercessory prayer was said by one person for for the well-being and recovery of the entire intervention group.

Main outcome measures: Mortality in hospital, length of stay in hospital and duration of fever.

Main results: Mortality was seen in 28.1% (475/1691) in the intervention group and 30.2% (514/1702) in the control group ($P = 0.4$). The length of stay in the hospital and duration of fever were significantly shorter in the intervention group ($P = 0.01$ and $P = 0.04$, respectively).

Conclusions: Remote, retroactive intercessory prayer said for bloodstream infected patients is associated with a shorter stay in the hospital and a shorter duration of fever.

Reference: Leibovici L 2001 Effects of remote, retroactive intercessory prayer on outcomes in patients with bloodstream infection: randomized controlled trial. British Medical Journal 323: 1450–1451

Quality scores: IV: 58%   EV: 14%   MV: 8.3%   JADAD: 4

Healing Touch can be Clinically Effective

Objective: To determine the clinical effectiveness of healing touch (HT) for improving health as well as to determine whether practitioner training levels moderate treatment effectiveness.

Design: Mixed method, quantitative as well as qualitative data, repeated measures design using naturalistic and quasi-experimental approaches.

Setting: Practitioner's offices.

Participants: Twenty-two clients who had never experienced HT but were familiar with the practitioners.

Intervention: Subjects received no treatment, 30 minutes of just lying on the table, then HT treatment was next for 30 minutes, and then a HT, plus music, plus guided imagery was the third treatment for 30 minutes. At least 1 day was allowed between each treatment and the three conditions for each client was completed within a 2-week time-frame.

Main outcome measures: Secretory immunoglobulin A (sIgA) concentrations in saliva, self-reports of stress, perceptions of health, and qualitative questions about individual effects from treatments.

Main results: Clients of practitioners with more training experienced statistically significant positive sIgA change over the HT treatments, while those with less experience did not. Clients reported a significant reduction of stress after both HT treatments. Enhancement in health was reported by 59% of clients. From the qualitative questions, themes of relaxation, enhanced awareness and connectedness were expressed.

Conclusions: The data support the clinical effectiveness of HT for health enhancement, for raising sIgA concentrations, reducing stress, and relieving pain.

Reference: Wilkinson D S, Knox P L, Chatman J E et al 2002 The clinical effectiveness of healing touch. Journal of Alternative and Complementary Medicine 8(1): 33–47

Quality scores: IV: 69%   EV: 52%   MV: 58%   JADAD: 1

There is a Need to Pursue Research on the Relationship between Therapeutic Touch and State Anxiety among Children with HIV

Objective: To determine whether therapeutic touch is associated with reductions in anxiety in children with HIV.

Design: A randomized controlled pilot study.

Setting: Two pediatric ambulatory care centers specializing in HIV disease during the months of January and September, 1997.

Patients: Twenty HIV-infected children aged 6–12 years, living in a north-eastern city, the majority being either African American or Hispanic and asymptomatic.

Intervention: Patients received either therapeutic touch from a trained nurse for 5–7 minutes or a mimic therapeutic touch which a naïve, inexperienced nursing student provided. This was to blind the children to what treatment they were receiving.

Main outcome measures: Children filled out the Peabody picture vocabulary test-revised (PPVT-R) to determine age appropriate ranges prior to study, and the A-state anxiety scale questions (STAIC) pre and post intervention.

Main results: Two failed to score the age-appropriate range of the PPVT-R at pre-test and so were excluded leaving only 20 children. Comparison of pre-test and post-test means between the therapeutic touch and mimic therapeutic touch groups showed a significant decrease in anxiety post-test in the therapeutic touch group ($P < 0.01$) compared to the control group ($P = 0.20$).

Conclusions: This pilot study implies that there is a need to further investigate the relationship between therapeutic touch and state anxiety among children with HIV infection. It supports the research available that this technique may help or improve the experience of those living with a chronic yet life-threatening disease such as AIDS.

Reference: Ireland M 1998 Therapeutic touch with HIV-infected children: a pilot study. Journal of the Association of Nurses in AIDS Care 9(4): 68–78

Quality scores: IV: 73.1   EV: 48.3   MV: 75.0   JAHAD: 3

A comprehensive bibliography of spiritual healing, 'energy' medicine, and intentionality research

Appendix 2

A comprehensive bibliography of spiritual healing, 'energy' medicine, and intentionality research

Cindy C Crawford and Wayne B Jonas

Randomized Clinical Studies

Abbot N C, Harkness E F, Stevinson C, Marshall F P, Conn D A, Ernst E 2001 Spiritual healing as a therapy for chronic pain: a randomized, clinical trial. Pain 91(1–2): 79–89

Angus J, Faux S 1989 The effect of music on adult postoperative patient pain during a nursing procedure. In: Funk S, Tornquist E, Champagne M (eds) Key aspects of comfort: management of pain, fatigue, and nausea. Springer, New York, pp. 166–172

Aviles J M, Whelan E, Hernke D A et al 2001 A study of intercessory prayer and cardiovascular disease progression in a coronary care unit population. Mayo Clinic Proceedings 76: 1192–1198

Barger D 1979 The effect of music and verbal suggestions on heart rate and self-reports. Journal of Music Therapy 11: 68–73

Beck S 1988 The effect of the therapeutic use of music on cancer-related pain. Unpublished dissertation, University of Utah, Salt Lake City, UT

Beck S 1991 The therapeutic use of music for cancer-related pain. Oncology Nursing Forum 18(8): 1327–1337

Beutler J J, Attevelt J T M, Geijskes G G, Schouten S A, Faber J A J, Dorhout Mees E J 1987 The effect of paranormal healing on hypertension. Journal of Hypertension 5: 551–552

Beutler J, Attevelt J, Schouten S et al 1988 Paranormal healing and hypertension. British Medical Journal (Clinical Research) 296(6635): 1491–1494

Braud W 1992 Remote mental influence of electrodermal activity. Journal of Indian Psychology 19(1): 1–10

Braud W, Schlitz M 1983 Psychokinetic influence on electrodermal activity. Journal of Parapsychology 47: 95–119

Burr H 1952 Electrometrics of atypical growth. Yale Journal of Biology Medicine 25: 67–75

Byrd R C 1988 Positive therapeutic effects of intercessory prayer in a coronary care unit population. Southern Medical Journal 81(7): 826–829

Bzkek V M 1986 Effects of therapeutic touch on tension headache pain. Nursing Research 35(2): 101–104

Castronova J, Oleson T 1991 A comparison of supportive psychotherapy and laying on of hands healing for chronic back pain patients. Alternative Medicine 3(4): 217–226

Cha K Y, Wirth D P, Lobo R A 2001 Does prayer influence the success of in vitro fertilization: embryo transfer? Journal of Reproductive Medicine 46(9): 781–787

Collipp P 1969 The efficacy of prayer: a triple blind study. Medical Times 97(5): 201–204

Dixon M 1998 Does healing benefit patients with chronic symptoms? A quasi-randomized trial in general practice. Journal of the Royal Society of Medicine 91: 183–188

Dressen L J, Singg S 1998 Effects of reiki on pain and selected affective and personality variables of chronically ill patients. Subtle Energies and Energy Medicine 9(1): 51–82

Ernst E 2001 [Science or quackery? Complementary medicine: mental healing]. MMW Fortschritte der Medizin 143(3): 40–41

Gagne D, Toye R 1994 The effects of therapeutic touch and relaxation therapy in reducing anxiety. Archives of Psychiatry and Nursing 8(3): 184–189

Gelade G, Harvie R 1975 Confidence ratings in an ESP task using affective stimuli. Journal of the Society for Psychical Research 48: 209–219

Giasson M, Bouchard L 1998 Effect of therapeutic touch on the well-being of persons with terminal cancer. Journal of Holistic Nursing 16(3): 383–398

Goldmeier D, Ivens D 2000 Distant healing. International Journal of STD and AIDS 11(3): 203

Gordon A, Merenstein J, D'Amico F, Hudgens D 1998 The effects of therapeutic touch on patients with osteoarthritis of the knee. Journal of Family Practice 47: 271–277

Grad B, Cadoret R J, Paul G I 1961 The influence of an unorthodox method of treatment on wound healing in mice. International Journal of Parapsychology 2: 5–19

Greyson B 1996 Distance healing of patients with major depression. Journal of Scientific Exploration 10: 447–465

Guerrero M 1986 The effects of therapeutic touch on state-trait anxiety level of oncology patients. Masters Abstracts International 24(3): 252

Hale E 1986 A study of the relationship between therapeutic touch and the anxiety levels of hospitalized adults. Dissertation Abstracts International 47: 1982b

Harkness E, Abbot N, Ernst E 2000 A randomized clinical trial of distant healing for peripheral common warts. American Journal of Medicine 108(6): 444–452

Harris W, Gowda M, Kolb J et al 1999 A randomized, controlled trial of the effects of remote, intercessory prayer on outcomes in patients admitted to the coronary care unit. Archives of Internal Medicine 159(19): 2773–2778

Heidt P 1979 An investigation of the effects of therapeutic touch and the anxiety levels of hospitalized patients. Dissertation Abstracts International 40: 52063–55207b

Honorton C, Berger R, Varvogles M et al 1990 Psi communication in the ganzfeld. Journal of Parapsychology 54: 99–139

Keller E, Bzdek V 1986 Effects of therapeutic touch on tension headache pain. Nursing Research 35(2): 101–106

Krieger D 1976 Healing by the laying on of hands as a faciliator of bio-energetic change: the response of in vivo human hemoglobin. Psychoenergetic Systems 1: 121–129

Krucoff M W, Crater S W, Green C L et al 2001 Integrative noetic therapies as adjuncts to percutaneous intervention during unstable coronary syndromes: monitoring and actualization of noetic training (MANTRA) feasibility pilot. American Heart Journal 142(5): 760–769

Lafreniere K, Mutus B, Cameron S et al 1999 Effects of therapeutic touch on biochemical and mood indicators in women. Journal of Alternative and Complementary Medicine 5(4): 367–370

Lianglun Z 1998 Effect and mechanism of mainly using Traditional Chinese Medicine of replenishing qi and nourishing yin in treating Graves disease. Chinese Journal of Internal Medicine 4(3): 178–181

Loscin R 1981 The effect of music on the pain of selected postoperative patients. Journal of Advanced Nursing 6(1): 19–25

Matthews W, Conti J, Sireci S 2001 The effects of intercessory prayer, positive visualization, and expectancy on the well-being of kidney dialysis patients. Alternative Therapies 7(5): 42–52

Meehan T 1985 The effect of therapeutic touch on the experience of acute pain in post-operative patients. Unpublished doctoral dissertation, New York University, New York

Meehan T 1992 Therapeutic touch and postoperative pain: a Rogerian research study. Nursing Science Quarterly 6(2): 69–78

Miller R 1982 Study on the effectiveness of remote mental healing. Medical Hypotheses 8(5): 481–490

Nash C B 1982 Psychokinetic control of bacterial growth. Journal of the American Society for Psychical Research 51: 217–221

Neil C, Harkness E, Stevinson C, Marshall F, Conn D, Ernst E 2001 Spiritual healing as a therapy for chronic pain: a randomized, clinical trial. Pain 91: 79–89

O'Laoire S 1997 An experimental study of the effects of distant, intercessory prayer on self-esteem, anxiety, and depression. Alternative Therapies in Health and Medicine 3(6): 38–53

Olson M, Sneed N 1995 Anxiety and therapeutic touch. Issues in Mental Health Nursing 16(2): 97–108

Olson M, Sneed N, LaVia M, Virella G, Bonadonna R, Michel Y 1997 Stress-induced immunosuppression and therapeutic touch. Alternative Therapies 3(2): 68–74

O'Mathuna D 2000 Therapeutic touch for acute wounds. Cochrane Database for Systematic Reviews 4(2)

Quinn J 1984 Therapeutic touch as energy exchange: testing the theory. Advances in Nursing Science 6(2): 42–49

Quinn J 1989 Therapeutic touch as energy exchange: replication and extension. Nursing Science Quarterly 2(2): 79–87

Randolph G 1984 Therapeutic and physical touch: physiological response to stressful stimuli. Nursing Research 33(1): 33–36

Rebman J, Wezelman R, Radin D, Stevens P, Hapke R, Gaughan K 1995 Remote influence of human physiology by a ritual healing technique. Subtle Energies 6(2): 111–134

Redner R, Briner B, Snellman L 1991 Effects of a bioenergy healing technique on chronic pain. Subtle Energies 2(3): 43–68

Reilly D T, Taylor M A, McSharry C, Aitchison T 1986 Is homoeopathy a placebo response? Controlled trial of homoeopathic potency, with pollen in hayfever as model. Lancet 2(8512): 881–886

Rider M S, Achterberg J 1989 Effect of music-associated imagery on neutrophils and lymphocytes. Biofeedback and Self-Regulation 14(3): 247–257

Ruegemar W, Silverman F 1956 Influence of gentling on the physiology of the rat. Paper presented at the Proceedings of the Society for Experimental Biology and Medicine

Schwartz S A, De Mattei R J, Brame Jr E G, Spottiswoode S J P 1990 Infrared spectra alteration in water proximate to the palms of therapeutic practitioners. Subtle Energies 1(1): 43–72

Sicher F, Targ E, Moore D, Smith H 1998 A randomized double-blind study of the effect of distant healing in a population with advanced AIDS: report of a small scale study. Western Journal of Medicine 169(6): 356–363

Simington J, Laing G 1993 Effects of therapeutic touch on anxiety in the institutionalized elderly. Clinical Nursing Research 2(4): 438–450

Smith J G, Fisher R 2000 The effect of remote intercessory prayer on clinical outcomes. Archives of Internal Medicine 160(12): 1876; discussion 1877–1878

Stanford R, Angelini R 1984 Effects of noise and the trait of absorption on ganzfeld ESP performance. Journal of Parapsychology 48(2): 85–99

Sundblom D M, Haikonen S, Niemi-Pynttari J, Tigerstedt I 1994 Effect of spiritual healing on chronic idiopathic pain: a medical and psychological study. Clinical Journal of Pain 10(4): 296–302

Turner J, Clark A, Gauthier D, Williams M 1998 The effect of therapeutic touch on pain and anxiety in burn patients. Journal of Advanced Nursing 28(1): 10–20

Walker S, Tonigan J, Miller W, Corner S, Kahlich L 1997 Intercessory prayer in the treatment of alcohol abuse and dependence: a pilot investigation. Alternative Therapies in Health and Medicine 3(6): 79–86

Wiesendanger H, Werthmuller L, Reuter K, Walach H 2001 Chronically ill patients treated by spiritual healing improve in quality of life: results of a randomized waiting-list controlled study. Journal of Alternative and Complementary Medicine 7(1): 45–51

Wirth D 1997 Multisite electromyographic analysis of therapeutic touch and qigong therapy. Journal of Alternative and Complementary Medicine 3: 109–118

Wirth D, Barrett M 1994 Complementary healing therapies. International Journal of Psychosomatic Research 41(2): 61–67

Wirth D, Cram J 1993 Multi-site surface electromyographic analysis of non-contact therapeutic touch. International Journal of Psychosomatics 40(1–4): 47–55

Wirth D, Cram J 1994 The psychophysiology of nontraditional prayer. International Journal of Psychosomatics 41(1–4): 68–75

Wirth D, Mitchell B 1994 Complementary healing therapy for patients with type 1 diabetes mellitus. Journal of Scientific Exploration 8(3): 350–361

Wirth D, Brenlan D, Levine R, Rodriguez C 1993 The effect of complementary healing therapy on postoperative pain after surgical removal of impacted third molar teeth. Complementary Therapies in Medicine 1: 133–138

Wirth D, Richardson J, Eidelman W, O'Malley A 1993 Full thickness dermal wounds treated with non contact therapeutic touch: a replication and extension. Complementary Therapies in Medicine 1: 127–132

Wirth D, Barrett M, Eidelman W 1994 Non-contact therapeutic touch and wound re-epithelialization: an extension of previous research. Complementary Therapies in Medicine 2: 187–192

Wirth D, Richardson J, Martinez R, Eidelman W, Lopez M 1996 Non-contact therapeutic touch intervention and full-thickness cutaneous wounds: a replication. Complementary Therapies in Medicine 4: 237–240

Wirth D, Chang R, Eidelman W, Paxton J 1996 Hematologic indicators of complementary healing intervention. Complementary Therapies in Medicine 4(1): 14–20

Wirth D P 1990 The effect of non-contact therapeutic touch on the healing of full thickness dermal wounds. Subtle Energies 1(1): 1–20

Woods D L, Craven R, Whitney J 1996 The effect of therapeutic touch and disruptive behaviors of individuals with dementia of the Alzheimer type. Alternative Therapies

Wu W, Bandilla E, Ciccone D et al 1999 Effects of qigong on late-stage complex regional pain syndrome. Alternative Therapies 5(1): 45–54

Zimmerman L, Pozehl B, Duncan K, Schmitz R 1989 Effects of music in patients who had chronic cancer pain. Western Journal of Nursing Research 11(3): 298–309

Zuckerman D M, Kasl S V, Ostfeld A M 1984 Psychosocial predictors of mortality among the elderly poor: the role of religion, well-being, and social contacts. American Journal of Epidemiology 119(3): 410–423

Basic and Laboratory Research

Adey W 1981 Tissue interactions with nonionizing electromagnetic fields. Physiological Reviews 61: 435–511

Ashton H, Dear P, Harley T, Sargent C 1981 A four-subject study of psi in the ganzfeld. Journal of the Society for Psychical Research 51: 12–21

Barry J 1968 General and comparative study of the psychokinetic effect on a fungus culture. Journal of Parapsychology 32: 237–243

Barry J 1968 PK on fungus growth. Journal of Parapsychology 32: 55

Bassett C, Pawluk R, Becker R 1964 Effects of electric currents on bone in vivo. Science 204: 652–654

Beloff J, Evans L 1961 A radioactivity test for PK. Journal of the Society for Psychical Research 41: 41–46

Braud W 1984 Further studies on the bio-PK effects: feedback, blocking, specificity/generality. Paper presented at the Fourth Annual Parapsychological Association Meeting

Braud W 1993 On the use of living target systems in distant mental influence research. In: Shapin B, Coly L (eds) Psi research methodology: a re-examination. Parapsychology Foundation, New York, pp. 149–188

Braud W, Braud L 1973 Preliminary explorations of psi-conducive states: progressive muscle relaxation. Journal of the American Society for Psychical Research 67: 27–46

Braud W G, Schlitz M J 1991 Consciousness interactions with remote biological systems: anomalous intentionality effects. Subtle Energies 2(1): 1–46

Braud W, Wood R, Braud L 1975 Free-response GESP performance during an experimental hypnagogic state induced by visual and acoustic ganzfeld techniques: a replication and extension. Journal of the American Society for Psychical Research 69: 105–113

Braud W G, Davis G, Wood R 1979 Experiments with Matthew Manning. Journal of the American Society for Psychical Research 50(782): 199–223

Braud W, Shafer D, Andrews C 1996 Further studies of autonomic detection of remote staring: replications, new control procedures, and personality correlates. In: Cook E (ed) Research in parapsychology 1992. Scarecrow Press, Lanham, MD

Brier R 1969 PK on a bio-electrical system. Journal of Parapsychology 33: 187–205

Brookes-Smith C 1973 Data-tape recorded experimental PK phenomena. Journal of the Society for Psychical Research 47: 69–89

Bunnell T 1996 The effect of hands-on healing on enzyme activity. International Journal of Research in Complementary Medicine 3: 265–340

Bunnell T 1999 The effect of 'healing with intent' on pepsin enzyme activity. Journal of Scientific Exploration 13(2): 139–148

Burr H, Mauro A 1949 Electrostatic fields of the sciatic nerve in the frog. Yale Journal of Biology and Medicine 21: 455–462

Burr H, Northrop F 1939 Evidence for the existence of an electrodynamic field in living organisms. Paper presented at the Proceedings of the National Academy of Science of the United States of America 24: 284–288

Campbell A 1968 Treatment of tumours by PK. Journal of the Society for Psychical Research 46(428)

Carpenter J 1988 Quasi-therapeutic group process and ESP. Journal of Parapsychology 52: 279–304

Chien C, Tsuei J, Lee S, Huang Y, Wei Y 1991 Effect of emitted bioenergy on biochemical functions of cells. American Journal of Chinese Medicine 19(3–4): 285–292

Cox W, Feather S, Carpenter J 1966 The effect of PK on electromechanical systems. II. Further experiments and analysis with the PK clocks machine. Journal of Parapsychology 30: 184–194

Dean D 1983 An examination of infra-red and ultra-violet techniques to test for changes in water following the laying-on-of-hands. Unpublished Doctoral dissertation, Saybrook Institute, San Francisco

Dean D, Brame E G 1975 Physical changes in water by laying on of hands. Paper presented at the Proceedings of the Second International Congress of Psychotronics. Psychotronics Association, pp 200–202

Dean E 1975 The effects of healers on biologically significant molecules. New Horizons 1(5): 215–219

Delanoy D, Parker A, Wilson K 1981 A three-subject study of psi in the ganzfeld. In: Roll W, Beloff J (eds) Research in parapsychology 1980. Scarecrow Press, Metuchen, NJ, pp. 86–88

Delanoy D, Morris R, Brady C, Roe A 1999 An EDA DMILS study exploring agent-receiver pairing. Paper presented at the Parapsychological Association 42nd Annual Convention, Durham, NC

Dennis M, Miledi R 1974 Electrically induced release of acetylcholine from denervated Schwann cells. Journal of Physiology 237: 431–452

Dibble W, Tiller W 1999 Electronic device-mediated pH changes in water. Journal of Scientific Exploration 13(2): 155–176

Dunne B, Nelson R, Jahn R 1988 Operator-related anomalies in a random mechanical cascade. Journal of Scientific Exploration 2(2): 155–179

Edge H 1980 The effect of laying on of hands on an enzyme: an attempted replication. In: Roll W (ed) Research in parapsychology 1979. Scarecrow Press, Metuchen, NJ, p. 137

Fahrion S 1992 Wirkus & Patricia Pooley EEG amplitude, brain mapping and synchrony in and between a bioenergy practitioner and client during healing. Subtle Energies 3(2): 19–52

Grad B 1964 A telekinetic effect on plant growth: 11. Experiments involving treatment of saline in stoppered bottles. International Journal of Parapsychology 6(Autumn): 473–498

Grad B 1965 A telekinetic effect on yeast activity. Journal of Parapsychology 29: 285–286

Grad B 1977 Laboratory evidence of 'laying on of hands'. In: Regush N (ed) Frontiers of healing. Avon Books, New York, pp. 203–213

Grad B 1996 Some heat experiments implicating the existence of a subtle energy. Subtle Energies 7(3): 239–262

Graham K, Watkins A 1971 Possible PK influence on the resuscitation of anesthetized mice. Journal of Parapsychology 35(4): 257–272

Green E, Parks P, Guyer P, Fahrion S, Coyne L 1991 Anomalous electrostatic phenomena in exceptional subjects. Subtle Energies 2(3): 69–94

Haraldsson E, Thorsteinsson T 1973 Psychokinetic effects on yeast: an exploratory experiment. In: Roll W, Morris R, Morris J (eds) Research in parapsychology 1972. Scarecrow Press, Metuchen, NJ

Harari S 1974 Exploratory study of PK effects on the growth of seedlings. Psychical Research Foundation, Durham, NC

Harary S 1975 A pilot study of the effects of psychically treated saline solution on the growth of seedlings. Psychical Research Foundation, Durham, NC

Hartwell W 1978 Contingent negative variation as an index of precognitive information. European Journal of Parapsychology 2: 83–103

Heaton E Mouse healing experiments. Foundation for Research on the Nature of Man, Durham, NC

Hickman J 1979 Plant growth experiments with Matthew Manning. In: Mishlove J (ed) A month with Matthew Manning: experiences and experiments in NC during May–June. Washington Research Center, San Francisco, pp. 74–76

Honorton C 1974 Apparent psychokinesis on static objects by a 'gifted' subject. In: Roll W, Morris R, Morris J (eds) Research in parapsychology 1973. Scarecrow Press, Metuchen, NJ, pp. 128–131

Jahn R, Dunne B, Nelson R, Dobyns Y, Bradish G 1997 Correlations of random binary sequences with pre-stated operator intention: a review of a 12 year program. Journal of Scientific Exploration 11(3): 345–367

Kaznacheev V P, Shurin S P et al 1976 Distant intercellular interactions in a system of two tissue cultures. Psychoenergetic Systems 1: 141–142

Kiang J, Marotta D, Wirkus M, Wirkus M, Jonas W 2002 External bioenergy increases intracellular free calcium concentration and reduces cellular response to heat stress. Journal of Investigative Medicine 50(1): 38–45

Kirkin A F 1981 Non-chemical distant interactions between cells in culture. Biofizika 26: 839–843

Klintman H 1983 Is there a paranormal (precognitive) influence in certain types of perceptual sequences? Part I. European Journal of Parapsychology 5: 19–49

Kmetz J 1979 PK experiments with cancer cells. Science Unlimited Research Foundation, San Antonio, TX

Kmetz J 1981 Effects of healing on cancer cells (Appendix). In: Kraft D (ed) Portrait of a psychic healer. Putnam, New York, pp. 181–185

Knowles F W 1959 Rat experiments and mesmerism. Journal of the American Society for Psychical Research 48

Krieger D 1972 The response of in vivo human hemoglobin to an active healing therapy by direct laying on of hands. Human Dimensions 1: 12–15

Krieger D 1973 Relationship of touch, with intent to help or heal to subjects in-vivo hemoglobin values: a study in personalized interactions. Paper presented at the Proceedings of the Ninth Nursing Research Conference, San Antonio, TX

Krippner S, Rhinehart L 1997 Scores of psychic claimants on the mari card test. Subtle Energies 8(2): 153–173

Lenington S 1979 Effects of holy water on the growth of radish plants. Psychological Reports 45: 381–382

Levengood W, Gedye J, Chir B 1997 Evidence for charge density pulses associated with bioelectric fields in living organisms. Subtle Energies and Energy Medicine 8(1): 33–54

Levy W 1974 Possible PK by rats to receive pleasurable brain stimulation. In: Roll W, Morris R, Morris J (eds) Research in parapsychology 1973. Scarecrow Press, Metuchen, NJ, pp. 78–81

Levy W, Andre E 1970 Possible PK by young chickens to obtain warmth. Journal of Parapsychology 34: 303

Lowry R 1981 Apparent PK effect on computer-generated random digit series. Journal of the American Society for Psychical Research 75: 209–220

May E, Radin D, Hubbard G, Humphrey B, Utts J 1996 Psi experiments with random number generators: an informational model. In: Weiner D, Radin D (eds) Research in parapsychology 1985. Scarecrow Press, Metuchen, NJ, pp. 119–120

Miller R The effect of thought upon the growth rate of remotely located plants. Journal of Pastoral Counsel 6(2): 62–63

Moss T 1969 ESP effects in artists contrasted with non-artists. Journal of Parapsychology 33: 57–69

Moss T, Gengerelli J 1968 ESP effects generated by affective states. Journal of Parapsychology 32: 90–100

Nash C 1944 PK tests of a large population. Journal of Parapsychology 8: 304–310

Nash C 1982 Test of psychokinetic control of bacterial mutation. Journal of the American Society for Psychical Research 51: 217–221

Nash C, Nash C 1967 The effect of paranormally conditioned solution on yeast fermentation. Journal of Parapsychology 31(314)

Nash C B 1982 Psychokinetic control of bacterial growth. Journal of the American Society for Psychical Research 51: 217–221

Nash C B 1984 Test of psychokinetic control of bacterial growth. Journal of the American Society for Psychical Research 78(2): 145–152

Nelson R, Mayer E 1996 A FieldREG application at the San Francisco Bay Revels. Internal Document PEAR 95004, Princeton Engineering Anomalies Research, Princeton University, December, 1995

Nelson R, Bradish G, Jahn R, Dunne B 1994 A linear pendulum experiment: effects of operator intention on damping rate. Journal of Scientific Exploration 8(4): 471–489

Nicholas C 1977 The effects of loving attention on plant growth. New England Journal of Parapsychology 1: 19–24

Null G, Stone C, Revici E, Bryan C, Berman V An experiment in paranormal healing: influence exerted by a parapsychological technique with cancerous ascites in mice. Nutrition Institute of America, New York

Olcese J, Reuss S, Semm P 1988 Geomagnetic field detection in rodents. Life Sciences 42(6): 605–613

Olson M, Sneed N, LaVia M, Virella G, Bonadonna R, Michel Y 1997 Stress-induced immunosuppression and therapeutic touch. Alternative Therapies 3(2): 68–74

Onetto B, Elguin G 1966 Psychokinesis in experimental tumorogenesis. Journal of Parapsychology 30: 220

Pauli E 1973 PK on living targets as related to sex, distance and time. In: Roll W, Morris R, Morris J (eds) Research in parapsychology 1972. Scarecrow Press, Metuchen, NJ, pp. 68–70

Radin D 1981 Mental influence on machine-generated random events: six experiments. In: White RA, Morris RL (eds) Research in Parapsychology. Scarecrow Press, Metuchen, NJ, pp. 141–142.

Radin D 1996 Towards a complex systems model of psi performance. Subtle Energies 7(1): 35–69

Radin D, Nelson R 1989 Consciousness related effects in random physical systems. Found Physics 19: 1400–1514

Radin D, Taylor R, Braud W 1995 Remote mental influence on human electrodermal activity: a pilot replication. European Journal of Parapsychology 11: 19–31

Rauscher E 1990 Human volitional effects on a model bacterial system. Subtle Energies 1(1): 21–41

Rauscher E, Rubik B 1980 Effects on motility behavior and growth of Salmonella typhimurium in the presence of a psychic subject. In: Roll W (ed) Research in parapsychology. Scarecrow Press, Metuchen, NJ

Reid G 1982 State, emotionality, belief, and absorption in ESP scoring. Journal of the Association for the Study of Perception 17: 28–39

Rein G 1993 Modulation of neurotransmitter function by quantum fields. In: Pribram K (ed) Rethinking neural networks: quantum fields and biological data. Lawrence Erlbaum, Hillsdale, NJ, pp. 379–388

Rein G, McCraty R 1994 Structural changes in water and DNA associated with new physiologically measurable states. Journal of Scientific Exploration 8(3): 438

Richards D, McMillin D, Nelson C, Mein E 1996 Improvement of circulation using the radial appliance. Subtle Energies and Energy Medicine 7(1): 71–88

Ruegemar W, Silverman F 1956 Influence of gentling on the physiology of the rat. Paper presented at the Proceedings of the Society for Experimental Biology and Medicine

Saklani A 1990 Psychokinesis effects on plant growth: further studies. In: Henkel L, Palmer J (eds) Research in parapsychology 1989. Scarecrow Press, Metuchen, NJ, pp. 37–41

Schlitz M 1982 PK on living systems: further studies with anesthetized mice. Journal of Parapsychology 46: 51–52

Schlitz M, Braud W 1985 Reiki-plus natural healing: an ethnographic and experimental study. In: Weiner D, Radin D (eds) Research in parapsychology. Scarecrow Press, Metuchen, NJ, pp. 17–18

Schlitz M, Gruber E 1980 Transcontinental remote viewing. Journal of Parapsychology 44(4): 305–317

Schmidt H 1971 Mental influence on random events. New Scientist and Science Journal: 757–758

Schmidt H 1973 PK tests with a high-speed random number generator. Journal of Parapsychology 37: 105–118

Schmidt H 1974 Comparison of PK on two different random number generators. Journal of Parapsychology 38: 47–55

Schmidt H 1985 Additional effects for PK on pre-recorded targets. Journal of Parapsychology 49: 229–244

Schmidt H 1990 PK tests with and without preobservation by animals. In: Henkel L, Palmer J (eds) Research in parapsychology 1989. Scarecrow Press, Metuchen, NJ, pp. 15–19

Schmidt H 1993 New PK tests with an independent observer. Journal of Parapsychology 57: 227–240

Schmidt H, Pantas L 1972 PSI tests with internally different machines. Journal of Parapsychology 36: 222–232

Schmidt H, Morris R, Rudolph L 1986 Channeling evidence for a PK effect to independent observers. Journal of Parapsychology 50 (March): 1–15

Schwartz G, Russek L, Beltran J 1995 Interpersonal hand-energy registration: evidence for implicit performance and perception. Subtle Energies 6(3): 183–200

Schwartz G, Russek L, She Z, Song L, Xin Y 1997 Anomalous organization of random events during an international qigong meeting: evidence for group consciousness or accumulated qi fields? Subtle Energies and Energy Medicine 8(1): 55–65

Semm P, Schenider T, Vollrath L 1980 Effect of an Earth strength magnetic field on electrical activity of pineal cells. Nature 288: 607–608

Shah S, Ogden A, Pettker C, Raffo A, Itescu S, Oz M 1999 A study of the effect of energy healing on in vitro tumor cell proliferation. Journal of Alternative and Complementary Medicine 5(4): 359–365

Singer M, Weckesser E, Geraudie J, Maier C, Singer J 1987 Open finger tip healing and replacement after distal amputation in Rhesus monkey with comparison to limb regeneration in lower vertebrates. Anatomy and Embryology 177: 29–36

Smith J 1972 Paranormal effects on enzyme activity through 'laying-on' of hands. Human Dimensions 1 (Spring–Summer): 15–19

Smith M 1973 Enzymes are activated by the laying on of hands. Human Dimensions 2: 46–48

Smith M J 1972 Paranormal effects on enzyme activity. Human Dimensions 1: 15–19

Snel F 1980 PK influence on malignant cell growth [research letter]. University of Utrecht 10: 19–27

Snel F, van der Sijde P 1990 The effect of retro-active distance healing on Babesia rodhani (rodent malaria) in rats. European Journal of Parapsychology 8: 123–130

Solfvin G 1982 Studies of the effects of mental healing and expectations on the growth of corn seedlings. European Journal of Parapsychology 4(3): 287–323

Solfvin G 1982 Studies of the effects of an induced expectancy structure on the growth of corn seedlings. European Journal of Parapsychology 4(3)

Solfvin G F 1982 Psi expectancy effects in psychic healing studies with malarial mice. European Journal of Parapsychology 4(2): 160–197

Thompson R 1991 Numerical analysis and theoretical modeling of causal effects of conscious intention. Subtle Energies 2(1): 47–70

Uhlenhuth E, Canter A, Neustadt J, Payson H 1959 The symptomatic relief of anxiety with meprobamate, phenobarbital and placebo. American Journal of Psychiatry 115: 905–910

Walleczek J, Shiu E, Hahn G 1999 Increase in radiation-induced HPRT gene mutation frequency after nonthermal exposure to nonionizing 60 Hz electromagnetic fields. Radiation Research 151(4): 489–497

Watkins G K, Watkins A M 1971 Possible PK influence on the resuscitation of anesthetized mice. Journal of Parapsychology 35(4): 257–272

Watkins G K, Watkins A M, Wells R A 1973 Further studies on the resuscitation of anesthetized mice. In: Roll W, Morris R, Morris J (eds) Research in parapsychology 1972. Scarecrow Press, Metuchen, NJ, pp. 157–159

Wells R, Klein J 1972 A replication of a psychic healing paradigm. Journal of Parapsychology 36: 144–149

Wirth D, Johnson C, Horvath J, MacGregor J 1992 The effect of alternative healing therapy on the regeneration rate of salamander forelimbs. Journal of Scientific Exploration 6(4): 375–391

Reviews, Systematic Reviews, and Meta-Analyses

Abbot N C 2000 Healing as a therapy for human disease: a systematic review. Journal of Alternative and Complementary Medicine 6(2): 159–169

Alcock J 1988 A comprehensive review of major empirical studies in parapsychology involving random event generators or remote viewing. In: Druckman D, Swets J (eds) Enhancing human performance: issues, theories, and techniques. National Academy Press, Washington, DC

Aldridge D 1993 Is there evidence for spiritual healing? Advances in Mind Body Health 9(4): 4–21

Aldridge D 1994 An overview of music therapy research. Complementary Therapies in Medicine 2(4): 204–216

Altshuler I 1954 The past, present, and future of music therapy. In: Podolsky E (ed) Music therapy. Philosophical Library, New York

Astin J The efficacy of spiritual healing: a systematic review of randomized trials. Stanford University School of Medicine, Stanford

Astin J, Harkness E, Ernst E 2000 The efficacy of 'distant healing': a systematic review of randomized trials. Annals of Internal Medicine 132: 903–910

Bailey S 1997 The arts in spiritual care. Seminars in Oncology Nursing 13(4): 242–247

Baldacchino D, Draper P 2001 Spiritual coping strategies: a review of the nursing research literature. Journal of Advanced Nursing 34(6): 833–841

Barnard D 1983 Religion and religious studies in health care and health education. Journal of Allied Health: 192–200

Bem D J, Honorton C 1994 Does psi exist? Replicable evidence for an anomalous information transfer. Psychological Bulletin 115(1): 4–18

Benor D 1984 Fields and energies related to healing: a review of Soviet and Western studies. Psi Research 3: 8–15

Benor D J 1990 Survey of spiritual healing research. Complementary Medicine Research 4(1): 9–33

Benor D J 1992 Lessons from spiritual healing research and practice. Subtle Energies 3(1): 77–92

Benor D J 1992 Intuitive diagnosis. Subtle Energies 3(2): 41–64

Bergin A 1983 Religiosity and mental health: a critical reevaluation and meta-analysis. Professional Psychology: Research Practice 14: 170–184

Blackmore S 1994 PSI in psychology. Skeptical Inquirer 18(Summer): 351–355

Braud W 1994 Empirical explorations of prayer, distant healing, and remote mental influence. Journal of Religion and Psychical Research 17(2): 62–73

Braud W 2000 Wellness implications of retroactive intentional influence: exploring an outrageous hypothesis. Alternative Therapies 6(1): 37–48

Bronner A 1964 Psychotherapy with religious patients (review of the literature). American Journal of Psychotherapy 18: 475–487

Brookes-Smith C, Hunt D 1970 Some experiments in psychokinesis. Journal of the Society for Psychical Research 45: 265–281

Browner W S, Goldman L 2000 Distant healing: an unlikely hypothesis. American Journal of Medicine 108(6): 507–508

Brown-Saltzman K 1997 Replenishing the spirit by meditative prayer and guided imagery. Seminars in Oncology Nursing 13(4): 255–259

Bullis R K 1991 The spiritual healing 'defense' in criminal prosecutions for crimes against children. Child Welfare 70(5): 541–555

Burton L A 1998 The spiritual dimension of palliative care. Seminars in Oncology Nursing 14(2): 121–128

Colwell J, Schroder S, Sladen D 2000 The ability to detect unseen staring: a literature review and empirical tests. British Journal of Psychology 91: 71–85

Cook J 1981 The therapeutic use of music: a literature review. Nursing Forum 20: 252–267

Craigie F C, Liu I Y, Larson D B, Lyons J S 1988 A systematic analysis of religious variables in the Journal of Family Practice, 1976–1986. Journal of Family Practice 27: 509–513

Craigie F C Jr, Hobbs R F 3rd 1999 Spiritual perspectives and practices of family physicians with an expressed interest in spirituality. Family Medicine 31(8): 578–585

Craigie F C Jr, Larson D B, Liu I Y 1990 References to religion in the Journal of Family Practice: dimensions and valence of spirituality. Journal of Family Practice 30(4): 477–480

Daley B 1997 Therapeutic touch, nursing practice and contemporary cutaneous wound healing research. Journal of Advanced Nursing 25: 1123–1132

DeGracia D 1999 Report of referee on 'the effect of "healing with intent" on pepsin enzyme activity'. Journal of Scientific Exploration 13(2): 149–153

Dillbeck M C, Orme-Johnson D W 1987 Physiological differences between transcendental meditation and rest. American Psychologist 42: 879–881

Dolin Y, Davydov V, Morozova E, Ye Shumov D 1993 Studies of a remote mental effect on plants with electrophysiological recording. Paper presented at the Proceedings of the 36th Annual Convention of the Parapsychological Association, Toronto, Canada

Donahue M 1985 Intrinsic and extrinsic religiousness: review and meta-analysis. Journal of Personality and Social Psychology 48(2): 400–419

Dossey L 1999 Controlled experimental trials of healing. In: Healing words: the power of prayer and the practice of medicine. Harper San Francisco, San Francisco, CA, pp. 211–235

Dwyer J, Clarke L, Miller M 1990 The effect of religious concentration and affiliation on county cancer mortality rates. Journal of Health and Social Behavior 31: 185–202

Dyson J, Cobb M, Forman D 1997 The meaning of spirituality: a literature review. Journal of Advanced Nursing 26(6): 1183–1188

Ebneter M, Binder M, Saller R 2001 Fernheilung und klinische forschung. Forschende Komplementarmedizin und Klassische Naturheilkunde 8: 274–287

Ellison C W 1983 Spiritual well-being: conceptualization and measurement. Journal of Psychology and Theology 11: 330–340

Eppley K R, Abrams A I, Shear J 1989 Differential effects of relaxation technique on trait anxiety: a meta-analysis. Journal of Clinical Psychology 45: 957–974

Gardner R 1983 Miracles of healing in Anglo-Celtic Northumbria as recorded by the Venerable Bede and his contemporaries: a reappraisal in the light of twentieth century experience. British Medical Journal 287: 1927–1933

Gartner J, Larson D, Allen G 1991 Religious commitment and mental health: a review of the empirical literature. Journal of Psychology and Theology 19: 6–25

Girden E 1962 A review of psychokinesis (PK). Psychological Bulletin 59: 353–388

Grad B 1965 Some biological effects of laying-on of hands: a review of experiments with animals and plants. Journal of the American Society for Psychical Research 59: 95–127

Grad B 1970 Healing by the laying on of hands: review of experiments and implications. Pastoral Psychology 21: 19–26

Greenberg R P, Bornstein R F, Greenberg M D, Fisher S 1992 A meta-analysis of antidepressant outcome under 'blinder' conditions. Journal of Consulting and Clinical Psychology 60(5): 664–669

Hadaway C 1978 Life satisfaction and religion: a reanalysis. Social Forces 57(2): 637–643

Halstead M T, Mickley J R 1997 Attempting to fathom the unfathomable: descriptive views of spirituality. Seminars in Oncology Nursing 13(4): 225–230

Hart D, Schneider D 1997 Spiritual care for children with cancer. Seminars in Oncology Nursing 13(4): 263–270

Hawks S R, Hull M L, Thalman R L, Richins P M 1995 Review of spiritual health: definition, role, and intervention strategies in health promotion. American Journal of Health Promotion 9(5): 371–378

Hodges R D, Scofield A M 1995 Is spiritual healing a valid and effective therapy? Journal of the Royal Society of Medicine 88(4): 203–207

Honorton C 1985 Meta-analysis of psi ganzfeld research: a response to Hyman. Journal of Parapsychology 49: 51–91

Honorton C, Ferrari D C 1989 'Future telling': a meta-analysis of forced-choice precognition experiments, 1935–1987. Journal of Parapsychology 53: 281–308

Honorton C, Ferrari D, Bem D 1990 Extraversion and ESP performance: a meta-analysis and a new confirmation. In: Association P (ed) Research in parapsychology 1990. Abstracts and Papers from the 33rd Annual Convention of the Parapsychological Association. Scarecrow Press, Metuchen, NJ, pp. 35–44

Idler E, Benyamini Y 1997 Self-reported health and mortality: a review of 27 community studies. Journal of Health and Social Behavior 38: 21–37

Keller E 1984 Therapeutic touch: a review of literature and implication of a holistic nursing modality. Journal of Holistic Nursing 2(1): 24–29

Kneafsey R 1997 The therapeutic use of music in a care of the elderly setting: a literature review. Journal of Clinical Nursing 6: 341–346

Koenig H 1990 Research on religion and mental health in later life: a review and commentary. Journal of Geriatric Psychiatry 23(1): 23–53

Koenig H, Smiley M, Gonzales J 1988 Religion, health, and aging: a review and theoretical integration. Greenwood Press, Westport, CT

Koenig H G, Larson D B, Weaver A J 1998 Research on religion and serious mental illness. New Directions in Mental Health Services 80: 81–95

Kress K 1999 Parapsychology in intelligence: a personal review and conclusion. Journal of Scientific Exploration 13(1): 69–85

Krieger D 1975 Therapeutic touch: the imprimatur of nursing. American Journal of Nursing 75(5): 784–787

Landau L 1987 Experimental tests of general quantum theories. Letters in Math and Physics 14: 33–40

Larson D B, Pattison M, Blazer D G, Omran A R, Kaplan B H 1986 Systematic analysis of research on religious variables in four major psychiatric journals, 1978–1982. American Journal of Psychiatry 143: 329–334

Larson D, Sherrill K, Lyons J et al 1992 Associations between dimensions of religious commitment and mental health reported in the American Journal of Psychiatry and Archives of General Psychiatry: 1978–1989. American Journal of Psychiatry 149: 557–559

Larson D, Sherrill K, Lyons J 1994 Neglect and misuse of the 'r' word: systematic reviews of religious measures in health, mental health, and aging. In: Levin J (ed) Religion in aging and health: theoretical foundations and methodological frontiers. Sage Publications, Thousand Oaks, CA, pp. 178–195

Levin J 1997 Religious research in gerontology, 1980–1994: a systematic review. Journal of Religious Gerontology 10(3): 3–31

Levin J, Vanderpool H 1987 Is frequent religious attendance really conducive to better health? Toward an epidemiology of religion. Social Science and Medicine 24: 589–600

Levin J, Vanderpool H 1989 Is religion therapeutically significant for hypertension? Social Science and Medicine 29(1): 69–78

Levin J, Larson D, Puchalski C 1997 Religion and spirituality in medicine: research and education. Journal of the American Medical Association 278(9): 792–793

Loh S-H 1999 Qigong therapy in the treatment of metastatic colon cancer. Alternative Therapies 5(4): 111, 112

Long J K 1977 Extrasensory ecology: a summary of the evidence. In: Long J K (ed) Extrasensory ecology. Scarecrow Press, London, pp. 371–396

Lukoff D, Turner R, Lu F 1993 Transpersonal psychology research review: psychospiritual dimensions of healing. Journal of Transpersonal Psychology 25: 11–28

Lukoff D, Provenzano R, Lu F, Turner R 1999 Religious and spiritual case reports on Medline: a systematic analysis of records from 1980 to 1996. Alternative Therapies 5(1): 64–70

Luskin F M, Newell K A, Griffith M et al 1998 A review of mind–body therapies in the treatment of cardiovascular disease. Part 1: Implications for the elderly. Alternative Therapies in Health and Medicine 4(3): 46–61

Luskin F, DiNucci E, Newell K 2000 A review of the effect of spiritual and religious factors on mortality and morbidity with a focus on cardiovascular and pulmonary disease. Journal of Cardiopulmonary Rehabilitation 20: 8–15

Luskin F M, Newell K A, Griffith M et al 2000 A review of mind/body therapies in the treatment of musculoskeletal disorders with implications for the elderly. Alternative Therapies in Health and Medicine 6(2): 46–56

Malmquist J 2000 [Scrutiny of alternative medicine. 'Distant healing' – a special kind of telemedicine]. Lakartidningen 97(51–52): 6050–6052

Mann S 2000 The mind/body link in essential hypertension: time for a new paradigm. Alternative Therapies 6(2): 39–45

Martsolf D S 1997 Cultural aspects of spirituality in cancer care. Seminars in Oncology Nursing 13(4): 231–236

Matthews D, McCullough M, Larson D, Koening H, Swyers J, Milano M 1998 Religious commitment and health status: a review of the research and implications for family medicine. Archives of Family Medicine 7: 118–124

Miller M A 1995 Culture, spirituality, and women's health. Journal of Obstetrics Gynecology and Neonatal Nursing 24(3): 257–263

Milton J, Wiseman R 1999 Does psi exist? Lack of replication of an anomalous process of information transfer. Psychological Bulletin 125(4): 387–391

Nadin R, Kihlstrom J 1987 Hypnosis, psi, and the psychology of anomalous experience. Behavioral and Brain Sciences 10(4): 597–599

Nelson R D 1990 Meta-analysis. The Explorer, Society for Scientific Exploration 6(2); Chantilly, VA

Nelson R, Jahn R, Dunne B, Dobyns Y, Bradish G 1998 FieldREG II: consciousness field effects: replications and explorations. Journal of Scientific Exploration 12(3): 425–454

O'Neill D P, Kenny E K 1998 Spirituality and chronic illness. Image – the Journal of Nursing Scholarship 30(3): 275–280

Payne I, Bergin A, Bielema K, Jenkins P 1991 Review of religion and mental health: prevention and the enhancement of psychosocial functioning. Preventive Human Services 9: 11–40

Persinger M A 1985 Geophysical variables and behavior: XXIX, intense paranormal experiences occur during days of quiet global geomagnetic activity. Perceptual Motor Skills 61: 320–322

Persinger M 1987 Spontaneous telepathic experiences from phantasms of the living and low global geomagnetic activity. Journal of the American Society for Psychical Research 81: 23–36

Persinger M 1988 Increased geomagnetic activity and the occurrence of bereavement hallucinations: evidence for melatonin-mediated microseizuring in the temporal lobe? Neuroscience Letters 88: 271–274

Persinger M A, Schaut G B 1988 Geomagnetic factors in subjective telepathic, precognitive and postmortem experiences. Journal of the American Society for Psychical Research 82(3): 217–235

Pollner M 1989 Divine relations, social relations, and well-being. Journal of Health and Social Behavior 30(1): 92–104

Quinn J 1988 Building a body of knowledge: research on therapeutic touch, 1974–1986. Journal of Holistic Nursing 6: 37–45

Radin D, Ferrari D 1991 Effects of consciousness on the fall of dice: a meta-analysis. Journal of Scientific Exploration 5: 1–24

Radin D, Nelson R 1989 Evidence for consciousness-related anomalies in random physical systems. Found Physics 19: 1499–1514

Radin D, Utts J 1989 Experiments investigating the influence of intention on random and pseudorandom events. Journal of Scientific Exploration 3: 65–79

Radin D, May E C, Thomson M J 1986 Psi experiments with random number generators. Meta-analysis Part I. In Weiner DH, Radin DI (eds) Research in Parapsychology, 1985, Metuchen, NJ: Scarecrow Press

Roberts A H, Kewman D G, Mercier L, Hovell M 1993 The power of nonspecific effects in healing: implications for psychological and biological treatments. Clinical Psychology Reviews 13: 373–391

Roberts L, Ahmed I, Hall S, Sargent C 1999 Intercessory prayer for the alleviation of ill health. Cochrane Database for Systematic Reviews 2(2)

Rosenthal R, Rubin D 1978 Interpersonal expectancy effects: the first 345 studies. Behavioral and Brain Sciences 3: 377–415

Sancier K 1996 Medical applications of qigong. Alternative Therapies 2(1): 40–46

Sancier K, Hu B 1991 Medical applications of qigong and emitted qi on humans, animals, cell cultures, and plants: review of selected scientific research. American Journal of Acupuncture 19(4): 367–377

Sanua V 1969 Religion, mental health, and personality: a review of empirical studies. American Journal of Psychiatry 125(9): 1203–1213

Schienle A, Stark R, Vaitl D 1998 Biological effects of very low frequency (VLF) atmospherics in humans: a review. Journal of Scientific Exploration 12(3): 455–468

Schiller P, Levin J 1988 Is there a religious factor in health care utilization? A review. Social Science and Medicine 27(12): 1369–1379

Schmidt H 1987 The strange properties of psychokinesis. Journal of Scientific Exploration 1(2): 103–118

Schmidt H 1993 Observation of a psychokinetic effect under highly controlled conditions. Journal of Parapsychology 57: 351–372

Schopler E 1987 Specific and nonspecific factors in the effectiveness of a treatment system. American Psychologist 42(4): 376–383

Schouten S A 1993 Applied parapsychology: studies of psychics and healers. Journal of Scientific Exploration 7(4): 375–401

Sheldrake R 1998 Experimenter effects in scientific research: how widely are they neglected? Journal of Scientific Exploration 12(1): 73–78

Spence C, Danielson T 1987 The faith assembly: a follow-up study of faith healing and mortality. Indiana Medicine 80: 238–240

Spottiswood S J P 1990 Geomagnetic activity and anomalous cognition: a preliminary report of new evidence. Subtle Energies 1(1): 91–102

Springer S, Eicher D 1999 Effects of a prayer circle on a moribund premature infant. Alternative Therapies 5(2): 115–118, 120

Stack S 1983 The effect of religious commitment on suicide: a cross-national analysis. Journal of Health and Social Behavior 24(4): 362–374

Standley J 1986 Music research in medical/dental treatment: meta-analysis and clinical applications. Journal of Music Therapy 23: 56–122

Stanford R 1974 An experimentally testable model for spontaneous psi events II. Psychokinetic events. Journal of the American Society for Psychical Research 68(4): 321–356

Tang K 1994 Qigong therapy – its effectiveness and regulation. American Journal of Chinese Medicine 22(3–4): 235–242

Targ E 1997 Evaluating distant healing: a research review. Alternative Therapies in Health and Medicine 3(6): 74–78

Tart C 1988 Geomagnetic effects on GESP: two studies. Journal of the American Society for Psychical Research 82(3): 193–216

Utts J 1996 An assessment of the evidence for psychic functioning. Journal of Scientific Exploration 10(1): 63–76

Wallis C 1996 Faith and healing: can prayer, faith, and spirituality really improve your physical health? A growing and surprising body of scientific evidence says they can. Time 147: 58–63

Warber S, Gillespie B, Kile G, Gorenflo D, Bolling S (2000) Meta-analysis of the effects of therapeutic touch on anxiety symptoms. Focus on Alternative and Complementary Therapies 5(1): 106 (abstract)

Winstead-Fry P, Kijek J 1999 An integrative review and meta-analysis of therapeutic touch research. Alternative Therapies 5(6): 58–67

Wirth D 1995 Complementary healing intervention and dermal wound reepithelialization: an overview. International Journal of Psychosomatics 42(1–4): 48–53

Wirth D, Richardson J, Eidelman W 1996 Wound healing and complementary therapies: a review. Journal of Alternative and Complementary Medicine 2(4): 493–502

Witter R, Stock R, Okun M, Haring M 1985 Religion and subjective well-being in adulthood: a quantitative synthesis. Review of Religious Research 26: 332–342

Observational Studies and Non-Randomized Clinical Trials

Arango M A, Persinger M A 1988 Geophysical variables and behavior: LII, decreased geomagnetic activity and spontaneous telepathic experiences from the Sidgwick collection. Perceptual Motor Skills 67: 907–910

Bearden T 1995 Simultaneous psychophysiological assessments of a Hawaiian healer and client during healing. Subtle Energies 6(3): 241–266

Berman B, Singh B 1997 Chronic low back pain: an outcome analysis of a mind-body intervention. Complementary Therapies in Medicine 5: 29–35

Biley F 1994 Exploring the therapeutic potential of background music. Complementary Therapies in Medicine 2: 221–224

Biller W, Olson P, Breen T 1974 The effect of happy versus sad music and participation on anxiety. Journal of Music Therapy 11: 68–73

Blazer D, Palmore E 1976 Religion and aging in a longitudinal panel. Gerontologist 16(1): 82–85

Bourguignon E 1976 The effectiveness of religious healing movements. Transpersonal Psychiatry Research Review 13: 5–21

Braud W G 1990 Distant mental influence of the rate of hemolysis of human red blood cells. Journal of the American Society for Psychical Research 84(1): 1–24

Braun C, Layton J, Braun J 1986 Therapeutic touch improves residents' sleep. American Health Care Association Journal 12(1): 48–49

Brewitt B, Vittetoe T, Hartwell B 1997 The efficacy of Reiki hands-on healing: improvements in spleen and nervous system function as quantified by electrodermal screening. Alternative Therapies 3: 89

Brickman P, Coates D 1978 Lottery winners and accident victims: is happiness relative? Journal of Personality and Social Psychology 36: 917–927

Casler L 1965 Effects of extra tactile stimulation on a group of institutionalized infants. Genetic and Psychology Monographs 71: 137–175

Cassileth B, Lusk E, Walsh W 1986 Anxiety levels in patients with malignant disease. Hospice Journal 2(2): 57–69

Chetta H 1981 The effect of music and desensitization on preoperative anxiety in children. Journal of Music Therapy 18(2): 74–87

Cohen J 1989 Spiritual healing in a medical context. Practitioner 233(1473): 1056–1057

Connell-Meehan T 1985 The effects of therapeutic touch on the experience of acute pain in post-operative patients. Unpublished doctoral dissertation, New York University, New York

Davis C, Cunningham S 1985 The physiological responses of patients in the coronary care unit to selected music. Heart Lung 14(3): 291–292

Dickman C 1977 Therapeutic effects of spirituality on alcoholism. Unpublished Master's thesis, University of Utah, Salt Lake City

Dolin Y, Dymov V, Khatchenkov N 1993 Preliminary study of a human operator's remote effect on the psychophysiological state of another individual with EEG recording. Paper presented at the Proceedings of the 36th Annual Convention of the Parapsychological Association, Toronto, Canada, pp. 24–40

Epstein G, Barrett E, Halper J, Seriff N, Phillips K, Lowenstein S 1997 Alleviating asthma with mental imagery: a phenomenological approach. Alternative and Complementary Therapies 3(1): 42–52

Fahrion S 1992 Mietek Wirkus and Patricia Pooley, EEG amplitude, brain mapping and synchrony in and between a bioenergy practitioner and client during healing. Subtle Energies 3(2): 19–52

Fedoruk R 1983 Transfer of the relaxation response: therapeutic touch B as a method for reduction of stress in premature neonates. Unpublished dissertation, University of Maryland

Frank J 1985 The effect of music therapy and guided visual imagery on chemotherapy-induced nausea and vomiting. Oncology Nursing Forum 12(5): 47–52

Glik D 1986 Psychosocial well-being among spiritual healing participants. Social Science and Medicine 22(5): 579–586

Glik D 1988 Symbolic, ritual and social dynamics of spiritual healing. Social Science and Medicine 27(11): 1197–1206

Goodman F D 1986 Body posture and the religious altered state of consciousness: an experimental investigation. Journal of Human Psychology 26(3): 81–118

Goodrich J 1974 Psychic healing: a pilot study. Unpublished Doctoral dissertation, Union Graduate School, Vermont

Goslen B 1988 Wound healing for the dermatologic surgeon. Journal of Dermatology and Surgical Oncology 14: 959–972

Grad B 1967 The 'laying on of hands': implications for psychotherapy, gentling, and the placebo effect. Journal of the American Society for Psychical Research 61(4): 286–305

Grad B 1976 The biological effects of the 'laying on of hands' on animals and plants: implications for biology. In: Schmeidler G (ed) Parapsychology: its relation to physics, biology, psychology, and psychiatry. Scarecrow Press, Metuchen, NJ., pp. 76–89

Gruber E 1979 A study of conformance behavior involving rats and mice. Paper presented at the meeting of the Society for Psychical Research, Edinburgh, Scotland

Gruber E 1979 Conformance behavior involving animal and human subjects. European Journal of Parapsychology 3(1): 36–50

Gruber E 1980 PK effects on pre-recorded group behavior of living systems. European Journal of Parapsychology 3(2): 167–175

Hall J, Kim C, McElroy B, Shimony A 1977 Wave-packet reduction as a medium of communication. Found Physics 7: 759–767

Heidt P 1981 Effective therapeutic touch on the anxiety level of hospitalized patients. Nursing Research 30(1): 32–37

Holmes D S 1984 Meditation and somatic arousal reduction: a review of the experimental evidence. American Psychology 39(1): 1–10

Honorton C 1986 Ganzfeld target retrieval with an automated testing system: a model for initial ganzfeld success. Research in parapsychology. Scarecrow Press, Metuchen, NJ, pp. 36–39

Isaacs J, Patten T 1991 A double-blind study of the biocircuit, a putative subtle-energy-based relaxation device. Subtle Energies 2(2): 1–28

Iwao M, Kajiyama S, Mori H, Oogaki K 1999 Effects of qigong walking on diabetic patients: a pilot study. Journal of Alternative and Complementary Medicine 5(4): 353–358

Jackson M, Franzoi S, Schmeidler G 1977 Effects of feedback on ESP: a curious partial replication. Journal of the American Society for Psychical Research 71: 147–155

Jing-ming Y, Mei-yu R, Dai-yu D, Li-ying X 1996 Invigorating qi and promoting blood circulation in treatment of chronic idiopathic thrombocytopenic purpura. Chinese Journal of Internal Medicine 2(1): 12–14

Joyce C R B, Welldon B 1965 The objective efficacy of prayer: a double-blind clinical trial. Journal of Chronic Diseases 18: 367–377

Jung C 1997 An observational study of human energy fields in infants and young children. Subtle Energies and Energy Medicine 8(3): 213–241

Kark J, Shemi G, Friedlander Y, Martin O, Manor O, Blondheim S 1996 Does religious observance promote health? Mortality in secular and religious kibbutzim in Israel. AJPH 86: 341–346.

Ke-qi J, Wan-chun C 1996 A preliminary observation on effect of qigong on electrocardiographic autopower spectrum function. Chinese Journal of Internal Medicine 2(1): 49–50

Kibler V, Rider M 1983 The effect of progressive muscle relaxation and music on stress as measured by finger temperature response. Journal of Clinical Psychology 39(2): 213–215

King S, Funkerstein D 1957 Religious practice and cardiovascular reaction during stress. Journal of Abnormal Social Psychology 55: 135–137

Koenig H, Pargament K, Nielsen J (in press) Religious coping and health status in medically ill hospitalized older adults. Journal of Nervous and Mental Disease

Koizumi H, Reeves A 1999 A pilot study of electroencephalographic changes associated with Ki. Journal of Alternative and Complementary Medicine 5(4): 349–352

Kramer N 1990 Comparison of therapeutic touch and casual touch in stress reduction of hospitalized children. Pediatric Nursing 16(5): 483–485

Krieger D, Peper E, Ancoli S 1979 Therapeutic touch: searching for evidence of physiological change. American Journal of Nursing 79: 660–662

Lamontagne L, Mason K, Hepworth J 1985 Effects of relaxation on anxiety in children: implications for coping with stress. Nursing Research 34: 289–292

Landreth J, Landreth H 1974 Effects of music on physiological response. Journal of Research in Music Education 22: 4–12

Levin J 1993 Age differences in mystical experience. Gerontologist 33(4): 507–513

Lim Y 1993 Effects of qigong on cardiorespiratory changes: a preliminary study. American Journal of Chinese Medicine 21(1): 1–6

Locsin R 1981 The effect of music on the pain of selected postoperative patients. Journal of Advanced Nursing 6: 19–25

Makarec K, Persinger M A 1987 Geophysical variables and behavior: XLIII, negative correlation between accuracy of card-guessing and geomagnetic activity: a case study. Perceptual Motor Skills 65: 105–106

Mansour A, Beuche M, Laing G, Leis A, Nurse J 1999 A study to test the effectiveness of placebo Reiki standardization procedures developed for a planned Reiki efficacy study. Journal of Alternative and Complementary Medicine 5(2): 153–164

Markides K 1983 Aging, religiosity and adjustment: a longitudinal analysis. Journal of Gerontology 38(5): 621–625

Matthews D, Marlowe S, MacNutt F 2000 Effects of intercessory prayer on patients with rheumatoid arthritis. Southern Medical Journal 93(12): 1177–1186

Medalie H, Goldhourt U 1976 Angina pectoris among 10 000 men II: psychosocial and other risk factors as evidence by a multivariate analysis of five-year incidence. American Journal of Medicine 60: 910–921

Meehan T, Mersmann C, Wiseman M, Wolff B, Malgady R 1990 The effect of therapeutic touch on postoperative pain. Paper presented at the Annual Meeting of Nurse Healers-Professional Association, Toronto, Canada

Metta L 1972 Psychokinesis on Lepidopterous larvae. Journal of Parapsychology 36: 213–221

Olson K, Hanson J 1997 Using Reiki to manage pain: a preliminary report. Cancer Prevention Control 1(2): 108–113

Olson M, Sneed N, Bonadonna R, Ratliff J, Dias J 1992 Therapeutic touch and post-hurricane Hugo stress. Journal of Holistic Nursing 10(2): 120–136

Parkes B 1986 Therapeutic touch as an intervention to reduce anxiety in elderly, hospitalized patients. Dissertation Abstracts International 47: 4755B

Poser E 1966 Effect of therapists' training on group therapeutic outcome. Journal of Consulting Psychology 13: 283–289

Pressman P, Lyons J, Larson D, Strain J 1990 Religious belief, depression, and ambulation status in elderly women with broken hips. American Journal of Psychiatry 147: 758–760

Prueter B, Mezzano J 1973 Effects of background music upon initial counseling interaction. Journal of Music Therapy 10: 205–212

Reuther I, Aldridge D 1998 Qigong Yangsheng as a complementary therapy in the management of asthma: a single-case appraisal. Journal of Alternative and Complementary Medicine 4(2): 173–183

Rhine L, Rhine J 1943 The psychokinetic effect. Journal of Parapsychology 7: 20–43

Rider M, Kibler V 1990 Treating arthritis and lupus patients with music-mediated imagery and group psychotherapy. Arts in Psychotherapy 17: 29–33

Rider M, Floyd J, Kirkpatrick J 1985 The effect of music, image and relaxation on adrenal corticosteroids and the re-entrainment of circadian rhythms. Journal of Music Therapy 22(1): 46–58

Riscalla L 1982 A study of religious healers and healees. Journal of the American Society for Psychosomatic and Dental Medicine 29(3): 97–103

Rosa L, Rosa E, Sarner L, Narrett S 1998 A close look at therapeutic touch. Journal of the American Medical Association 279: 1005–1010

Ross C 1990 Religion and psychological distress. Journal of Scientific Studies and Religion 29(2): 236–245

Sancier K 1994 The effect of qigong on therapeutic balancing measured by electroacupuncture according to voll (EAV): a preliminary study. Acupuncture and Electrotherapeutics Research 19: 119–127

Scartelli J 1984 The effect of EMG biofeedback and sedative music only on frontalis muscle relaxation ability. Journal of Music Therapy 21(2): 67–87

Schlitz M J, Honorton C 1992 Ganzfeld psi performance within an artistically gifted population. Journal of the American Society for Psychical Research 86(2): 83–98

Schmidt H 1976 PK effects on pre-recorded targets. Journal of the American Society for Psychical Research 70: 267–291

Schmidt H 1997 Random generators and living systems as targets in retro-PK experiments. Journal of the American Society for Psychical Research 91(1): 1–13

Schmidt H, Braud W 1993 New PK tests with an independent observer. Journal of Parapsychology 57: 227–240

Schmidt H, Stapp H 1993 PK with prerecorded random events and the effects of preobservation. Journal of Parapsychology 57: 331–349

Schwartz G, Russek L 1999 Registration of actual and intended eye gaze: correlation with spiritual beliefs and experiences. Journal of Scientific Exploration 13(2): 213–229

Sears W 1958 The effect of music on muscle tonus. In: Gaston E (ed) Music therapy 1957. Allen Press, Lawrence, KS

Stack S 1983 The effect of the decline in institutionalized religion on suicide 1954–78. Journal of the Scientific Study of Religion 22(3): 239–252

Strauch I 1963 Medical aspects of 'mental' healing. International Journal for Parapsychology 5: 135–166

Streng F 1970 The objective study of religion and the unique quality of religiousness. Religious Studies 6: 209–219

Syldona A, Rein G 1999 The use of DC electrodermal potential measurements and healer's felt sense to assess the energetic nature of qi. Journal of Alternative and Complementary Medicine 5(4): 329–347

Takegawa Y 2000 Combined Kampo with radiation therapy prolongs survival in patients with cervical cancer. Journal of Traditional Medicine 17(3): 108–114

Uhlenhuth E H, Rickels K, Fisher S, Park L C, Lipman R S, Mock J 1966 Drug, doctor's verbal attitude and clinical setting in the symptomatic response to pharmacotherapy. Psychopharmacologia 9: 392–418

Wirth D 1995 The significance of belief and expectancy within the spiritual healing encounter. Social Science and Medicine 41(2): 249–260

Wright S, Pratt C, Schmall V 1985 Spiritual support for caregivers of dementia patients. Journal of Religious Health 24(1): 31–38

Zimmy G, Weidenfeller E 1963 Effect of music upon GSR and heartrate. American Journal of Psychology 76: 311–314

Descriptive Studies and Case Reports, Surveys

Appelbaum S A 1993 The laying on of health: personality patterns of psychic healers. Bulletin of the Menninger Clinic 57(1): 33–40

Armstrong D 2001 Exploring fathers' experiences of pregnancy after a prior perinatal loss. MCN. American Journal of Maternal Child Nursing 26(3): 147–153

Asser S M, Swan R 1998 Child fatalities from religion-motivated medical neglect. Pediatrics 101(4/1): 625–629

Astin J A 1998 Why patients use alternative medicine: results of a national study. Journal of the American Medical Association 279(19): 1548–1553

Asuni T 1979 The dilemma of traditional healing with special reference to Nigeria. Social Science and Medicine [Med Anthropol] 13B(1): 33–39

Attevelt H 1981 A statistical survey of the patients of paranormal healers. Netherlands Federation for Paranormal and Naturopathic Healers, Amsterdam

Avants S K, Warburton L A, Margolin A 2001 Spiritual and religious support in recovery from addiction among HIV-positive injection drug users. Journal of Psychoactive Drugs 33(1): 39–45

Backus C J, Backus W, Page D I 1995 Spirituality of EMTs: a study of the spiritual nature of EMS workers and its effects on perceived happiness and prayers for patients. Prehospital Disaster Medicine 10(3): 168–173

Bailey L 1983 The effects of live music versus tape-recorded music on hospitalized cancer patients. Music Therapy 3: 17–28

Barrington R 1994 A naturalistic inquiry of postoperative pain after therapeutic touch. In: Gaut D, Boykin A (eds) Caring as healing: renewal through hope. National League for Nursing Press, New York

Barroso J 1999 Long-term nonprogressors with HIV disease. Nursing Research 48(5): 242–249

Bearon L, Koenig H 1990 Religious cognitions and use of prayer in health and illness. Gerontologist 30(2): 249–253

Benko M A, da Silva M J 1996 [Considering spirituality in undergraduate nursing education]. Review Latin American Enfermagem 4(1): 71–85

Benson H, Dusek J A 1999 Self-reported health, and illness and the use of conventional and unconventional medicine and mind/body healing by Christian Scientists and others. Journal of Nervous and Mental Disease 187(9): 539–548

Bergin A, Jensen J 1990 Religiosity of psychotherapists: a national study. Psychotherapy 27(1): 3–7

Bergin A, Masters K, Richards P 1987 Religiousness and mental health reconsidered: a study of an intrinsically religious sample. Journal of Counsel Psychology 34(2): 197–204

Boutell K A, Bozett F W 1990 Nurses' assessment of patients' spirituality: continuing education implications. Journal of Continuing Education and Nursing 21(4): 172–176

Braam A, Beekman A, Deeg D, Smit J, van Tilburg W 1997 Religiosity as a protective or prognostic factor of depression in later life: results from the community survey in the Netherlands. Acta Psychiatrica Scandinavica 96: 199–205

Brown C 1995 Spirituality in a general practice: a quality of life questionnaire to measure outcome. Complementary Therapies in Medicine 3: 230–233

Butler M H, Gardner B C, Bird M H 1998 Not just a time-out: change dynamics of prayer for religious couples in conflict situations. Family Process 37(4): 451–478

Byers A 1992 The normalization of a personality through neurofeedback therapy. Subtle Energies 3(1): 1–17

Campion J, Bhugra D 1997 Experiences of religious healing in psychiatric patients in south India. Social Psychiatry and Psychiatric Epidemiology 32(4): 215–221

Carroll S 1993 Spirituality and purpose in life in alcoholism recovery. Journal of Studies on Alcohol 54(3): 297–301

Cesarman F 1957 Religious conversion of sex offenders during psychotherapy: two cases. Journal of Pastoral Care 11: 25–35

Chang B H, Noonan A E, Tennstedt S L 1998 The role of religion/spirituality in coping with caregiving for disabled elders. Gerontologist 38(4): 463–470

Chang S O 2001 The conceptual structure of physical touch in caring. Journal of Advanced Nursing 33(6): 820–827

Chiu L 2001 Spiritual resources of Chinese immigrants with breast cancer in the USA. International Journal of Nursing Studies 38(2): 175–184

Christo G, Franey C 1995 Drug users' spiritual beliefs, locus of control and the disease concept in relation to Narcotics Anonymous attendance and six-month outcomes. Drug and Alcohol Dependence 38(1): 51–56

Cole B, Pargament K 1999 Re-creating your life: a spiritual/psychotherapeutic intervention for people diagnosed with cancer. Psycho-oncology 8(5): 395–407

Coleman C L, Holzemer W L 1999 Spirituality, psychological well-being, and HIV symptoms for African Americans living with HIV disease. Journal of the Association of Nurses in AIDS Care 10(1): 42–50

Cooper-Effa M, Blount W, Kaslow N, Rothenberg R, Eckman J 2001 Role of spirituality in patients with sickle cell disease. Journal of the American Board of Family Practice 14(2): 116–122

Cooperstein A 1990 The myths of healing: a descriptive analysis and taxonomy of transpersonal healing experiences. Unpublished Doctoral dissertation, Saybrook Institute, San Francisco, CA

Cooperstein M 1995 Healing myths: a study of the inner world of transpersonal healers. Radionics Quarterly 40(4): 7–14

Corrington J 1989 Spirituality and recovery: relationships between levels of spirituality, contentment and stress during recovery from alcoholism in AA. Alcohol Treatment Quarterly 6(3/4): 151–165

Craigie F C Jr, Hobbs R F 3rd 1999 Spiritual perspectives and practices of family physicians with an expressed interest in spirituality. Family Medicine 31(8): 578–585

Craigie F C, Jr, Larson D B, Liu I Y 1990 References to religion in the Journal of Family Practice: dimensions and valence of spirituality. Journal of Family Practice 30(4): 477–480

Croog S, Levine S 1972 Religious identity and response to serious illness: a report on heart patients. Social Science and Medicine 6: 17–32

Curtis S 1986 The effect of the music on pain relief and relaxation of the terminally ill. Journal of Music Therapy 23: 10–24

Daaleman T, Nease D 1994 Patient attitudes regarding physician inquiry into spiritual and religious issues. Journal of Family Practice 39(6): 564–568

Draucker C B 1992 The healing process of female adult incest survivors: constructing a personal residence. Image – the Journal of Nursing Scholarship 24(1): 4–8

Dunne B 1998 Gender differences in human/machine anomalies. Journal of Scientific Exploration 12(1): 3–55

Ehman J W, Ott B B, Short T H, Ciampa R C, Hansen-Flaschen J 1999 Do patients want physicians to inquire about their spiritual or religious beliefs if they become gravely ill? Archives of Internal Medicine 159(15): 1803–1806

Elkins D, Hedstrom L, Hughes L, Leaf J, Saunders C 1988 Toward a humanistic-phenomenological spirituality. Journal of Humanistic Psychology 28(4): 5–18

Ellis J B, Smith P C 1991 Spiritual well-being, social desirability and reasons for living: is there a connection? International Journal of Social Psychiatry 37(1): 57–63

Ellis M R, Vinson D C, Ewigman B 1999 Addressing spiritual concerns of patients: family physicians' attitudes and practices. Journal of Family Practice 48(2): 105–109

Ellison C 1991 Religious involvement and subjective well-being. Journal of Health and Social Behavior 32: 80–89

Ellison C, Gay D, Glass T 1989 Does religious commitment contribute to individual life satisfaction? Social Forces 68: 100–123

Emblen J D, Halstead L 1993 Spiritual needs and interventions: comparing the views of patients, nurses, and chaplains. Clinical Nurse Spectrum 7(4): 175–182

Engquist D E, Short-DeGraff M, Gliner J, Oltjenbruns K 1997 Occupational therapists' beliefs and practices with regard to spirituality and therapy. American Journal of Occupational Therapy 51(3): 173–180

Enstrom J 1975 Cancer mortality among Mormons. Cancer 36: 825–841

Enstrom J 1978 Cancer and total mortality among active Mormons. Cancer 42: 1943–1951

Everett D 1999 Forget me not: the spiritual care of people with Alzheimer's disease. Journal of Health Care Chaplain 8(1–2): 77–88

Faulkner J, DeJong G 1966 Religiosity in 5-D: an empirical analysis. Social Forces 45: 246–254

Fehring R J, Brennan P F, Keller M L 1987 Psychological and spiritual well-being in college students. Research in Nursing and Health 10(6): 391–398

Finney J, Lee G 1977 Age differences on five dimensions of religious involvement. Review of Religious Research 18: 173–179

Foley L, Wagner J, Waskel S A 1998 Spirituality in the lives of older women. Journal of Women Aging 10(2): 85–91

Foster D F, Phillips R S, Hamel M B, Eisenberg D M 2000 Alternative medicine use in older Americans. Journal of the American Geriatric Society 48(12): 1560–1565

France N 1991 A phenomenological inquiry on the child's lived experience of perceiving the human energy field using therapeutic touch. Unpublished dissertation, University of Colorado, Denver, CO

Frankel B, Hewitt W 1994 Religion and well-being among Canadian university students: the role of faith groups on campus. Journal of Scientific Studies and Religion 33: 62–73

Fryback P B, Reinert B R 1999 Spirituality and people with potentially fatal diagnoses. Nursing Forum 34(1): 13–22

Fulton R A, Moore C M 1995 Spiritual care of the school-age child with a chronic condition. Journal of Pediatric Nursing 10(4): 224–231

Gabbard G, Twemlow S, Jones F 1982 Differential diagnosis of altered mind/body perception. Psychiatry 45: 361–369

Gangdev P S 1998 Faith-assisted cognitive therapy of obsessive-compulsive disorder. Australian and New Zealand Journal of Psychiatry 32(4): 575–578

Ganje-Fling M, McCarthy P 1991 A comparative analysis of spiritual direction and psychotherapy. Journal of Psychology and Theology 19(1): 103–117

Gardner J, Lyon J 1982 Cancer in Utah Mormon women by church activity level. American Journal of Epidemiology 116(2): 258–265

Gardner J, Lyon J 1982 Cancer in Utah Mormon men by lay priesthood level. American Journal of Epidemiology 116(2): 243–257

Gardner R 1983 Miracles of healing in Anglo-Celtic Northumbria as recorded by the Venerable Bede and his contemporaries: a reappraisal in the light of twentieth century experience. British Medical Journal 287: 1927–1933

George L 1981 A survey of research into the relationships between imagery and psi. Journal of Parapsychology 45: 121–146

Gettig E 1987 Faith healing: a case presentation. Birth Defects Orig Artic Serv 23(6): 267–270

Ginn D R, Aliff L 1998 The northeast Tennessee spirituality and end of life issues survey. Tennessee Medicine 91(11): 425–430

Gioiella M E, Berkman B, Robinson M 1998 Spirituality and quality of life in gynecologic oncology patients. Cancer Practice 6(6): 333–338

Glik D 1984 Illness, wellness, and healing: subjective correlates of healer utilization. Johns Hopkins University, Baltimore, MD

Glik D 1985 Fieldwork in the research paradigm: observations and selected findings from a survey of spiritual healing adherents. Paper presented at the American Sociological Association Annual Meeting, Washington, DC

Glik D 1986 Psychosocial well-being among spiritual healing participants. Social Science and Medicine 22(5): 579–586

Graham T, Kaplan B, Cornoni-Huntley J 1978 Frequency of church attendance and blood pressure elevation. Journal of Behavioral Medicine 1: 37–43

Graham-Pole J 2001 'Physician, heal thyself': how teaching holistic medicine differs from teaching CAM. Academic Medicine 76(6): 662–664

Greasley P, Chiu L F, Gartland M 2001 The concept of spiritual care in mental health nursing. Journal of Advanced Nursing 33(5): 629–637

Greenfield S 1992 Spirits and spiritist therapy in southern Brazil: a case study of an innovative syncretic healing group. Culture, Medicine and Psychiatry 16: 23–51

Griffith E, Young J, Smith D 1984 An analysis of the therapeutic elements in a black church service. Hospitals and Community Psychiatry 35: 464–469

Guillory J A, Sowell R, Moneyham L, Seals B 1997 An exploration of the meaning and use of spirituality among women with HIV/AIDS. Alternative Therapies in Health and Medicine 3(5): 55–60

Guy R 1982 Religion, physical disabilities, and life satisfaction in older age cohorts. International Journal of Aging and Human Development 15: 225–232

Hall B A 1998 Patterns of spirituality in persons with advanced HIV disease. Research in Nursing and Health 21(2): 143–153

Halstead M T, Fernsler J I 1994 Coping strategies of long-term cancer survivors. Cancer Nursing 17(2): 94–100

Haraldsson E, Olafsson O 1980 A survey of psychic healing in Iceland. Christian Parapsychologist 3(8): 276–279

Hatch R L, Burg M A, Naberhaus D S, Hellmich L K 1998 The spiritual involvement and beliefs scale. Development and testing of a new instrument. Journal of Family Practice 46(6): 476–486

Heidt P 1990 Openness: a qualitative analysis of nurses' and patients' experiences of therapeutic touch. Journal of Nursing Scholarship 22(3): 180–186

Heidt P 1991 Helping patients to rest: clinical studies in therapeutic touch. Holistic Nursing Practice 5(4): 57–66

Heiligman R, Lee L, Kramer D 1983 Pain relief associated with a religious visitation: a case report. Journal of Family Practice 16(2): 299–302

Hendlin S 1985 The spiritual emergency patient: concept and example. In: Stern E (ed) Psychotherapy in the religiously committed patient. Haworth Press, New York, pp. 79–88

Hermann C P 2001 Spiritual needs of dying patients: a qualitative study. Oncology Nursing Forum 28(1): 67–72

Highfield M, Cason C 1983 Spiritual needs of patients: are they recognized? Cancer Nursing 6: 187–192

Hinkle L E, Wolff H G 1958 Ecological investigations of the relationship between illness, life experiences and the social environment. Annals of Internal Medicine 49: 1373–1388

Hood R 1975 The construction and preliminary validation of a measure of reported religious experience. Journal of the Scientific Study of Religion 14: 29–41

Hughes C E 1997 Prayer and healing: a case study. Journal of Holistic Nursing 15(3): 318–324; discussion 325–316

Hughes C B, Caliandro G 2000 Empowerment: a case study of a grandmother caring for her HIV-positive grandchild. Journal of the Association of Nurses in AIDS Care 11(5): 29–38

Hummer R, Rogers R, Nam C, Ellison C 1999 Religious involvement and US adult mortality. Demography 36: 273–285

Hunglemann J, Kenkl-Ross E, Klasser L, Stollenwerk R 1985 Spiritual well-being in older adults: harmonious interconnectedness. Journal of Religion and Health 24: 147–153

Hunsberger B 1985 Religion, age, life satisfaction, and perceived sources of religiousness: a study of older persons. Journal of Gerontology 40(4): 615–620

Hunt L M, Arar N H, Akana L L 2000 Herbs, prayer, and insulin: use of medical and alternative treatments by a group of Mexican American diabetes patients. Journal of Family Practice 49(3): 216–223

Idler E 1987 Religious involvement and the health of the elderly: some hypotheses and an initial test. Social Forces 66: 226–238

Idler E, Kasl S 1997 Religion among disabled and nondisabled persons I: cross-sectional patterns in health practices, social activities, and well-being. Journal of Gerontology: Social Sciences 52B(6): S294–S305

Idler E, Kasl S 1997 Religion among disabled and nondisabled persons II: attendance at religious services as a predictor of the course of disability. Journal of Gerontology: Social Sciences 52B(6): S306–S316

Janin P 1975 Psychocinese dans le passé? Une experience exploratoire. Revue Metapsychique 1(21–22): 71–96

Jimenez M 1993 The spiritual healing of post-traumatic stress disorder at the Menlo Park Veteran's Hospital. Stud Format Spiritual 14: 175–187

Johnson C D, Hathaway D K 1996 The lived experience of end-stage liver failure and liver transplantation. Journal of Transpl Coord 6(3): 130–133

Johnson D, Mullins L 1989 Subjective and social dimensions of religiosity and loneliness among the well elderly. Review of Religious Research 31: 3–15

Johnson D, Williams J, Bromley D 1986 Religion, health and healing: findings from a southern city. Sociological Analysis 47: 66–73

Juchli L 1991 The spiritual dimension of depression. Schweizerische Rundschau fur Medizin Praxis 80(38): 980–983

Kaczorowski J 1987 State-trait anxiety and spiritual well-being in adults who have been diagnosed with cancer. Unpublished Master's thesis, Rutgers, the State University of New Jersey

Kaczorowski J M 1989 Spiritual well-being and anxiety in adults diagnosed with cancer. Hospital Journal 5(3–4): 105–116

Kahn D L, Steeves R H, Benoliel J Q 1994 Nurses' views of the coping of patients. Social Science and Medicine 38(10): 1423–1430

Kass J, Friedman R, Leserman J, Zuttermeister P, Benson H 1991 Health outcomes and a new index of spiritual experience. Journal of Scientific Studies and Religion 30(2): 203–211

Kaye J, Robinson K M 1994 Spirituality among caregivers. Image – the Journal of Nursing Scholarship 26(3): 218–221

Kendler K, Gardner C, Prescott C 1997 Religion, psychopathology, and substance use and abuse: a multimeasure, genetic-epidemiologic study. American Journal of Psychiatry 154(3): 322–329

Kennedy G, Kelman H, Thomas C, Chen J 1996 The relation of religious preference and practice to depressive symptoms among 1855 older adults. Journal of Gerontology 51B(6): P301–P308

King D, Bushwick B 1994 Beliefs and attitudes of hospital patients about faith healing and prayer. Journal of Family Practice 39: 349–352

King D, Sobal J, DeForge B 1988 Family practice patients' experiences and beliefs in faith healing. Journal of Family Practice 27(5): 505–508

King D E, Sobal J, Haggerty J 3rd, Dent M, Patton D 1992 Experiences and attitudes about faith healing among family physicians. Journal of Family Practice 35(2): 158–162

King M, Hunt R 1975 Measuring the religious variable: national replication. Journal of Scientific Studies and Religion 14: 13–22

King M, Speck P, Thomas A 1995 The Royal Free interview of religious and spiritual beliefs: development and standardization. Psychological Medicine 25: 1125–1134

Kirschling J, Pittman J 1989 Measurement of spiritual well-being: a hospice caregiver sample. Hospice Journal 5(2): 1–11

Koenig H, George L, Siegler I 1988 The use of religion and other emotion-regulating coping strategies among older adults. Gerontologist 28(3): 303–310

Koenig H, Kvale J, Ferrel C 1988 Religion and well-being in later life. Gerontologist 28: 18–28

Koenig H, Meador K, Cohen H, Blazer D 1988 Depression in elderly hospitalized patients with medical illness. Archives of Internal Medicine 148: 1929–1936

Koenig H, Bearon L, Dayringer R 1989 Physician perspectives on the role of religion in the physician–older patient relationship. Journal of Family Practice 28(4): 441–448

Koenig H, Cohen H, Blazer D et al 1992 Religious coping and depression among elderly, hospitalized medically ill men. American Journal of Psychiatry 149(12): 1693–1700

Koenig H, George L, Meador K, Blazer D, Dyck P 1994 Religious affiliation and psychiatric disorder among protestant baby boomers. Hospital and Community Psychiatry 45(6): 586–596

Koenig H, Hays J, George L, Blazer D, Larson D, Landerman L 1997 Modeling the cross-sectional relationships between religion, physical health, social support, and depressive symptoms. American Journal of Geriatric Psychiatry 5: 131–143

Koenig H, George L, Meador K, Blazer D, Ford S 1994 Religious practices and alcoholism in a southern adult population. Hospital and Community Psychiatry 45(3): 225–231

Koenig H, George L, Peterson B 1998 Religiosity and remission from depression in medically ill older patients. American Journal of Psychiatry 155: 536–542

Koenig H, George L, Hays J, Larson D, Cohen H, Blazer D 1998 The relationship between religious activities and blood pressure in older adults. International Journal of Psychiatry and Medicine 28(2): 189–213

Koenig H, George L, Blazer D, Meador K, Pritchett J (in press) The relationship between religion and anxiety in a sample of community-dwelling older adults. Journal of Geriatric Psychiatry

Koenig H, George L, Cohen H, Hays J, Larson D, Blazer D (in press) The relationship between religious activities and cigarette smoking in elderly adults. Journal of Gerontology

Koenig H G 1998 Religious attitudes and practices of hospitalized medically ill older adults. International Journal of Geriatric Psychiatry 13(4): 213–224

Koenig H G, Larson D B 1998 Use of hospital services, religious attendance, and religious affiliation. Southern Medical Journal 91(10): 925–932

Krause N, Tran T 1989 Stress and religious involvement among elderly black adults. Journal of Gerontology (Social Sciences) 44: 4–13

Krippner S 1990 A questionnaire study of experiential reactions to a Brazilian healer. Journal of the Society for Psychical Research 56(820): 208–216

Krippner S 1995 A cross-cultural comparison of four healing models. Alternative Therapies in Health and Medicine 1(1): 21–29

Kristeller J L, Zumbrun C S, Schilling R F 1999 'I would if I could': how oncologists and oncology nurses address spiritual distress in cancer patients. Psychooncology 8(5): 451–458

Kroll J, Sheehan W 1989 Religious beliefs and practices among 52 psychiatric inpatients in Minnesota. American Journal of Psychiatry 146(1): 67–72

Larson D, Koenig H, Kaplan B, Greenberg R, Logue E, Tyroler H 1989 The impact of religion on blood pressure status in men. Journal of Religion and Health 28(4): 265–278

Larson D, Thielman S, Greenwold M et al 1993 Religious content in the DSM-III-R glossary of technical terms. American Journal of Psychiatry 150: 1884–1885

Lehna C R 1998 A childhood cancer sibling's oral history. Journal of Pediatric Oncology Nursing 15(3): 163–171

Levin J, Markides K 1986 Religious attendance and subjective health. Journal of Scientific Studies and Religion 25(1): 31–40

Levin J, Markides K 1988 Religious attendance and psychological well-being in Mexican Americans. Sociological Analysis 49: 66–72

Levin J, Lyons J, Larson D 1993 Prayer and health during pregnancy: findings from the Galveston low birthweight survey. Southern Medical Journal 86: 1022–1027

Levin J, Chatters J, Taylor R 1995 Religious effects on health status and life satisfaction among black Americans. Journal of Gerontology (Social Sciences) 50B(3): S154–S163

Levin J, Wichramasekera I, Hirshberg C 1998 Is religiousness a correlate of absorption? Implications for psychophysiology, coping, and morbidity. Alternative Therapies 4(6): 72–76

Loh S-H 1999 Qigong therapy in the treatment of metastatic colon cancer. Alternative Therapies 5(4): 112

Lowis M J, Hughes J 1997 A comparison of the effects of sacred and secular music on elderly people. Journal of Psychology 131(1): 45–55

Lubchansky I, Egri G, Strokes I 1970 Puerto Rican spiritualists view mental illness: the faith healer as a paraprofessional. American Journal of Psychiatry 127: 312–321

Lyon J, Klauber M, Gardner J 1976 Cancer incidence in Mormons and non-Mormons in Utah, 1966–1970. New England Journal of Medicine 294: 129–133

Lyon J, Wetzler H, Gardner J 1978 Cardiovascular mortality in Mormons and non-Mormons in Utah, 1969–1971. American Journal of Epidemiology 108: 357–366

Lyon J, Gardner J, West D 1980 Cancer in Utah: risk by religion and place of residence. Journal of National Cancer Institute 65: 1063–1071

Lyon J, Gardner J, West D 1980 Cancer incidence in Mormons and non-Mormons in Utah during 1967–1975. Journal of National Cancer Institute 65: 1055–1061

McBride J L, Arthur G, Brooks R, Pilkington L 1998 The relationship between a patient's spirituality and health experiences. Family Medicine 30(2): 122–126

McColl M A, Bickenbach J, Johnston J et al 2000 Spiritual issues associated with traumatic-onset disability. Disability and Rehabilitation 22(12): 555–564

McColl M A, Bickenbach J, Johnston J et al 2000 Changes in spiritual beliefs after traumatic disability. Archives of Physical Medicine and Rehabilitation 81(6): 817–823

McCraty R, Atkinson M, Tomasino K D, Tiller W 1996 The electricity of touch: detection and measurement of cardiac energy exchange between people. Paper presented at the Proceedings of the Fifth Appalachian Conference on Neurobehavioral Dynamics: Brain and Values, Radford, VA. Lawrence Erlbaum Assoc., Mahwah, NJ

McCurdy D B 1998 Personhood, spirituality, and hope in the care of human beings with dementia. Journal of Clinical Ethics 9(1): 81–91

McDowell D, Galanter M, Goldfarb L, Lifshutz H 1996 Spirituality and the treatment of the dually diagnosed: an investigation of patient and staff attitudes. Journal of Addictive Diseases 15(2): 55–68

Mackenzie E R, Rajagopal D E, Meibohm M, Lavizzo-Mourey R 2000 Spiritual support and psychological well-being: older adults' perceptions of the religion and health connection. Alternative Therapies in Health and Medicine 6(6): 37–45

McSherry W 1998 Nurses' perceptions of spirituality and spiritual care. Nursing Standards 13(4): 36–40

Mailloux N, Ancona L 1960 A clinical study of religious attitudes and a new approach to psychopathology. In: David H, Brengelman J (eds) Perspectives in personality research. Crosby Lockwood, London

Mansour A, Laing G, Leis A, Nurse J 1998 The experience of Reiki as perceived by middle-aged women in the Midwest. Journal of Alternative and Complementary Therapies 4: 211–217

Markides K, Levin J, Ray L 1987 Religion, aging, and life satisfaction: an eight-year, three-wave longitudinal study. Gerontologist 27(5): 660–665

Massey P, Kisling G 1999 A single case report of healing through specific martial art therapy: comparison of MRI to clinical resolution in severe cervical stenosis: a case report. Journal of Alternative and Complementary Medicine 5(1): 75–79

Mathew R J, Mathew V G, Wilson W H, Georgi J M 1995 Measurement of materialism and spiritualism in substance abuse research. Journal of Studies on Alcohol 56(4): 470–475

Mathew R J, Georgi J, Wilson W H, Mathew V G 1996 A retrospective study of the concept of spirituality as understood by recovering individuals. Journal of Substance Abuse Treatment 13(1): 67–73

Maton K 1989 The stress-buffering role of spiritual support: cross-sectional and prospective investigations. Journal of Scientific Studies and Religion 28(3): 310–323

Maugans T, Wadland W 1991 Religion and family medicine: a survey of physicians and patients. Journal of Family Practice 32: 210–213

Meador K, Koenig H, Hughes D, Blazer D, Turnbull J, George L 1992 Religious affiliation and major depression. Hospital and Community Psychiatry 43(12): 1204–1208

Mechanic D 1963 Religion, religiosity, and illness behavior: the special case of the Jews. Human Organ 22: 202–208

Messerli-Rohrbach V 2000 Personal values and medical preferences: postmaterialism, spirituality, and the use of complementary medicine. Forschende Komplementarmedizin Klass Naturheilkd 7(4): 183–189

Michel D, Chesky K 1995 A survey of music therapists using music for pain relief. Arts in Psychotherapy 22: 49–51

Miller J 1985 Assessment of loneliness and spiritual well-being in chronically ill and healthy adults. Journal of Professional Nursing 1: 79–85

Millison M B, Dudley J R 1990 The importance of spirituality in hospice work: a study of hospice professionals. Hospice Journal 6(3): 63–78

Millison M, Dudley J R 1992 Providing spiritual support: a job for all hospice professionals. Hospice Journal 8(4): 49–66

Moller M D 1999 Meeting spiritual needs on an inpatient unit. Journal of Psychosocial Nursing and Mental Health Services 37(11): 5–10

Moon M 1975 Artists contrasted with non-artists concerning belief in ESP: a poll. Journal of the American Society for Psychical Research 69(2): 161–166

Munro S, Mount B 1978 Music therapy in palliative care. Canadian Medical Association Journal 119: 1029–1034

Narayanasamy A, Owens J 2001 A critical incident study of nurses' responses to the spiritual needs of their patients. Journal of Advanced Nursing 33(4): 446–455

Nealon-Woods M A, Ferrari J R, Jason L A 1995 Twelve-step program use among Oxford House residents: spirituality or social support in sobriety? Journal of Substance Abuse 7(3): 311–318

Nelson B 1976 How graduate nurses in maternal child health (MCH) perceive their role in the spiritual dimension of nursing care: a survey. Unpublished Master's thesis, Boston University

Nelson F 1977 Religiosity and self-destructive crises in the institutionalized elderly. Suicide and Life Threatening Behavior 7(2): 67–73

Ness R 1980 The impact of indigenous healing activity: an empirical study of two fundamentalist churches. Social Science and Medicine 14B: 167–180

Newell S, Sanson-Fisher R W 2000 Australian oncologists' self-reported knowledge and attitudes about non-traditional therapies used by cancer patients. Medical Journal of Australia 172(3): 110–113

O'Connor T S, Meakes E, McCarroll-Butler P, Gadowsky S, O'Neill K 1997 Making the most and making sense: ethnographic research on spirituality in palliative care. Journal of Pastoral Care 51(1): 25–36

Olson K, Hanson J 1997 The effect of Reiki in the management of pain: a preliminary report. Cancer Prevention Control 1: 108–113

Olson L, Reis J, Murphy L, Gehar J 1988 The religious community as a partner in health care. Journal of Community Health 13(4): 249

Oman D, Reed D 1998 Religion and mortality among the community-dwelling elderly. American Journal of Public Health 88: 1469–1475

Oxman T, Freeman D, Manheimer E 1995 Lack of social participation or religious strength and comfort as risk factors for death after cardiac surgery in the elderly. Journal of Psychosomatic Medicine 57(1): 5–15

Paproski D L 1997 Healing experiences of British Columbia First Nations women: moving beyond suicidal ideation and intention. Canadian Journal of Community and Mental Health 16(2): 69–89

Park C, Cohen L 1993 Religious and nonreligious coping with the death of a friend. Cognitive Therapy Research 17(6): 561–577

Pattison E, Lapins N, Doerr H 1973 Faith healing: a study of personality and function. Journal of Nervous and Mental Diseases 157(6): 397–409

Payne M 1989 The use of therapeutic touch with rehabilitation clients. Rehabilitative Nursing 14(2): 69–72

Pehler S R 1997 Children's spiritual response: validation of the nursing diagnosis spiritual distress. Nursing Diagnosis 8(2): 55–66

Persinger M 1987 Spontaneous telepathic experiences from phantasms of the living and low global geomagnetic activity. Journal of the American Society for Psychical Research 81: 23–36

Persinger M, Krippner S 1989 Dream ESP experiments and geomagnetic activity. Journal of the American Society for Psychical Research 83: 101–116

Peteet J 1993 A closer look at the role of a spiritual approach in addictions treatment. Journal of Substance Abuse Treatment 10: 263–267

Petersen L, Roy A 1985 Religiosity, anxiety and meaning and purpose: religion's consequences for psychological well-being. Review of Religious Research 27: 49–62

Phillips L 1995 Churches of all faiths help connect health and spirit. Volunteer Leader 36(3): 5–7

Poloma M, Gallup G 1991 Varieties of prayer: a survey report. Trinity Press, Philadelphia, PA

Prezioso F A 1987 Spirituality in the recovery process. Journal of Substance Abuse Treatment 4(3–4): 233–238

Pullen L, Modrcin-Talbott M A, West W R, Muenchen R 1999 Spiritual high vs high on spirits: is religiosity related to adolescent alcohol and drug abuse? Journal of Psychiatric and Mental Health Nursing 6(1): 3–8

Reed P 1986 Religiousness among terminally ill and healthy adults. Research in Nursing and Health 9: 35–41

Reed P 1987 Spirituality and well-being in terminally ill hospitalized adults. Research in Nursing and Health 10: 335–344

Reese D J, Brown D R 1997 Psychosocial and spiritual care in hospice: differences between nursing, social work, and clergy. Hospital Journal 12(1): 29–41

Richards T A, Folkman S 1997 Spiritual aspects of loss at the time of a partner's death from AIDS. Death Studies 21(6): 527–552

Richards T A, Acree M, Folkman S 1999 Spiritual aspects of loss among partners of men with AIDS: postbereavement follow-up. Death Studies 23(2): 105–127

Rider M 1987 Treating chronic disease and pain with music mediated imagery. Arts in Psychotherapy 14: 113–120

Rider M, Kibler V 1990 Treating arthritis and lupus patients with music-mediated imagery and group psychotherapy. Arts in Psychotherapy 17: 29–33

Roberson M 1985 The influence of religious beliefs on health choices of Afro-Americans. Topics in Clinical Nursing 7(3): 57–63

Rosa L 1994 Survey of research on therapeutic touch: a report to the therapeutic touch review committee, Health Sciences Center, University of Colorado. University of Colorado, Loveland, CO

Rosen C 1982 Ethnic differences among impoverished rural elderly in use of religion as a coping mechanism. Journal of the Rural Community for Psychology 3(2): 27–34

Rosenberg M 1962 The dissonant religious context and emotional disturbance. American Journal of Sociology 68(1): 1–10

Samarel N 1992 The experience of receiving therapeutic touch. Journal of Advanced Nursing 17: 651–657

Sansone R, Khatain K, Rodenhauser P 1990 The role of religion in psychiatric education: a national survey. Academic Psychiatry 14: 34–38

Schiller P, Levin J 1988 Is there a religious factor in health care utilization? A review. Social Science and Medicine 27(12): 1369–1379

Schwarz B E 1964 Possible telesomatic reactions. Journal of the Medical Society for NJ 64(1): 600–603

Sellers S C, Haag B A 1998 Spiritual nursing interventions. Journal of Holistic Nursing 16(3): 338–354

Seltzer A 1983 Psychodynamics of spirit possession among the Inuit. Canadian Journal of Psychiatry 28: 52–56

Shafranske E, Gorsuch R 1984 Factors associated with the perception of spirituality in psychotherapy. Journal of Transpersonal Psychology 16(2): 231–241

Shafranske E, Malony H 1990 Clinical psychologists' religious and spiritual orientations and their practice of psychotherapy. Psychotherapy 27: 72–78

Shaver P, Lenauer M, Sadd S 1980 Religiousness, conversion, and subjective well-being: The 'healthy-minded' religion of modern American women. American Journal of Psychiatry 137(5): 1563–1568

Shih F J, Gau M L, Mao H C, Chen C H 1999 Taiwanese nurses' appraisal of a lecture on spiritual care for patients in critical care units. Intensive Critical Care Nursing 15(2): 83–94

Shuler P, Gelberg L, Brown M 1994 The effects of spiritual/religious practices on psychological well-being

among inner city homeless women. Nursing Practice Forum 5: 106–113

Silber T, Reilly M 1985 Spiritual and religious concerns of the hospitalized adolescent. Adolescence 20(77): 217–223

Silverman H D 1997 Creating a spirituality curriculum for family practice residents. Alternative Therapies in Health and Medicine 3(6): 54–61

Skokan L, Bader D 2000 Spirituality and healing. Health Progress 81(1): 38–42

Smith D 1986 Safety of faith healing. Lancet 1: 621

Smith D W 1995 Power and spirituality in polio survivors: a study based on Rogers' science. Nursing Science Quarterly 8(3): 133–139

Smith G R, McKenzie J M, Marmer D J, Steele R W 1985 Psychological modulation of the human immune system response to varicella zoster. Archives of Internal Medicine 145: 2110–2112

Sneed N, Olson M, Bonadonna R 1997 The experience of therapeutic touch for novice recipients. Journal of Holistic Nursing 15(3): 243–253

Somlai A M, Kelly J A, Kalichman S C et al 1996 An empirical investigation of the relationship between spirituality, coping, and emotional distress in people living with HIV infection and AIDS. Journal of Pastoral Care 50(2): 181–191

Sorajjakool S 1998 Gerontology, spirituality, and religion. Journal of Pastoral Care 52(2): 147–156

Springer S, Eicher D 1999 Effects of a prayer circle on a moribund premature infant. Alternative Therapies 5(2): 115–118, 120

Stack S 1983 The effect of religious commitment on suicide: a cross-national analysis. Journal of Health and Social Behavior 24(4): 362–374

Stranahan S 2001 Spiritual perception, attitudes about spiritual care, and spiritual care practices among nurse practitioners. Western Journal of Nursing Research 23(1): 90–104

Strawbridge W, Cohen R, Shema S, Kaplan G 1997 Frequent attendance at religious services and mortality over 28 years. American Journal of Public Health 87(6): 957–961

Strayhorn J, Weidman C, Larson D 1990 A measure of religiousness and its relation to parent and child mental health variables. Journal of Community Psychology 18: 34–43

Subach R A, Abul-Ezz S R 1999 Religious reasons for discontinuation of immunosuppressive medications after renal transplant. Renal Failure 21(2): 223–226

Suhr G, Lushington J, Brogdon B 1991 A miraculous cure: spontaneous disappearance of abdominal tumor after 'laying on of hands'. American Journal of Roentgenology 157(6): 1355

Sullivan W P 1998 Recoiling, regrouping, and recovering: first-person accounts of the role of spirituality in the course of serious mental illness. New Directions for Mental Health Services (80): 25–33

Sutton T D, Murphy S P 1989 Stressors and patterns of coping in renal transplant patients. Nursing Research 38(1): 46–49

Tamburrino M, Franco K, Campbell N, Pentz J, Evans C, Jurs S 1990 Post-abortion dysphoria and religion. Southern Medical Journal 83: 736–738

Taylor E, Mitchell J E, Kenan S, Tacker R 2000 Attitudes of occupational therapists toward spirituality in practice. American Journal of Occupational Therapy 54(4): 421–426

Taylor E J, Amenta M, Highfield M 1995 Spiritual care practices of oncology nurses. Oncology Nursing Forum 22(1): 31–39

Taylor E J, Highfield M F, Amenta M 1999 Predictors of oncology and hospice nurses' spiritual care perspectives and practices. Applied Nursing Research 12(1): 30–37

Taylor E J, Outlaw F H, Bernardo T R, Roy A 1999 Spiritual conflicts associated with praying about cancer. Psycho-oncology 8(5): 386–394

Taylor R 1986 Religious participation among elderly blacks. Gerontologist 26: 630–636

Thomas J, Retsas A 1999 Transacting self-preservation: a grounded theory of the spiritual dimensions of people with terminal cancer. International Journal for Nursing Studies 36(3): 191–201

Tomenius L 1986 50-Hz electromagnetic environment and the incidence of childhood tumors in Stockholm County. Bioelectromagnetics 7: 191–207

Waldfogel S, Wolpe P 1993 Using awareness of religious factors to enhance interventions in consultation-liaison psychiatry. Hospital and Community Psychiatry 44(5): 473–559

Walton J 1999 Spirituality of patients recovering from an acute myocardial infarction: a grounded theory study. Journal of Holistic Nursing 17(1): 34–53

Weiner E L, Swain G R, Wolf B, Gottlieb M 2001 A qualitative study of physicians' own wellness-promotion practices. Western Journal of Medicine 174(1): 19–23

West D, Lyon J, Gardner J 1980 Cancer risk factors: an analysis of Utah Mormons and non-Mormons. Journal of National Cancer Institute 65: 1083–1095

Westerbeke P, Gover J, Krippner S 1977 Subjective reactions to the Philippino 'healers': a questionnaire study. Research in Parapsychology 1976: 70–71

Williams D, Larson D, Buckler R, Heckmann R, Pyle C 1991 Religion and psychological distress in a community sample. Social Science and Medicine 32(11): 1257–1262

Wilson K, Lipscomb L D, Ward K, Replogle W H, Hill K 2000 Prayer in medicine: a survey of primary care physicians. Journal of the Mississippi State Medical Association 41(12): 817–822

Wilson W 1972 Mental health benefits of religious salvation. Disease and Nervous System 33: 382–386

Winkelman M 1990 Shaman and other magico-religious healers: a cross-cultural study of their origins, nature, and social transformations. Ethos 18(3): 308–352

Wirth D 1987 Healing expectations: a study of the significance of expectation within the healing encounter. Unpublished Master's thesis, John F. Kennedy University, Orinda, CA

Wirth D 1997 Menstruation and spiritual healing. Alternative and Complementary Therapies 3(2): 115–121

Wolfe D 1978 Pain rehabilitation and music therapy. Journal of Music Therapy 15(4): 162–178

Woods T, Antoni M, Ironson G, Kling D 1999 Religiosity is associated with affective and immune status in symptomatic HIV-infected gay men. Journal of Psychosomatic Research 46(2): 165–176

Yamashita H, Tsukayama H, Hori N, Kimura T, Tanno Y 2000 Incidence of adverse reactions associated with acupuncture. Journal of Alternative and Complementary Medicine 6(4): 345–350

Yanni M, Nelson M 1987 Relationship between the spiritual well-being and perceived quality of life of adult cancer patients. Unpublished Doctoral research, Rutgers, the State University of New Jersey

Yates J, Chalmers B, St James P, Follansbee M, McKegney F 1981 Religion in patients with advanced cancer. Medical and Pediatric Oncology 9: 121–128

Zaldivar A, Smolowitz J 1994 Perceptions of the importance placed on religion and folk medicine by non-Mexican-American Hispanic adults with diabetes. Diabetes Education 20(4): 303–306

Zorn C R, Johnson M T 1997 Religious well-being in noninstitutionalized elderly women. Health Care for Women International 18(3): 209–219

Others (includes: Opinions, Claims, Anecdotes, Letters to Editors, Commentaries, Critiques, and Meeting Reports)

Anon. 1958 Professor Huntingdon and the press release on the statistics of ESP. Parapsychology Bulletin (47)

Anon. 1981 How is healing accomplished? Heal Light 1(3): 4–5

Anon. 1985 Exploring the effectiveness of healing. Lancet 2(8465): 1177–1178

Anon. 1986 Divine healing. Journal of the Royal College of General Practitioners 36(286): 223–224

Anon. 1988 Emotion, illness and healing in Middle Eastern societies. Culture, Medicine, and Psychiatry 12(1): 1–135

Anon. 1989 Spirituality and healing. Holistic Nursing Practice 3(3): v–x, 1–77

Anon. 1989 Spirituality within the science of unitary human beings. Members' forum. Rogerian Nursing Science News 2(2): 2–5

Anon. 1991 True or false: design promotes healing. Contract Design 33(2): 45

Anon. 1993 Healing advances: New York Hospital. Interiors 152(1): 75

Anon. 1994 HIV/AIDS and spirituality: selected bibliography. Pediatrics, AIDS and HIV Infection 5(6): 400

Anon. 1994 Portrait of a reader. Ursula Zawada: more spirituality in care. Pflege Z 47(9): 484

Anon. 1996 Toward a philosophy of science in women's health research. Journal of Scientific Exploration 10(4): 535–545

Anon. 1997 Sacred spaces. Nursing Times 93(38): 22–23

Anon. 1998 Faith and healing: making a place for spirituality. Harvard Health Letters 23(4): 1–3

Anon. 1998 Religion: faith in managed care. Hospitals and Health Networks 72(4): 22

Anon. 2001 A White Paper. Professional chaplaincy: its role and importance in health care. Journal of Pastoral Care 55(1): 81–97

Achterberg J 1996 What is medicine? Alternative Therapies in Health and Medicine 2(3): 58–61

Achterberg J, Dossey L, Gordon J 1993 Report of the panel on mind/body interventions. Office of Alternative Medicine, National Institutes of Health, Bethesda, MD

Achterberg J, Dossey L, Gordon J 1993 Mind body interventions. Alternative medicine expanding medical horizons. NIH report on alternative medical systems and practices in the US. Bethesda, MA, pp. 3–45

Adair R 1991 Constraints on biological effects of weak extremely-low frequency electromagnetic fields. Physical Review A 43: 1039–1048

Adams M 1985 Variability in remote viewing performance: possible relationship to the geomagnetic field. Paper presented at the 27th Annual Convention of the Parapsychological Society

Adams M 1986 Persistent temporal relationships of ganzfeld results to geomagnetic activity, appropriateness of using standard geomagnetic indices. Paper presented at the 28th Annual Convention of the Parapsychological Society

Adams P 1998 When healing is more than simply clowning around. Journal of the American Medical Association 279(5): 401

Adams R, Brittain J 1987 Functional status and church participation of the elderly: theoretical and practical implications. Journal of Religion and Aging 3(3/4): 35–48

Agnew M 1999 The spiritual side of illness: spirit care process implements a systematic approach to spiritual health care. Health Progress 80(4): 66–67

Ainlay S, Smith D 1984 Aging and religious participation. Journal of Gerontology 39: 357–363

Ainlay S, Singleton R, Swigert V 1992 Aging and religious participation: reconsidering the effects of health. Journal of Scientific Studies and Religion 31: 175–188

Akyeampong E 1995 Alcoholism in Ghana – a socio-cultural exploration. Culture, Medicine, and Psychiatry 19(2): 261–280

Alandydy P, Alandydy K 1999 Using Reiki to support surgical patients. Journal of Nursing Care Quality 13(4): 89–91

Alcock J 1987 Parapsychology: science of the anomalous or search for the soul? Behavioral and Brain Sciences 10: 553–565

Aldridge D 1991 Spirituality, healing and medicine. British Journal of General Practice 41: 425–427

Aldridge D 1991 Healing and medicine. Journal of the Royal Society of Medicine 84: 516–518

Aldridge D 1993 Patients and their spiritual needs. Advanced Journal of Mind Body Health 9(4): 82–85

Aldridge D 1999 Music therapy in palliative care: new voices. Jessica Kingsley, London

Alexander F, Duff R 1991 Influence of religiosity and alcohol use on personal well-being. Journal of Religion and Gerontology 8(2): 11–25

Alexander F, Duff R 1992 Religion and drinking in the retirement community. Journal of Religion and Gerontology 8(4): 27–44

Alfaro de Sanchez A M, Gomes Pinal L, de Castro A D, Pineda Moreno A, Lopez Sandoval J 1980 Christian spirituality challenge to the nurse. Nouvelles – Comité International Catholique des Infirmières et Assistantes Medico-sociales [News-International Committee of Catholic Nurses and Medico-social Workers] (2): 38–42

Alhauser R 1990 Paradox in popular religion: the limits of instrumental faith. Social Forces 69: 585–602

Allen C 1991 Spirituality: the inner light. Nursing Standards 5(20): 52–53

Allison P C, Barnes M, Burnett J et al 1998 The anatomy of a healing garden. Journal of Healthcare Design 10: 101–112

Almeida A M, Almeida T M, Gollner A M 2000 [Spiritual surgery: an investigation]. Revista da Associacao Medica Brasileira 46(3): 194–200

Alonso Y 1993 Geophysical variables and behavior: LXII. Barometric pressure, lunar cycle, and traffic accidents. Perceptual and Motor Skills 77: 371–376

Alston J 1973 Perceived strength of religious beliefs. Journal of Scientific Studies and Religion 12: 109–111

Altshuler I 1945 The past, present, and future of music therapy. Education Music Magazine 24: 16

Altshuler I 1948 A psychiatrist's experience with music as a therapeutic agent. In: Schullian D, Schoen M (eds) Music as medicine. Henry Schuman, New York

Ameling A, Povilonis M 2001 Spirituality, meaning, mental health, and nursing. Journal of Psychosocial Nursing and Mental Health Services 39(4): 14–20

Anandarajah G 1999 Spirituality and medicine. Journal of Family Practice 48(5): 389

Anandarajah G, Hight E 2001 Spirituality and medical practice: using the HOPE questions as a practical tool for spiritual assessment. American Family Physician 63(1): 81–89

Anandarajah G, Long R, Smith M 2001 Integrating spirituality into the family medicine residency curriculum. Academic Medicine 76(5): 519–520

Anderson D 1986 A different approach to traditional nursing goals. RN 49(11): 98–108

Anderson D A, Worthen D 1997 Exploring a fourth dimension: spirituality as a resource for the couple therapist. Journal of Marital and Family Therapy 23(1): 3–12

Anderson M 1962 The relations of psi to creativity. Journal of Parapsychology 26: 277–292

Anderson M 1966 The use of fantasy in testing for extrasensory perception. Journal of the American Society for Psychical Research 60: 150–163

Andrews A, Pinch W 1991 Ethical decision-making and spirituality. Nebraska Nurse 24(1): 6–7

Andrus V, Lunt J 1997 Bringing holistic nursing into the new millennium. Alternative & Complementary Therapies 3(1): 24–28.

Angell M 1985 Disease as a reflection of the psyche. New England Journal of Medicine 312: 1570–1572.

Angelucci P A 1999 Spirituality and the use of an intensive care unit on-staff/on-site chaplain. Critical Care Nurse 19(4): 62–65.

Anson O, Antonovsky A, Sagy S 1990 Religiosity and well-being among retirees: a question of causality. Behavior, Health, and Aging 1: 86–97

Anson O, Carmel S, Bonneh D, Levenson A, Maoz B 1990 Recent life events, religiosity, and health: an individual or collective effect. Human Relations 43: 1051–1066

Anson O, Levenson A, Maoz B, Bonneh D 1991 Religious community, individual religiosity, and health: a tale of two kibbutzim. Sociology 25: 119–132

Aponte H J 1996 Political bias, moral values, and spirituality in the training of psychotherapists. Bulletin of the Menninger Clinic 60(4): 488–502

Arieti S 1980 Man's spirituality and potential for creativity as revealed in mental illness. Comprehensive Psychiatry 21(6): 436–443

Armstrong P, Crowe B, Wright S 1999 Spirituality: record breakers. Nursing Times 95(36): 34–35

Armstrong D L 2000 A community diabetes education and gardening project to improve diabetes care in a Northwest American Indian tribe. Diabetes Education 26(1): 113–120

Aspect S, Dalibard A, Roger G 1982 Experimental test of Bell's inequalities using time-varying analyzers. Physical Review Letters 49(25): 1804–1807

Astrow A B, Puchalski C M, Sulmasy D P 2001 Religion, spirituality, and health care: social, ethical, and practical considerations. American Journal of Medicine 110(4): 283–287

Atmanspacher H 1999 Guest editorial: data analysis in mind–matter research. Journal of Scientific Exploration 13(4): 557–560

Attevelt J 1988 Paranormal healing. Unpublished Doctoral dissertation, State University Utrecht, Utrecht, Netherlands

Auerbach T, von Ludwiger I 1992 Heim's theory of elementary particle structures. Journal of Scientific Exploration 6(3): 217

Avery T L 1997 Spirituality and psychiatry. Australian and New Zealand Journal of Psychiatry 31(4): 606–607

Baasher T 1982 The healing power of faith. World Health 9(10): 5–7

Backus C, Page D 1994 Prehospital prayer? Emergency Medical Services 23(9): 47–49

Bacon J 1995 Healing prayer: the risks and rewards. Journal of Christian Nursing 12(1): 14–17

Bailey L 1983 Music therapy as an intervention in pain management. Handbook on interventions in Pain management. Cancer Nursing Regional Committee, New York–New Jersey, vol. 2, pp. 39–46

Bailey L 1986 Music therapy in pain management. Journal of Pain and Symptomatic Management 1: 25–28

Baker M, Gorsuch R 1982 Trait anxiety and intrinsic–extrinsic religiousness. Journal of Scientific Studies and Religion 21: 119–122

Baker D C 1998 A response to Larry Dossey: prayer, medicine, and science: the new dialogue. Journal of Health Care and Chaplaincy 7(1–2): 97–104

Balducci L, Meyer R 2001 Spirituality and medicine: a proposal. Cancer Control 8(4): 368–376

Ball T, Alexander D 1998 Catching up with eighteenth century science in the evaluation of therapeutic touch. Skeptical Inquirer 22: 31–34

Bandura A 1977 Self-efficacy: towards a unifying theory of behavioral change. Psychological Reviews 84: 191–215

Banks R 1980 Health and the spiritual dimensions: relationship and implications for professional preparation programs. Journal of School Health 50: 195

Barinaga M 1992 Giving personal magnetism a whole new meaning. Science 256: 967

Barnard D, Dayringer R, Cassel C 1995 Toward a person centered medicine: religious studies in the medical curriculum. Academic Medicine 70: 806–813

Barnes N J 1989 Lady Rokujo's ghost: spirit possession, Buddhism, and healing in Japanese literature. Literature and Medicine 8: 106–121

Barnes L L, Plotnikoff G A, Fox K, Pendleton S 2000 Spirituality, religion, and pediatrics: intersecting worlds of healing. Pediatrics 106 (4 Suppl.): 899–908.

Barnett K 1972 A theoretical construct of the concepts of touch as they relate to nursing. Nursing Research 21: 102–110

Barnhouse R 1985 Secular and religious models of care. In: Griffiss J (ed) Anglican theology and pastoral care. Morehouse Barlow, Wilton, CT

Barthwell A G 1995 Alcoholism in the family: a multicultural exploration. Recent Developments in Alcoholism 12: 387–407

Basmajian J V 1999 The third therapeutic revolution: behavioral medicine. Applied Psychophysiology Biofeedback 24(2): 107–116

Bass L 1975 A quantum-mechanical mind-body interaction. Found Physics 5: 159–172

Bastis M K 1998 A Buddhist response to Larry Dossey. Journal of Health Care and Chaplaincy 7(1–2): 87–96

Batcheldor K 1979 PK in sitter groups. Psychoenergetic Systems 3: 77–93

Batten M, Oltjenbruns K A 1999 Adolescent sibling bereavement as a catalyst for spiritual development: a model for understanding. Death Studies 23(6): 529–546

Battin M P 1995 Christian Science's right to refuse. Hastings Center Reports 25(4): 2–3

Baum G 1997 Health care, social justice and spirituality. CHAC Review 25(2): 20–25

Bazan W, Dwyer D 1998 Assessing spirituality: health care organizations must address their employees' spiritual needs. Health Progress 79(2): 20–24

Bearden T 1989 On rotary permanent magnet motors and free energy. Raum und Zeit 1(3): 43–53

Bechterev W 1948 Direct influence of a person upon the behavior of animals. Journal of Parapsychology 13: 166–176

Beck F, Eccles J 1992 Quantum aspects of brain activity and the role of consciousness. Proceedings of the National Academy of Science USA 89: 11357–11361

Becker R 1963 The geomagnetic environment and its relationship to human biology. New York State Journal of Medicine 63: 2215–2219

Becker R 1990 The machine brain and properties of the mind. Subtle Energies 1(2): 79–87

Becker R 1991 Evidence for a primitive DC electrical analog system controlling brain function. Subtle Energies 2(1): 71–88

Becker R 1992 Modern bioelectromagnetics and functions of the central nervous system. Subtle Energies 3(1): 53–72

Becker R 1982 Electrical control systems and regenerative growth. Journal of Bioelectricity 1: 267–277

Becker R 1984 Electromagnetic controls over biological growth processes. Journal of Bioelectricity 3: 105–118

Becker R, Esper C 1981 Electrostimulation and undetected malignant tumors. Clinical Orthopedics and Related Research 161: 336–339

Becker R, Murray D 1970 The electrical control system regulating fracture healing in amphibians. Clinical Orthopedics and Related Research 73: 169–173

Becker A 1990 Geomagnetic activity and violent behavior. Subtle Energies 1(2): 65–77

Beecher H K 1955 The powerful placebo. Journal of the American Medical Association 159(17): 1602–1606

Beeny J 1990 Primary health care: health visiting: spiritual healing. Nursing Standards 5(11): 48–49

Begay D H, Maryboy N C 2000 The whole universe is my cathedral: a contemporary Navajo spiritual synthesis. Medical Anthropology Quarterly 14(4): 498–520

Bejenaru F 1983 [Indispensable values of the spirituality of our people: dignity and national pride]. Revista Medico-Chirurgicala a Societatii de Medici si Naturalisti din Iasi 87(4): 665–666

Belcher A E, Dettmore D, Holzemer S P 1989 Spirituality and sense of well-being in persons with AIDS. Holistic Nursing Practice 3(4): 16–25

Bell J S 1964 Physics 1: 195

Bell L 1973 Foreword. In: Frazier C (ed) Faith healing: finger of God? Or scientific curiosity? Thomas Nelson, New York, pp. 7–8

Bell H 1985 The spiritual care component of palliative care. Seminars in Oncology 12: 482–485

Benett I 1992 Spirituality, healing and medicine. British Journal of General Practice 42(354): 39

Bennett C, Brassard C, Crepeau R, Jozsa R, Peres A, Wooters W 1993 Teleporting an unknown quantum state via dual classical and EPR channels. Physical Review Letters 70: 1895–1899

Benor D 1982 An annotated bibliography of psychic healing. Albert Einstein Medical Center

Benor D J 1991 Spiritual healing in clinical practice. Nursing Times 87(44): 35–37

Benor D 1993 Healers and a changing medical paradigm. Center for Frontier Sciences 3(2): 38–40

Benor D 1993 1st World Congress on the instantaneous healing of the deliberately caused bodily damage phenomena and the unconventional healing methods. Paper presented at the 1st World Congress on the Instantaneous Healing of the Deliberately Caused Bodily Damage Phenomena and the Unconventional Healing Methods. Paramann Programme Laboratories, Baghdad

Benor D 1994 Healing: hands-on help. Nursing Times 90(44): 28–29

Benor D 1996 Intention: an experimental focus. Advances: The Journal of Mind-Body Health 12(3): 4–8

Benor D J 1996 Spiritual healing for infertility, pregnancy, labour, and delivery. Complementary Therapies and Nursing Midwifery 2(4): 106–109

Benor D, Benor R 1993 Spiritual healing, assuming the spiritual is real. Advanced Journal of Mind Body Health 9(4): 22–30

Benson H 1993 Powers of the mind. Interview by Joe Flower. Health Forum Journal 36(6): 64–69

Benson H, Epstein M D 1975 The placebo effect: a neglected asset in the care of patients. Journal of the American Medical Association 232(12): 1225–1227

Benya J R 1989 Lighting for healing. Journal of Health Care Interior Design 1: 55–58

Benzein E, Norberg A, Saveman B I 1998 Hope: future imagined reality. The meaning of hope as described by a group of healthy Pentecostalists. Journal of Advanced Nursing 28(5): 1063–1070

Berg E P 1980 Faith healing. Australian Family Physician 9(5): 303–307

Berger R 1989 A critical examination of the Blackmore psi experiments. Journal of the American Society for Psychical Research 83: 123–144

Berger R, Persinger M 1991 Geophysical variables and behavior: LXVII. Quieter annual geomagnetic activity and larger effect size for experimental psi (ESP) studies over six decades. Perceptual and Motor Skills 73: 1219–1223

Berger J A 2001 Living the discipline on a stem cell transplant unit: spiritual care outcomes among bone marrow transplant survivors. Journal of Health Care and Chaplaincy 11(1): 83–93

Berggren-Thomas P, Griggs M J 1995 Spirituality in aging: spiritual need or spiritual journey? Journal of Gerontology and Nursing 21(3): 5–10

Bergin A 1980 Psychotherapy and religious values. Journal of Consulting and Clinical Psychology 48(1): 95–105

Bergin A, Masters K, Stinchfield R et al 1990 Religious life-styles and mental health. In: Brown L, Malony H (eds) Religion, personality, and mental health. Springer, New York

Berman A 1974 Belief in afterlife, religion, religiosity, and life-threatening experiences. OMEGA 5: 127–135

Bessinger C D Jr 1996 Reflections on reality, healing, and consciousness. Alternative Therapies in Health and Medicine 2(2): 40–45

Bhandari B, Mandowara S L, Gupta N M 1985 Management of protein energy malnutrition by 'faith healers'. Indian Pediatrics 22(5): 345–348

Bierman D 1995 The Amsterdam ganzfeld series III and IV: target clip emotionality, effect sizes and openness. Paper presented at the Proceedings of Presented Papers, 38th Annual Parapsychological Association Convention, Fairhaven, MA, pp 27–37

Bierman D 1996 Exploring correlations between local emotional and global emotional events and the behavior of a random number generator. Journal of Scientific Exploration 10(3): 363–374

Bierman D J, Radin D I 1997 Anomalous anticipatory response on randomized future conditions. Perceptual and Motor Skills 84(2): 689–690

Biersdorf J, Johnson J 1968 Religious factors in physical disability and rehabilitation. In: Palmer C (ed) Religion and rehabilitation. Charles C Thomas, Springfield, Illinois

Biley R 1996 Rogerian science, phantoms and therapeutic touch: exploring potentials. Nursing Science Quarterly 9(4): 165–169

Bilkis M R, Mark K A 1998 Mind-body medicine: practical applications in dermatology. Archives of Dermatology 134(11): 1437–1441

Birckhead L M 1982 Nurses, spirituality, and clients. Part I: The spiritual aspect of nursing care. Assertive Nurse 5(1): 10–15

Bishop E 1996 Reader questions discussion of therapeutic touch. Oncology Nursing Forum 23(8): 1165

Blackmore S 1980 The extent of selective reporting of ESP ganzfeld studies. European Journal of Parapsychology 3: 213–219

Blackmore S 1994 PSI in psychology. Skeptical Inquirer 18 (Summer): 351–355

Blackmore S 1996 Reply to 'Do you believe in psychic phenomena?' Times Higher Education Supplement: 5

Blumenthal H E 1990 I am a hospital chaplain who happens to be a Jewish woman. Journal of Health Care and Chaplaincy 3(1): 93–103

Board C I 1958 The church's ministry of healing: report of the Archbiship's commission. London

Boderman A 1972 Touch me, like me: testing an encounter group assumption. Journal of Applied Behavior Science 8: 527–533

Bodey G P 2001 Physicians and patient spirituality. Annals of Internal Medicine 135(3): 220

Boguslawski M 1979 The use of therapeutic touch in nursing. Journal of Continuing Education for Nursing 10(4): 9–15

Boguslawski M 1980 Therapeutic touch: a facilitator of pain relief. Topics in Clinical Nursing 2: 27–37

Bohm D 1986 A new theory of the relationship of mind and matter. Journal of the American Society for Psychical Research 80: 113–136

Boland C S 1998 Parish nursing: addressing the significance of social support and spirituality for sustained health-promoting behaviors in the elderly. Journal of Holistic Nursing 16(3): 355–368

Bolletino R C 2001 A model of spirituality for psychotherapy and other fields of mind-body medicine. Advances in Mind Body Medicine 17(2): 90–101, 104–107

Bollwinkel E M 1994 Role of spirituality in hospice care. Annals of Academic Medicine Singapore 23(2): 261–263

Bolton J 2000 Trust and the healing encounter: an examination of an unorthodox healing performance. Theoretical Medicine and Bioethics 21(4): 305–319

Bonny H, Pahnke W 1972 The use of music in psychedelic (LSD) psychotherapy. Journal of Music Therapy 9: 64

Bonny H, Cistrunk M, Makuch R, Stevens E, Tally J 1965 Some effects of music on verbal interaction in groups. Journal of Music Therapy 2: 61–63

Boon H 1998 Canadian naturopathic practitioners: holistic and scientific world views. Social Science and Medicine 46(9): 1213–1225

Boring E 1955 The present status of parapsychology. American Scientist 43: 108–116

Boring E 1966 Paranormal phenomena: evidence, specification, and chance. [Introduction.] In: Hansel C (ed) ESP: a scientific evaluation. Scribner, New York

Borrie R A 1990 The use of restricted environmental stimulation therapy in treating addictive behaviors. International Journal of Addiction 25(7A–8A): 995–1015

Boubakeur D 1999 [Spiritual needs at the end of life]. Bulletin of Academic National Medicine 183(5): 929–933

Boucher F 1980 The cadences of healing: perceived benefits from treatment among the clientele of psychic healers. Unpublished Doctoral dissertation, University of California, Davis, CA

Bowers C 1987 Spiritual dimensions of the rehabilitation journey. Rehabilitation Nursing 12(2): 81, 90–91

Bradford D 1985 A therapy of religious imagery for paranoid schizophrenic psychosis. In: Spero M (ed) Psychotherapy of the religious patient. Charles C Thomas, Springfield, IL

Bram J 1958 Spirits, mediums and believers in contemporary Puerto Rico. Transactions of the New York Academic Science 20: 340–347

Branch M 1995 Spirituality: the missing dimension in nursing care. Journal of Cultural Diversity 2(4): 99–100

Brand P, Yancey P 1985 The miracle of everyday healing: expecting the extraordinary can be dangerous. Journal of Christian Nursing 2(2): 4–8

Braud W 1978 Allobiofeedback: immediate feedback for a psychokinetic influence upon another person's physiology. In: Roll W (ed) Research in parapsychol 1977. Scarecrow Press, Metuchen, NJ

Braud W 1979 Conformance behavior involving living systems. In: Cook EW, Delanoy D L (eds) Research in Parapsychology 1978. Scarecrow Press, Metuchen, NJ, pp. 11–5

Braud W 1981 Psi performance and autonomic nervous system activity. Journal of the American Society for Psychical Research 75: 1–35

Braud W, Jackson M 1982 Use of ideomotor reactions as psi indicators. Parapsychology Reviews 13: 10–11

Braud W 1985 ESP, PK and sympathetic nervous system activity. Parapsychology Reviews 16(2): 8–11

Braud W, Schlitz M, Schmidt H 1989 Remote mental influence of animate and inanimate target systems: a method of comparison and preliminary findings. Paper presented at the Proceedings of the Annual Meeting of the Parapsychological Association 32: 12–25

Braud W, Schlitz M 1989 A methodology for the objective study of transpersonal imagery. Journal of Scientific Exploration 3(1): 43–63

Braud W, Schlitz M 1989 Possible role of intuitive data sorting in electrodermal biological psychokinesis (Bio-PK). Journal of the American Society for Psychical Research 83: 289–302

Braud W, Dennis S 1989 Geophysical variables and behavior: LVIII. Autonomic activity, hemolysis, and biological psychokinesis: possible relationships with geomagnetic field activity. Perceptual and Motor Skills 68: 1243–1254

Braud W, Shafer D, Andrews S 1990 Electrodermal correlates of remote attention: autonomic reactions to an unseen gaze. Paper presented at the Proceedings of the Annual Meeting of Parapsychology Association 33: 14–28

Braud W 1990 Implications and applications of laboratory psi findings. European Journal of Parapsychology 8: 57–65

Braverman E R 1987 The religious medical model: holy medicine and the spiritual behavior inventory. Southern Medical Journal 80(4): 415–420, 425

Brennan B 1993 Light emerging. Journal of Personality and Health

Bright R 1974 Music in geriatric care. St Martin, NY

British Medical Association 1956 Divine healing and cooperation between doctor and clergy. BMA, London.

Brittain J, Boozer J 1987 Spiritual care: integration into a collegiate nursing curriculum. Journal of Nursing Education 26(4): 155–160

Bronheim H E 1994 Psychoanalysis and faith. Journal of the American Academy of Psychoanalysis 22(4): 681–697

Brooker S 1994 Healing: centre of balance. Interview by Irene Heywood Jones. Nursing Times 90(44): 32

Brooks H 1973 The role of music in a community drug abuse prevention program. Journal of Music Therapy 10: 3

Brown C, Fischer R, Wagman A, Horrom N, Marks P 1978 The EEG in meditation and therapeutic touch healing. Journal of Altered States of Consciousness 3: 169–180

Brown D, LE G 1987 Stressful life events, social support networks, and physical and mental health of urban black adults. Journal of Human Stress 13: 165–174

Brown C 1989 Spiritual healing in general practice. Journal of the Royal College of General Practice 39: 466–467

Brown H, Peterson J 1991 Assessing spirituality in addiction treatment and follow-up: development of the Brown-Peterson recovery progress inventory (B-PRPI). Alcohol Treatment Quarterly 8(2): 21–50

Brown C K 1992 Spirituality, healing and medicine. British Journal of General Practice 42(354): 39

Brown C K 1995 Is spiritual healing a valid and effective therapy? Journal of the Royal Society of Medicine 88(12): 722

Brown C 1998 Natural born healers. Nursing Standards 12(17): 18

Brown C 2000 Colloquium on spiritual healing. Journal of Alternative and Complementary Medicine 6: 157

Brown C K 2000 Methodological problems of clinical research into spiritual healing: the healer's perspective. Journal of Alternative and Complementary Medicine 6(2): 171–176

Browner W S, Goldman L 2000 Distant healing: an unlikely hypothesis. American Journal of Medicine 108(6): 507–508

Bruder E 1952 Psychotherapy and some of its religious implications. Journal of Pastoral Care 6: 28–38

Brunk D 1996 The power of faith: spirituality plays a key rôle in residents' lives. Contemporary Long-term Care 19(5): 40–41, 43, 45 passim

Brush B L, Daly P R 2000 Assessing spirituality in primary care practice: is there time? Clinical Excellence in Nurse Practitioner 4(2): 67–71

Bryrne J, Price J 1979 In sickness and in health: the effects of religion. Health Education 10: 6–10

Buchanan R, Ripley H 1964 Religiosity in paranoid schizophrenia. Paper presented at the 120th Annual Meeting of the American Psychiatric Association, Los Angeles

Buehler J 1975 What contributes to hope in the cancer patient? American Journal of Nursing 75: 1353–1356

Bulbrook M J 1984 Bulbrook's model of therapeutic touch: one form of health and healing in the future. Canadian Nurse 80(11): 32–34

Bullough V, Bullough B 1993 Therapeutic touch: why do nurses believe? Skeptical Inquirer 17: 169–174

Bunnell T 1997 A tentative mechanism for healing. Positive Health 23: 5–9

Burke B K 1993 Wellness in the healing ministry. Health Progress 74(7): 34–37

Burkett S 1977 Religion, parental influence, and adolescent alcohol and marijuana use. Journal of Drug Issues 7: 263–273

Burkhardt M A 1989 Spirituality: an analysis of the concept. Holistic Nursing Practice 3(3): 69–77

Burkhardt M A 1998 Reintegrating spirituality into health care. Alternative Therapies in Health and Medicine 4(2): 128, 127

Burkhardt M A, Nagai–Jacobson M G 1994 Reawakening spirit in clinical practice. Journal of Holistic Nursing 12(1): 9–21

Burnard P 1987 Spiritual distress and the nursing response: theoretical considerations and counselling skills. Journal of Advanced Nursing 12: 377–382

Burns C 1982 Hands on or hands off? Dolores Krieger's therapeutic touch stirs a medical debate. People 17: 77–78

Burns C R 1986 Traditions of health in Western culture. Second Opinion (2): 120–136

Burns S 1991 The spirituality of dying: pastoral care's holistic approach is crucial in hospice. Health Progress 72(7): 48–52, 54

Burns P 1991 Elements of spirituality and Watson's theory of transpersonal caring: expansion of focus. NLN Publications (15–2392): 141–153

Burns N V 1998 Spirituality and healing in EMS. Emergency Medical Services 27(8): 45–46, 52

Burnside I 1973 Caring for the aged: touching is talking. American Journal of Nursing 73(12): 2060–2063

Burr H, Northrop F 1935 The electro-dynamic theory of life. Quarterly Review of Biology 10: 322–333

Burr H, Northrop F 1939 Evidence for the existence of an electrodynamic field in living organisms. Paper presented at the Proceedings of the National Academy of Science of the United States of America 24: 284–288

Burton A, Heller L 1964 Touching of the body. Psychoanalytic Review 51: 127–133

Buxton M E, Smith D E, Seymour R B 1987 Spirituality and other points of resistance to the 12-step recovery process. Journal of Psychoactive Drugs 19(3): 275–286

Cai W 1992 Acupuncture and the nervous system. American Journal of Chinese Medicine 20(3–4): 331–337

Cairns A B 1999 Spirituality and religiosity in palliative care. Home Health-care Nurse 17(7): 450–455

Callahan S 1993 Ethical issues of unconventional therapies. Health Progress 74(7): 42–43

Calvert R 1994 Dolores Krieger, PhD and her therapeutic touch. Massage 47: 56–60

Calvert R 1994 Research on the energy component of massage related to therapeutic touch. Massage 47: 57

Camstra B 1973 PK conditioning. In: Roll W, Morris R, Morris J (eds) Research in Parapsychology 1972. Scarecrow Press, Metuchen, NJ, pp. 25–27

Capps D 1985 Religion and psychological well-being. Hammond, pp. 237–258

Capps D 1992 Religion and child abuse: perfect together. Journal of Scientific Studies and Religion 31(1): 1–14

Capurso A 1952 Music and your emotions. Liverright, New York

Carmichael V 1995 Using creative imagery to help heal the body. California Hospital 9(2): 13–14

Carroll J L, Dimmer S 1989 Humor for the health of it. Michigan Hospital 25(5): 22–25

Carson V 1993 Prayer, meditation, exercise, and special diets: behaviors of the hardy person with HIV/AIDS. Journal of the Association of Nurses in AIDS Care 4: 18–28

Carson V, Soeken K, Grimm P 1988 Hope and its relationship to spiritual well-being. Journal of Psychology and Theology 16(2): 159–167

Casey R 1943 Religion and psychoanalysis. Psychiatry 6: 291–302

Cassidy J 1996 Holistic center stresses spiritual healing: a team approach to therapy helps clients tap their inner healing powers. Health Progress 77(3): 39, 49

Castledine G 2000 Spirituality and being a 'friend of the patient'. British Journal of Nursing 9(1): 62

Cerrato P L 1998 Alternatives: complementary therapies – spirituality and healing. RN 61(2): 49–50

Chalmers D 1995 The puzzle of conscious experience. Scientific American

Chandler E 1999 Spirituality. Hospice Journal 14(3–4): 63–74

Chappel J 1990 Spirituality is not necessarily religion: a commentary on divine intervention and the treatment of chemical dependency. Journal of Substance Abuse 2: 481–483

Chari C 1977 Some generalized theories and models of psi: a critical evaluation. In: Wolman B (ed) Handbook of parapsychology. Wiley, New York, pp. 803–822

Charlton R 1992 Spiritual need of the dying and bereaved – views from the UK and New Zealand. Journal of Palliative Care 8(4): 38–40

Charman R A 2000 Placing healers, healees, and healing into a wider research context. Journal of Alternative and Complementary Medicine 6(2): 177–180

Chiaramonte D 1997 Mind-body therapies for primary care physicians. Primary Care 24(4): 787–804

Chibnall J T, Duckro P N 2000 Does exposure to issues of spirituality predict medical students' attitudes toward spirituality in medicine? Academic Medicine 75(6): 661

Chibnall J T, Jeral J M, Cerullo M A 2001 Experiments on distant intercessory prayer: God, science and the lesson of Massah. Archives of Internal Medicine 161(21): 1–13

Childs-Clarke A, Sharpe J 1991 Keeping the faith: religion in the healing of phobic anxiety. Journal of Psychosocial Nursing and Mental Health Services 29(2): 22–24

Chin W L 2001 More on spirituality. Journal of the American Osteopathic Association 101(5): 269–270

Christensen C 1959 Faith, its genesis and its function in psychotherapy. Journal of Pastoral Care 13: 133–143

Christensen C 1963 Religious conversion. Archives of General Psychiatry 9: 207–216

Churchland P 1986 Neurophilosophy: towards a unified science of the mind/brain. MIT Press, Cambridge

Claman H 1994 Report of the Chancellor's Committee on Therapeutic Touch. University of Colorado Health Sciences Center, Denver, CO

Clark M 1984 Therapeutic touch: is there a scientific basis for practice? Reply. Nursing Research 33(5): 296–297

Clark M, McCarkle R, Williams S 1981 Music therapy-assisted labor and delivery. Journal of Music Therapy 18(2): 88–100

Clark C C 1997 Recognizing spiritual needs of orthopaedic patients. Orthopedic Nursing 16(6): 27–32

Clifford M, Gruca J 1987 Facilitating spiritual care in the rehabilitation setting. Rehabilitation Nursing 12(6): 331–333

Clouser K D, Hufford D J 1993 Nonorthodox healing systems and their knowledge claims. Journal of Medical Philosophy 18(2): 101–106

Coakley D V, McKenna G W 1986 Safety of faith healing. Lancet 1(8478): 444

Coe R M 1997 The magic of science and the science of magic: an essay on the process of healing. Journal of Health and Social Behavior 38(1): 1–8

Cohen D 1975 Magnetic fields of the human body. Physics Today 28: 34–43

Cohen M 1995 Expanding legal paradigms to incorporate subtle energies. Subtle Energies 6(1): 99–109

Cohen C B, Wheeler S E, Scott D A, Edwards B S, Lusk P 2000 Prayer as therapy: a challenge to both religious belief and professional ethics. Anglican Working Group in Bioethics. Hastings Center Report 30(3): 40–47

Collins H 1987 Scientific knowledge and scientific criticism. Parapsychological Reviews 18

Collins H, Pinch T 1979 The construction of the paranormal: nothing unscientific is happening. Sociological Review Monograph 27: 237–270

Colliton M 1988 The spiritual dimension of nursing. In: Beland I, Passos J (eds) Clinical nursing: pathophysiological and psychosocial approaches. Macmillan, New York

Colon K 1996 The healing power of spirituality. Minnesota Medicine 79(12): 12–18

Comstock G, Partridge K 1972 Church attendance and health. Journal of Chronic Disease 25: 665–672

Conrad N L 1985 Spiritual support for the dying. Nursing Clinics of North America 20(2): 415–426

Conrad M, Home D, Josephson B 1988 Beyond quantum theory: a realist psycho-biological interpretation of the quantum theory. In: Tarozzi G, van der Merwe A, Selleri F (eds) Microphysical reality and quantum formalism. Kluwer Academic, Dordrecht, Netherlands, vol. 1, pp. 285–293

Cook M, Freethy M 1973 Use of music as a positive reinforcer to eliminate complaining behavior. Journal of Music Therapy 10: 213–216

Cooperstein M 1993 The myths of healing: a summary of research into transpersonal healing experience. Australian Parapsychology Review 17: 3–7

Cooperstein M 1994 Healing myths. Christian Parapsychologist 10(6): 197–204

Cooperstein A 1996 Consciousness and cognition in alternative healers: an interim report on research into the relationship of belief, healing, and purported subtle energies. Subtle Energies 7(3): 185–237

Corcoran E 1993 Spirituality: an important aspect of emergency nursing. Journal of Emergency Nursing 19(3): 183–184

Corin M 1993 Healing and forgiveness. Christian Nurse International 9(2): 9

Coughlin D M 1996 Honoring the spirituality of grieving parents. Home Care Providing 1(2): 62–66

Courcey K 1999 Religiosity and health. Scientific Review of Alternative Medicine 3(2): 70–76

Cousins N 1976 Anatomy of an illness. New England Journal of Medicine 295: 1458–1463

Cousins N 1979 Anatomy of an illness as perceived by a patient: reflections on healing and recuperation. Norton, New York

Cousins N 1989 Belief becomes biology. Advances 6(3): 20–29

Cowens D 1996 A gift for healing: how you can use therapeutic touch. Crown Trade Paperbacks, New York

Cramond W A 1970 Psychotherapy of the dying patient. British Medical Journal 3(719): 389–393

Crawford P R 1993 A national laughter day: are you serious? Journal of Canadian and Dental Association 59(7): 569

Croll-Young C 1985 The door to a healing lifestyle: therapeutic touch and the new physics. Theosophical Research Journal 2: 72–81

Crombez J C, Dubreuco J L 1991 Can one die healed? Journal of Palliative Care 7(2): 39–43

Crossley D 1995 Religious experience within mental illness: opening the door on research. British Journal of Psychiatry 166: 284–286

Csordas T J 2000 The Navajo healing project. Medical Anthropology Quarterly 14(4): 463–475

Cumes D 1998 Nature as medicine: the healing power of the wilderness. Alternative Therapies in Health and Medicine 4(2): 79–86

Cutting M 1998 Response to Larry Dossey. Journal of Health Care and Chaplaincy 7(1–2): 45–61

Daaleman T P, Frey B 1998 Association between spirituality and health hard to measure. Family Medicine 30(7): 470–471

Daaleman T P, VandeCreek L 2000 Placing religion and spirituality in end-of-life care. Journal of the American Medical Association 284(19): 2514–2517

Dacher E S 1999 Loving openness and the healing relationship. Advances in Mind Body Medicine 15(1): 24–27; discussion 32–43

Dainow E 1977 Physical effects and motor responses to music. Journal of Research in Music Education 25: 211–221

Daniel R 2000 The place of healing in medicine today. Healing Today, pp. 8–13

Daniels G, McCabe P 1994 Nursing diagnosis and natural therapies: a symbiotic relationship. Journal of Holistic Nursing 12(2): 184–192

Daugherty J D 2001 The discipline for doing spiritual care: variations on a theme. Journal of Health Care and Chaplaincy 11(1): 143–147

Davidson J 1972 Religious belief as an independent variable. Journal of Scientific Studies and Religion 11: 67–75

Davies G 1980 The hands of the healer: has faith a place? Journal of Medical Ethics 6(4): 185–189

Davis V 1984 Individual health and social health: expanding the concept of holistic medicine. Paper presented at the South Anthropological Society, Atlanta, Georgia

Davis T 1986 Can prayer facilitate healing and growth? Southern Medical Journal 79(6): 733–735

Dawson P J 1997 A reply to Goddard's 'spirituality as integrative energy'. Journal of Advanced Nursing 25(2): 282–289

Day C 1993 Healing environments: the human experience. Journal of Health-care Design 5: 181–186

De Marco D G 2000 Medicine and spirituality. Annals of Internal Medicine 133(11): 920–921

Dean D 1962 The plethysmograph as an indicator of ESP. Journal of the Society for Psychical Research 41: 351–353

Dean D 1966 Plethysmograph recordings as ESP responses. International Journal of Neuropsychiatry 2: 439–446

Dean E 1975 Molecular effects of healers. Paper presented at the Proceedings of the First Canadian Conference on Psychokinesis and Related Phenomena, New Horizons Research Foundation Toronto

DeBoer K F, Waagen G N 1987 Portrait of the healer as an artist. Journal of Manipulative Physiological Therapy 10(4): 201–203

Decter B 1995 The art of healing. Interview by Vivian Carmichael. California Hospital 9(2): 13

DeFord H A 2001 Medicine and spirituality. Texas Medicine 97(4): 10

DeGracia D 1999 Report of referee on 'the effect of "healing with intent" on pepsin enzyme activity'. Journal of Scientific Exploration 13(2): 149–153

Delaney G 1984 Creativity in music. Paper presented at the Proceedings of the Association for the Anthropological Study of Consciousness

Delanoy D 1982 The training of psi in the ganzfeld. In: Roll W, Morris R, White R (eds) Research in Parapsychology 1981. Scarecrow Press, Metuchen, NJ, pp. 157–159

Delanoy D, Sha S 1994 Cognitive and physiological psi responses to remote positive and neutral emotional states. Paper presented at the Proceedings of Presented Papers, 37th Annual Parapsychological Association Convention, Fairhaven, MA, pp 128–137

Deloney L A, Graham C J, Erwin D O 2000 Presenting cultural diversity and spirituality to first-year medical students. Academic Medicine 75(5): 513–514

DeLong W R 1998 A response to Larry Dossey: the prayers of the faithful: prayer as a metaphor for medicine and healing. Journal of Health Care and Chaplaincy 7(1–2): 63–71

Denys J G 1997 The religiosity variable and personal empowerment in pastoral counseling. Journal of Pastoral Care 51(2): 165–175

Derrickson B S 1996 The spiritual work of the dying: a framework and case studies. Hospice Journal 11(2): 11–30

Devine B 1980 Attitudes of the elderly toward religion. Journal of Gerontology and Nursing 6: 679–687

Dewitt B, Graham R 1971 Resource letter IQM-1 on the interpretation of quantum mechanics. American Journal of Physics 39: 724–725

Dieppe P 2000 The role of complementary medicine in our society and the implications that this has for research. Focus on Alternative and Complementary Therapies 5(2): 109–110

DiLorenzo P, Johnson R, Bussey M 2001 The role of spirituality in the recovery process. Child Welfare 80(2): 257–273

Dittes J 1971 Two issues in measuring religion. In: Strommen M (ed) Research on religious development: a comprehensive handbook. Hawthorn Books, New York

Dixon M 1991 A healer in the practice. British Journal of General Practice 45: 396

Dixon M 1993–4 A healer in GP practice. Doctor-Healer Network Newsletter Winter (7): 6–7

do Rozario L 1997 Spirituality in the lives of people with disability and chronic illness: a creative paradigm of wholeness and reconstitution. Disability and Rehabilitation 19(10): 427–434

Dobyns Y 1992 On the Bayesian analysis of REG data. Journal of Scientific Exploration 6(1): 23–45

Dobyns Y 1996 Selection vs influence revisited: new methods and conclusions. Journal of Scientific Exploration 10(2): 253–268

Dolan M 1973 Music therapy: an explanation. Journal of Music Therapy 10(4): 172–176

Dolan M B 1994 Laughter: a daily trip to your internal pharmacy. Caring 13(12): 38–40

Donahue M 1985 Intrinsic and extrinsic religiousness: the empirical research. Journal of Scientific Studies and Religion 24: 418–423

Donald M 1991 Quantum theory and the brain. Proceedings of the Royal Society of London 427A: 43–93

Doniger S (ed) 1957 Healing: human and divine. Man's search for health and wholeness through science, faith and prayer. Association Press, New York

Dopson L 1988 Spiritual healing. Nursing Times 84(51): 43–45

Dossey L 1989 Recovering the soul: a scientific and spiritual search. Bantam Books, New York

Dossey L 1991 Meaning and medicine: a doctor's tales of breakthrough and healing. Bantam Books, New York

Dossey L 1992 But is it energy? Reflections on consciousness, healing and the new paradigm. Subtle Energies 3(3): 69–82

Dossey L 1993 The integration of healing and modern medicine. American Society for Psychical Research News 18(2): 1–4

Dossey L 1994 Healing and the mind: is there a dark side? Journal of Scientific Exploration 8(1): 73–90

Dossey L 1994 Prayer and health: research and theological implications. Paper presented at the Examining research assumptions in alternative medical systems, NIH Bethesda, MD

Dossey L 1994 Healing, energy, and consciousness: into the future or a retreat to the past? Subtle Energies 5(1): 1–33

Dossey L 1996 Distant intentionality: an idea whose time has come. Advances: the Journal of Mind-Body Health 12(3): 9–13

Dossey L 1996 In praise of unhappiness. Alternative Therapies 2(1): 7–10

Dossey L 1997 The forces of healing: reflections on energy, consciousness, and the beef Stroganoff principle [editorial]. Alternative Therapies in Health and Medicine 3(5): 8–14

Dossey L 1997 The return of prayer. Alternative Therapies 3(6): 10–17, 113–120

Dossey L 1997 Lessons from twins: of nature, nurture, and consciousness. Alternative Therapies in Health and Medicine 3(3): 8–15

Dossey L 1997 Prayer is good medicine: how to reap the healing benefits of prayer. HarperCollins, New York

Dossey L 1998 Prayer, medicine, and science: the new dialogue. Journal of Health Care and Chaplaincy 7(1–2): 7–37

Dossey L 1999 Dreams and healing: reclaiming a lost tradition. Alternative Therapies 5(6): 12–20, 120

Dossey L 1999 Do religion and spirituality matter in health? A response to the recent article in the Lancet. Alternative Therapies 5(3): 16–18

Dossey L 1999 Healing and the nonlocal mind. Interview by Bonnie Horrigan. Alternative Therapies in Health and Medicine 5(6): 84–93

Dossey L 2000 Prayer and medical science: a commentary on the prayer study by Harris et al and a response to critics. Archives of Internal Medicine 160: 1735–1738

Dossey L, Holman G, Capra F 1982 Space, time and medicine. Bantam Books, New York

Dossey L, Kabat-Zinn J, Rinpoche S, Kornfield J, Toms M 1997 The power of meditation and prayer. Hay House, CA

Dossey B 1999 Barbara Dossey, RN, MS on holistic nursing, Florence Nightingale, and healing rituals. Interview by Bonnie Horrigan. Alternative Therapies in Health and Medicine 5(1): 78–86

Drane J, Reich G 1999 The spirit of healing: treating the whole patient. New Jersey Medicine 96(9): 41–43

Dreher H 1993 Mind–body research and its detractors. Advances 9(1): 59–62

Dugan D O 1989 Laughter and tears: best medicine for stress. Nursing Forum 24(1): 18–26

Dulnev G, Prokopenko V, Polyakova O 1993 Optical methods for the study of psi phenomena. Parapsikhologiya i Psikhofizika 1(9): 39–44

Dunne B 1993 Co-operator experiments with an REG device. In: Rao K (ed) Cultivating consciousness: enhancing human potential, wellness, and healing. Praeger, Westport, CT

Dunne B, Jahn R 1992 Experiments in remote human/machine interaction. Journal of Scientific Exploration 6(4): 311–332

Dunphy R 1987 Helping persons with AIDS find meaning and hope. Health Progress 68(4): 58–63

Durkin M B 1992 A community of caring: patients in a rehabilitation unit experience holistic healing through a spiritual support group. Health Progress 73(8): 48–53, 70

Easterbrook G 1997 Science and God: a warming trend? Science 277: 890–893

Eaves L, Martin N, Heath A 1990 Religious affiliation in twins and their parents: testing a model of cultural inheritance. Behavior Genetics 20: 1–22

Eccles J 1977 The human person in its two-way relationship to the brain. In: Morris J, Roll W, Morris R (eds) Research in parapsychology 1976. Scarecrow Press, Metuchen, NJ, pp. 251–262

Eckert R M 2001 Spirituality is valuable. Texas Medicine 97(6): 9

Edelberg R 1972 Electrical activity of the skin: its measurement and uses in psychophysiology. In: Greenfield N, Sternback R (eds) Handbook of psychophysiology Holt, Rinehart, and Winston, New York, pp. 368–418

Editorial 1998 Healing powers. Journal of the Royal Society of Medicine 91: 177

Edmunds V, Scorer C 1956 Some thoughts on faith healing. Tyndale Press, London

Ehrenwald J 1972 A neurophysiological model of psi phenomena. Journal of Nervous and Mental Disease 154(6): 406–418

Ehrenwald J 1977 Parapsychology and the healing arts. In: Wolman B (ed) Handbook of parapsychology. Van Nostrand Reinhold, New York

Einstein A, Podolsky B, Rosen N 1935 Can quantum-mechanical description of physical reality be considered complete? Physical Reviews 47: 770–780

Eisenberg H, Donderi D 1979 Telepathic transfer of emotional information in humans. Journal of Psychology and Theology 103: 19–43

Ekstein R 1956 A clinical note on the therapeutic use of a quasi-religious experience. Journal of the American Psychoanalytic Association 4: 304–313

el-Bakkali-Bellini F 1997 [A communication tool that permits us to keep up hope: spirituality: the fourth dimension of care]. Krankenpflege Soins Infirmiers 90(7): 54–58

Elliot H 1997 Religion, spirituality and dementia: pastoring to sufferers of Alzheimer's disease and other associated forms of dementia. Disability and Rehabilitation 19(10): 435–441

Ellison C, George L 1992 Religious involvement, social ties, and social support in a southeastern community. Journal of Scientific Studies and Religion 33: 46–61

Ellison C 1994 Religion, the life stress paradigm, and the study of depression. In: Levin J (ed) Religion in aging and health: theoretical foundations and methodological frontiers. Sage Publications, Thousand Oaks, CA, pp. 78–121

Ellison C, Levin J 1998 The religion-health connection: evidence, theory and future directions. Health Education and Behavior 25: 700–720

Elsdon R 1995 Spiritual pain in dying people: the nurse's role. Professional Nurse 10(10): 641–643

Emblen J D 1992 Religion and spirituality defined according to current use in nursing literature. Journal of Professional Nursing 8(1): 41–47

Emdon T 1997 Spirituality: cry freedom. Nursing Times 93(40): 35–38

Emmer R, Browne P 1984 Program helps nurses develop spiritual care skills. Hospital Progress 65(2): 64–66

Engebretson J 1996 Considerations in diagnosing in the spiritual domain. Nursing Diagnosis 7(3): 100–107

Engel H 1978 Energy healing. Research Report on Ernest Holmes Research Foundation, Los Angeles, CA

Ercums J 1998 Nursing's caring paradigm: a story of mutuality and transcendent healing. Alternative and Complementary Therapies 4(1): 68–72

Ernst E 1999 Healing. Health Which? (Oct): 28–29

Fahlberg L L, Fahlberg L A 1991 Exploring spirituality and consciousness with an expanded science: beyond the ego with empiricism, phenomenology, and contemplation. American Journal of Health Promotion 5(4): 273–281

Fahrion S 1991 Inside out, outside in. Subtle Energies 2(2): i–iv

Fahrion S 1992 The power of two: polarity and perception. Subtle Energies 3(2): i–iii

Fahrion S 1992 The power of one: participation in learning from individual case studies. Subtle Energies 3(1): i–iv

Fahrion S 1994 Laws of form. Subtle Energies 5(3): i–iii

Fahrion S 1995 Empirical observation. Subtle Energies 6(2): i–iii

Fahrion S 1995 The clinical face of energy medicine. Subtle Energies 6(1): i–iii

Fahrion S 1996 Dream emergence. Subtle Energies 7(3): i–iii

Fahrion S 1997 Intention. Subtle Energies 8(2): i–iii

Fallot R D 1998 Recommendations for integrating spirituality in mental health services. New Directions for Mental Health Services (80): 97–100

Fallot R D 1998 Spiritual and religious dimensions of mental illness recovery narratives. New Directions for Mental Health Services (80): 35–44

Fallot R D 1998 The place of spirituality and religion in mental health services. New Directions for Mental Health Services (80): 3–12

Fallot R D 1998 Assessment of spirituality and implications for service planning. New Directions for Mental Health Services (80): 13–23

Fanslow C 1983 Therapeutic touch: a healing modality throughout life. Topics in Clinical Nursing 5: 73–79

Fanslow C 1989 Therapeutic touch: compassion awakened for dying persons and their families. Cooperative Connection. Nurse Healers – Professional Associates, New York, vol. 10, pp. 11–17

Favazza A 1982 Modern Christian healing of mental illness. American Journal of Psychiatry 139: 728–735

Feifel H 1958 Symposium on relationships between religion and mental health. American Psychologist 13: 565–579

Feifel H 1974 Religious conviction and the fear of death among the healthy and the terminally ill. Journal of Scientific Studies and Religion 13: 353–360

Ferguson C 1986 Subjective experience of therapeutic touch survey (SETTS): psychometric examination of an instrument. Unpublished Doctoral dissertation, University of Texas at Austin, Austin, TX

Ferngren G B 1992 Early Christianity as a religion of healing. Bulletin of the History of Medicine 66(1): 1–15

Fersurella S, Mancini M 1987 [Therapeutic aspects of a current religious phenomenon]. Minerva Psichiatry 28(4): 353–355

Fichter J, Maddox G 1965 Religion in the south old and new. In: McKinney J, Thompson E (eds) The south in continuity and change. Duke University Press, Durham, NC

Finkler K 1984 The nonsharing of medical knowledge among spiritualist healers and their patients: a contribution to the study of intra-cultural diversity and practitioner-patient relationship. Medical Anthropology 8(3): 195–209

Finkler K 1985 Spiritual healers in Mexico. Bergin and Garvey, South Hadley, MA

Fins J J, Schwager Guest R, Acres C A 2000 Gaining insight into the care of hospitalized dying patients: an interpretative narrative analysis. Journal of Pain and Symptom Management 20(6): 399–407

Finucane R C 1973 Faith healing in medieval England: miracles at saints' shrines. Psychiatry 36(3): 341–346

Fish S 1993 Therapeutic touch: can we trust the data? Journal of Christian Nursing 10(3): 6–8

Fish S 1995 Can research prove that God answers prayer? Journal of Christian Nursing 12(1): 24–27, 46

Fish S 1996 Therapeutic touch: healing science or metaphysical fraud? Journal of Christian Nursing 13(3): 4–10

Fish S, Shelly J 1978 Spiritual care: the nurse's role. Intervarsity, Downers Grove

Fisher S, Greenberg R 1972 Selective effects upon women of exciting and calm music. Perceptual and Motor Skills 34: 987–990

Fishman R Spiritualism in Western New York: a study in ritual healing. Medical Anthropology 3: 1–22

Fisk G, Mitchell A 1953 The application of differential scoring methods to PK tests. Journal of the Society for Psychical Research 37: 45–60

Focht S 1998 Spirituality becomes a prominent component of holistic care. Oncology Nursing Forum 25(6): 988–990

Foglio J, Brody H 1988 Religion, faith, and family medicine. Journal of Family Practice 27(5): 473–474

Foltz-Gray D 1998 Make 'em laugh: humor programs can help residents heal – seriously. Contemporary Long-term Care 21(9): 44–46, 48, 50

Ford C, Benett N, Biles J, Randolph G 1982 Healing effects on a self-organizing system. Journal of Holistic Medicine.

Forrest C 1972 Music and the psychiatric nurse. Nursing Times 68: 410–411

Fox B 1983 Current theory of psychogenic effects on cancer incidence and prognosis. Journal of Psychosocial Oncology 1: 17–31

Fox R 1998 Healing powers. Journal of the Royal Society of Medicine 91(4): 177

Frank J 1975 Mind-body relationships in illness and healing. Journal of the International Academy of Preventive Medicine 2: 46–59

Frank J 1975 The faith that heals. Johns Hopkins Medical Journal 137: 127–131

Frank J 1977 Nature and functions of belief systems: humanism and transcendental religion. American Psychology 32: 555–559

Frauchiger U 1999 [The body – music – the 'soul']. Schweiz Rundschau fur Medizin Praxis 88(21): 965–967

Freeman D W, Wolfson R, Affolter H U 1998 Spiritual dimensions of a mind-body group for people with severe mental illness. New Directions in Mental Health Services (80): 57–67

Friedemann M L 1994 [A plea for spirituality in care. The hidden gold in a seemingly useless life]. Krankenpflege Soins Infirmiers 87(1): 10–15

Friedman H 1963 Geomagnetic parameters and psychiatric hospital admissions. Nature 200 (626)

Friedman H 1965 Psychiatric ward behavior and geophysical parameters. Nature 205 (1050)

Fry A 1998 Spirituality, communication and mental health nursing: the tacit interdiction. Australian and New Zealand Journal of Mental Health and Nursing 7(1): 25–32

Galanter M 1997 Spiritual recovery movements and contemporary medical care. Psychiatry 60: 211–223

Galbraith J, Hodges D 1998 Healing research in general practice. Journal of the Royal Society of Medicine 91(10): 561

Galishoff M L 2000 God, prayer, and coronary care unit outcomes: faith vs works? Archives of Internal Medicine 160(12): 1877; discussion 1877–1878

Galton F 1872 Statistical inquiries into the efficacy of prayer. Fortnightly Review 12: 125–135

Gardner W, Licklider J, Weisz A 1960 Suppression of pain by sound. Science 132: 32–33

Gardner J, Lyon J 1977 Low incidence of cervical cancer in Utah. Gynecologic Oncology 5: 68–80

Garrity J F 2000 Jesus, peyote, and the holy people: alcohol abuse and the ethos of power in Navajo healing. Medical Anthropology Quarterly 14(4): 521–542

Gaston E 1968 Man and music. In: Gaston E (ed) Music in therapy. Macmillan, New York

Gatling W, Rhine J 1946 Two groups of PK subjects compared. Journal of Parapsychology 10: 120–125

Gau J V 2000 The gestalt of emptiness/receptivity: Christian spirituality and psychotherapy. Journal of Pastoral Care 54(4): 403–409

Gaynor M 1998 Mitchell Gaynor, MD the capacity to heal. Interview by Bonnie Horrigan. Alternative Therapies in Health and Medicine 4(2): 72–78

Gelo F 1995 Spirituality: a vital component of health counseling. Journal of the American College Health 44(1): 38–40

George L, Larson D, Koenig H, McCullough M 2000 Spirituality and health: what we know, what we need to know. Journal of Social and Clinical Psychology 19(1): 102–116

Georgi J M 1998 The spiritual platform: spirituality and psychotherapy in addiction medicine. North Carolina Medical Journal 59(3): 168–171

Gibbs H, Achterberg-Lawlis J 1978 Spiritual values and death anxiety: implications for counseling with terminal cancer patients. Journal of Counseling Psychology 25: 563–569

Gibbs S 2000 Losing touch with the healing art: dermatology and the decline of pastoral doctoring. Journal of the American Academy of Dermatology 43(5/1): 875–878

Girard J 1954 Music therapy in the anxiety states. In: Poldolsky E (ed) Music therapy. Philosophical Library, New York

Girardin D W 2000 Integration of complementary disciplines into the oncology clinic. Part VI. Implications for spirituality with oncology patients. Current Problems in Cancer 24(5): 268–279

Girden E 1962 A review of psychokinesis (PK). Psychological Bulletin 59: 353–388

Girden E, Girden E 1985 Psychokinesis: fifty years afterward. In: Kurtz P (ed) A skeptic's handbook of parapsychology. Prometheus Books, Buffalo, NY

Girden E, Murphy G, Beloff J et al 1964 A discussion of 'A review of psychokinesis (PK)'. International JP 6: 26–137

Gissurarson L 1990 Some PK attitudes as determinants of PK performance. European Journal of Parapsychology 8: 112–122

Gissurarson L 1992 The psychokinesis effect: geomagnetic influence, age and sex differences. Journal of Scientific Exploration 6(2): 157–166

Gissurarson L, Morris R 1990 Volition and psychokinesis: attempts to enhance PK performance through the practice of imagery strategies. Journal of Parapsychology 54: 331–370

Glik D 1984 Personality differences between meta-physical and charismatic spiritual healing adherents. Paper presented at the American Psychological Association Annual Meeting, Toronto, Canada

Glock C, Stark R 1965 Religion and society in tension. Rand McNally, Chicago, Ill

Goddard H 1899 The effects of the mind on the body as evidenced by faith cures. American Journal of Psychology 10: 431–502

Goddard N C 1995 'Spirituality as integrative energy': a philosophical analysis as requisite precursor to holistic nursing practice. Journal of Advanced Nursing 22(4): 808–815

Goddard N C 2000 A response to Dawson's critical analysis of 'spirituality as "integrative energy"'. Journal of Advanced Nursing 31(4): 968–979

Godin A 1961 Mental health in Christian life. Journal of Religion and Health 1: 41–51

Goldberg D 1978 The nature of psychological healing. In: Gaind R, Hudson B (eds) Current themes in psychiatry I. Macmillan, London

Goldfarb L M, Galanter M, McDowell D, Lifshutz H, Dermatis H 1996 Medical student and patient attitudes toward religion and spirituality in the recovery process. American Journal of Drug and Alcohol Abuse 22(4): 549–561

Goldstein J 2000 Waiving informed consent for research on spiritual matters? Archives of Internal Medicine 160(12): 1870–1871

Goleman D 1985 Vital lies, simple truths: the psychology of self-deception. Touchstone, New York

Gordon R 1995 The healing event in Graeco-Roman folk-medicine. Clio Medica 28: 363–376

Gordon D 2000 When faith-healing fails: the Oregon legislature has drawn a fine line between punishing devout parents and ensuring necessary medical care for youngsters. State Legislation 26(3): 26–27

Gorgun S 1998 Studies on the interaction between electromagnetic fields and living matter neoplastic cellular culture. Center for Frontier Sciences 7(2): 44–59

Gorsuch R 1984 Measurement: the boon and bane of investigating religion. American Psychology 39: 228–236

Goswami A 1989 The idealistic interpretation of quantum mechanics. Physics Essays 2(4): 385–400

Gough W, Shacklett R 1993 The science of connectiveness. Part I: Modeling a greater unity. Subtle Energies 4(1): 66

Gough W, Shacklett R 1993 The science of connectiveness. Part II: Mapping beyond space-time. Subtle Energies 4(2): 99–123

Gough W, Shacklett R 1993 The science of connectiveness. Part III: The human experience. Subtle Energies 4(3): 187–214

Gough W 1997 The cellular communication process and alternative modes of healing. Subtle Energies 8(2): 67–101

Govier I 2000 Spiritual care in nursing: a systematic approach. Nursing Standards 14(17): 32–36

Graber D R, Johnson J A 2001 Spirituality and health care organizations. Journal of Health Care Management 46(1): 39–50; discussion 50–32

Grad B 1963 A telekinetic effect on plant growth. International Journal of Parapsychology 5(Spring): 117–133

Grad B 1964 A telekinetic effect on plant growth. III. Stimulating and inhibiting effects. Oxford University, Oxford, England

Grad B 1991 The laying on of hands: some clinical and experimental concerns. Theta 17: 13–17

Graner J 2000 Physicians and patient spirituality. Annals of Internal Medicine 133(9): 748–749

Graner J 2001 Physicians and patient spirituality. Annals of Internal Medicine 135(3): 220

Granstrom S 1985 Spiritual nursing care for oncology patients. Topics in Clinical Nursing 7: 39–45

Gray R E, Doan B D 1990 Heroic self-healing and cancer: clinical issues for the health professions. Journal of Palliative Care 6(1): 32–42

Greeley A 1987 Mysticism goes mainstream. American Health 7: 47–49

Greeley A 1991 The paranormal is normal: a sociologist looks at parapsychology. Journal of the American Society of Psychical Research 85: 367–374

Green R 1986 Healing and spirituality. Practitioner 230(1422): 1087–1093

Green E 1990 Psychophysiologic self-regulation and human potential. Subtle Energies 1(1): 73–89

Green E 1993 Mind over matter: volition and the cosmic connection in yogic theory. Subtle Energies 4(2): 151–170

Green E, Green A 1992 Healing: self-reliance versus intervention. International Society for the Study of Subtle Energy News 3(1): 1, 4–8

Green A 1995 Biofeedback methodology in psychophysiologic self-regulation. Subtle Energies 6(3): 227–240

Green J, Shellenberger R 1996 The healing energy of love. Alternative Therapies in Health and Medicine 2(3): 46–56

Green L L, Fullilove M T, Fullilove R E 1998 Stories of spiritual awakening: the nature of spirituality in recovery. Journal of Substance Abuse and Treatment 15(4): 325–331

Greenberg D, Witzum E 1991 Problems in the treatment of religious patients. American Journal of Psychotherapy 45: 554–565

Greenberg L A 1998 In God we trust: faith healing subject to liability. Journal of Contemporary Health Law Policy 14(2): 451–476

Grey A 1994 The spiritual component of palliative care. Palliative Medicine 8(3): 215–221

Griffin D 2000 Parapsychology, science and religion. Religion and scientific naturalism: overcoming the conflicts SUNY, Albany, NY, pp. 179–240

Griffith E 1983 The impact of socio-cultural factors on a church-based healing model. American Journal of Orthopsychiatry 53: 291–302

Griffith E, English T, Mayfield V 1980 Possession, prayer, and testimony: therapeutic aspects of the Wednesday night meeting in a black church. Psychiatry 35: 464–469

Griffith E, Mahy G 1984 Psychological benefits of spiritual Baptist mourning. American Journal of Psychiatry 141: 769–773

Griffith P 2000 Spirituality in medicine. Western Indian Medical Journal 49(2): 108–109

Grinberg-Zylberbaum J 1982 Psychophysiological correlates of communication, gravitation and unity. Psychoenergetics 4: 227–256

Groer M W, O'Connor B, Droppleman P G 1996 A course in health care spirituality. Journal of Nursing Education 35(8): 375–377

Gula R M 2000 Spirituality and ethics in health care: the two do not inhabit separate spheres, but are connected. Health Progress 81(4): 17–19

Gundersen L 2000 Faith and healing. Annals of Internal Medicine 132: 169–172

Gutterman L 1990 A day treatment program for persons with AIDS. American Journal of Occupational Therapy 44(3): 234–237

Hagen P S 1995 A quiet healing. Journal of Christian Nursing 12(1): 18–20

Haight W L 1998 'Gathering the spirit' at First Baptist Church: spirituality as a protective factor in the lives of African American Children. Social Work 43(3): 213–221

Hall B A 1997 Spirituality in terminal illness: an alternative view of theory. Journal of Holistic Nursing 15(1): 82–96

Hall J M 1997 Safe closure of therapeutic relationships with abuse survivors. Journal of Psychosocial Nursing and Mental Health Services 35(11): 7–13

Hall S E 1997 Spiritual diversity: a challenge for hospice chaplains. American Journal of Hospice and Palliative Care 14(5): 221–223

Hamadeh G 1987 Religion, magic, and medicine. Journal of Family Practice 25(6): 561–568

Hameroff S 1994 Quantum coherence in microtubules: a neural basis for emergent consciousness? Journal of Consciousness Studies 1(1): 91–118

Hamilton D G 1998 Believing in patients' beliefs: physician attunement to the spiritual dimension as a positive factor inpatient healing and health. American Journal of Hospice and Palliative Care 15(5): 276–279

Hamilton J 1999 Yes, religion and spirituality do matter in health. Alternative Therapies in Health and Medicine 5(4): 18

Hamm R M 2000 No effect of intercessory prayer has been proven. Archives of Internal Medicine 160(12): 1872–1873; discussion 1877–1878

Hammell K W 2001 Intrinsicality: reconsidering spirituality, meaning(s) and mandates. Canadian Journal of Occupational Therapy 68(3): 186–194

Hammerschmidt D E 2000 Ethical and practical problems in studying prayer. Archives of Internal Medicine 160(12): 1874; discussion 1877–1878

Hammond P 1994 Healing is believing. Nursing Times 90(40): 55

Hancock B 2000 Are nursing theories holistic? Nursing Standards 14(17): 37–41

Hannay D 1980 Religion and health. Social Science and Medicine 14A: 683–685

Hanson M J 1998 The religious difference in clinical health care. Cambridge Quarterly of HealthCare Ethics 7(1): 57–67

Haraldsson E, Gissuarson L 1987 Does geomagnetic activity effect extrasensory perception? Personal and Individual Differences 8: 745–747

Hardy R 1996 Living spirituality: the essence of being human. CHAC Review 24(2): 3–7

Harmon R L, Myers M A 1999 Prayer and meditation as medical therapies. Physical Medicine and Rehabilitation Clinics of North America 10(3): 651–662

Harrison J 1992 Spirituality needs more attention. Nursing Times 88(43): 58

Harrison R L 1997 Spirituality and hope: nursing implications for people with HIV disease. Holistic Nursing Practice 12(1): 9–16

Harsham P 1982 Physicians treat, God heals: here's an inside look at whole person medicine. Medical Economy 59(11): 198, 201–192

Hassed C 1999 Spirituality and health. Australian Family Physician 28(4): 387–388

Hassed C S 2000 Depression: dispirited or spiritually deprived? Medical Journal of Australia 173(10): 545–547

Hatch J, Lovelace K 1980 Involving the southern rural church and students of the health professions in health education. Public Health Reports 95: 23–25

Hatch R L 1998 Relationship between spirituality and health is important. Family Medicine 30(6): 399–400

Hatgidakis J, Timko E R, Plotnikoff G A, Gale C 1997 Spirituality and practice: stories, barriers and opportunities. Interview by Laurence A Savett. Creative Nursing 3(4): 7–11, 16

Haviland D 1986 Safety of faith healing. Lancet 1(8482): 684

Hay M 1989 Principles in building spiritual assessment tools. American Journal of Hospice Care 7: 25–31

Haynes R 1977 Faith healing and psychic healing: are they the same? Parapsychology Review July–August

Hebard A C 1988 Spiritual aid for dying patients. Iowa Medicine 78(8): 365–366

Hegde B M 2000 The healer inside a physician. Journal of the Association of Physicians India 48(2): 234–235

Heilig J S 1997 Testing the power of belief. Science 276(5314): 881

Heliker D 1992 Reevaluation of a nursing diagnosis: spiritual distress. Nursing Forum 27(4): 15–20

Henry J 1982 The relation of social to biological processes in disease. Social Science and Medicine 16: 369–380

Henson H 1925 Notes on spiritual healing. Williams and Norgate

Heriot C S 1992 Spirituality and aging. Holistic Nursing Practice 7(1): 22–31

Herman E 1954 Music therapy in depression. In: Poldolsky E (ed) Music therapy. Philosophical Library, New York

Herth K 1978 The therapeutic use of music. Supervised Nursing 78(10): 22–23

Heyes T G 1992 Spirituality, healing and medicine. British Journal of General Practice 42(355): 81

Hiatt J F 1986 Spirituality, medicine, and healing. Southern Medical Journal 79(6): 736–743

Hicks T J Jr 1999 Spirituality and the elderly: nursing implications with nursing home residents. Geriatric Nursing 20(3): 144–146

Highfield M E 2000 Providing spiritual care to patients with cancer. Clinical Journal of Oncology Nursing 4(3): 115–120

Hilsman G J 1997 The place of spirituality in managed care: attending to spiritual needs can help managed care systems achieve their goals. Health Progress 78(1): 43–46

Hinds P 1980 Music: a milieu factor with implications for the nurse therapist. Journal of Psychosocial Nursing and Mental Health Services 18: 28–33

Hittle J M 1994 Death and spirituality: a nurse's perspective. American Journal of Hospice and Palliative Care 11(5): 23–24

Hodge D R 2000 Spiritual ecomaps: a new diagrammatic tool for assessing marital and family spirituality. Journal of Marital and Family Therapy 26(2): 217–228

Holt-Ashley M 2000 Nurses pray: use of prayer and spirituality as a complementary therapy in the intensive care setting. AACN Clinical Issues 11(1): 60–67

Honorton C 1970 Effects of feedback on discrimination between correct and incorrect ESP responses. Journal of the American Society for Psychical Research 64: 404–410

Honorton C 1977 Psi and internal attention states. In: Wolman B (ed) Handbook of parapsychology. Van Nostrand Reinhold, New York

Honorton C 1993 Rhetoric over substance: the impoverished state of skepticism. Journal of Parapsychology 57(2): 191–214

Honorton C, Barksdale W 1972 PK performance with waking suggestions for muscle tension versus relaxation. Journal of the American Society for Psychical Research 66: 208–214

Hoover D R, Margolick J B 2000 Questions on the design and findings of a randomized, controlled trial of the effects of remote, intercessory prayer on outcomes in patients admitted to the coronary care unit. Archives of Internal Medicine 160(12): 1875–1876; discussion 1877–1878

Hopkins P E 1999 Pastoral counseling as spiritual healing: a credo. Journal of Pastoral Care 53(2): 145–151

Horowitz S 1998 The power of more than one: the role of support groups in mind-body healing. Alternative and Complementary Therapies 4(2): 84–88

Horrigan B 1998 Eugene Taylor, PhD on spiritual healing and the American visionary tradition. Alternative Therapies 4(6): 79–87

Horrigan B 1998 Dolores Krieger, RN, PhD healing with therapeutic touch. Alternative Therapies 4(1): 87–92

Horrigan B 1999 Barbara Dossey, RN, MS on holistic nursing, Florence Nightingale, and healing rituals. Alternative Therapies 5(1): 79–86

Horrigan B 2000 Earl E Bakken building a healing hospital. Alternative Therapies 6(2): 83–89

Horrigan B, Krieger D 1998 Healing with therapeutic touch. Alternative Therapies 4: 87–92

Horrigan B, Quinn J 1996 Therapeutic touch and a healing way. Alternative Therapies 2: 70

Horsburgh M 1997 Towards an inclusive spirituality: wholeness, interdependence and waiting. Disability and Rehabilitation 19(10): 398–406

Horton J G 2001 More on spirituality. Journal of the American Osteopathic Association 101(5): 269

Hover-Kramer D 1989 Creating a context for self-healing: the transpersonal perspective. Holistic Nursing Practice 3(3): 27–34

Howard B S, Howard J R 1997 Occupation as spiritual activity. American Journal of Occupational Therapy 51(3): 181–185

Howitt J 1967 An evaluation of audio-analgesia effects. Journal of Dentistry for Child 34(5): 406–411

Hubbard G, May E 1986 Aspects of measurement and applications of geomagnetic indices and extremely low frequency electromagnetic radiation for use in parapsychology. Paper presented at the 29th Annual Convention of the Parapsychological Association

Hubbard G, Vincent W 1988 Electromagnetic measurements of the shielded room at UC Davis. Journal of the American Society for Psychical Research 82: 147–152

Hubbert M 1963 Spiritual care for every patient. Journal of Nursing Education 2(2): 9–11, 29–31

Hudesman J, Schmeidler G 1971 ESP scores following therapeutic sessions. Journal of the American Society for Psychical Research 65: 215–222

Hudesman J, Schmeidler G 1976 Changes in ESP scores after therapy sessions. Journal of the American Society for Psychical Research 70: 371–380

Hudleson I M 1977 Mental energy: a new dimension for nursing. Virginia Nurse Q 45(1): 7–9, 11

Hufford D 1977 Christian religious healing. Journal of Operational Psychiatry 8(2): 22–27

Hufford D 1987 Appendix: The love of God's mysterious will: suffering and the popular theology of healing. Listening: Journal of Religion and Culture 22: 225–239

Hufford D J 1993 Epistemologies in religious healing. Journal of Medical Philosophy 18(2): 175–194

Hull S K, DiLalla L F, Dorsey J K 2001 Student attitudes toward wellness, empathy, and spirituality in the curriculum. Academic Medicine 76(5): 520

Humphrey B 1947 Simultaneous high and low aim in PK tests. Journal of Parapsychology 11: 160–174

Hunsberger B 1991 Empirical work in the psychology of religion. Canadian Psychology 32: 497–504

Huntington E 1938 Is it chance or ESP? American Scholar 7: 201–210

Huston P 1995 China, chi, chicanery: examining traditional Chinese medicine and chi theory. Skeptical Inquirer 19(5): 38–42, 58

Hutch R, Brurg M, Naberhaus D, Hellmich L 1998 The spiritual involvement and beliefs scale. Journal of Family Practice 46: 476–486

Hutchings D 1991 Spirituality in the face of death. Canadian Nurse 87(5): 30–31

Hyman R 1985 A critical overview of parapsychology. In: Kurtz P (ed) A skeptic's handbook of parapsychology. Prometheus Books, Buffalo, NY, pp 1–96

Hyman R 1985 The ganzfeld psi experiment: a critical appraisal. Journal of Parapsychology 49: 3–49

Hyman R 1996 Evaluation of anomalous mental phenomena. Journal of Scientific Exploration 10(1): 31–58

Hyman R, Honorton C 1986 A joint communiqué: the psi ganzfeld controversy. Journal of Parapsychology 50: 351–364

Idler E, Kasl S 1992 Religion, disability, depression, and the timing of death. American Journal of Sociology 97: 1052–1079

Ingbar D, Brody R, Pearson C 1982 Music therapy: a tune-up for mind and body. Science Digest 9(1): 78

Irwin H 1985 Parapsychological phenomena and the absorption domain. Journal of the American Society for Psychical Research 79(1): 1–11

Irwin H 1994 The phenomenology of parapsychological experience. In: Krippner S (ed) Advances in parapsychological research. McFarland, Jefferson, NC, vol. 7, pp. 10–76

Isaacs K, Alexander J, Haggard E 1963 Faith, trust, and gullibility. International Journal of Psychoanalysis 44: 461–469

Iwao M 1997 The clinical use of qigong walking. The 2nd World Congress on Qigong. Paper presented at the 1st American Qigong Association Conference, San Francisco

Jacobson J, Yamanaski W 1994 A possible physical mechanism in the treatment of neurologic disorders with externally applied picotesla magnetic fields. Subtle Energies 5(3): 239–252

Jahn R 1982 The persistent paradox of psychic phenomena: an engineering perspective. Paper presented at the Proceedings of the IEEE, pp. 136–170

Jahn R 1989 Anomalies: analysis and aesthetics. Journal of Scientific Exploration 3(1): 15–26

Jahn R G 1996 Consciousness, information and health. Alternative Therapies 2(3): 32–38

Jahn R, Dunne B 1986 On the quantum mechanics of consciousness, with application to anomalous phenomena. Found Physics 16(8): 721–772

Jahn R, Dunne B 1997 Science of the subjective. Journal of Scientific Exploration 11(2): 201–224

Jahn R G, Dunne B J, Nelson R D 1987 Engineering anomalies research. Journal of Scientific Exploration 1(1): 21–50

Jahn R, Dobyns Y, Dunne B 1991 Count population profiles in engineering anomalies experiments. Journal of Scientific Exploration 5(2): 205–232

James W 1996 1896 Society for Psychical Research, president's address. Subtle Energies and Energy Medicine 7(1): 23–33

Jamison J E 1995 Spirituality and medical ethics. American Journal of Hospice and Palliative Care 12(3): 41–45

Janin P 1973 Nouvelles perspectives sur les relations entre la psyche et le cosmos. Revue Metapsychique

Jaroff L 1994 A no-touch therapy. Time vol. 89

Jarvis G, Northcutt H 1987 Religious differences in morbidity and mortality. Social Science and Medicine 25: 813–824

Jealous J 1997 Jim Jealous, DO: healing and the natural world. Interview by Bonnie Horrigan. Alternative Therapies in Health and Medicine 3(1): 68–76

Jealous J 1998 The other pair of hands. Alternative Therapies in Health and Medicine 4(1): 108, 107

John C C 1988 Faith, hope, and love in medicine. Pharos Alpha Omega Alpha Honor Medical Society 51(4): 12–17

Johnson B A 1997 Spirituality and aging. Journal of Gerontological Nursing 23(7): 7–8

Jonas W B 2001 The middle way: realistic randomized controlled trials for the evaluation of spiritual healing. Journal of Alternative and Complementary Medicine 7(1): 5–7

Jones J 1993 Living on the boundary between psychology and religion. Psychological Religious Newsletter 18(4): 1–7

Josephson B, Pallikari-Viras F 1991 Biological utilization of quantum nonlocality. Found Physics 21: 197–207

Jung C Psychology and spiritualism. Subtle Energies 8(3): 243–248

Jurgens A, Connell-Meehan T, Lavaughan-Wilson H 1987 Therapeutic touch as a nursing intervention. Holistic Nursing Practice 2(1): 1–13

Kaelin J 1998 Spirituality in medical training: where biography meets biology. Continuum 18(5): 14–18

Kaiser L R 2000 Spirituality and the physician executive. Physician Executive 26(2): 6–13

Kane J 1998 Another take on the forces of healing. Alternative Therapies in Health and Medicine 4(2): 19–20

Kaplan B 1976 A note on religious beliefs and coronary heart disease. Journal of South Carolina Medical Association (Suppl.): 60–64

Karagulla S 1977 Seminar presentation. Dynamics of energy fields in health and disease. Theosophical Society of America, Wheaton, IL

Karis R, Karis D 2000 Intercessory prayer. Archives of Internal Medicine 160(12): 1870; discussion 1877–1878

Kavanaugh K M 1997 The importance of spirituality. Journal of Long Term Care Administration 24(4): 29–31

Kehoe N C, Gutheil T G 1994 Neglect of religious issues in scale-based assessment of suicidal patients. Hospital Community Psychiatry 45(4): 366–369

Keil H, Herbert B, Ullman M, Pratt J 1976 Directly observable voluntary PK effects. Proceedings of Social Psychology Research 56(210): 197–235

Kellehear A 2000 Spirituality and palliative care: a model of needs. Palliative Medicine 14(2): 149–155

Kelly M, Varvoglis M, Keane P 1979 Physiological response during psi and sensory presentation of an arousing stimulus. In: Roll W (ed) Research in Parapsychology 1978. Scarecrow Press, Metuchen, NJ, pp. 40–41

Kelly J 1997 Revealing and healing illness with art therapy. Alternative and Complementary Therapies 3(2): 107–114

Kendall J 1994 Wellness spirituality in homosexual men with HIV infection. Journal of the Association of Nurses in AIDS Care 5(4): 28–34

Kendall M L 1999 A holistic nursing model for spiritual care of the terminally ill. American Journal of Hospice and Palliative Care 16(2): 473–476

Kennedy J 1979 Methodological problems in free-response ESP experiments. Journal of the American Society for Psychical Research 73(1): 1–15

Kennedy J 1995 Methods for investigating goal-oriented PSI. Journal of Parapsychology 59: 47–62

Kennedy M 1997 Natural-borne healers. Wisconsin Medical Journal 96(3): 21–27

Kennison M 1987 Faith: an untapped health resource. Journal of Psychosocial Nursing 25(10): 28–30

Kenny G 1999 The iron cage and the spider's web: children's spirituality and the hospital environment. Paediatric Nursing 11(5): 20–23

Kenny G 1999 Assessing children's spirituality: what is the way forward? British Journal of Nursing 8(1): 28, 30–22

Kenosian C 1995 Wound healing with noncontact therapeutic touch used as an adjunct therapy. Journal of Wound, Ostomy and Continence Nursing 22(2): 95–99

Kerfoot K 1995 Keeping spirituality in managed care: the nurse manager's challenge. Nurs Econ 13(1): 49–51

Kernberg O 1980 Internal world and external reality. Aronson, New York

Kettle P R 1992 Spirituality, healing and medicine. British Journal of General Practice 42(354): 38

Kief H 1973 A method for measuring PK ability with enzymes. In: Roll W, Morris R, Morris J (eds) Research in parapsychology 1972. Scarecrow Press, Metuchen, NJ

Kiev A 1969 Primitive religious rites and behavior: clinical considerations. In: Pattison E (ed) Clinical psychiatry and religion. Little Brown, Boston, pp. 119–131

Kilwein J H 1990 Health, illness and willpower. Journal of Clinical Pharmacy and Therapeutics 15(3): 165–168

Kimball E 1983 Oral Roberts' city of faith: does prayer heal? Canadian Medical Association Journal 128(9): 1114–1117

King H, Diamond E, Bailar J 1965 Cancer mortality and religious preference: a suggested method in research. Milbank Memorial Fund Quarterly 43: 349–358

King M, Speck P, Thomas A 1994 Spiritual and religious beliefs in acute illness – is this a feasible area for study? Social Science and Medicine 38: 631–636

Kirkpatrick H, Landeen J, Woodside H, Byrne C 2001 How people with schizophrenia build their hope. Journal of Psychosocial Nursing and Mental Health Services 39(1): 46–53

Kirk-Smith M 1998 Healing and expectation. Journal of the Royal Society of Medicine 91(7): 400

Kittelson R 1977 The healing touch. Australian Nurses Journal 7(1): 41

Kleindienst M J 1998 Spirituality – where there is hope, there is life. American Nephrology Nurses Association (ANNA) Journal 25(4): 442

Kleinman A, Sung L 1979 Why do indigenous practitioners successfully heal? Social Science and Medicine 13: 7–26

Kleinman A, Eisenberg H, Good B 1978 Culture, illness, and care: clinical lessons from anthropologic and cross-cultural research. Annals of Internal Medicine 88: 251–258

Knodt H 1978 Counseling through prayer: avenues of divine healing in pastoral care. Bulletin – American Protestant Hospital Association 42(2): 116–119

Knowles F W 1954 Some investigations into psychic healing. Journal of American Society for Psychical Res 48: 21–26

Knowles F W 1956 Psychic healing in organic disease. Journal of American Society for Psychical Research 50: 110–117

Koch M 1982 Nurses, spirituality, and clients. Part 3. Healing with love and light. Assertive Nurse 5(1): 17–18

Koenig H 1990 Research on religion and mental health in later life: a review and commentary. Journal of Geriatric Psychiatry 23(1): 23–53

Koenig H 1992 Religious affiliation and major depression. Hospital and Community Psychiatry 43(12): 1204

Koenig H 1994 Religion and hope for the disabled elder. In: Levin J (ed) Religion in aging and health: theoretical foundations and methodological frontiers. Sage Publications, Thousand Oaks, CA, pp. 18–51

Koenig H 1999 Letter to the editor. Scientific Review of Alternative Medicine 3(1)

Koenig H 1999 Exploring links between religion/spirituality and health. Scientific Review of Alternative Medicine 3(1): 52–55

Koenig H G 1999 How does religious faith contribute to recovery from depression? Harvard Mental Health Letter 15(8): 8

Koenig H G 2000 MSJAMA: religion, spirituality, and medicine: application to clinical practice. Journal of the American Medical Association 284(13): 1708

Koenig H G 2000 Should doctors prescribe religion? Interview by Anita J Slomski. Medical Economics 77(1): 144–146, 151, 155

Koenig H G 2000 Religion and medicine I: historical background and reasons for separation. International Journal of Psychiatry in Medicine 30(4): 385–398

Koenig H G, Seeber J J 1987 Religion, spirituality, and aging. Journal of the American Geriatrics Society 35(5): 472

Koenig H, Moberg D, Kvale J 1988 Religious activities and attitudes of elderly people in a geriatric assessment clinic. Journal of the American Geriatrics Society 36: 362–374

Koenig H G, Idler E, Kasl S et al 1999 Religion, spirituality, and medicine: a rebuttal to skeptics. International Journal of Psychiatry in Medicine 29(2): 123–131

Kohane M, Tiller W 1999 Energy, fitness and electromagnetic fields in Drosophila melanogaster. Journal of Scientific Exploration (in press)

Kohler C 1999 The nursing diagnosis of 'spiritual distress', a necessary re-evaluation. Recherche en Soins Infirmiers (56): 12–72

Koizumi H 1995 Ki-energy: conversation between self and universe. Proceedings of Intersymp '95, Annual Meeting of the International Institute for Advanced Studies in Systems Research and Cybernetics

Kolata G 1981 Drug found to help heart attack survivors. Science 214: 774–775

Kortman L 1977 The use of music as a program tool with regressed geriatric patients. Journal of Gerontology and Nursing 3: 4

Krause N 1992 Stress, religiosity, and psychological well-being among older blacks. Journal of Aging and Health 4: 412–439

Kreidler M C 1995 Victims of family abuse: the need for spiritual healing. Journal of Holistic Nursing 13(1): 30–36

Kreisman S 1988 Religion and medicine. Southern Medical Journal 81(12): 1598

Kreitzer M J 1999 Creating healing environments. Creative Nursing 5(2): 16

Kreitzer M J, Jensen D 2000 Healing practices: trends, challenges, and opportunities for nurses in acute and critical care. AACN Clinical Issues 11(1): 7–16; quiz 155–156

Kress K 1999 Parapsychology in intelligence: a personal review and conclusion. Journal of Scientific Exploration 13(1): 69–85

Krieger D 1975 Therapeutic touch: an ancient but unorthodox nursing intervention. Journal of New York State Nursing Association 6(2): 6–10

Krieger D 1976 Alternative medicine: therapeutic touch. Nursing Times 72(15): 572–574

Krieger D 1978 The potential use of therapeutic touch in healing. In: Kasloff J (ed) Wholistic dimensions in healing a resource guide. Doubleday, Garden City, pp. 182–183

Krieger D 1979 Physiologic indices of TT. American Journal of Nursing 79(4): 660–662

Krieger D 1990 Therapeutic touch: two decades of research, teaching, and clinical practice. Imprint 3: 83–88

Krieger D 1997 A yoga of healing: the perspective of a therapeutic touch therapist. Subtle Energies and Energy Medicine 8(1): 21–31

Krippner S 1963 Creativity and psychic phenomena. Indian Journal of Parapsychology 4: 1–20

Krippner S 1988 Energy medicine in indigenous healing systems. In: Srinivasan T (ed) Energy medicine around the world. Gabriel Press, Phoenix, AZ, p. 34

Krippner S 1991 Learning guide for systems of healing. Saybrook Institute, San Francisco

Krippner S, Achterberg J 2000 Anomalous healing experiences. In: Cardena E, Lynn S, Krippner S (eds)

Varieties of anomalous experiences: examining the scientific evidence. American Psychological Association, Washington, DC, pp. 353–395

Krippner S, George L 1986 Psi phenomena as related to altered states of consciousness. In: Wolman B, Ullman M (eds) Handbook of states of consciousness. Van Nostrand, New York

Krucoff M W 1999 Mitchell W. Krucoff, MD. The MANTRA study project. Interview by Bonnie Horrigan. Alternative Therapies in Health and Medicine 5(3): 74–82

Krucoff M, Crater S, Green C, Maas A, Seskevich J 2001 Integrative noetic therapies as adjuncts to percutaneous intervention during unstable coronary syndromes: Monitoring and Actualization of Noetic Training (MANTRA) feasibility pilot. American Heart Journal 142(5): 760–769

Krystal S, Zweben J E 1988 The use of visualization as a means of integrating the spiritual dimension into treatment: a practical guide. Journal of Substance Abuse and Treatment 5(4): 229–238

Kubie L 1963 Medicine as a spiritual challenge. Journal of Religion and Health 3: 39–55

Kuhn C C 1988 A spiritual inventory of the medically ill patient. Psychiatric Medicine 6(2): 87–100

Kumasaka L 1996 My pain is God's will. American Journal of Nursing 96(6): 45–47

Kvale J, Koenig H, Ferrel C, Moore H 1989 Life satisfaction of the aging woman religious. Journal of Religion and Aging 5(4): 59–71

Labun E 1988 Spiritual care: an element in nursing care planning. Journal of Advanced Nursing 13(3): 314–320

Landauer R 1996 Minimal energy requirements in communication. Science 272: 1914–18

Landis B 1996 Uncertainty, spiritual well-being, and psychosocial adjustment to chronic illness. Issues in Mental Health Nursing 17: 217–231

Lane J 1987 The care of the human spirit. Journal of Professional Nursing 3: 332–337

LaPierre L L 1994 The spirituality and religiosity of veterans. Journal of Health Care and Chaplaincy 6(1): 73–82

Larson D, Larson S 1991 Religious commitment and health: valuing the relationship. Second Opinion: Health, Faith, and Ethics 17(1): 26–40

Larson D, Milano M 1995 Are religion and spirituality clinically relevant in health care? Mind/Body Medicine 1: 147–157

Larson D, Donahue M, Lyons J et al 1989 Religious affiliations in mental health research samples as compared with national samples. Journal of Nervous and Mental Disease 177(2): 109–111

Larson D, Lu F, Swyers J 1996 Model curriculum for psychiatry residency training programs: religion and spirituality in clinical practice. National Institute for Healthcare Research, Rockville, MD

Larson D, Swyers J, McCullough M 1997 Scientific research on spirituality and health: a consensus report. National Institute for Health Care Research, Rockville, MD

Larson E, Witham L 1997 Scientists are still keeping the faith. Nature 386: 435–436

Larson S, Larson D 1992 Clinical religious research: how to enhance risk of disease: don't go to church. Christian Medical Dental Society Journal 23: 14–19

Larson T J 1997 Resuscitating and transforming hospice volunteer services. American Journal of Hospice and Palliative Care 14(6): 308–310

Larson D B, Koenig H G 2000 Is God good for your health? The role of spirituality in medical care. Cleveland Clinical Journal of Medicine 67(2): 80, 83–84

Laszlo E 1997 Energy talk. Science and Medicine Network Review 63

Laukhuf G, Werner H 1998 Spirituality: the missing link. Journal of Neuroscience Nursing 30(1): 60–67

Lauver D R 2000 Commonalities in women's spirituality and women's health. ANS Advanced Nursing in Science 22(3): 76–88

Lavine R, Buchsbaum M, Poncy M 1976 Analgesia: somatosensory evoked response and subjective pain rating. Psychophysiology 13(2): 140–148

Lea G 1982 Religion, mental health and clinical issues. Journal of Religion and Health 21: 336–351

Lebacqz K 1986 Faith dimensions in medical practice. Primary Care 13 (2): 263–270

Lemieux L 1999 [Spirituality and nursing care]. Infirmière du Quebec 6(6): 31–37

LeShan L 1973 What is important about the paranormal? In: Ornstein R (ed) The nature of human consciousness: a book of readings. Viking, New York, pp. 458–467

Leskowitz E 1997 Phantom limb pain: subtle energy perspectives. Subtle Energies 8(2): 125–152

Lettieri A 1996 Toward a philosophy of science in women's health research. Journal of Scientific Exploration 10(4): 535–545

Levesque-Barbes H 1984 Therapeutic touch: origin, basis, education. Infirmière Canadienne 26(11): 17–19

Levin J 1989 Religious factors in aging, adjustment, and health: a theoretical overview. In: Clements W (ed) Religion, aging and health: a global perspective. Hawthorn Press, New York, pp. 133–146

Levin J 1993 Esoteric vs. exoteric explanations for findings linking spirituality and health. Advanced Journal of Mind Body Health 9(4): 54–56

Levin J 1994 Religion and health: is there an association, is it valid, and is it causal? Social Science and Medicine 38(11): 1475–1482

Levin J 1994 Investigating the epidemiologic effects of religious experience: findings, explanations, and barriers. In: Levin J (ed) Religion in aging and health: theoretical foundations and methodological frontiers. Sage Publications, Thousand Oaks, CA, pp. 3–17

Levin J 1996 How religion influences morbidity and health: reflections on natural history, salutogenesis and host resistance. Social Science and Medicine 43(5): 849–864

Levin J 1996 How prayer heals: a theoretical model. Alternative Therapies 2(1): 66–73

Levin J 1999 Jeff Levin, MPH, PhD. The power of love. Interview by Bonnie Horrigan. Alternative Therapies in Health and Medicine 5(4): 78–86

Levin J, Markides K 1985 Religion and health in Mexican Americans. Journal of Religion and Health 24: 60–69

Levin J, Schiller P 1987 Is there a religious factor in health? Journal of Religion and Health 26: 9–39

Levin J, Tobin S 1995 Religion and psychological well-being. In: Kimble M, McFadden S, Ellor J, Seeber J (eds) Aging, spirituality, and religion: a handbook. Fortress Press, Minneapolis, Minn, pp. 30–46

Levin J, Vanderpool H 1992 Religious factors in physical health and the prevention of illness. In: Pargament K, Maton K, Hess R (eds) Religion and prevention in mental health: research, vision, and action. Haworth Press, New York, pp. 83–103

Levin J, Chatters L, Ellison C, Taylor R 1996 Religious involvement, health outcomes, and public health practice. Current Issues in Public Health 2: 220–225

Levin J S 1996 How prayer heals: a theoretical model. Alternative Therapies in Health and Medicine 2(1): 66–73

Levin J S, Larson D B, Puchalski C M 1997 Religion and spirituality in medicine: research and education. Journal of the American Medical Association 278(9): 792–793

Levin M 1993 Current and potential applications of bioelectromagnetics in medicine. Subtle Energies 4: 77–85

Levin J, Coreil J 1986 New age healing in the US. Social Science and Medicine 23: 889–897

Levy W 1971 Possible PK by chicken embryos to obtain warmth. Proceedings from the Parapsychology Association 8: 25–27

Levy W, Davis J 1974 A potential animal model for parapsychological interaction between organisms. In: Roll W, Morris R, Morris J (eds) Research in parapsychology 1973. Scarecrow Press, Metuchen, NJ, pp. 78–81

Levy-Suhl M 1946 The role of ethics and religion in psychoanalytic theory and therapy. International Journal of Psychoanalysis 27: 81–95

Ley D C, Corless I B 1988 Spirituality and hospice care. Death Studies 12(2): 101–110

Libet B 1994 A testable field theory of mind-brain interaction. Journal of Consciousness Studies 1(1): 119–126

Liboff A 1997 Bioelectromagnetic fields and acupuncture. Journal of Alternative and Complementary Medicine 3: S77–S87

Lieban R 1982 Urban Philippine healers and their contrasting clienteles. Culture, Medicine and Psychiatry 5: 217–231

Lili C 1989 Fitness and health through qigong. Beijing Review April 24–30: 20–26

Lindenthal J, Myers J, Pepper M, Stern M 1970 Mental status and religious behavior. Journal of Scientific Studies in Religion 9(2): 143–149

Lingle E A 1996 Treating children by faith: colliding constitutional issues. Journal of Legal Medicine 17(2): 301–330

Linton P E 1993 Healing environments: creating a total healing environment. Journal of Healthcare Design 5: 167–174

Lintz K C, Penson R T, Chabner B A, Lynch T J 1998 Schwartz Center rounds: a staff dialogue on caring for an intensely spiritual patient: psychosocial issues faced by patients, their families, and caregivers. Oncologist 3(6): 439–445

Lionberger H 1985 An interpretive study of nurses' practice of therapeutic touch. Unpublished Doctoral dissertation, University of California, San Francisco

Livingston M 1979 Music for the childbearing family. Journal of Obstetrics and Gynecologic Nursing 8: 363–367

Loftin R 1990 Auras: searching for the light. Skeptical Inquirer 4: 403–409

Loftus J A 1988 Spirituality and wellness for the caregiver. CHAC Review 16(3): 16–23

Long A 1997 Nursing: a spiritual perspective. Nursing Ethics 4(6): 496–510

Long J K 1977 Parapsychology in anthropology. In: Long J K (ed) Extrasensory Ecology. Scarecrow Press, London, pp. 1–11

Lowenthal R M 1989 Can cancer be cured by meditation and 'natural therapy'? A critical review of the book You can conquer cancer by Ian Gawler. Medican Journal of Australia 151(11–12): 710–715

Lucadou W 1987 A multivariate PK experiment, Part I. An approach combining physical and psychological conditions of the PK process. European Journal of Parapsychology 6: 305–346

Lucadou W 1987 A multivariate PK experiment, Part II. Is PK a real force? The results and their interpretation. European Journal of Parapsychology 6: 369–428

Lucadou W, Lay B, Kunzmann H 1987 A multivariate PK experiment, Part II. Relationships between psychological variables. European Journal of Parapsychology 6: 305–346

Ludwig A M 1968 The influence of nonspecific healing techniques with chronic schizophrenics. American Journal of Psychotherapy 22(3): 382–404

Lukoff D 2000 David Lukoff, PhD. The importance of spirituality in mental health. Interview by Bonnie Horrigan. Alternative Therapies in Health and Medicine 6(6): 80–87

Lukoff D, Turner R, Lu F 1992 Transpersonal psychology research review: psychoreligious dimensions of healing. Journal of Transpersonal Psychology 24(1): 41–60

Lukoff D, Lu F, Turner R 1992 Toward a more culturally sensitive DSM-IV: psychoreligious and psychospiritual problems. Journal of Nervous and Mental Disease 180(11): 673–682

Lukoff D, Lu F, Turner R 1995 Cultural considerations in the assessment and treatment of religious and spiritual problems. Psychiatric Clinics of North America 18: 467–485

Lukoff D, Lu F, Turner R 1998 From spiritual emergency to spiritual problem: the transpersonal roots of the new DSM-IV category. Journal of Humanistic Psychology 38(2): 21–50

Lumby J 1993 'A New Zealand spirituality'. Interview by Kathy Stodart. Nursing in New Zealand 1(3): 19

Lustig-Juon E 1983 [Alternative medicine. The determining factor is the intention]. Krankenpflege Soins Infirmiers 76(12): 56–58

McBride J L 1998 The new focus on spirituality in medicine. Journal of the Medical Association of Georgia 87(4): 281–284

McBride J L 1999 The family practice residency curriculum: is there any place for spirituality and religion? Family Medicine 31(10): 685–686

McBride J L, Pilkington L, Arthur G 1998 Development of brief pictorial instruments for assessing spirituality in primary care. Journal of Ambulatory Care Management 21(4): 53–61

McClelland D 1979 Music in the operating room. AORN Journal 29: 252–260

McConnell R 1955 Remote night tests for PK. Journal of the American Society for Psychical Research 49: 99–108

McCormick D P, Holder B, Wetsel M A, Cawthon T W 2001 Spirituality and HIV disease: an integrated perspective. Journal of the Association of Nurses and AIDS Care 12(3): 58–65

MacDonald R, Hickman J, Dakin G 1977 Preliminary physical measurements of psychophysical effects associated with three alleged psychic healers. In: Morris J, Roll W, Morris R (eds) Research in Parapsychology. Scarecrow Press, Metuchen, NJ

McFadden S 1996 Religion, spirituality, and aging. In: Birren J, Schaie K (eds) Handbook of the psychology of aging, 4th edn. Academic Press, San Diego, CA, pp. 162–177

McFadden S 1996 Religion and spirituality. In: Birren J (ed) Encyclopedia of gerontology: age, aging, and the aged. Academic Press, San Diego, CA, vol. 2, pp. 387–397

McGlone M E 1990 Healing the spirit. Holistic Nursing Practice 4(4): 77–84

McGrath P 1997 Putting spirituality on the agenda: hospice research findings on the 'ignored' dimension. Hospice Journal 12(4): 1–14

McGrath P 1997 Spirituality and discourse: a postmodern approach to hospice research. Australian Health Review 20(2): 116–128

McGuire M 1993 Health and spirituality as contemporary concerns. Annals of the American Academy of Political and Social Sciences 527: 144–154

McIntosh D, Silver R, Wortman C 1991 Religion's role in adjustment to a negative life event: coping with the loss of a child. Denver

McKee D D, Chappel J N 1992 Spirituality and medical practice. Journal of Family Practice 35(2): 201, 205–208

Mackereth P, Wright J 1997 Therapeutic touch: nursing activity or form of spiritual healing? Complementary Therapies in Nursing Midwifery 3(4): 106–110

Mackey R 1995 Discover the healing power of therapeutic touch. American Journal of Nursing 5(1): 27–33

McLain M V 1998 Religion, spirituality, and AIDS. World (82): 5

MacLennan S, Tsai S 1995 A nursing perspective on spiritual healing. Perspectives 19(1): 9–13

McNichol T 1996 The new faith in medicine. USA Today: 4

Macrae J 1979 Therapeutic touch in practice. American Journal of Nursing 79(1): 664–665

Macrae J 1981 Therapeutic touch: a way of life. In: Borelli M, Heidt P (eds) Therapeutic touch: a book of readings. Springer Publishing, New York, pp. 56–84

McSherry E 1983 The spiritual dimension of elder health care. Generations 8(1): 18–21

McSherry W, Draper P 1998 The debates emerging from the literature surrounding the concept of spirituality as applied to nursing. Journal of Advanced Nursing 27(4): 683–691

Magana A, Clark N M 1995 Examining a paradox: does religiosity contribute to positive birth outcomes in Mexican American populations? Health Education Quarterly 22(1): 96–109

Magarey C 1981 Healing and meditation in medical practice. Medical Journal of Australia 1(7): 338, 340–331

Maltby J, Day L 2001 The relationship between spirituality and Eysenck's personality dimensions: a replication among English adults. Journal of Genetic Psychology 162(1): 119–122

Mandell A 1980 Toward a psychobiology of transcendence: God in the brain. In: Davidson J, Davidson R (eds) The psychobiology of consciousness. Plenum, New York, pp. 379–464

Mann S 2000 The mind/body link in essential hypertension: time for a new paradigm. Alternative Therapies 6(2): 39–45

Markov M, Pilla A, Wang S 1993 Effects of weak low frequency sinusoidal and DC magnetic fields on myosin phosphorylation in a cell-free preparation. Biochemistry and Bioenergetics 30 (119)

Marks D 1981 On the review of The psychology of the psychic: a reply to Dr Morris. Journal of the American Society for Psychical Research 75: 197–203

Marks D 1986 Investigating the paranormal. Nature 320: 119–124

Marrone J 1968 Suppression of pain by sound. Psychology Reports 22: 1055–1056

Marrone R 1999 Dying, mourning, and spirituality: a psychological perspective. Death Studies 23(6): 495–519

Martsolf D S, Mickley J R 1998 The concept of spirituality in nursing theories: differing world-views and extent of focus. Journal of Advanced Nursing 27(2): 294–303

Marty M E 1998 The science of spirituality in medicine. Administration and Radiology Journal 17(11): 24–26

Marwick C 1995 Should physicians prescribe prayer for health? Spiritual aspects of well-being considered. Journal of the American Medical Association 273(20): 1561–1562

Mathias J M 1999 Mind-body-spirit healing in the OR. OR Manager 15(1): 18–22

Matthews D, Larson D 1997 Faith and medicine: reconciling the twin traditions of healing. Mind/Body Medicine 2: 3–6

Matthews D A 2000 Prayer and spirituality. Rheumatic Diseases Clinics of North America 26(1): 177–187, xi

Mattuck R 1977 Random fluctuation theory of psychokinesis: thermal noise model. In: Morris J, Roll W, Morris R (eds) Research in parapsychology. Scarecrow Press, Mehichen, NJ, pp. 191–195

Maugans T A 1996 The spiritual history. Archives of Family Medicine 5(1): 11–16

Maves P 1960 Aging, religion, and the church. In: Tibbitts C (ed) Handbook of social gerontology: societal aspects of aging. University of Chicago Press, Chicago

Maxey E 1990 Electromagnetic fields. Subtle Energies 1(1): 103–106

Maxey E 1991 A lethal subtle energy. Subtle Energies 2(2): 55–72

May E, Utts J, Spottiswoode S 1995 Decision augmentation theory: toward a model of anomalous mental phenomena. Journal of Parapsychology 59: 195–220

Mayer M 1999 Qigong and hypertension: a critique of research. Journal of Alternative and Complementary Medicine 5(4): 371–382

Meehan T C 1996 Encouraging and preserving spirituality. Image – the Journal of Nursing Scholarship 28(2): 92

Meehl P, Scriven M 1956 Compatibility of science and ESP. Science 123: 14–15

Megregian P S 1998 Response to Larry Dossey: prayer, medicine, and science: the new dialogue. Journal of Health Care and Chaplaincy 7(1–2): 105–116

Melzack R, Weisz A, Sprague L 1963 Stratagems for controlling pain: contributions of auditory stimulation and suggestion. Experimental Neurology 8(3): 239–247

Mentgen J L 1989 Therapeutic touch: a healing art. Journal of the Association of Pediatric Oncology Nurses 6(2): 29–30

Mentgen J 1996 The clinical practice of healing touch. Imprint 43(5): 33–36

Meraviglia M G 1999 Critical analysis of spirituality and its empirical indicators. Prayer and meaning in life. Journal of Holistic Nursing 17(1): 18–33

Merrill G G 1981 Health, healing and religion. Maryland State Medical Journal 30(12): 45–47

Mickley J R, Carson V, Soeken K L 1995 Religion and adult mental health: state of the science in nursing. Issues in Mental Health and Nursing 16(4): 345–360

Miller R 1976 Research into healing energies. Science Mind Bulletin 49(1)

Miller R 1977 Methods of detecting and measuring healing energies. In: White J, Krippner S (eds) Future science. Doubleday, Garden City, NY, pp. 431–444

Miller L 1979 An explanation of therapeutic touch using the science of unitary man. Nursing Forum 18: 278–287

Miller W 1990 Spirituality: the silent dimension in addiction research. Drug and Alcohol Review 9: 259–266

Miller W R 1998 Researching the spiritual dimensions of alcohol and other drug problems. Addiction 93(7): 979–990

Millison M B 1995 A review of the research on spiritual care and hospice. Hospice Journal 10(4): 3–18

Milstein J M, Little T H 2000 Invoking spirituality in medical care. Alternative Therapies in Health and Medicine 6(6): 120, 118–129

Minarik P A 1993 Mind–body connection: enhancing healing through imagery. Clinical Nurse Specialist 7(4): 169

Mindel C, Vaughan C 1978 A multidimensional approach to religiosity and disengagement. Journal of Gerontology 33: 103–108

Miners S 1997 Comments on the nature of prayer research. Alternative Therapies in Health and Medicine 3(4): 19–20, 22

Mintz E 1969 On the rationale of touch in psychotherapy. Psychotherapy Theory and Research Practice 6(4): 232–234

Mischel F 1959 Faith healing and medical practice in the southern Caribbean. Southwest Journal of Anthropology 15: 407–417

Mison K 1968 Statistical processing of diagnostics done by subject and by physician. Paper presented at the Proceedings of the 6th International Conference on Psychotronics Research. Psychotronics Association, pp 137–8

Moberg D 1965 Religiosity in old age. Gerontologist 5(2): 78–87

Moberg D 1970 Religion in the later years. In: Hoffman A (ed) The daily needs and interests of older persons. Charles C Thomas, Springfield, IL

Moberg D 1971 Spiritual well-being: background and issues. Paper presented at the White House Conference on Aging, Washington, DC

Moberg D, Brusek P 1978 Spiritual well-being: a neglected subject in quality of life research. Social Indicators Research 5: 303–323

Moberg D, Taves M 1965 Church participation and adjustment in old age. In: Rose A, Peterson W (eds) Older people and their social worlds. FA Davis, Philadelphia

Monckton J 1998 Spirituality and medicine. Complementary Therapy and Nursing Midwifery 4(4): 93–94

Montgomery R A 1986 Modernizing medicine with lessons from an ancient healing art. Pharos Alpha Omega Alpha Honor Medical Society 49(3): 6–11

Moore N G 1996 Spirituality in medicine. Alternative Therapies in Health and Medicine 2(6): 24–26, 103–105

Morell C 1996 Radicalizing recovery: addiction, spirituality, and politics. Social Work 41(3): 306–312

Morgan P P, Cohen L 1994 Spirituality slowly gaining recognition among North American psychiatrists. Canadian Medical Association Journal 150(4): 582–585

Moriarty A, Murphy G 1967 Some thoughts about prerequisite conditions or states in creativity and paranormal experience. Journal of the American Society for Psychical Research 61: 203–218

Morris L E 1996 A spiritual well-being model: use with older women who experience depression. Issues in Mental Health and Nursing 17(5): 439–455

Morris Owen R M 1980 The medicine of self-healing. Lancet 2(8196): 698

Morse C, Wisocki P 1987 Importance of religiosity to elderly adjustment. Journal of Religion and Aging 4(1): 15–26

Mosely E 1997 The pen can heal. Disability and Rehabilitation 19(10): 452–455

Mulloney S, Wells-Federman C 1996 Therapeutic touch: a healing modality. Journal of Cardiovascular Nursing 10(3): 27–49

Mungiu O C 1995 Spirituality and material reality in medical education in Iasi. Revista Medico-Chirurgicala a Societatii de Medici si Naturalisti din Iasi 99(1–2): 203–205

Murphy D 2000 Developing research methodology in spiritual healing: definitions, scope, and limitations. Journal of Alternative and Complementary Medicine 6(4): 299–302

Myers S S, Benson H 1993 Psychological factors in healing: a new perspective on an old debate. Behavioral Medicine 18: 5–11

Mytko J J, Knight S J 1999 Body, mind and spirit: towards the integration of religiosity and spirituality in cancer quality of life research. Psycho-oncology 8(5): 439–450

Nadin R, Kihlstrom J 1987 Hypnosis, psi, and the psychology of anomalous experience. Behavioral and Brain Sciences 10(4): 597–599

Nagai-Jacobson M, Burkhardt M 1989 Spirituality: cornerstone of holistic nursing practice. Holistic Nursing Practice 3(3): 18–26

Narayanasamy A 1999 Learning spiritual dimensions of care from a historical perspective. Nurse Education Today 19(5): 386–395

Narayanasamy A 1999 ASSET: a model for actioning spirituality and spiritual care education and training in nursing. Nurse Education Today 19(4): 274–285

Nash C 1951 Psychokinesis reconsidered. Journal of the American Society for Psychical Research 35: 62–68

Nash C 1961 The unorthodox science of parapsychology. International Journal of Parapsychology 3: 5–24

Nash C B, Nash C S 1981 Psi-influenced movement of chicks and mice onto a visual cliff. In: Roll W, Beloff J, McAllister J (eds) Research in Parapsychology 1980. Scarecrow Press, Metuchen, NJ, pp. 109–110

Nelson R 1989 Statistically robust anomalous effects: replication in random event generator experiments. In: Henckle L, Berger R (eds) Research in Parapsychology 1988. Scarecrow Press, Metuchen, NJ, pp. 23–26

Nelson R, Dunne B 1986 Attempted correlation of engineering anomalies with global geomagnetic activity. Paper presented at the 29th Annual Convention of the Parapsychological Association

Nelson R, Radin D 1987 When immovable objections meet irresistible evidence. Behavioral and Brain Sciences 10: 600–601

Nelson R D, Bradish G J, Dobyns Y H, Dunne B J, Jahn R G 1996 Field REG anomalies in group situations. Journal of Scientific Exploration 10: 111–114

Neubert R 1987 Reiki: the radiance technique. New Realities 7(4): 18–22

Newshan G 1989 Therapeutic touch for symptom control in persons with AIDS. Holistic Nursing Practice 3(4): 45–51

Newshan G 1998 Transcending the physical: spiritual aspects of pain in patients with HIV and/or cancer. Journal of Advanced Nursing 28(6): 1236–1241

Nobel K 1987 Psychological health and the experience of transcendence. Counseling Psychology 15: 601–614

Nolan P, Crawford P 1997 Towards a rhetoric of spirituality in mental health care. Journal of Advanced Nursing 26(2): 289–294

Nordlicht S 1981 Symposium on medicine and religion. New York State Journal of Medicine 81: 1855–1856

Norris P 1997 Psychophysiology, psychosynthesis and the search for self. Subtle Energies and Energy Medicine 8(1): 1–19

Norton C 2000 Guilty conscience can damage your immune system. Paper presented at the British Psychological Society Annual Conference, UK

Nott P 1988 Partnership of medicine and religion. British Medical Journal 297: 1680–1681

Novey S 1960 Considerations on religion in relation to psychoanalysis and psychotherapy. Journal of Nervous and Mental Disease 130: 315–322

Nucci A 1978 The use of music in individual psychotherapy. Unpublished Doctoral dissertation, New York University, New York

Null G 1981 Healers of hustlers: IV. Self Help Update 18.

O'Brien M 1982 Religious faith and adjustment to long-term hemodialysis. Journal of Religion and Health 21: 68–80

O'Brien M E 1999 Sacred covenants: exploring spirituality in nursing. AWHONN Lifelines 3(2): 72, 69–71

O'Connell L J 1996 Changing the culture of dying: a new awakening of spirituality in America heightens sensitivity to needs of dying persons. Health Progress 77(6): 16–20

O'Connor C I 2001 Characteristics of spirituality, assessment, and prayer in holistic nursing. Nursing Clinics of North America 36(1): 33–46

O'Donohue J 1998 Spirituality and leadership: genuine leaders recognize the sacredness of the human presence. Health Progress 79(6): 31–34, 42

O'Kane P 1996 Spirituality in the chronos of AIDS. Journal of the Association of Nurses and AIDS Care 7(4): 17–18

Olcese J, Reuss S, Vollrath L 1985 Evidence for the involvement of the visual system in mediating magnetic field effects on pineal melatonin synthesis in the rat. Brain Research 33: 382–384

Oldnall A 1996 A critical analysis of nursing: meeting the spiritual needs of patients. Journal of Advanced Nursing 23(1): 138–144

O'Mathuna D 1998 Therapeutic touch and wound healing. Alternative Medicine Alert 1(5): 49–52

O'Mathuna D 1998 Therapeutic touch: what could be the harm? Scientific Review of Alternative Medicine 2(1): 56–62

O'Mathuna D P 1998 The subtle allure of therapeutic touch. Journal of Christian Nursing 15(1): 4–7, 9–10, 12–13

O'Regan B 1985 Placebo: the hidden asset in healing. Investigations: Institute of Noetic Sciences 2: 1–32

Orme-Johnson D, Dillbeck M, Wallace R, Landrith G 1982 Intersubject EEG coherence: is consciousness a field? International Journal of Neuroscience 16: 203–209

Orme-Johnson D W, Alexander C N 1992 Critique of the National Research Council's report on mediation. MIU, Fairfield, IA

Osler W 1910 The faith that heals. British Medical Journal: 1470–1471

Otani S 1955 Relations of mental set and change of skin resistance to ESP score. Journal of Parapsychology 19(3): 164–170

Ott C 1997 Spirituality and the nurse. Nebraska Nurses 30(3): 34–35

PadField A 1976 Music as sedation for local anesthesia. Anesthesiology 31: 300–301

Palmer C 2001 A disciplined approach to spiritual care giving for adults living with cystic fibrosis. Journal of Health Care and Chaplaincy 11(1): 95–102

Paloutzian R, Ellison C 1982 Loneliness, spiritual well-being, and quality of life. In: Peplau L, Perlmen D (eds) Loneliness: a sourcebook of current theory, research, and therapy. Wiley Interscience, New York, pp. 224–237

Pande P 2000 Does prayer need testing? Archives of Internal Medicine 160(12): 1873–1874

Pardini D A, Plante T G, Sherman A, Stump J E 2000 Religious faith and spirituality in substance abuse recovery: determining the mental health benefits. Journal of Substance Abuse and Treatment 19(4): 347–354

Pargament K, Hahn J 1986 God and the just world: causal and coping attributions to God in health situations. Journal of Scientific Studies in Religion 25(2): 193–207

Parker M W, Fuller G F, Koenig H G et al 2001 Soldier and family wellness across the life course: a developmental model of successful aging, spirituality, and health promotion, Part II. Military Medicine 166(7): 561–570

Parriott S 1969 Music as therapy. American Journal of Nursing 69: 1723–1726

Parsons T 1960 Mental illness and 'spiritual malaise': the role of the psychiatrist and of the minister of religion. In: Hofman H (ed) The ministry and mental health. Association Press, New York

Patrovsky V 1988 Objective evaluation of so-called therapeutic energy. Casopis Lekaur Ceskych 127(23): 726–727

Patterson E 1998 The philosophy and physics of holistic health care: spiritual healing as a workable interpretation. Journal of Advanced Nursing 27: 287–293

Patterson J, Hayworth M, Turner C, Raskin M 2000 Spiritual issues in family therapy: a graduate-level course. Journal of Marital and Family Therapy 26(2): 199–210

Pattison E 1966 Social and psychological aspects of religion in psychotherapy. Journal of Nervous and Mental Disease 141(5): 586–597

Pattison E 1977 Religion, faith, and healing. In: Pattison E (ed) The experience of dying. Prentice-Hall, Englewood Cliffs, NJ

Pattison E (in press) Ideological support for the marginal middle class: faith healing and glossolalia. In: Zaretsky I, Leone M (eds) Pragmatic religion: marginal religious movements in America today. Princeton University Press, Princeton, NJ

Pattison E, Casey R 1969 Glossolallia: a contemporary mystical experience. In: Pattison E (ed) Clinical psychiatry and religion. Little, Brown, Boston, pp. 133–148

Paulsen A 1926 Religious healing. Journal of the American Medical Association 36: 1519–1524, 1617–1623, 1969–11697

Payne F E 1999 Research on spirituality: dangerous and deceptive ground? Journal of Family Practice 48(7): 501–503

Payne D 2001 Holy water not always a blessing. British Medical Journal 322: 190

Peat F 1993 Towards a process theory of healing: energy, activity, and global form. Subtle Energies 3(2): 1–40

Peck M L 1981 The therapeutic effect of faith. Nursing Forum 20(2): 153–166

Peretti M 1983 The effect of musical preference on anxiety as determined by GSR. Acta Psychaetric – Belgium 83(5): 437–442

Peri T A 1995 Promoting spirituality in persons with acquired immunodeficiency syndrome: a nursing intervention. Holistic Nursing Practice 10(1): 68–76

Persinger M A 1979 ELF field mediation in spontaneous psi events: direct information transfer of conditioned elicitation? In: Tart C, Puthoff H, Targ R (eds) Mind at large. Praeger, New York, pp. 191–204

Persinger M 1989 Psi phenomena and temporal lobe activity: the geomagnetic factor. In: Henkel L, Berger R (eds) Research in parapsychology. Scarecrow Press, Metuchen, NJ

Peteet J 1985 Religious issues presented by cancer patients in psychiatric consultation. Journal of Psychosocial Oncology 3(1): 53–66

Peters D 2000 Colloquium on spiritual healing. Meeting summary: major themes. Journal of Alternative and Complementary Medicine 6(2): 187–188

Peterson E, Nelson K 1987 How to meet your clients' spiritual needs. Journal of Psychosocial Nursing 25: 34–39

Peterson L, Roy A 1985 Religiosity, anxiety and meaning and purpose: religion's consequences for psychological well-being. Review of Religious Research 27: 49–62

Pethig R 1988 Electrical properties of biological tissue. In: Marino A (ed) Modern bioelectricity. Marcel Dekker, New York

Pettitt G A 1988 Changes of heart: the role of love and will in illness and wellness: Part 3. New Zealand Medical Journal 101(853): 573–574

Phelan E, Simpleman R 1994 Pastoral care's role in a reformed system: pastoral care professionals need to promote the spiritual dimension of healing throughout the continuum of care. Health Progress 75(6): 64–66

Pierce L L 2001 Caring and expressions of spirituality by urban caregivers of people with stroke in African American families. Quality Health Research 11(3): 339–352

Plotnikoff G A 2000 In search of a good death: the spiritual dimension. Minnesota Medicine 83(5): 50–51

Poetter L, Stewart H 1975 Fundamental values, the work ethic, and spirituality are basic for the therapeutic program at Anneewakee. Adolescence 10(38): 247–252

Poloma M 1994 Evidence of prayer's healing power: a sociological perspective. Second Opinion 20(1): 82–86

Pomerhn A 1987 The effect of therapeutic touch on nursing students' perceptions of stress during clinical experiences. Masters Abstracts International 25(4): 362

Popp F 1993 Electromagnetism and living systems. In: Popp F, Ho M, Warnke U (eds) Bioelectrodynamics and biocommunications. World Scientific Publishing, River Edge, NJ, pp. 33–80

Posner G 2000 Another controversial effort to establish the medical efficacy of intercessory prayer. Scientific Review of Alternative Medicine 4: 15–17

Post S G, Whitehouse P J 1999 Spirituality, religion, and Alzheimer's disease. Journal of Health Care and Chaplaincy 8(1–2): 45–57

Post S G, Puchalski C M, Larson D B 2000 Physicians and patient spirituality: professional boundaries, competency, and ethics. Annals of Internal Medicine 132(7): 578–583

Price J M 2000 Does prayer really set one apart? Archives of Internal Medicine 160(12): 1873; discussion 1877–1878

Primus H 1996 Synchronizitat und Zufall. Zeitschrift fur Parapsychologie und Grenzgebiete der Psychologie 38: 61–91

Pritchard S 1997 Spirituality can mean many different things. Nursing Times 93(40): 8–9

Pryjmachuk S, O'Mathuna D, Spencer W, Stanwick M, Matthiesen S 1998 Therapeutic touch: misusing science to justify non science. Submitted to Research in Nursing and Health

Puchalski C M, Larson D B 1998 Developing curricula in spirituality and medicine. Academic Medicine 73(9): 970–974

Puchalski C M, Larson D B, Post S G 2000 Physicians and patient spirituality. Annals of Internal Medicine 133(9): 748–749

Puharich A 1977 On the possible usefulness of extrasensory perception in psychological warfare. Washington Post, August

Quinn J The healing arts in modern health care. American Theosophist 72: 198–203

Quinn J 1979 One nurse's evolution as a healer. American Journal of Nursing 79(4): 662–664

Quinn J 1987 TT and anxiety in pre-op cardiac patients. Unpublished research grant funded by health and human services, 1984–1987, University of Colorado

Quinn J 1989 Future directions for therapeutic touch research. Journal of Holistic Nursing 7(1): 19–25

Quinn J 1992 The senior's therapeutic touch education program. Holistic Nursing Practice 7(1): 32–37

Quinn J 1992 Holding sacred space: the nurse as healing environment. Holistic Nursing Practice 6(4): 26–36

Quinn J, Strelkauskas A 1993 Psychoimmunologic effect of therapeutic touch on practitioners and recently bereaved recipients: a pilot study. Advances in Nursing Science 15(4): 13–26

Radin D 1982 Experimental attempts to influence pseudorandom number sequences. Journal of the American Society for Psychical Research 76: 359–374

Radin D 1989 Searching for 'signatures' in anomalous human–machine interaction research: a neural network approach. Journal of Scientific Exploration 3: 185–200

Radin D 1990 Testing the plausibility of psi-mediated computer system failures. Journal of Parapsychology 54: 1–19

Radin D 1992 Beyond belief: exploring interactions among mind, body and environment. Subtle Energies 2(3): 1–40

Radin D 1993 Environmental modulation and statistical equilibrium in mind–matter interaction. Subtle Energies 4(1): 1–30

Radin D 1993 Neural network analyses of consciousness-related patterns in random sequences. Journal of Scientific Exploration 7(4): 355–374

Radin D 1998 Further investigation of unconscious differential anticipatory responses to future emotions. Proceedings of Presented Papers: 41st Annual Convention of the Parapsychological Association. Parapsychological association, Halifax, Nova Scotia, Canada, pp. 163–183

Radin D, Nelson R 1988 Repeatable evidence for anomalous human–machine interactions. In: Albertson M, Ward D, Freeman K (eds) Paranormal research. Rocky Mountain Research Institute, Fort Collins, CO, pp. 307–317

Raloff J 1998 Electromagnetic fields may trigger enzymes. Science News 123 (February 12): 119

Raloff J 1998 EMFs' biological influences: electromagnetic fields exert effects on and through hormones. Science News 153 (January 10): 29–31

Rancour P 1991 Guided imagery: healing when curing is out of the question. Perspectives in Psychiatric Care 27(4): 30–33

Randall J 1970 An attempt to detect psi effects with protozoa. Journal of the Society for Psychical Research 45.

Randolph G 1980 The difference in physiological response of female college students exposed to stressful stimulus, when simultaneously treated by either therapeutic touch or casual touch. Unpublished Dissertations Abstracts International, New York University, New York

Rankin-Box D 1998 Personal account: defining spirituality. Complementary Therapies and Nursing Midwifery 4(4): 107

Rao K R 1993 Charles Honorton: a savant of his own kind. Journal of Parapsychology 57(2): 1–6

Rassool G H 2000 The crescent and Islam: healing, nursing and the spiritual dimension: some considerations towards an understanding of the Islamic perspectives on caring. Journal of Advanced Nursing 32(6): 1476–1484

Rauscher E 1984 Application of human volition mind/matter interactions. Archaes Journal 2 (71)

Ravitz L 1950 Electro-metric correlates of the hypnotic state. Science 112: 341–342

Ravitz L 1959 Application of the electro-dynamic field theory in biology, psychiatry, medicine and hypnosis. I. General Survey. American Journal of Clinical Hypnosis 1: 135–150

Ravitz L 1962 History, measurements and applicability of periodic changes in the electromagnetic field in health and disease. Annals of the New York Academy of Science 98: 1145–1201

Rea W, Fan Y, Fenyves E et al 1991 Electromagnetic field sensitivity. Journal of Bioelectricity 10 (241)

Reading M 1998 Qigong shows promise: needs controlled research studies. Journal of Alternative and Complementary Medicine 2: 117–119

Rebman J, Radin D, Hapke R, Gaughan K 1996 Remote influence of the autonomic nervous system by a ritual healing technique. Paper presented at the Parapsychological Association 39th Annual Convention, Durham, NC. Parapsychological Association, Durham, NC

Reed P G 1992 An emerging paradigm for the investigation of spirituality in nursing. Research in Nursing and Health 15(5): 349–357

Reed G, Kemeny M, Taylor S, Wang H, Visscher B 1994 Realistic acceptance as a predictor of decreases survival time in gay men with AIDS. Health Psychology 13: 299–307

Rehder H 1955 Wunderheilungen, ein experiment. Hippokrates 26: 577–580

Rein G 1986 A psychokinetic effect of neurotransmitter metabolism: alterations in the degradative enzyme monoamine oxidase. Research in Parapsychology 1985: 77–80

Rein G 1992 The scientific basis for healing with subtle energies. In: Laskow L (ed) Healing with love: a physician's breakthrough mind/body medical guide for healing yourself and others. The art of holoenergetic healing. HarperCollins, New York, vol. 1, pp. 279–319

Rein G 1998 Biological effects of quantum fields and their role in the natural healing process. Frontier Perspectives 7: 16–23

Remen N 1993 On defining spirit. Noetic Sciences Review 27: 41

Reynolds M 1982 Religious institutions and the prevention of mental illness. Journal of Religion and Health 21(3): 245–253

Rhine J 1944 Mind over matter or the PK effect. Journal of the American Society for Psychical Research 38: 185–201

Richards H 1982 God's principles of health. Your Life and Health 97(4): 12–13

Richmond N 1952 Two series of PK tests on paramecia. Journal of the American Society for Psychical Research 36: 577–578

Rickel W 1961 Is psychotherapy a religious process? In: Oates W (ed) The minister's own mental health. Channel Press, Great Neck, NY

Riley D S 1997 The mystery of health: reclaiming medicine's soul. Alternative Therapies in Health and Medicine 3(2): 128, 127

Riley D 2000 The mind/body continuum. Alternative Therapies 6(2): 34

Rinpoche S 1999 The spiritual heart of Tibetan medicine: its contribution to the modern world. Alternative Therapies 5(3): 70–72

Ritchie K 1991 Guilt and the cancer patient. Cancer Bulletin 43(5): 430–432

Robbins A 1985 Reiki therapy and the hands-on approach. Dance Magazine 59(2): 88

Robinson D 1970 Is there a correlation between rhythmic response and emotional disturbance? Journal of Music Therapy 7: 54

Robinson A 1994 Spirituality and risk: toward an understanding. Holistic Nursing Practice 8(2): 1–7

Roche J 1989 Spirituality and the ALS patient. Rehabilitation and Nursing 14(3): 139–141

Roessler S 1982 The role of spiritual values in the recovery of alcoholics. Unpublished dissertation, Wesley Theological Seminary, Washington, DC

Rogers M 1987 Rogers' science of unitary human beings. In: Parse R, Saunders W (eds) Nursing sciences: major paradigms, theories, and critiques. Philadelphia

Rogers M 1988 Nursing science and art: a prospective. Nursing and Science Quarterly 1(3): 99–102

Roland C 1970 Does prayer preserve? Archives of Internal Medicine 125: 580–587

Romeira O 1998 [Spirituality 'importance for care']. Servir 46(3): 127–128

Roney-Dougal S, Vogl G 1993 Some speculations on the effect of geomagnetism on the pineal gland. Journal of the Society for Psychical Research 59(830): 1–15

Rosa L 1994 Therapeutic touch: skeptics in hand to hand combat over the latest New Age health fad. Skeptical Inquirer 3(1): 40–49

Rosa E, Rosa L, Sarner L 1996 Investigation into therapeutic touch: perceptibility of a therapeutic field.

Rose L 1954 Some aspects of paranormal healing. British Medical Journal 2: 13–29

Rosenthal R 1986 Meta-analytic procedures and the nature of replication: the ganzfeld debate. Journal of Parapsychology 50: 315–336

Rosner F 1975 The efficacy of prayer: scientific v. religious evidence. Journal of Religion and Health 14(4): 294–298

Rothman K 1988 Inferring causal connections – habit, faith or logic? In: Rothman K (ed) Causal inference. Epidemiology Resources, Chestnut Hill, MA

Rothrock J C 1994 The meaning of spirituality to perioperative nurses and their patients. AORN Journal 60(6): 894, 896

Roud P 1990 Making miracles: an exploration into the dynamics of self-healing. Warner Books, Wellingborough, England

Roush W 1997 Herbert Benson: mind-body maverick pushes the envelope. Science 276: 357–359

Rousseau P 2000 Spirituality and the dying patient. Journal of Clinical Oncology 18(9): 2000–2002

Rowan A 1996 Religious beliefs and health psychology: empirical foundations. Health Psychology 18: 16–17

Roy D 1987 Editorial. The spiritual need of the dying. Journal of Palliative Care 2: 3–4

Royce J 1985 What do you mean spiritual illness? Alcoholism: The National Magazine, vol. 5

Ruffing-Rahal M 1984 The spiritual dimension of well-being implications for the elderly. Home Healthcare Nurse March/April: 12–13, 16

Rutte M 1998 Spirituality in the health care workplace. Aspens Advisor for Nurse Executives 13(6): 1, 3–5

Sabatino F 1993 New concepts of health and healing may affect hospitals' approach to care. Trustee 46(3): 8–10

Salzman L 1957 Spiritual and faith healing. Journal of Pastoral Care 11: 146–155

Salzman L 1986 Religion as metaphor in mental illness. In: Robinson L (ed) Psychiatry and religion: overlapping concerns. American Psychiatric Press, Washington, DC

Sandroff R 1980 A skeptic's guide to therapeutic touch. RN 43(6): 25–30, 82ff

Sanua V 1969 Religion, mental health, and personality: a review of empirical studies. American Journal of Psychiatry 125(9): 1203–1213

Saudia T L, Kinney M R, Brown K C, Young-Ward L 1991 Health locus of control and the helpfulness of prayer. Heart Lung 20: 60–65

Saunders J, Retsas A 1998 Spirituality and nursing: toward an ontological understanding. Collegian 5(1): 16–19

Savva S 1991 Comments on the 'IR spectra alteration in water proximate to the palms of therapeutic practitioners'. Subtle Energies 2(2): 73–84

Sayre-Adams J 1992 Therapeutic touch: research and reality. Nursing Standards 2: 50–53

Sayre-Adams J 1993 Therapeutic touch: principles and practice. Complementary Therapies in Medicine 1(2): 96–99

Schaffner M 1981 Faith and the healing process. Your Life and Health 96(11): 21–23

Schaut G, Persinger M 1985 Geophysical variables and behavior: XXXI. Global geomagnetic activity during spontaneous paranormal experiences: a replication. Perceptual and Motor Skills 61: 412–414

Scheiber B 1993 Colorado board of nursing supports therapeutic touch, skeptics continue challenge. Skeptical Inquirer 17(3): 327–330

Scheiber B 1994 University of Colorado report critical of therapeutic touch. Skeptical Inquirer 18(3): 232–234

Scheiber B 1997 Therapeutic touch: evaluating the 'growing body of evidence' claim. Scientific Review of Alternative Medicine 1(1): 13–15

Scheiber B, Selby C 1997 UAB final report of therapeutic touch: an appraisal. Skeptical Inquirer 21(3): 53–54

Schlitz M 1982 Psi induction rituals. In: Roll W, Morris R, White R (eds) Research in parapsychology 1981. Scarecrow Press, Metuchen, NJ, pp. 39–40

Schlitz M 1996 Intentionality: a program of study. Advances: the Journal of Mind-Body Health 12(3): 31–32

Schlitz M, Braud W 1997 Distant intentionality and healing: assessing the evidence. Alternative Therapies in Health and Medicine 3(6): 62–73

Schlitz M, LaBerge S 1994 Autonomic nervous system detection of remote observation. Paper presented at the Proceedings of the 37th Annual Convention of the Parapsychological Associations, Amsterdam, Netherlands

Schlotfeldt R 1973 Critique of the relationship of touch with intent to help or heal to subjects' in-vivo hemoglobin values: a study in personalized interaction. Paper presented at the Proceedings of the Ninth ANA Nursing Research Conference, NY, for the American Nursing Association, pp 59–65

Schmidt H 1970 Quantum mechanical random number generator. Journal of Applied Physics 41: 462–468

Schmidt H 1975 Toward a mathematical theory of psi. Journal of the American Society for Psychical Research 69(4): 301–319

Schmidt H 1978 Can an effect precede its cause? A model of a noncausal world. Found Physics 8(5/6): 463–480

Schmidt H 1981 PK test with pre-inspected and prerecorded seed numbers. Journal of Parapsychology 45: 87–98

Schmidt H 1982 Collapse of the state vector and psychokinetic effects. Found Physics 12(6): 565–581

Schmidt H 1984 Superposition of PK efforts by man and dog. In: White R, Broughton R (eds) Research in parapsychology 1983. Scarecrow Press, Metuchen, NJ, pp. 96–98

Schmidt H 1991 Search for a correlation between PK performance and heart rate. Journal of the American Society for Psychical Research 85(2): 101–118

Schmidt H 1994 Thoughts and experiments on mind-matter interactions. Center for Frontier Sciences 4(1): 22–24

Schmidt H, Braud W 1992 New PK tests with an outside observer. Journal of Parapsychology 57: 227–240

Schneider R, Binder M, Walach H (2000) Examining the role of neutral versus personal experimenter–participant interactions: An EDA-DMILS experiment. Journal of Parapsychology 64: 181–194

Schoenberger L, Braswell C 1971 Music therapy in rehabilitation. Journal of Rehabilitation 37: 30

Schopenhauer A 1974 Transcendent speculation on the apparent deliberateness in the fate of the individual. In: Payne E (ed) Pererga and paralipomena: short philosophical essays. Clarendon Press, Oxford, England, pp. 201–223

Schopler E 1962 The development of body image and symbol formation through body contact with an autistic child. Journal of Child Psychology 3: 191–202

Schorr J 1993 Music and pattern change in chronic pain. Advances in Nursing Science 15: 27–36

Schouten S A 1993 Psychic healing and complementary medicine. European Journal of Parapsychology 9: 35–92

Schreiber K 1991 Religion in the physician–patient relationship. Journal of the American Medical Association 266(21): 3062–3064

Schuetz B 1995 Spirituality and palliative care. Australian Family Physician 24(5): 775–777

Schult, A 1991 Self-care activating support: therapeutic touch and chronic skin disease. Dermatologic Nursing 3: 335–339

Schultz-Ross R A, Gutheil T G 1997 Difficulties in integrating spirituality into psychotherapy. Journal of Psychotherapy Practice and Research 6(2): 130–138

Schuster S J 1997 Wholistic care: healing a 'sick' system. Nursing Management 28(6): 56–59; quiz 60

Schwartz S 1990 Creativity, intuition, and innovation. Subtle Energies 1(2): i–x

Schwartz S 1990 Therapeutic intent and the art of observation. Subtle Energies 1(1): ii–viii.

Schwartz S 1991 The challenge and the promise of subtle energies and energy medicine research. Subtle Energies 2(1): i–xv

Schwartz G, Brame E, Spottiswoode J 1991 Response to the Savva critique. Subtle Energies 2(2): 76–82

Schwartz G E, Russek L G, Shapiro L, Harada P 1999 Loving openness as a meta-world hypothesis: expanding our vision of mind and medicine. Advances in Mind Body Medicine 15(1): 5–19

Schwartz J 1979 Human energy systems: a way of good health using our electromagnetic fields. Arkana, New York

Schwartz M D, Hughes C, Roth J et al 2000 Spiritual faith and genetic testing decisions among high-risk breast cancer probands. Cancer Epidemiology, Biomarkers and Prevention 9(4): 381–385

Seaward B 2000 Stress and human spitituality 2000: at the cross roads of physics and metaphysics. Applied Psychophysiology and Biofeedback 25(4): 241–246

Seaward B L 2000 Stress and human spirituality: at the crossroads of mind–body–spirit healing. Journal of the Michigan Dental Association 82(4): 28–32, 34

Sedei G, Cheryl A 1987 The use of music therapy in pain clinics. Music Therapy Perspectives 4: 24–28

Seiden H M 1996 The healing presence: Part I. The witness as self-object function. Psychoanalysis Review 83(5): 685–693

Seiden H M 1997 The healing presence, Part II. What the analyst says. Psychoanalysis Review 84(1): 17–26

Seidl L G 1993 The value of spiritual health. Health Progress 74(7): 48–50

Selby C, Scheiber B 1996 Science or pseudoscience? Pentagon grant funds alternative health study. Skeptical Inquirer 20(2): 15–17

Selm M 1991 Chronic pain: three issues in treatment and implications for music therapy. Music Therapy Perspectives 9: 91–97

Sevensky R 1981 Religion and illness: an outline of their relationship. Southern Medical Journal 74: 745–750

Sevensky R 1983 The religious foundations of health care: a conceptual approach. Journal of Medical Ethics 9: 165–169

Shaara L, Strathern A 1992 A preliminary analysis of the relationship between altered states of consciousness, healing, and social structure. University of Pittsburgh, Department of Anthropology, Pittsburgh

Shacklett R, Gough W 1991 The unification of mind and matter: a proposed scientific model. Foundation for Mind–Being Research, Los Altos CA

Shealy C N 1975 The role of psychics in medical diagnosis. In: Carlson R (ed) Frontiers of science and medicine. Contemporary Books, New York

Shealy C N 1988 Clairvoyant diagnosis. In: Srinivasan T M (ed) Energy medicine around the world. Gabriel Press, Phoenix, AZ

Sheldon M G 1992 Spirituality, healing and medicine. British Journal of General Practice 42(354): 38

Sheldrake R 1994 Prayer: a challenge for science. Noetic Sciences Review 30: 5–6

Sheldrake R 1998 Experimenter effects in scientific research: how widely are they neglected? Journal of Scientific Exploration 12(1): 73–78

Sherrill K, Larson D 1988 Adult burn patients: the role of religion in recovery. Southern Medical Journal 81(7): 821–825

Sherill K, Larson D 1994 The anti-tenure factor in religious research in clinical epidemiology and aging. In: Levin J (ed) Religion in aging and health: theoretical foundations and methodological frontiers. Sage Publishers, Thousand Oaks, CA, pp. 149–177

Shinagawa Y 1990 Ki and image. In: Yuasa Y (ed) Ki and human science. Hirakawa Shuppan, Tokyo

Sieggreen M 1987 Healing of physical wounds. Nursing Clinics of North America 22: 439–447

Silva M C, DeLashmutt M 1998 Spirituality and prayer: a new age paradigm for ethics. Nursing Connections 11(2): 13–17

Skelly C, Haslerud G 1954 Music and general activity in apathetic schizophrenics. In Podolsky E (ed.), Music Therapy. Philosophical Library, New York.

Skultans O 1976 Empathy and healing. In: Landon I (ed) Social anthropology and medicine. Academic Press, New York

Sloan R, Bagiella E 2000 Data without a prayer. Archives of Internal Medicine 160(12): 1870

Sloan R, Bagiella E, Powell T 1999 Religion, spirituality, and medicine. Lancet 353(9153): 664–667

Sloan R, Bagiella E, Vandecreek L, Hover M, Casalone C 2000 Sounding board: should physicians prescribe religious activities? New England Journal of Medicine 342(25): 1913–1916

Slomski A 2000 Should doctors prescribe religion? Medical Economics 77(1): 145–159

Smet W 1954 Religious experience in client-centered therapy. In: Arnold M, Gasson J (eds) The human person. Ronald Press, New York

Smith C 1998 Is a living system a macroscopic quantum system? Frontier Perspectives 7(1): 9

Smith C 1994 Electromagnetic bio-information and water. In: Endler PC, Schulte J (Eds) Ultra high dilutions – physiology and physics. Kluwer Academic, London

Smith D E 1994 AA recovery and spirituality: an addiction medicine perspective. Journal of Substance Abuse and Treatment 11(2): 111–112

Smith I W, Airey S, Salmond S W 1990 CE feature. Part 2. Nontechnologic strategies for coping with chronic low back pain. Orthopedic Nursing 9(4): 26–34

Smith M 1972 The influence on enzyme growth by the 'laying on of hands'. The dimensions of healing: a symposium. Academy of Parapsychology and Medicine, Los Altos, CA, pp. 110–120

Smith M 1977 The influence of 'laying-on' of hands. In: Regush N (ed) Frontiers of healing. Avon Books, New York

Smucker C J 1998 Nursing, healing and spirituality. Complementary Therapies and Nursing Midwifery 4(4): 95–97

Smyth P, Bellemare D 1988 Spirituality, pastoral care, and religion: the need for clear distinctions. Journal of Palliative Care 4(1–2): 86–88

Sneider R 1998 Asking the hard questions about prayer. Alternative Therapies in Health and Medicine 4(2): 20–22

Snell J 1965 The use of music in group psychotherapy. In: Masserman J (ed) Current psychiatric therapies. Grune, New York

Sobel D S 1993 Mind matters, money matters: the cost-effectiveness of clinical behavioral medicine. Mental Medicine Update Special Report, pp. 1–8

Soeken K L, Carson V J 1987 Responding to the spiritual needs of the chronically ill. Nursing Clinics of North America 22(3): 603–611

Solfvin G 1983 Towards a model for mental healing studies in real life settings. In: Roll W, Beloff J, White R (eds) Research in parapsychology 1982. Scarecrow Press, Metuchen, NJ, pp. 210–214

Solfvin J 1984 Mental healing. In: Krippner S (ed) Advances in parapsychology research. McFarland, Jefferson, NC, vol. 4, p. 31

Solzhenitsyn A 1978 A world split apart: the world demands from us a spiritual blaze. Vital Speeches of the Day 45: 678–684

Spero M 1982 Identity and individuality in the nouveau-religious patient: theoretical and clinical aspects. Psychiatry 50: 55–71

Spiegel D 1990 Can psychotherapy prolong cancer survival? Psychosomatics 31(4): 361–366

Spindrift I 1993 The Spindrift papers. Spindrift, Lansdale, PA

Spivak C Hebrew prayers for the sick. Annals of Medical History 83–85

Srinivasan T 1993 The unity of one. Subtle Energies 4(3): i–v

Srinivasan T 1993 The paradox of holism. Subtle Energies 4(3): 215–230

Srinivasan T 1993 The matter of energy. Subtle Energies 4(2): i–iv

Stallwook J, Part C 1975 Spiritual dimensions of nursing practice. In: Beland I, Passos J (eds) Clinical nursing: pathophysiological and psychosocial approaches. Macmillan, New York

Stanford R G 1993 Learning to lure the rabbit: Charles Honorton's process-relevent ESP research. Journal of Parapsychology 57(2): 129–175

Stark R 1984 Religion and conformity: reaffirming a sociology of religion. Soci Anal 45: 273–282

Stark R, Bainbridge W 1980 Towards a theory of religious commitment. Journal of the Scientific Study of Religion 19: 114–128

Stark R, Doyle D, Rushing J 1983 Beyond Durkheim: religion and suicide. Journal of the Scientific Study of Religion 22(2): 120–131

Stefanatos J 1997 Introduction to bioenergetic medicine. In: Schoen A, Wynn S (eds) Complementary and alternative veterinary medicine: principles and practice. Mosby-Year Book, St Louis, MO

Steinitz L 1980 Religiosity, well-being, and Weltanschauung among the elderly. Journal of the Scientific Study of Religion 19: 60–67

Stenger V 1999 Bioenergetic fields. Scientific Review of Alternative Medicine 3(1): 16–21

Stern K 1955 Some spiritual aspects of psychotherapy. In: Braceland F (ed) Faith, reason, and modern psychiatry. Kennedy, New York

Stoll R 1979 Guidelines for spiritual assessment. American Journal of Nursing 9: 1574–1577

Stolley J M, Koenig H 1997 Religion/spirituality and health among elderly African Americans and Hispanics. Journal of Psychosocial Nursing and Mental Health Services 35(11): 32–38

Strang S, Strang P 2001 Spiritual thoughts, coping and 'sense of coherence' in brain tumour patients and their spouses. Palliative Medicine 15(2): 127–134

Struzzo J A 1989 Pastoral counseling and homosexuality. Journal of Homosexuality 18(3–4): 195–222

Stuart E M, Deckro J P, Mandle C L 1989 Spirituality in health and healing: a clinical program. Holistic Nursing Practice 3(3): 35–46

Sugerman D 1996 Healing body and spirit. Minnesota Medicine 79(12): 8–9, 44–45

Sulmasy D P 1999 Is medicine a spiritual practice? Academic Medicine 74(9): 1002–1005

Swan R 1983 Faith healing, Christian science, and the medical care of children. New England Journal of Medicine 309(26): 1639–1641

Targ E 1996 The continuum of intention. Advances: the Journal of Mind-Body Health 12(3): 32–35

Targ E, Thomson K 1997 Can prayer and intentionality be researched? Should they be? Alternative Therapies in Health and Medicine 3: 92–96

Targ R 1996 Remote viewing at Stanford Research Institute in the 1970s: a memoir. Journal of Scientific Exploration 10(1): 77–88

Targ R, Katra J 2001 The scientific and spiritual implications of psychic abilities. Alternative Therapies in Health and Medicine 7(3): 143–149

Tart C 1988 Geomagnetic effects on GESP: two studies. Journal of the American Society for Psychical Research 82(3): 193–216

Tauber A I 1991 On pigeons, physicians and placebos. Journal of the Royal Society of Medicine 84: 328–331

Taylor R 1985 The reiki touch. The Movement Newspaper, October p. 3

Taylor E 1998 Eugene Taylor, PhD on spiritual healing and the American visionary tradition. Interview by Bonnie Horrigan. Alternative Therapies in Health and Medicine 4(6): 78–87

Taylor E 2000 Retroactive intentional influence: a new science based on a new psychology? Alternative Therapies 6(1): 34–36

Taylor E J, Amenta M 1994 Midwifery to the soul while the body dies: spiritual care among hospice nurses. American Journal of Hospice and Palliative Care 11(6): 28–35

Taylor T K 1978 The laying on of hands. Australian and New Zealand Journal of Medicine 8(6): 587–588

Tedder W, Monty M 1981 Exploration of long-distance PK: a conceptual replication of the influence on a biological system. Research in Parapsychology 1980. Scarcrow Press, Metuchen, NJ, pp. 90–93

Tesla N 1904 Transmission of energy without wires. Scientific American 57: (Suppl.): 237

Thomas J, Schrot J, Liboff A 1986 Low-intensity magnetic fields alter operant behavior in rats. Bioelectromagnetics 7(4): 349–357

Thomas S A 1989 Spirituality: an essential dimension in the treatment of hypertension. Holistic Nursing Practice 3(3): 47–55

Thomas-Beckett J 1991 Attitudes toward therapeutic touch: a pilot study of women with breast cancer. Unpublished Master's thesis, Michigan State University

Thomason C L, Brody H 1999 Inclusive spirituality. Journal of Family Practice 48(2): 96–97

Thompson B 1985 The mysterious healing power of reiki. East-West Journal, pp. 50–54

Thomsen R J 1998 Spirituality in medical practice. Archives of Dermatology 134(11): 1443–1446

Thomson J E 2000 The place of spiritual well-being in hospice patients' overall quality of life. Hospice Journal 15(2): 13–27

Thomson K 1997 Miracles on demand: prayer and the causation of healing [editorial]. Alternative Therapies in Health and Medicine 3: 92–96

Thornton L 1996 A study of Reiki, an energy treatment, using Roger's science. Rogerian Nursing Science News 8: 14–15

Thorson J, Powell F 1991 Life, death, and life after death: meanings of the relationship between death anxiety and religion. Journal of Religion and Gerontology 8(1): 41–56

Tibesar L J 1986 AIDS: responding to the crisis. Pastoral care: helping patients on an inward journey. Health Progress 67(4): 41–47

Tickle L 2000 Positive thinking can kill cancer cells, say psychologists. UK News, April 16, p. 3

Tieman J 2001 Healing through nature: hospitals cultivate medical, financial interest in on-site gardens. Modern Healthcare 31(2): 34–35

Tiller W 1982 Explanation of electrodermal diagnostic and treatment instruments: Part I. Electrical behavior of human skin. Journal of Holistic Medicine 4(2): 105–127

Tiller W 1993 What are subtle energies? Journal of Scientific Exploration 7: 293

Tiller W 1994 But is it energy? Reflections on consciousness, healing and the new paradigm. Subtle Energies 5(3): 253–271

Tiller W 1995 Towards explaining anomalously large body voltage surges on exceptional subjects, Part I. The electrostatic approximation. Journal of Scientific Exploration 8(3): 438

Tiller W 1999 Towards a predictive model of subtle domain connections to the physical domain aspect of reality: the origins of wave-particle duality, electric-magnetic monopoles and the mirror principle. Journal of Scientific Exploration 13(1): 41–67

Tiller W, Dibble W, Kohane M 1997 Towards objectifying intention via electronic devices. Subtle Energies 8(2): 103–122

Tilley C 1996 Advanced Institute stresses personal assessment, spirituality. Health Progress 77(4): 90

Tilley J 1989 A phenomenology of the Christian healer's experience (faith healing). Unpublished Doctoral dissertation, Fuller Theological Seminary, Pasadena, CA

Tobin S 1991 Preserving the self through religion. In: Tobin S (ed) Personhood in advanced old age: implications for practice. Springer, New York, Ch. 6, pp. 119–133

Toperzer R 1998 Considering the dangers and opportunities of pastoral care and medicine: a search for vitality, accountability and balance. Journal of Health Care and Chaplaincy 7(1–2): 117–122

Travaline J M, D'Alonzo G E 2000 Spirituality in medicine. Journal of American Osteopathic Association 100(12): 775

Troyer H 1988 Review of cancer among 4 religious sects: evidence that life-styles are distinctive sets of risk factors. Social Science and Medicine 26: 1007–1017

Tuck I, Wallace D, Pullen L 2001 Spirituality and spiritual care provided by parish nurses. Western Journal of Nursing Research 23(5): 441–453; discussion 454–462

Turner R, Lukoff D, Barnhouse R, Lu F 1995 Religious or spiritual problem: a culturally sensitive diagnostic category in the DSM-IV. Journal of Nervous and Mental Disease 183: 435–444

Tyagotin Y, Bondarenko Y 1991 A study of peculiarities of growth of hybrid cells after they are affected by biofield of a human operator. In: Kogan I (ed) Mezhregionalnaya nauchnaya konferentsiya: problemy biopolya. AS Popov Society, Russia

Ulett G 1997 Therapeutic touch: tracing back to Mesmer. Scientific Review of Alternative Medicine 1(1): 16–18

Underwood-Gordon L, Peters D J, Bijur P, Fuhrer M 1997 Roles of religiousness and spirituality in medical rehabilitation and the lives of persons with disabilities: a commentary. American Journal of Physical and Medical Rehabilitation 76(3): 255–257

Upledger J 1995 Craniosacral therapy: Part I. Its origins and development. Subtle Energies 6(1): 1–53

Upledger J 1995 Craniosacral therapy: Part III. In the future. Subtle Energies 6(3): 201–216

Utts J 1991 Replication and meta-analysis in parapsychology. Statistical Science 6(4): 363–403

Utts J 1999 The significance of statistics in mind–matter research. Journal of Scientific Exploration 13(4): 615–638

Valentine J 1982 Towards a physics of consciousness. Psychoenergetics 4: 257–274

Van der Does W 2000 A randomized, controlled trial of prayer? Archives of Internal Medicine 160(12): 1871–1872

Van Tilburg E 1991 Meditation and palliative care. CHAC Review 19(2): 9–12

Vanderpool H, Levin J 1990 Religion and medicine: how are they related? Journal of Religion and Health 29: 9–20

Vandragt B 1980 Paranormal healing: a phenomenology of the healer's experience. Fuller Theological Seminary, Pasadena, CA, vols 1–2

Vaughan A, Houck J 1991 Software for training anomalous cognition: a preliminary report. Subtle Energies 2(2): 29–53

Vaughan F 1991 Spiritual issues in psychotherapy. Journal of Transpersonal Psychology 23(2): 104–119

Vaughan S 1995 The gentle touch. Journal of Clinical Nursing 4: 359–368

Vaux K 1976 Religion and health. Preventive Medicine 5: 522–536

Vecsey G 1978 Spiritual healing gaining ground with Catholics and Episcopalians. New York Times, June 18, pp. 1, 20

Vilenskaya L, May E 1993 Anomalous mental phenomena research in Russia and the former soviet union: a follow-up. Subtle Energies 4(3): 231–250

Voljc B 1997 On the spirituality of the doctor–patient relationship. Annals of New York Academy of Science 809: 80–82

Walach H, Romer H 2000 Complementarity is a useful concept for consciousness studies: a reminder. Neuroendocrinology Letters 21: 221–232

Waldfogel S 1997 Spirituality in medicine. Primary Care 24(4): 963–976

Waldram J B 1993 Aboriginal spirituality: symbolic healing in Canadian prisons. Culture, Medicine and Psychiatry 17(3): 345–362

Walike, Bruno, Donaldson et al 1975 Letter. American Journal of Nursing 75(8): 1275, 1278, 1292

Walker E 1975 Foundations of parapsychical and parapsychological phenomena. In: Oteri L (ed) Quantum Physics in Parapsychology. Parapsychology Foundation, New York, NY, pp. 1–53

Walker E H 1977 The complete quantum mechanical anthropologist: the physical basis for paranormal events. In: Long J K (ed) Extrasensory ecology. Scarecrow Press, London, pp. 53–95

Walker E 1979 The quantum theory of psi phenomena. Psychoenergetic Systems 3: 259–299

Walleczek J 1993 Bioelectromagnetics and the question of subtle energies. Noetic Sciences Review 28: 33–36

Walsh A 1980 The prophylactic effect of religion on blood pressure levels among a sample of immigrants. Social Science and Medicine 14B: 56–63

Walters O 1964 Religion and psychopathology. Comprehensive Psychiatry 5: 24–35

Walton J, St Clair K 2000 'A beacon of light': spirituality in the heart transplant patient. Critical Care Nursing Clinics of North America 12(1): 87–101

Wardwell W 1965 Christian science healing. Journal of the Scientific Study of Religion 4: 175–181

Washburn T C 1991 Humor can facilitate health. Archives of Internal Medicine 151(6): 1237

Wasserman N 1972 Music therapy for the emotionally disturbed in a private hospital. Journal of Music Therapy 9(2): 99

Watkins A 1996 Intention and the electromagnetic activity of the heart. Advances: the Journal of Mind–Body Health 12(3): 35

Watt C, Ravenscroft J, McDermott Z 1999 Exploring the limits of direct mental influence: two studies comparing blocking and co-operating strategies. Journal of Scientific Exploration 13: 515–535

Weaver J, Astumain R 1990 The response of living cells to very weak electric fields: the thermal noise limit. Science 247: 459–462

Weaver A J, Flannelly L T, Flannelly K J, Koenig H G, Larson D B 1998 An analysis of research on religious and spiritual variables in three major mental health nursing journals, 1991–1995. Issues in Mental Health Nursing 19(3): 263–276

Weber R 1984 Philosophical foundations and framework for healing. American Theosophist 72: 176–189

Weber C 1997 From hospital to holistic nursing practice. Alternative and Complementary Therapies 3(1): 64–66

Weil A, Smith H 1995 Roots of healing: the new medicine. Alternative Therapies in Health and Medicine 1(2): 46–52

Weiss S 1979 The language of touch. Nursing Research 28: 76–80

Wells R, Watkins G 1975 Linger effects in several PK experiments. Research in Parapsychology 1974. Scarecrow Press, Metuthen, NJ, pp. 143–147

Wertheimer N, Leeper E 1979 Electrical wiring configuration and childhood cancer. American Journal of Epidemiology 109(3): 273–284

Wesch J 1996 After the white crow: integrating science and anomalous experience. Subtle Energies and Energy Medicine 7(1): 1–22

Westlake C, Dracup K 2001 Role of spirituality in adjustment of patients with advanced heart failure. Progress in Cardiovascular Nursing 16(3): 119–125

Wetzel M 1989 Reiki healing: a physiologic perspective. Journal of Holistic Nursing 7(1): 47–53

Wigner E 1962 Remark on the mind body problem. In: Good I (ed) Scientific Speculates. Basic Books, New York, pp. 284–302

Williams D 1994 The measurement of religion in epidemiologic studies. In: Levin J (ed) Religion, aging and health. Sage, London, pp. 125–148

Williams M E 1991 Spirituality of the elderly. AARN News Letters 47(4): 25–27

Wilson J 1978 The measurement of religiosity. In: Wilson J (ed) Religion in American society. Prentice-Hall, Englewood Cliffs, NJ

Wilson J S Jr 1998 Miracles: quirks of nature or the hand of God. Journal of the Medical Association of Georgia 87(4): 291–293

Wilson W 1988 Religion in healing. Southern Medical Journal 81(7): 819–820

Wilson B, Wright C, Morris J et al 1990 Evidence of an effect of ELF electromagnetic fields on human pineal gland function. Journal of Pineal Research 9: 259–269

Winkelman M 1986 Magico-religious practitioner types and socioeconomic conditions. Behavioral Sciences Research 20: 17–46

Winkelman M 1990 Physiological and therapeutic aspects of shamanistic healing. Subtle Energies 1(2): 1–18

Winstead-Fry P 1987 Therapeutic touch during childbirth preparation by the Lamaze method and its relation to marital satisfaction and state anxiety of the married couple. In: Krieger D (ed) Living the therapeutic touch. Dodd, Mead and Co., New York, pp. 157–188

Wirth D 1993 Implementing spiritual healing in modern medical practice. Advances: the Journal of Mind-Body Health 9(4): 69–81

Wirth D 1994 The cultural significance of belief and expectancy within the spiritual healing encounter

Wootton J 1999 Qigong and energy medicine: a challenge to the peer-review process. Journal of Alternative and Complementary Medicine 5(4): 317

Wootton J 1999 The role of traditional healers in the fight against AIDS in Africa. Journal of Alternative and Complementary Medicine 5(3): 225–228

Worthington E 1989 Religious faith across the life span: implications for counseling and research. Counseling Psychologist 17(4): 555–612

Wright S 1987 The use of therapeutic touch in the management of pain. Nursing Clinics of North America 22(3): 705–714

Wright S 1994 Therapeutic touch and healing touch: what is the difference? Cooperative Connection: Newsletter of the Nurse Healers-Professional Associates 15: 1–3

Wytias C 1994 Therapeutic touch in primary care. Nursing Practice Forum 5(2): 91–97

Xu S 1994 Psychophysiological reactions associated with qigong therapy. Chinese Medical Journal (Engl) 107: 230–233

Yan X, Li S, Lu Z 1988 Laser raman observation on tap water, saline, glucose and medemycine solutions under the influence of the external qi of qigong. Chongqing Institute of Chinese Medicine, Qing Hua University Institute of High Energy Physics, Sichuan, China

Yan X, Zheng C, Zhou G, Lu Z 1988 The observation of the effect of the external qi of qigong on the ultraviolet absorption of nucleic acid solutions. Chongqing Institute of Traditional Chinese Medicine, Qinghua University Institute of High Energy Physics, Sichuan, China

Yan Z, Lu Z, Yan S, Li S 1988 Measurement of the effects of external qi on the polarization plane of a linearly polarized laser beam. Chongqing Institute of Traditional Chinese Medicine, Institute of High Energy Physics Qinghua University, Sichuan, China

Yates P, Beadle G, Clavarino A, Najman J, Thomson D, Wiliams G 1993 Patients with terminal cancer who use alternative therapies: their beliefs and practices. Sociology Health Illness 15(2): 205–216

Yauger R 1976 A note on religious beliefs and coronary heart disease. Journal of South Carolina Medical Association Supplement (February): 60–64

Young C 1993 Spirituality and the chronically ill Christian elderly. Geriatric Nursing 14(6): 298–303

Zefron L 1975 The history of the laying-on of hands in nursing. Nursing Forum 15: 350–363

Ziegler J 1998 Spirituality returns to the fold in medical practice. Journal of the National Cancer Institute 90(17): 1255–1257

Zimmerman J 1985 New technologies detect effects of healing hands. Brain/Mind Bulletin 10: 16

Zinnbauer B, Pargament K, Cowell B, Rye M, Scott A 1997 Religion and spirituality: unfuzzing the fuzzy. Journal of the Scientific Study of Religion 38: 412–423

Zlokazov V, Pushkin V, Shevchik E 1982 Bioenergetic aspects of the relationship between the image of perception and the perceived object. Psi Research 1(3): 11–21

Zylberbaum J, Ramos J 1987 Patterns of interhemispheric correlates during human communication. International Journal of Neuroscience 36: 41–53

Selected Books

Achterberg J 1985 Imagery in healing: shamanism and modern medicine. Shambhala, Boston

Alcock J 1981 Parapsychology: science or magic? A psychological perspective. Pergamon Press, Elmsford, NY

Aldridge D 2000 Music therapy in dementia care. Jessica Kingsley, London

Aldridge D 2000 Spirituality, healing and medicine: return to the science. Jessica Kingsley, London

Allport G 1950 The individual and his religion. Macmillan, New York

Alvin J 1966 Music therapy. Hutchison, New York

Angelo J 1991 Spiritual healing: energy medicine for today. Element, Shaftesbury

Arnold L, Nevius S 1982 The reiki handbook: a manual for students and therapists. PSI Press, Harrisburg, PA

Baginski B, Shanamon S 1988 Reiki: universal life energy. Life Rhythm Publishers, Mendocino, CA

Barnett L, Chambers M, Davidson S 1996 Reiki: energy medicine, bringing healing touch into home, hospital, and practice. Healing Arts Press, Rochester, VT

Barrow J, Tipler F 1986 The anthropic cosmological principle. Oxford University Press, Oxford, England

Batson C, Ventis W 1982 The religious experience. Oxford University Press, New York

Becker R 1990 Cross currents: the promise of electro-medicine Los Angeles, CA

Becker R, Marino A 1982 Electomagnetism and life. SUNY Press, New York, NY

Becker R, Selden G 1985 The body electric: electromagnetism and the foundation of life. William Morrow, New York

Benor D 1994 Healing research: holistic energy medicine and spirituality. Helix Verlag, Munich, Germany

Benor D 2001 Spiritual healing: Scientific validation of a healing revolution. Vision, Southfield, MI

Benor D J 1993 Research in healing. Helix Books, England, vol. 1

Benor D J (ed) 1993 Healing research. Helix Verlag, Munich, Germany

Berkman L, Breslow L 1983 Health and ways of living: the Alameda County study. Oxford University Press, New York

Bohm D 1980 Wholeness and the implicate order. Routledge and Kegan Paul, London

Borelli M, Heidt P (eds) 1981 Therapeutic touch: a book of readings. Springer, New York

Borysenko J 1993 Fire in the soul: a new psychology of spiritual optimism. Warner Books, New York

Bowles N, Hynds F, Maxwell J 1978 Psi search. Harper and Row, San Francisco, CA

Bragdon E 1990 The call of spiritual emergency: from personal crisis to personal transformation. Harper and Row, San Francisco, CA

Brennen B 1988 Hands of light: a guide to healing through the human energy field. Bantam New Age Books, New York

Briggs J, Peat F D 1989 Turbulent mirror. Harper and Row, New York

Broad C 1953 Religion, philosophy and psychical research. Harcourt Brace, New York

Broughton R S 1991 Parapsychology: the controversial science. Ballantine Books, New York

Bullough V, Bullough B 1978 Care of the sick: the emergence of modern nursing. Science History/Prodist Books, New York

Burr H 1972 The fields of life: our links to the universe. Ballantine Books, New York

Capra F 1975 The Tao of Physics. Shambhala Publications, Berkeley, CA

Cardena E, Lynn S, Krippner S Varieties of anomalous experience. American Psychological Association, Washington, DC

Carson V 1989 Spiritual dimensions of nursing practice. Saunders, Philadelphia

Casdorph R 1976 The miracles. Logos International, Plainfield, New Jersey

Chopra D 1990 Quantum healing: exploring the frontiers of mind/body medicine. Bantam Books, New York

Chuen L 1991 The way of energy. Gaia Books, London

Church D, Serr A (eds) 1987 The heart of the healer. Aslan Publishing, New York

Churchland P 1984 Matter and consciousness: a contemporary introduction to the philosophy of mind. MIT Press, Bradford Books, Cambridge

Clements W 1989 Religion, aging, and health: a global perspective. Haworth Press, New York

Cohen K 1997 The way of qigong. Ballantine Books, New York

Coles R 1990 The spiritual life of children. Houghton Mifflin, Boston

Collins G 1977 The rebuilding of psychology: an integration of psychology and Christianity. Tyndale House, Wheaton, IL

Collins H 1982 Frames of meaning: the social construction of extraordinary science. Routledge and Kegan Paul, Boston

Cooper J 1979 The ancient teaching of yoga and the spiritual evolution of man. Research, London

Crick F 1994 The astonishing hypothesis: the scientific search for the soul. Simon and Simon, London

Critchley M, Henson R (eds) 1977 Music and the brain: studies in the neurology of music. Heinemann, London

Crossan J D 1992 The historical Jesus. HarperCollins, New York

Dean D 1986 The mystery of healing. Search, Buffalo, NY

Dethlefsen T, Dahlke R 1990 The healing power of illness. Element Press, Longmead, England

Doka K, Morgan J 1993 Death and spirituality. Baywood, Amityville, NY

Dollard J 1983 Toward spirituality: the inner journey. Hazelden, Center City, NM

Dossey L 1993 Healing words: the power of prayer and the practice of medicine. HarperSanFrancisco, San Francisco, CA

Dossey L 1998 Be careful what you pray for ... you just might get it. HarperCollins, New York

Dossey L 1999 Reinventing medicine: beyond mind–body to a new era of healing. HarperCollins, New York

Druckman D, Swets J A (eds) 1988 Enhancing human performance: issues, theories, and techniques. National Academy Press, Washington, DC

Eddy M 1971 Science and health with key to the scriptures. First Church of Christ Scientist, Boston, MA

Edge H, Morris R, Rush J, Palmer J 1986 Foundations of parapsychology. Routledge and Kegan Paul, New York

Edmunds V, Scorer G 1979 Some thoughts on faith healing, 3rd edn. Christian Medical Fellowship Publications, London

Edwards H 1945 The science of spiritual healing. Rider, London, UK

Eeman L 1947 Cooperative healing. Frederick Muller, London

Eisenbud J 1982 Paranormal foreknowledge. Human Sciences Press, New York

Eliade M 1958 Yoga: immortality and freedom. Princeton University Press, New York

Eliade M 1970 Shamanism. Routledge and Kegan Paul, London

Evans D 1993 Spirituality and human nature. SUNY, Albany, NY

Eysenk H, Sargent C 1982 Explaining the unexplained. Weidenfeld and Nicolson, London

Fadiman A 1998 The spirit catches you and you fall down. Farrar Straus and Giroux, New York

Feltman J (ed) 1991 Hands on healing. Rodeo Press, Pennsylvania

Fleischman P 1990 The healing spirit. Paragon House, New York

Foster D, Marty M, Vaux K 1982 Religion and medicine: the physicians' perspective. Fortress Press, Philadelphia

Fowler J 1981 Stages in faith. Harper and Row, San Francisco

Francis B 1993 Opening the energy gates of your body. North Atlantic Books, Berkeley, CA

Frank J 1961 Persuasion and healing. Johns Hopkins University Press, Baltimore, MD

Frank J 1973 Persuasion and healing, 2nd edn. Johns Hopkins University Press, Baltimore, MD

Gerber R 1988 Vibrational medicine: new choices for healing ourselves. Bear, Santa Fe, NM

Gersten D, Dossey L 1998 Are you getting enlightened or losing your mind?: how to master everyday and extraordinary spiritual experiences. Three Rivers Press, New York

Goldberg S 1999 Seduced by science: how American religion has lost its way. New York University Press, New York

Govinda A 1976 Creative meditation and multidimensional consciousness. Quest Books, Wheaton, IL

Greeley A 1975 The sociology of the paranormal: a reconnaissance. Sage, Beverly Hills, CA

Griffin D 1997 Parapsychology, philosophy, and spirituality: a postmodern exploration. State University of New York Press, Albany, NY

Grof C 1993 Thirst for wholeness: attachment, addiction, and the spiritual path. HarperCollins, San Francisco, CA

Grof S, Grof C (eds) 1989 Spiritual emergency: when personal transformation becomes a crisis. Tarcher, Los Angeles, NV

Gundling D 1996 Musical massage sound therapy. Morris Publishing, Kearney, NE

Haberly H 1990 Reiki: the Hawayo Takatas story. Archedign Publishers, CA

Hagelin J 1987 Is consciousness the unified field? A field theorist's perspective. Maharishi International University, Iowa

Hamburg D, Elliott G, Parron D (eds) 1982 Health and behavior: frontiers of research in the biobehavioral sciences. National Academy Press, Washington, DC

Harman W, DeQuincey C 1994 The scientific exploration of consciousness: toward an adequate epistemology. Institute of Noetic Sciences, Sausalito, CA

Harman W W 1991 A re-examination of the metaphysical foundations of modern science. Institute of Noetic Sciences, Sausalito, CA

Harner M 1980 The way of the shaman. Harper and Row, New York

Harvey D 1983 The power to heal: an investigation of healing and the healing experience. Aquarian, Wellingborough, England

Heim B 1989 (revised) Elementarstrukturen der Materie. Resch Verlag, Innsbruck, Austria

Herbert N 1987 Quantum reality. Anchor Books, New York

Herbert N 1993 Elemental mind: human consciousness and the new physics. Dutton, New York

Hirschberg C, Barasch M 1995 Remarkable recovery: what extraordinary healings tell us about getting well and staying well. Putnam, New York

Hutschnecker A 1953 The will to live. Putnam, New York

Hyman R 1987 Shifting worlds, changing minds. Shambhala, Boston

Inglis B 1989 The unknown guest: the mystery of intuition. Coronet/Hodder and Stoughton, Sevenoaks, England

Inglis B 1992 Natural and supernatural: a history of the paranormal. Prism, Bridport, England

Jaffe E 1980 Healing from within. Knopf, New York

Jahn R, Dunne B 1987 Margins of reality: the role of consciousness in the physical world. Harcourt Brace Jovanovich, New York

James W 1917 The varieties of religious experience: a study in human nature. Longmans, Green, New York

James W 1961 The varieties of religious experience. Collier, New York

Jeans J 1948 The mysterious universe. Cambridge University Press, Cambridge, England

Joy W 1979 Joy's way: a map for the transformational journey: an introduction to the potentials for healing with body energies. Jeremy P Tarcher, New York

Jung C 1960 The structure and dynamics of the psyche. Collected works, vols. 2 and 8. Trevor Hull, London

Kabat-Zinn J 1990 Full catastophe living: using the wisdom of your body and mind to face stress, pain and illness. Delacorte Press, New York

Karagulla S, Kunz D 1989 The chakras and the human energy fields. Theosophical Publishing House, Wheaton, IL

Kelsey M T 1973 Healing and Christianity. Harper and Row, New York

Kiev A (ed) 1964 Magic, faith and healing. Free Press of Glencoe, New York

Klausner S 1964 Psychiatry and religion: a sociological study of the new alliance of ministers and psychiatrists. Free Press of Glencoe, New York

Kleinman A 1980 Patients and healers in the context of culture. University of California Press, Berkeley, CA

Koenig H 1994 Aging and God: spiritual pathways to mental health in midlife and later years. Haworth Press, New York

Koenig H 1997 Is religion good for your health?: the effects of religion on physical and mental health. Haworth Press, New York

Koenig H, Smiley M, Gonzales J 1988 Religion, health, and aging: a review and theoretical integration. Greenwood Press, Westport, CT

Kornfield J 1993 A path with heart. Bantam, New York

Krieger D 1979 The therapeutic touch: how to use your hands to help or to heal. Prentice-Hall, Englewood Cliffs, NJ

Krieger D 1981 Foundations for holistic health nursing practices: the renaissance nurse. JB Lippincott, Philadelphia, PA

Krieger D 1987 Living the therapeutic touch: healing as a lifestyle. Dodd, Mead and Co., New York

Krieger D 1993 Accepting your power to heal: the personal practice of therapeutic touch. Bear and Co, Santa Fe, NM

Krieger D 1993 Research backs therapeutic touch. Bristol Press

Krieger D 1997 Therapeutic touch inner workbook: ventures in transpersonal healing. Bear and Co, Santa Fe, NM

Krippner S (ed) 1984 Advances in parapsychological research. McFarland, Jefferson, NC

Krippner S, Villoldo A 1976 The realms of healing. Celestial Arts, Millbrae, CA

Krippner S, Welch P 1992 Spiritual dimensions of healing: from native shamanism to contemporary health care. Irvington, New York

Kunz D 1985 Spiritual aspects of the healing arts. Theosophical Publishing House, Wheaton, IL

Kunz D 1991 The personal aura. Quest/Theosophical, Wheaton, IL

Lambert H 1933 Cure through suggestion. Moss and Kamin, New York

Lansdowne Z 1986 The chakras and esoteric healing. Samuel Weiser, York Beach, MA

Laskow L 1992 Healing with love. Harper, San Francisco, CA

Lawlis G 1996 Transpersonal medicine: a new approach to healing body-mind-spirit. Shambhala, Boston, MA

Lawlis G, Dossey L 1996 Transpersonal medicine: the new approach to healing body-mind-spirit. Shambhala, Boston, MA

Leninger M 1978 Transcultural nursing: concepts, theories and practices. Wiley, New York

LeShan L 1969 Toward a general theory of the paranormal. Parapsychology Foundation, New York

LeShan L 1974 The medium, the mystic, and the physicist. Viking, New York

LeShan L 1984 From Newton to ESP. Aquarian Press, Wellingborough, Northamptonshire, England

LeShan L 1987 The science of the paranormal. Aquarian Press, Wellingborough, Northhamptonshire, England

Levin J S (ed) 1993 Religion in aging and health: theoretical foundations and methodological frontiers. Sage Publications, Los Angeles, CA

Lewis C S 1960 Miracles. Collier/Macmillan, New York

Lewis I 1971 Ecstatic religion: an anthropological study of spirit possession and shamanism. Penguin Books, Middlesex

Locke S, Colligan D 1986 The healer within: the new medicine of mind and body. E P Dutton, New York

Loehr F 1969 The power of prayer on plants. Signet, New York

Lohrey A 1997 The meaning of consciousness. University of Michigan Press, Ann Arbor, MI

Lovinger R 1984 Working with religious issues in therapy. Aronson, New York

Lowen A 1975 Bioenergetics. Penguin Books, New York

Machi Y 1993 Science of Ki. Tokyo Electric University Press, Tokyo

McDonald R, Hickman J, Dakin H 1976 Preliminary physical measurements of psychophysical effects associated with three alleged psychic healers. Washington Research Center, San Francisco, CA

McGuire M 1988 Ritual healing in suburban America. Rutgers University Press, New Brunswick, NJ

McMillin D, Richards D 1995 The radial appliance and wet cell battery: two electrotherapeutic devices recommended by Edgar Cayce. Lifeline Press, Virginia Beach, VA

MacNutt F 1974 Healing. Ave Maria Press, Notre Dame, Ind

MacNutt F 1977 The power to heal. Ave Maria Press, Notre Dame, Ind.

Macrae J 1988 Therapeutic touch: a practical guide. Alfred Knopf, New York

Maisel E 1963 Tai chi for health. Dell, New York

Majno G 1975 The healing hand: man and wound in the ancient world. Harvard University Press, Cambridge, MA

Malinski V M 1986 Explorations on Martha Rogers' science of unitary human beings. Appleton-Century-Crofts, Corwalk, Connecticut

Marty M, Vaux K (eds) 1982 Health/medicine and the faith traditions: an inquiry into religion and medicine. Fortress Press, Philadelphia, PA

Matthews D, Clark C 1998 The faith factor: proof of the healing power of prayer. Penguin Group, New York

May W 1983 The physicians' covenant: images of the healer in medical ethics. Westminster Press, Philadelphia, PA

Meek G 1977 Healers and the healing process. Theosophical Publishing House, Wheaton, IL

Meerloo J A M 1964 Hidden communion. Garrett, New York

Menninger K 1963 The vital balance: the life process in mental health and illness. Viking Press, New York

Motoyama H 1981 Theories of the chakras: bridge to higher consciousness. Theosophical Publishing House, Wheaton, IL

Motoyama H 1991 The correlation between psi energy and ki: unification of religion and science. Human Science Press, Tokyo, Japan

Motoyama H 1997 Measurements of ki energy diagnosis and treatment. Human Science Press, Tokyo, Japan

Mowrer O 1961 The crisis in psychiatry and religion. Van Nostrand, Princeton, NJ

Muktananda S 1971 Guru: Chitshaktivilas; the play of consciousness. Harper and Row, New York

Myers D 1978 The human puzzle: psychological research and Christian belief. Harper and Row, New York

Myss C 1996 Anatomy of the spirit: the seven stages of power and healing. Harmony Books, New York

Nelson R, Dunne B, Jahn R 1984 An REG experiment with large database capability: III: operator related anomalies: Technical Note PEAR 84003. Princeton Engineering Anomalies Research Laboratory, Princeton University School of Engineering/Applied Science, Princeton, NJ

Nelson R, Dobyns Y, Dunne B, Jahn R 1991 Analysis of variance of REG experiments; operator intention, secondary parameters, database structure: Technical Note PEAR 91004. Princeton Engineering Anomalies Research Laboratory, Princeton University School of Engineering/Applied Science, Princeton, NJ

Newman M 1986 Health as expanding consciousness. CV Mosby Company, St Louis

Nolen W 1974 Healing: a doctor in search of a miracle. Fawcett Publications, Greenwich, Connecticut

Nordoff P, Robbins C 1971 Music therapy in special education. John Day, New York

Nordoff P, Robbins C 1972 Therapy in music for handicapped children. St Martin's Press, New York

Numbers R, Amundsen D (eds) 1986 Caring and curing: health and medicine in the Western religious traditions. Macmillan, New York

O'Dea T 1966 The sociology of religion. Prentice-Hall, New Jersey

Oman M, Dossey L, Lama D 2000 Prayers for healing: 365 blessings, poems, and meditations from around the world. Conari Press, Berkeley, CA

O'Regan B 1987 Healing, remission and miracle cures. Institute of Noetic Sciences, Sausalito, CA

O'Regan B, Hirshberg C 1993 Spontaneous remission: an annotated bibliography. Institute of Noetic Sciences, Sausalito, CA

Park R 2000 Voodoo science: the road from foolishness to fraud. Oxford University Press, Oxford

Parker R 1957 Prayer can change your life. Prentice-Hall, Englewood Cliffs, NJ

Patten L, Patten T 1988 Biocircuits: amazing new tools for energy health. M J Kramer, Tiburon, CA

Peale N 1956 The power of positive thinking. CR Gibson, Norwalk, CT

Pearsall P 1998 The heart's code: tapping the wisdom and power of our heart energy. Broadway Books, New York

Peat F 1987 Synchronicity: the bridge between matter and mind. Bantam, New York

Peck M 1978 The road less traveled: a new psychology of love, traditional values, and spiritual growth. Simon and Schuster, New York

Pelletier K 1982 Mind as healer, mind as slayer. Dell, New York

Penfield W 1975 The mystery of the mind: a critical study of consciousness and the human brain. Princeton University Press, Princeton, NJ

Penrose R 1994 Shadows of the mind. Oxford University Press, Oxford

Penrose R T 1989 The emperor's new mind: concerning compters, minds, and the laws of physics. Oxford University Press, Oxford

Podolsky B (ed) 1954 Music therapy. Philosophical Library, New York

Podolsky E 1945 Music for your health. Bernard Acherman, New York

Polk C, Postow E (eds) 1986 CRC handbook of biological effects of electromagnetic fields. CRC Press, Boca Raton, FL

Polkinghorne J 1989 Science and providence: God's interaction with the world. New Science Library, Boston, MA

Poloma M, Gallup G 1991 Varieties of prayer: a survey report. Trinity Press, Philadelphia, PA

Pribram K 1977 Languages of the brain. Wadsworth Publishing, Monterey, CA

[Psychiatry] Gap Committee on Psychiatry and Religion 1976 Mysticism: Spiritual quest or psychic disorder, vol. 9. New York

Radin D 1997 The conscious universe: the scientific truth of psychic phenomena. HarperSan Francisco, San Francisco, CA

Radin D, Machado F, Zangari W 1998 Effects of distant healing intention through time and space: two exploratory studies. Proceedings of presented papers. The 41st Annual Convention of the Parapsychological Association. parapsychological Association, Halifax, Nova Scotia, Canada

Rama S 1981 Energy of consciousness in the human personality. Plenum Press, New York

Raso J, Barrett S 1993 Mystical diets: paranormal, spiritual, and occult nutrition practices. Consumer Health Library. Prometheus Books, Amherst, NY

Ray B 1985 The reiki factor. Radiance Associates, St Petersburg, FL

Ray B, Carrington Y 1982 The official reiki handbook. American-International Reiki Association, Atlanta, GA

Rhine L 1961 Hidden channels of the mind. Willian Sloane, New York

Roederer J 1973 Introduction to the physics and psychophysics of music. Springer Verlag, New York

Rogers M 1970 Introduction to the theoretical basis of nursing. FA Davis, Philadelphia, PA

Roll W (ed) 1980 Research in parapsychology 1979. Scarecrow Press, Metuchen, NJ

Roll WG, Morris RL, Morris JD (eds) 1974 Research in parapsychology 1973. Scarecrow Press, Metuchen, NJ

Rose L 1968 Faith healing. Gollancz, London Rosenthal R 1984 Meta-analytical procedures for social research. Sage, Beverly Hills, CA

Salisbury W 1964 Religion in American culture. Dorsey Press, Homewood, Illinois

Sanford A 1976 The healing light. Trumpet Books, New York

Schmidt H, Morris R, Hardin C 1990 Channeling evidence for a psychokinetic effect to independent observers: an attempted replication. Mind Science Foundation research report. Mind Science Foundation, San Antonio, TX

Schmidt H, Schlitz M 1988 A large scale pilot PK experiment with pre-recorded random events. Mind Science Foundation research report. Mind Science Foundation, San Antonio, TX

Schrodinger E 1969 What is life? and mind and matter. Cambridge University Press, London

Schullian D, Schoen M (eds) 1948 Music as medicine. Henry Schuman, New York

Scorer C 1979 Healing: biblical, medical and pastoral. Christian Medical Fellowship Publications, London

Seem M, Kaplan J 1987 Body/mind energetics. Thorsons, Wellingborough, England

Shealy C N, Myss C M 1988 The creation of health: merging traditional medicine with intuitive diagnosis. Stillpoint, Walole, NH

Sheikh A A, Sheikh K S (eds) 1989 Eastern and Western approaches to healing: ancient wisdom and modern knowledge. Wiley, New York

Sheldrake P 1992 Spirituality and history: questions of interpretation and method. Crossroads, New York

Sheldrake R 1988 The presence of the past: morphic resonance and the habits of nature. New York Times Books, New York

Sherman H 1967 Wonder healers of the Philippines. DeVorss, Los Angeles, CA

Sherwood K 1985 The art of spiritual healing. Llewellyn, St Paul, MN

Siegel B 1986 Love, medicine, and miracles. Harper and Row, New York

Siegel B 1989 Peace, love and healing. Harper and Row, New York

Singer J 1972 Boundaries of the soul: the practice of Jung's psychology. Anchor/Doubleday, New York

Srinivasan T M 1988 Energy medicine around the world. Gabriel Press, Phoenix, AZ

Stapleton R 1979 The experience of inner healing. Word Books, Waco, TX

Stapp H 1993 Mind, matter and quantum mechanics. Springer Verlag, Heidelberg, Germany

Stenger V 1990 Physics and psychics: the search for a world beyond the senses. Prometheus Books, Amherst, NY

Stevenson I 1970 Telepathic impressions: a review of 35 new cases. University Press of Virginia, Charlottesville, VA

Stokes D 1997 The nature of mind: parapsychology and the role of consciousness in the physical world. McFarland, Jefferson

Strommen M 1971 Research on religious development: a comprehensive handbook. Hawthorn Books, New York

Sulmasy D 1997 The healer's calling: a spirituality for physicians and other health care professionals. Paulist Press, New York

Szasz T 1978 The myth of psychotherapy: mental healing as religion, rhetoric, and repression. Doubleday, Garden City, NY

Talbot M 1991 The holographic universe. HarperCollins, New York

Tame D 1984 The secret power of music. Destiny Books, New York

Targ R, Katra J 1998 Miracles of mind: exploring nonlocal consciousness and spiritual healing. New World Library, Novato, CA

Targ R, Cole P, Puthoff H 1974 Development of techniques to enhance man/machine communication. SRI International, Menlo Park, CA

Tart C 1997 Body, mind, spirit: exploring the parapsychology of spirituality. Hampton Roads, Charlottesville, Va

Tart C, Puthoff H, Targ R (eds) 1979 Mind at large. Praeger, New York

Teresa M, Stern A, Dossey L 2000 Everything starts from prayer: Mother Teresa's meditations on spiritual life for people. SCB International, Arlington, VA

Thorson J, Cook T (eds) 1980 Spiritual well-being of the elderly. Charles C Thomas, Springfield

Tiller W 1997 Science and human transformation: subtle energies, intentionality and consciousness. Pavior Publishing, Walnut Creek, CA

Ulanov A, Ulanov B 1982 Primary speech: a psychology of prayer. John Knox Press, Atlanta, GA

Vandecreek L, Dossey L 1998 Scientific and pastoral perspectives on intercessory prayer: an exchange between Larry Dossey, MD and health care chaplains. Harrington Park Press

Vasiliev L 1976 Experiments in distant influence. Dutton, New York

Vitz P 1977 Psychology as religion: the cult of self-worship. Eerdmans, Grand Rapids, Mich

Waldrop M M 1992 Complexity: the emerging science at the edge of order and chaos. Simon and Schuster, New York

Wallace A 1966 Religion: an anthropological view. Random House, New York

Weatherhead L 1951 Psychology, religion, and healing. Abingdon, Nashville, Tennessee

Weber M 1922 The sociology of religion. Beacon Press, New York

Wilson W 1984 The grace to grow: the power of Christian faith in emotional healing. Word Books, Waco, TX

Wolfe D, Burns S, Stoll M, Wichmann K 1974 Analysis of music therapy group procedures. Golden Valley Health Center, Minneapolis

Worrall A, Worrall O 1970 The healing touch. Harper and Row, New York

Yasuo Y 1987 The body: toward and Eastern mind–bodytheory. State University of New York Press, Albany, NY

Yogananda P 1925 Science of religion. Sat-Sanga, Boston, MA

Yogananda P 1962 Scientific healing affirmations: theory and practice of concentration. Self-Realization Fellowship, Los Angeles, CA

Young R, Dossey L 1997 Paths of a prodigal: exploring the deeper reaches of spiritual living. Larson

Yuasa Y 1993 The body, self-cultivation, and ki-energy. State University of New York, Albany, NY

Index